Renal Pharmacotherapy

D0763137

Larry K. Golightly • Isaac Teitelbaum
Tyree H. Kiser • Dimitriy A. Levin
Gerard R. Barber • Michael A. Jones
Nancy M. Stolpman • Katherine S. Lundin
Editors

Renal Pharmacotherapy

Dosage Adjustment of Medications Eliminated by the Kidneys

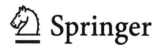 Springer

Editors

Larry K. Golightly, PharmD, BCPS
Medication Use Evaluation/
Adverse Drug Reaction Coordinator
University of Colorado Hospital and
Clinical Assistant Professor
University of Colorado Skaggs School of
Pharmacy and Pharmaceutical Sciences
Aurora, Colorado
USA

Gerard R. Barber, RPh, MPH, FASHP
Coordinator, P&T and Clinical Pharmacy Services
Co-Chair, Pharmacy and Therapeutics Committee
University of Colorado Hospital and
Clinical Assistant Professor
University of Colorado Skaggs School of
Pharmacy and Pharmaceutical Sciences
Aurora, Colorado
USA

Isaac Teitelbaum, MD, FACP
Director, Acute and Home Dialysis Programs
University of Colorado Hospital and
Professor of Medicine
Renal Medicine and Hypertension Section
Division of General Internal Medicine
University of Colorado School of Medicine
Aurora, Colorado
USA

Michael A. Jones, BS, PharmD
Informatics Pharmacist - Clinical
Decision Support
University of Colorado Hospital and
Clinical Associate Professor
University of Colorado Skaggs School of
Pharmacy and Pharmaceutical Sciences
Aurora, Colorado
USA

Tyree H. Kiser, PharmD, BCPS
Assistant Professor
Department of Clinical Pharmacy
University of Colorado Skaggs School of
Pharmacy and Pharmaceutical Sciences and
Critical Care Clinical Pharmacy Specialist
University of Colorado Hospital
Aurora, Colorado
USA

Nancy M. Stolpman, PharmD, PhD
Pharmacy Director
University of Colorado Hospital
Aurora, Colorado
USA

Katherine S. Lundin, PharmD
Internal Medicine Clinical Pharmacy Specialist
University of Colorado Hospital
Aurora, Colorado
USA

Dimitriy A. Levin, MD
Director, Hospitalist Oncology Service
University of Colorado Hospital and
Assistant Professor of Medicine
Hospital Medicine Section
Division of General Internal Medicine
University of Colorado School of Medicine
Aurora, Colorado
USA

ISBN 978-1-4614-5799-2   ISBN 978-1-4614-5800-5   (eBook)
DOI 10.1007/978-1-4614-5800-5
Springer New York Heidelberg Dordrecht London

Library of Congress Control Number: 2013932847

Printed on acid-free paper

Springer is part of Springer Science+Business Media (www.springer.com)

Preface

For optimal effectiveness and safety, medications used to manage both acute and chronic diseases must be administered in dosages carefully tailored according to patient-specific metabolic and excretory functional capacity. Due to variably compromised ability to eliminate certain drugs from the body, patients with kidney disease often present with complex and potentially challenging clinical issues related to adjustment of drug dosages. In these patients, provision of effective and safe pharmacotherapy depends upon not only understanding the pharmacokinetic and pharmacodynamic actions of all prescribed medications but also comprehensive appreciation of each patient's current clinical status.

In this regard, additional challenges have been recently realized. As of 2009, clinical laboratories in North America and elsewhere are expected to report serum creatinine (SCr) concentrations that are consistent with reference values obtained by isotope dilution mass spectrometry [1]. For most laboratories, this has necessitated recalibration of autoanalyzers. Depending on analyzer manufacturer and model, recalibrated SCr levels are known to be 5–20 % lower than values reported prior to recalibration [2]. Use of recalibrated SCr values with the Cockroft-Gault equation [3] to calculate estimated creatinine clearance (CrCL) often results in a compounded error leading to a numerically exaggerated estimate of excretory kidney function. If this CrCL value is used as currently recommended by the US Food and Drug Administration [4] for the purpose of determining drug dosages for persons with renal impairment, risk for medication error and drug overdose is increased.

In order to improve the accuracy of measures of kidney function used for staging severity of kidney disease, clinical laboratories now are encouraged to utilize recalibrated SCr concentrations with the 4-variable Modification of Diet in Renal Disease (MDRD) equation [5] or the Chronic Kidney Disease Epidemiological (CKDepi) equation [6] to calculate estimated glomerular filtration rate (eGFR) in mL/min/1.73 m^2 and to report this number along with the SCr value to clinicians [1, 7]. Although this measure of excretory kidney function often is readily available, it is not fully compatible with FDA-mandated product labeling related to drug dosage adjustment in patients with renal insufficiency. These inconsistencies may lead to further confusion and additional potential errors.

Available resources for adjustment of dosages of drugs in patients with renal insufficiency have been found to be broadly inconsistent and imprecise. A systematic review of dosage recommendations for 100 commonly prescribed medications listed in four widely used compendia found disparities in all of these resources in their recommendations for adjustments of dosage and dosage interval [8]. These differences ranged from minor disagreement regarding suggested dosage amount for a specific medication to divergence as broad and conflicting as no adjustment needed versus contraindicated. The four sources varied in their definitions of renal impairment, and some were found to be qualitative and unclear. In response, authorities conceded that "despite numerous secondary sources of drug dosing information, drug prescribing in renal failure remains imprecise and relies on interpolation, extrapolation, and estimation" [9]. In similar fashion, frequent inconsistencies have been found not only among FDA-approved prescribing information concerning recommended dose adjustments for recently marketed medications but also clinicians' methods for interpretation and application of these recommendations [10].

Additional resource-related issues may be problematic concerning efforts to provide optimal drug therapy for patients with abnormal or rapidly changing renal function. At least as important as use of inconsistent or discrepant information concerning drug dosing is inability or failure to recognize disparate dosage recommendations. Clinicians should be provided with convenient access to at least two reputable, reliable, and evidence-based sources of information on renal drug dosing, thereby allowing individualized selection of the most relevant regimen based on clinical judgment in light of pharmacological concerns weighted for safety and effectiveness. We sought to satisfy this requirement by compiling a listing of dosing suggestions comprised of official and alternative recommendations.

Methods

Conduct oversight for this project was provided by the Colorado Multiple Institutional Review Board (COMIRB, Protocol № 10-1105). Our objective, based on a review of available resources, was to compile a comprehensive tabular listing of dosage recommendations for patients with compromised renal function.

Information concerning adjustment of selected drug dosages that is compatible with conventional and revised measures of kidney function was obtained from available tertiary, secondary, and primary literature sources. This information was compiled into an alphabetical listing according to the approved generic drug name. Information on drug dosage adjustment was included in the listing if, in the opinion of the authors, such adjustment is necessary.

For all medications included in the listing, FDA-mandated product information was obtained from the package insert. In every instance, careful attempt was made to directly quote or to remain entirely faithful to the actual language and/or meaning within the product information. Alternative dosage adjustment information routinely was obtained from commonly used compendia. Most often, this consisted of GFR-based adjustment recommendations taken from the professional standard *Drug Prescribing in Renal Failure* [11] (with permission) or any of its various derivatives [12–15]. In most cases, other tertiary [16–21], secondary [22–25], and primary references (or available Internet-based counterparts of these print media) were used. Use of these alternatives often was necessary to supply or, more commonly, to corroborate and/or expand evidence-based dosing information for antimicrobials, newly marketed medications, and drugs used in patients receiving renal replacement therapy. Specialized alternative resources also were used for certain drugs for which information other than that provided in standard compendia was considered preferable.

The primary literature related to drug dosing in kidney disease was reviewed for all renally eliminated medications. In the event that alternative dose recommendations differed from those provided by the manufacturer, information selected and subsequently included in the listing was believed to be the most clinically relevant based on original clinical research and experience. The primary literature also was utilized for all medications for which proprietary dosing information was believed to be inadequate or outmoded and in need of change. This was most often necessary for dose adjustment of medications used for patients receiving renal replacement therapy. Searches for information contained in the primary literature were performed with the US National Library of Medicine's PubMed indexing system and Elsevier's Embase using nonproprietary or preferred drug names.

Results

A review of available resources disclosed 349 medications that require or suggest need for dosage adjustment when administered to patients with acute or chronic kidney disease and 769 drug entities that normally do not require dose adjustment for renal impairment. From this review, salient data for each medication was extracted and incorporated into a pre-formatted computer file. This file comprises the listings shown below.

Discussion

To promote effectiveness and minimize possible toxicity, the dosage of certain medications must be adjusted in persons with compromised kidney function. Convenient and comprehensive evidence-based resources are needed to enable consistent application of such adjustments.

Failure to enjoin appropriate dosage adjustments in patients with abnormal or rapidly changing kidney function continues to lead to reports of drug toxicity involving a broad array of renally eliminated medications [26–37]. Better resources clearly are needed to facilitate dose optimization. Means to ensure that patients whose current medications need adjustment are consistently identified also are vitally necessary.

Computerized assessment and consequent-directed recommendations concerning drug dosage have proven capable of improving prescribing patterns. A recent meta-analysis that evaluated 26 controlled comparisons of behavioral prescriber changes and/or health outcomes of patients associated with computerized interventions targeted to affect prescribing documented significant benefit of computerized advice by increasing the initial dose, increasing serum drug concentrations, reducing the time to therapeutic stabilization, reducing the risk of toxic drug levels, and reducing the length of hospital stay [38]. In patients with renal insufficiency, automated clinical decision support (CDS) systems have proven capable of detecting potentially dangerous and costly exposure to excess dosages of antimicrobial and other drugs that occurs frequently despite the intensive monitoring afforded to critically ill patients [39] and those attended in the emergency department [40]. Perhaps most convincing of the value of CDS are data showing that, as compared with pre-implementation figures, implementation of a CDS system was associated with a statistically and clinically significant 39 % increase in the fraction of delivered prescriptions for renally eliminated or nephrotoxic medications deemed appropriate according to previously published and/or expert evaluation standards when the system was applied to approximately 100,000 orders for these medications in hospitalized patients with renal insufficiency [41]. CDS systems for renally eliminated medications may be most effective if supplemented with academic detailing [42].

The appendant listing was designed to close some identified gaps in information concerning dosage adjustment of medications eliminated by the kidneys. More importantly, it was composed with the intent that this was to be adapted and used as part of an automated system that would display each patient's identification, location, and kidney function. Ultimately, the listing is to be used with CDS as described above, thereby enabling provider alerting to need for attention based on determination of specific clinically relevant dosing cusps or breakpoints for prescribed medications with individualized information displayed concerning suggested dose modifications and recommended actions.

This resource listing displays several strengths including alphabetical format, completeness, referencing, and, when available, dosage recommendations based on eGFR [43]. In glaring contrast, it also has significant weaknesses and limitations. First and foremost, we fully understand and appreciate that no single reference related to medication management in patients with kidney disease can provide truly comprehensive, completely accurate, totally unbiased, and thoroughly evidence-based recommendations. Secondly, our information was largely compiled with use of secondary or tertiary data sources with corroboration of the primary literature. Thirdly, alternative dosage adjustment recommendations that include breakpoints set in terms of eGFR often are listed in our information. The authors of the original guidelines in which this standard was established concede that calculated CrCL, an approximation useful in clinical dosimetry, may be used to simulate GFR [44]. These measures of kidney function thusly were considered essentially interchangeable, as demonstrated in earlier clinical investigations [45], and this bias currently persists in the dosing guidelines used as our foremost source of alternative dosage adjustment recommendations [11]. This relationship likely will not hold true if currently available measures of SCr are used to calculate CrCL or if eGFR is not corrected for body surface area in unusually small or large adults. Lastly, other than an informal acceptability survey of clinicians at the University of Colorado Hospital, the utility of this resource has not been clinically tested. Nonetheless, the appendant listing is believed to satisfy some, if not most, of the dosing information needs of busy clinicians involved in pharmacotherapy for patients with kidney disease.

References

1. Myers GL, Miller WG, Coresh J, et al. Recommendations for improving serum creatinine measurement: a report from the Laboratory Working Group of the National Kidney Disease Education Program. Clin Chem. 2006;52:5–18.

2. Miller WG, Myers GL, Ashwood ER, et al. Creatinine measurement: state of the art in accuracy and interlaboratory harmonization. Arch Pathol Lab Med. 2005;129:297–304.

3. Cockroft DW, Gault MH. Prediction of creatinine clearance from serum creatinine. Nephron. 1976;16:31–41.

4. US Department of Health and Human Services, Food and Drug Administration. Guidance for industry. Pharmacokinetics in patients with impaired renal function: study design, data analysis, and impact on drug dosing and labeling. http://www.fda.gov/downloads/Drugs/GuidanceComplianceRegulatoryInformation/Guidances/ucm072127.pdf. Accessed 25 June 2010.

5. Levey AS, Greene T, Kusek JW, Beck G. A simplified equation to predict glomerular filtration rate from serum creatinine [abstract]. J Am Soc Nephrol. 2000;11:155A.

6. Levey AS, Stevens LA, Schmid CH, et al. A new equation to estimate glomerular filtration rate. Ann Intern Med. 2009;150:604–12.

7. National Kidney Disease Education Program. Laboratory professionals creatinine standardization program. http://www.nkdep.nih.gov/labprofessionals/creatinine_standardization.htm. Accessed 25 June 2010.

8. Vidal L, Shavit M, Fraser A, Paul M, Leibovici L. Systematic comparison of four sources of drug information regarding adjustment of dose for renal function. BMJ. 2005;331:263–5.

9. Aronoff GA. Dose adjustment in renal impairment: response from Drug Prescribing in Renal Failure [letter]. BMJ. 2005;331:293–4.

10. Dowling TC, Matzke GR, Murphy JE, Burckhart GJ. Evaluation of renal drug dosing: prescribing information and clinical pharmacist approaches. Pharmacotherapy. 2010;30:776–86.

11. Aronoff GA, Bennett WM, Berns JS, et al. Drug prescribing in renal failure: dosing guidelines for adults and children. 5th ed. Philadelphia: American College of Physicians; 2007.

12. Olyaei AJ, DeMattos AM, Bennett WM. Use of drugs in patients with renal failure. In: Schrier RW, editor. Diseases of the kidney and urinary tract. 8th ed. Philadelphia: Lippincott Williams & Wilkins; 2007. p. 2765–807.

13. Olyaei AJ, Bennett WM. Pharmacologic approach to renal insufficiency. In: Dale DC, Federman DD, Antman K, editors. ACP Medicine, WebMD June 2007 update. Hamilton: BC Decker; 2007; NEPHROLOGY IX: Appendix A1–25.

14. McIntyre CW, Owen PJ. Prescribing drugs in kidney disease. In: Brenner BM, editor. Brenner and Rector's the kidney. 8th ed. Philadelphia: Saunders Elsevier; 2008. p. 1930–55.

15. Olyaei AJ, Bennett WM. Drug dosing in elderly patients with chronic kidney disease. Clin Geriatr Med. 2009;25:459–527.

16. Lacy CF, Armstrong LL, Goldman MP, Lance LL, editors. Drug information handbook: a comprehensive source for all clinicians and healthcare professionals. 20th ed. Hudson: Lexi-Comp/American Pharmacists Association; 2011.

17. McEvoy GK, Snow EL, Miller J, et al. American hospital formulary service: drug information 2010. Bethesda: American Society of Health-System Pharmacists; 2010.

18. Kastrup ER, Meives CA, Johnson PB, et al. Drug facts and comparisons 2011. St Louis: Wolters Kluwer Health; 2010.

19. Fotsch E, Tanzer D, Côté C, et al. Physicians' desk reference 2011. 65th ed. Montvale: PDR Network; 2010.

20. Amsden GW. Tables of antimicrobial agent pharmacology. In: Mandell GL, Bennett JE, Dolin R, editors. Mandell, Douglas, and Bennett's principles and practice of infectious diseases, vol 1. 6th ed. Philadelphia: Elsevier; 2005. p. 634–700.

21. Abramowicz M, Zuccotti G, Pflomm J-M, et al., editors. Handbook of antimicrobial therapy. 19th ed. New Rochelle: The Medical Letter; 2011.

22. Munar MY, Singh H. Drug dosing adjustments in patients with chronic kidney disease. Am Fam Physician. 2007;75:487–96.

23. Heintz BH, Matzke GR, Dager WE. Antimicrobial dosing concepts and recommendations for critically ill adult patients receiving continuous renal replacement therapy or intermittent hemodialysis. Pharmacotherapy. 2009;29:562–77.

24. Trotman RL, Williamson JC, Shoemaker DM, Salzer WL. Antibiotic dosing in critically ill adult patients receiving continuous renal replacement therapy. Clin Infect Dis. 2005;41:1159–66.

25. Choi G, Gomersall CD, Tian Q, Joynt GM, Freebairn R, Lipman J. Principles of antibacterial dosing in continuous renal replacement therapy. Crit Care Med. 2009;37:2268–82.

26. Onuigbo MA, Nye D, Ilianya PC. Drug-induced encephalopathy secondary to non-renal dosing of common medications in two dialysis patients. Adv Perit Dial. 2009;25:89–91.

27. Bagon JA. Neuropsychiatric complications following quinolone overdose in renal failure [letter]. Nephrol Dial Transplant. 1999;14:1337.

28. Yoo L, Matalon D, Hoffman RS, Goldfarb DS. Treatment of pregabalin toxicity by hemodialysis in a patient with kidney failure. Am J Kidney Dis. 2009;54:1127–30.

29. Pierce DA, Holt SR, Reeves-Daniel A. A probable case of gabapentin-related reversible hearing loss in a patient with acute renal failure. Clin Ther. 2008;30:1681–4.

30. Nakata M, Ito S, Shirai Hattori T. Severe reversible neurological complications following amantadine treatment in three elderly patients with renal insufficiency. Eur Neurol. 2006;56:59–61.

31. Psaty BM, Psaty SE. Flecainide toxicity in an older adult [letter]. J Am Geriatr Soc. 2009;57:751–3.

32. Talbert Estlin KA, Sadun AA. Risk factors for ethambutol optic toxicity. Int Ophthalmol. 2010;30:63–72.

33. Barraclough K, Harris M, Montessori V, Levin A. An unusual case of acute injury due to vancomycin—lessons learnt from reliance on eGFR. Nephrol Dial Transplant. 2007;22:2391–4.

34. Vulliemoz S, Iwanowski P, Landis T, Jallon P. Levetiracetam accumulation in renal failure causing myoclonic encephalopathy with triphasic waves. Seizure. 2009;18:376–8.

35. Asahi T, Tsutsui M, Wakasugi M, et al. Valacyclovir neurotoxicity: clinical experience and a review of the literature. Eur J Neurol. 2009;16:457–60.

36. Boykin KM, Kernan W, Tarchini G, Lurix E. Neurotoxicity associated with standard doses of valacyclovir in renal insufficiency. Hosp Pharm. 2011;46:774–8.

37. Tourret J, Tostivint I, Tézenas Du Montcel S, et al. Antiretroviral drug dosing errors in HIV-infected patients undergoing hemodialysis. Clin Infect Dis. 2007;4:775–84.

38. Durieux P, Trinquart L, Colombet I, et al. Computerized advice on drug dosage to improve prescribing practice (review). Cochrane Database Syst Rev. 2008;(3):CD 002894. doi: 10.1002/14651858.CD002894.pub.2.

39. Helmons PJ, Groulis RJ, Roos AN, et al. Using a clinical decision support system to determine the quality of antimicrobial dosing in intensive care patients with renal insufficiency. Qual Saf Health Care. 2010;19:22–6.

40. Terrell KM, Perkins AJ, Hui SL, Callahan CM, Dexter PR, Miller DK. Computerized support for medication dosing in renal insufficiency: a randomized, controlled trial. Ann Emerg Med. 2010;56:623–9.

41. Chertow GM, Lee J, Kuperman GJ, et al. Guided medication dosing for inpatients with renal insufficiency. JAMA. 2001;286:2839–44.

42. Roberts GW, Farmer CJ, Cheney PC, et al. Clinical decision support implemented with academic detailing improves prescribing of key renally cleared drugs in the hospital setting. J Am Med Inform Assoc. 2010;17:308–12.

43. Stevens LA, Levey AS. Use of the MDRD Study Equation to estimate kidney function for drug dosing. Clin Pharmacol Ther. 2009;86:465–7.

44. Swan SK, Bennett WM. Dosing guidelines in patients with renal failure. West J Med. 1992;156:633–8.

45. Bennett WM, Porter GA. Endogenous creatinine clearance as a clinical marker of glomerular filtration rate. Br Med J. 1971;4:84–6.

Aurora, Colorado, USA   Larry K. Golightly, PharmD, BCPS

Contents

Disclaimer

Information presented is designed to facilitate clinical assessment of drug therapy and to enable discernment and determination of optimal drug dosing in persons with kidney disease. This information is intended to aid clinical decision making. This information must not be substituted for sound clinical judgment. Rather, it should be used with comprehensive understanding of pathological, pharmacological, and patient-specific clinical issues in order to provide the best treatment for seriously ill patients.

This document was originally designed for use by those who are competent healthcare professionals employed by or directly connected and having privileges with University of Colorado Hospital who rely on their clinical judgment and discretion. User assumes full responsibility for ensuring the appropriate use and reliance upon the information in view of all attendant circumstances, indications, and contraindications.

Abbreviations and Keys

CAPD	Chronic ambulatory peritoneal dialysis
CrCL	Creatinine clearance (mL/min)
CRRT	Continuous renal replacement therapy
CVVH	Continuous venovenous hemofiltration
CVVHD	Continuous venovenous hemodialysis
CVVHDF	Continuous venovenous hemodiafiltration
dL	Deciliter
doi	Digital object identifier
eCrCL	Estimated CrCL in mL/min using the Cockroft-Gault equation $CrCL = (140 - age) \times Weight/(72 \times SCr)$ for males and $0.85 \times CrCL$ for females where SCr is derived from rSCr in our hospital as follows: $SCr = (rSCr + 0.07)/0.99$; alternatively, this value may be approximated by increasing rSCr by 8 %. This may facilitate use of CrCL equations that were developed prior to availability and reporting of rSCr by clinical laboratories. In many patients, this may be closely approximated by eGFR with correction for body surface area [$eGFR \times (1.73 \text{ m}^2/BSA)$]. Other laboratories differ.
eGFR	Estimated GFR as calculated by the clinical laboratory using the 4-variable MDRD equation
ESRD	End-stage renal disease
FDA	United States Food and Drug Administration
g	Gram
GFR	Glomerular filtration rate in mL/min, usually determined by iohexol or ^{125}I-iothalamate clearance
IM	Intramuscular
IV	Intravenous
kg	Kilogram (actual body weight unless otherwise specified)
L	Liter
mg	Milligram
mL	Milliliter
NR	Non-renal
PRN	Pro re nata (as occasion requires; as necessary)
rSCr	Recalibrated serum creatinine (traceable to IDMS reference standard, mg/dL)
℞	Treatment
SCr	Serum creatinine (mg/dL)

Common systemic medications that normally do not require significant downward dose adjustment in the presence of renal impairment in adults (NR). Cautions are described if present in proprietary information.

Abacavir/Ziagen®
Abatacept/Orencia®
Abciximab/ReoPro®
Abiraterone/Zytiga™
AbobotulinumtoxinA/Dysport™
Acetylcysteine/Acetadote®
Adalimumab/Humira®
Adenosine/Adenocard®, Adenoscan®
Aflibercept (intravitreal)/Eylea™
Agalsidase beta/Fabrazyme®
Albendazole/Albenza®
Albumin/Albuminar®
Albuterol/Proventil®
Aldesleukin/Proleukin®
Alefacept/Amevive®
Alemtuzumab/Campath®
Alfentanil/Alfenta®
Alglucerase/Ceredase®
Alglucosidase alfa/Lumizyme™, Myozyme®
Alosetron/Lotronex®
Alpha₁-Proteinase Inhibitor (Alpha₁ Antitripsin)/Prolastin® C
Alpha galactosidase/Beano®
Alprazolam/Xanax®
Alprostadil/Caverject®
Alteplase/Activase®
Altretamine/Hexalen®
Aluminum hydroxide/Amphogel®, Alternagel®
Aluminum hydroxide and magnesium trisilicate or carbonate and alginic acid/Gaviscon®—Caution, contains small amounts of magnesium
Alvimopan/Entereg®
Ambenonium/Mytelase®
Ambrisentan/Letairis®
Amifostine/Ethyol®
Aminobenzoate potassium/Potaba®
Aminocaproic acid/Amicar®
Aminohippurate sodium
Aminolevulinic acid/Levulan®, Kerastick®
Aminophylline
Amiodarone/Cordarone®, Nexterone®
Amitriptyline/Elavil®
Amlodipine/Norvasc®
Amobarbital/Amytal®
Amoxapine/Asendin®

Amphotericin B/Fungizone®
Amphotericin B liposome/Ambisome®
Amyl nitrate
Anagrelide/Agrylin®
Anastrozole/Arimidex®
Anidulafungin/Eraxis™
Antihemophilic factor, human/ Monoclate P®, Koate DVI®
Antihemophilic factor, recombinant/ Recombinate®, Hexilate®
Antihemophilic factor/von Willebrand factor complex/Humate-P®
Anti-inhibitor coagulant complex/ Feiba NF
Antithrombin III/Thrombate III®
Antithymocyte globulin, equine/ Atgam®
Antithymocyte globulin, rabbit/ Thymoglobulin®
Antivenin lactrodectus mactans
Aprepitant/Emend®
Argatroban
Arginine/R-gene®
Aripiprazole/Abilify®
Artemether and lumefantrine/ Coartem®—Caution in severe renal impairment
Articaine 4 % and epinephrine/ Orabloc™, Septocaine®
Ascorbic acid/Vitamin C
Asenapine/Saphris®
Asparaginase/Elspar®
Asparaginase *Erwinia chrysanthemi*/ Erwinase™
Atomoxetine/Strattera®
Atorvastatin/Lipitor®
Atovaquone/Mepron®
Atracurium
Atropine
Avanafil/Stendra™
Axitinib/Inlyta®
Azficel-T/LaViv®
Azilsartan/Edarbi™
Azithromycin/Zithromax®—Caution in severe renal impairment (GFR < 10 mL/min)
Baclofen/Lioresal®—Caution in severe renal impairment
Balsalazide/Colazal®—Caution in severe renal impairment

Barium sulfate/Barobag™, Barosperse™, Cheetah™, Enhancer™, Entrobar™, HD 85™, HD™ 200 Plus, Intropaste™, Prepcat™, Scan C™, Tonojug™, Tonopaque™
Basiliximab/Simulect®
Beclomethasone/QVAR®, Beconase®
Belatacept/Nulojix®
Belimumab/Benlysta®
Belladonna and opium/B&O®
Benzphetamine/Didrex®
Benzonatate/Tessalon®
Benztropine/Cogentin®
Beta-carotene
Betamethasone/Celestone®
Betaxolol/Kerlone®—Caution, reduce dose in severe renal impairment
Bethanechol/Urecholine®
Bevacizumab/Avastin®
Bexarotene/Targretin®—Caution in severe renal impairment
Bicalutamide/Casodex®
Bisacodyl/Dulcolax®
Boceprevir/Victrelis™
Bortezomib/Velcade®
Bosentan/Tracleer®
Brentuximab/Adcetris™—Caution, the effects or risks imposed by renal impairment have not been determined
Bromocriptine/Cycloset®, Parlodel®
Brompheniramine/Brovex™
Budesonide/Entocort®
Bumetanide/Bumex®
Bupivacaine/Marcaine®
Buprenorphine/Buprenex®
Bupropion/Wellbutrin®—Caution in severe renal impairment
Busulfan/Myleran®
Butabarbital/Butisol®
C1 esterase inhibitor/Berinert®, Cinryze™
Cabazitaxel/Jevtana®—Caution in severe renal impairment
Cabergoline/Dostinex®
Caffeine sodium benzoate
Calcitonin/Miacalcin®
Calcitriol/Rocaltrol®
Calcium acetate/PhosLo®

Calcium carbonate/Tums®
Calcium citrate/Citracal®
Calcium polycarbophil/FiberCon®
Candesartan/Atacand®
Carbamazepine/Tegretol®
Carbidopa/Lodosyn®
Carbinoxamine/Palgic®
Carboprost/Hemabate®
Carisoprodol/Soma®
Carvedilol/Coreg®
Cascara sagrada
Caspofungin/Cancidas®
Castor oil
Cefaclor/Ceclor®
Ceftriaxone/Rocephin®
Certolizumab/Cimzia®—Caution,
    inadequate data to recommend
    dose in renal impairment
Cetrorelix/Cetrotide®
Cetuximab/Erbitux®
Cevimeline/Evoxac®
Chloramphenicol/Chloromycetin®—
    Caution in severe renal
    impairment
Chlordiazepoxide/Librium®
Chloroprocaine/Nesacaine®
Chloroquine/Aralen®
Chlorpheniramine/Chlor-trimeton®
Chlorpromazine/Thorazine®
Chlorzoxazone/Parafon®
Cholecalciferol/Vitamin D₃
Cholestyramine/Questran®
Choline magnesium trisalicylate/
    Trilisate®—Caution, monitor
    salicylate levels
Cilostazol/Pletal®—Caution in severe
    renal impairment (GFR < 25 mL/
    min)
Cinacalcet/Sensipar®
Cisatracurium/Nimbex®
Citalopram/Celexa®
Citric acid, sodium, and potassium
    citrate/Polycitra®—Caution with
    low urine output
Clemastine/Tavist®
Clevidipine/Cleviprex™
Clidinium and chlordiazepoxide/
    Librax®
Clindamycin/Cleocin®
Clobazam/Onfi™—Caution, no
    experience in severe renal
    impairment
Clomiphene/Clomid®, Serophene®

Clonazepam/Klonopin®
Clonidine/Catapres®
Clopidogrel/Plavix®
Clorazepate/Tranxene®
Cocaine
Collagenase *Clostridium histolyticum*
    injection/Xiaflex™
Colesevelam/Welchol®
Colestipol/Colestid®
Corticorelin/Acthrel®
Cortisone acetate
Cosyntropin/Cortrosyn®
Crizotinib/Xalkori®
Cromolyn/Gastrocrom®—Caution,
    consider dose reduction
Cyanocobalamin/Vitamin B₁₂
Cyclobenzaprine/Flexeril®
Cyclophosphamide/Cytoxan®—
    Caution, consider dose reduction
    in severe renal impairment
    (GFR < 10 mL/min) and/or
    chronic oral administration
Cyclosporine/Gengraf®, Neoral®,
    Sandimmune®
Cyproheptadine/Periactin®
Cytarabine/Cytosar®
Cytomegalovirus immune globulin/
    Cytogam®
Dacarbazine/DTIC®
Daclizumab/Zenapax®
Dactinomycin/Cosmegen®
Danazol/Cyclomen®
Dantrolene/Dantrium®
Dapsone
Darbepoetin alfa/Aranesp®
Darifenacin/Enablex®
Darunavir/Prezista®
Dasatinib/Sprycel®
Decitabine/Dacogen™
Deferiprone/Ferriprox®—Caution, not
    evaluated in patients with kidney
    disease
Degarelix/Firmagon®—Caution in
    severe renal impairment
Delavirdine/Rescriptor®
Denileukin/Ontak®
Denosumab/Prolia™, Xgeva™—
    Caution, patients with
    CrCL < 30 mL/min or on
    hemodialysis are at increased risk
    for hypocalcemia
Desflurane/Suprane®
Desipramine/Norpramin®

Desloratadine/Clarinex®—Caution in
    renal impairment, consider
    initiation with 5 mg every 48 h
Dexamethasone/Decadron®
Dexlansoprazole/Kapidex™
Dexmedetomidine/Precedex®
Dexmethylphenidate/Focalin®
Dextran 40/Gentran®—Caution in
    renal impairment
Dextroamphetamine/Dexedrine®
Dextroamphetamine and
    amphetamine/Adderall®
Dextromethorphan/Robitussin DM®
Diatrizoate/Gastrografin™,
    MD-Gastroview®
Diazepam/Valium®
Diazoxide/Proglycem®—Caution,
    consider reduced dosage in renal
    impairment
Dicloxacillin/Pathocil®
Dicyclomine/Bentyl®
Diethylpropion/Tenuate®
Diflunisal—Caution, no data in renal
    impairment
Digoxin immune Fab/Digibind®
Dihydrotachysterol/DHT™
Diltiazem/Cardizem®, Cartia®,
    Dilacor®, Taztia®, Tiazac®
Dimenhydrinate/Dramamine®
Dimercaprol/BAL®
Dinoprostone/Cervidil®, Prepidil®,
    Prostin E₂®
Diphenhydramine/Benadryl®
Diphenoxin and atropine/Motofen®
Diphenoxylate and atropine/Lomotil®
Diphtheria and tetanus toxoids and
    acellular pertussis vaccine/
    Adacel®, Boostrix®
Dipyridamole/Persantine®
Disulfiram/Antabuse®
Divalproex/Depakote®
Dobutamine/Dobutrex®
Docetaxel/Taxotere®
Docusate/Colace®
Dolasetron/Anzemet®
Donepezil/Aricept®
Dopamine/Intropin®
Doxapram/Dopram®
Doxazosin/Cardura®
Doxepin/Sinequan®
Doxercalciferol/Hectorol®
Doxorubicin/Adriamycin®
Doxylamine/Unisom®

Doxycycline/Vibramycin®
Dronabinol/Marinol®
Dronedarone/Multaq®
Droperidol/Inapsine®
Drotrecogin alfa/Xigris®
Dutasteride/Avodart®
Ecallantide/Kalbitor®—Caution, no
    data in renal impairment
Eculizumab/Soliris®
Edrophonium/Enlon®
Efalizumab/Raptiva®
Eletriptan/Relpax®
Eltrombopag/Promacta®—Caution, no
    data in renal impairment; monitor
    closely
Enflurane/Ethrane®
Enfuvirtide/Fuzeon®
Entacapone/Comtan®
Ephedrine
Epinephrine/Adrenalin®
Epirubicin/Ellence®
Epoetin alfa/Epogen®, Procrit®
Epoprostenol/Flolan®
Eprosartan/Teveten®
Ergocalciferol/Drisdol®
Ergoloid mesylates
Ergonovine/Ergotrate®
Ergotamine/Ergotrate®
Erlotinib/Tarceva™—Caution, no data
    in renal impairment
Erythromycin/EES®, Erythrocin®
Escitalopram/Lexapro®—Caution in
    severe renal impairment
Esmolol/Brevibloc®
Esomeprazole/Nexium®
Estazolam/ProSom®
Estradiol/Estrace®
Estramustine/Emcyt®
Estrogens, conjugated/Premarin®
Estrogens, esterified/Menest®
Estropipate/Ogen®
Eszopiclone/Lunesta®
Etanercept/Enbrel®
Ethanolamine/Ethamolin®
Ethinyl estradiol/Estinyl®
Ethosuximide/Zarontin®
Ethotoin/Peganone®
Ethosuximide/Zarontin®—Caution in
    patients with known renal disease
Etidronate/Didronel®—Caution,
    consider dosage decrease with
    reduction in GFR
Etomidate/Amidate®

Etravirine/Intelence™
Everolimus/Afinitor®, Zortress®
Exemestane/Aromasin®
Ezetemibe/Zetia®
Ezogabine/Potiga™—Caution, dose
    initiation should follow a
    conservative approach
Factor VIIa (recombinant)/
    NovoSeven®
Factor IX complex, human/Profilnine®
Fat emulsion/Intralipid®
Febuxostat/Uloric®—Caution in severe
    renal impairment
Felodipine/Plendil®
Fenoldopam/Corlopam®
Fentanyl/Sublimaze®, Subsys™
Ferric gluconate/Ferrlecit®
Ferrous sulfate/Feosol®
Ferumoxsil/GastroMARK™
    Ferumoxytol/Feraheme™
Fesoterodine/Toviaz™—Caution, in
    severe renal impairment
    (CrCL < 30 mL/min) max
    dose = 4 mg/day
Fidaxomicin/Dificid™
Filgrastim/Neupogen®
Finasteride/Proscar®
Fingolimod/Gilenya™
Flavoxate/Urispas®
Floxuridine/FUDR®
Fludrocortisone/Florinef®
Flumazenil/Romazicon®
Fluorescein/AK-Fluor®, Fluorescite®
Fluorouracil/Adrucil®—Caution in
    severe renal impairment
Fluoxetine/Prozac®
Fluoxymesterone/Androxy®
Fluphenazine/Prolixin®
Flurazepam/Dalmane®
Flurbiprofen/Ansaid®
Fluvastatin/Lescol®—Caution in
    severe renal impairment
Fulvestrant/Faslodex®
Fluvoxamine/Luvox®
Folic acid/Folvite®
Follitropin alfa/Gonal-f®
Fosamprenavir/Lexiva®
Fosaprepitant/Emend®
Fosinopril/Monopril®
Fosphenytoin/Cerebyx®—Caution,
    see phenytoin
Fospropofol/Lusedra™
Frovatriptan/Frova®

Furosemide/Lasix®
Galsulfase/Naglazyme®
Ganirelix
Gefitinib/Iressa®
Gemcitabine/Gemzar®—Caution, no
    data in severe renal impairment
Gemtuzumab/Mylotarg®—Caution, no
    data in renal impairment
Glatiramer/Copaxone®—Caution, no
    data in renal impairment
Glimepiride/Amaryl®
Glucagon
Glucarpidase/Voraxaze®
Glutamine/Sympt-X®
Glycerin
Glycopyrrolate/Robinul®
Golimumab/Simponi™—Caution, no
    data in renal impairment
Goserelin/Zoladex®
Granisetron/Kytril®
Griseofulvin/Grifulvin®
Guaifenesin/Robitussin®
Guanabenz/Wytensin®
Guanfacine/Tenex®
Haloperidol/Haldol®
Hemin/Panhematin®
Heparin—Caution, monitor carefully;
    renal dysfunction may reduce
    clearance
Hepatitis B immune globulin/
    HepaGam B™
Hepatitis B vaccine (recombinant)/
    Engerix-B®
Histrelin/Vantas™
Human chorionic gonadotropin/Pregnyl®
Hyaluronate/Hylaform®, Juvederm®,
    Orthovisc®, Restylane®,
    Supartz™, Synvisc®
Hydralazine/Apresoline®
Hydrocodone and acetaminophen/
    Vicodin®
Hydrocortisone/Cortef®, Solu-Cortef®
Hydromorphone/Dilaudid®
Hydroxocobalamin/Cyanokit®
Hydroxychloroquine/Plaquenil®
Hydroxyzine/Atarax®, Vistaril®
Hyoscyamine/Levsin®
Hyoscyamine, atropine, scopolamine,
    and phenobarbital/Donnatal®
Ibritumomab/Zevalin®
Ibuprofen/Motrin®, Advil®—Caution,
    no data in advanced renal disease;
    not recommended

Ibutilide/Corvert®
Icatibant/Firazyr®
Iloperidone/Fanapt™
Iloprost/Ventavis®
Imiglucerase/Cerezyme®
Imipramine/Tofranil®
Immune globulin/Gamastan®,
    Flebogamma®, Gammagard®,
    Gamunex®, Octagam®,
    Vivaglobin®
Indinavir/Crixivan®
Indocyanine green
Indigo Carmine
Infliximab/Remicade®
Influenza virus vaccine (inactivated)/
    Fluarix®, Fluzone®
Interferon alfa-2B/Intron® A
Interferon alfacon-1/Infergen®—
    Caution, no data available in
    patients with renal impairment
Interferon beta-1a/Avonex®, Rebif®
Interferon beta-1b/Betaseron®
Interferon beta-1b/Extavia®
Interferon gamma-1b/Actimmune®
Iodipamide meglumine/Cholografin™
Iodixanol/Visipaque®—Caution,
    possible contrast induced
    nephropathy
Iodoquinol/Yodoxin®
Iopamidol/Isovue®—Caution, possible
    contrast induced nephropathy
Iothalamate ¹²⁵I/Glofil®-125
Iothalamate meglumine/Conray®,
    Cysto-Conray™—Caution,
    possible contrast induced
    nephropathy
Ipecac
Ipilimumab/Yervoy™
Irbesartan/Avapro®
Irinotecan/Camptosar®—Caution, no
    data in renal impairment; not
    recommended in hemodialysis
Iron dextran/Dexferrum®, INFeD®
Iron sucrose/Venofer®
Isoniazid/Nydrazid®
Isoflurane/Forane®
Isoproterenol/Isuprel®
Isosorbide dinitrate/Isordil®
Isosorbide mononitrate/Imdur®
Isotretinoin/Accutane®
Isradipine/DynaCirc®—Caution, in
    renal impairment; starting dose is
    5 mg daily

Ivacaftor/Kalydeco™
Ivermectin/Stromectol®
Ixabepilone/Ixempra®
Japanese encephalitis virus vaccine/
    JE-Vax®
Ketamine/Ketalar®
Ketoconazole/Nizoral®
Labetalol/Trandate®
Lactulose/Enulose®
Lamotrigine/Lamictal®—Caution,
    minimal data available in patients
    with renal impairment
Lansoprazole/Prevacid®
Lanthanum/Fosrenol®
Lapatinib/Tykerb®
Leflunomide/Arava®—Caution in renal
    impairment
Letrozole/Femara®—No dosage
    adjustment required if CrCL
    ≥10 mL/min
Leucovorin calcium
Leuprolide/Lupron®
Levocarnitine/Carnitor®
Levodopa/Larodopa®
Levoleucovorin/Fusilev™
Levonorgestrel/Plan B®
Levorphanol/Levo-Dromoran®
Levothyroxine/Synthroid®
Lidocaine/Xylocaine®
Linagliptin/Tradjenta™
Linezolid/Zyvox®
Liothyronine/Cytomel®
Liotrix/Thyrolar®
Liraglutide/Victoza®
Lisdexamfetamine/Vyvanse™
Loperamide/Imodium®
Lopinavir and ritonavir/Kaletra®
Loratadine/Claritin®—Caution, if
    GFR < 30 mL/min starting dose is
    10 mg every other day
Lorazepam/Ativan®—Caution, renal
    impairment contributes to risk of
    propylene glycol accumulation in
    patients receiving high-dose
    continuous infusion
Losartan/Cozaar®
Lovastatin/Mevacor®
Loxapine/Loxitane®
Lubiprostone/Amitiza®—Caution, no
    data in renal impairment
Maprotiline/Ludiomil®
Measles, mumps, and rubella virus
    vaccine/MMR® II

Mebendazole/Vermox®
Mechlorethamine/Mustargen®
Meclizine/Antivert®
Medroxyprogesterone/Provera®
Mefloquine/Lariam®
Megestrol/Megace®—Caution, no data
    in renal impairment
Menotropins/Repronex®
Mephobarbital/Mebaral®—Caution,
    reduce dose in renal impairment
Mepivacaine/Carbocaine®
Mesalamine/Asacol®, Pentasa®,
    Rowasa™—Caution, renal
    impairment may increase risk for
    blood and kidney problems;
    monitor blood counts and renal
    function
Mesna/Mesnex®—Caution, no data in
    renal impairment
Metaproterenol/Alupent®
Methamphetamine/Desoxyn®—
    Caution in renal impairment
Methimazole/Tapazole®
Methocarbamol (oral)/Robaxin®
Methoxsalen/Oxsoralen®
Methsuximide/Celontin®
Methyclothiazide/Enduron®
Methylene blue
Methylergonovine/Methergine®
Methylphenidate/Methylin™, Ritalin®
Methylprednisolone/Solu-Medrol®,
    Depo-Medrol®
Metolazone/Zaroxolyn®
Metoprolol/Lopressor®, Toprol-XL®
Metronidazole/Flagyl®
Metyrosine/Demser®
Mexiletine/Mexitil®
Micafungin/Mycamine®
Midazolam/Versed®
Mifepristone/Mifeprex®, Korlym™
Minocycline/Minocin®
Minoxidil/Loniten®
Mirtazapine/Remeron®—Caution,
    consider dose reduction in renal
    impairment; clearance is
    decreased 50 % if CrCL is
    <10 mL/min
Misoprostol/Cytotec®
Mitotane/Lysodren®
Mitoxantrone/Novantrone®—Caution,
    no data in renal impairment
Modafinil/Provigil®—Safety not
    established in renal impairment

Molindone/Moban®

Montelukast/Singulair®

Moxifloxacin/Avelox®

Multivitamins/Hexavitamin

Muromonab-CD3/Orthoclone OKT3®

Nabilone/Cesamet™—Caution, no data in renal impairment

Nafarelin/Synarel®

Nafcillin/Unipen®

Nalbuphine/Nubain®—Caution in renal impairment; consider use of reduced doses

Nalmefene/Revex®

Naloxone/Narcan®

Naltrexone/ReVia®

Natalizumab/Tysabri®

Nateglinide/Starlix®

Nefazodone/Serzone®

Nelarabine/Arranon®

Nelfinavir/Viracept®

Nesiritide/Natrecor®

Nevirapine/Viramune®

Niacin/Niaspan®—Caution in renal disease

Nicardipine/Cardene®—Caution, in renal insufficiency initiate oral therapy with 20 mg three times daily or extended release 30 mg twice daily

Nicotine/Nicorette®, Nicoderm®

Nifedipine/Procardia®, Adalat®

Nilotinib/Tasigna®

Nilutamide/Nilandron®

Nimodipine/Nimotop®

Nisoldipine/Sular®

Nitazoxanide/Alinia®—Caution, no data in renal impairment

Nitroglycerin/Nitrostat®

Nitroprusside/Nitropress®

Norepinephrine/Levophed®

Norethindrone/Aygestin®

Nortriptyline/Pamelor®

Nystatin/Nilstat®, Mycostatin®

Octreotide/Sandostatin®

Ofatumumab/Arzerra™

Olanzapine/Zyprexa®

Olmesartan/Benicar®

Olsalazine/Dipentum®—Caution, monitor renal function

Omalizumab/Xolair®

Omega-3-acid esters/Lovaza®

Omeprazole/Prilosec®

Omeprazole and sodium bicarbonate/ Zegerid®

OnabotulinumtoxinA/Botox®

Ondansetron/Zofran®

Opium tincture

Orlistat/Xenical®, Alli™

Orphenadrine/Norflex™

Oxaliplatin/Eloxatin®—Caution in renal impairment; safety not established

Oxandrolone/Oxandrin®

Oxazepam/Serax®

Oxybutynin/Ditropan®

Oxycodone/Roxicodone®, Oxecta™, OxyContin®

Oxymetholone/Anadrol®-50

Oxytocin/Pitocin®

Paclitaxel/Taxol®

Palifermin/Kepivance®

Palivizumab/Synagis®

Palonosetron/Aloxi®

Pancrelipase/Creon®, Zenpep®

Panitumumab/Vectibix®—Caution, no data in renal impairment

Pantoprazole/Protonix®

Papaverine

Papillomavirus vaccine, human, recombinant/Gardasil®

Paregoric

Paricalcitol/Zemplar®

Paromomycin/Humatin®

Pazopanib/Votrient™

Pegaptanib/Macugen®

Pegaspargase/Oncaspar®

Pegfilgrastim/Neulasta®

Peginesatide/Omontys®—Caution, not indicated in patients with chronic kidney disease not on dialysis

Pegloticase/Krystexxa™

Pegvisomant/Somavert®—Caution, no data in renal impairment

Penbutolol/Levatol®

Penicillin G benzathine/Bicillin LA®

Penicillin G procaine/Wycillin®

Penicillin V potassium/Pen VK®

Pentamidine (inhaled)/Nebupent®

Pentobarbital/Nembutal®

Pentosan polysulfate/Elmiron®

Perphenazine/Trilafon®

Pertuzumab/Perjeta™

Phenelzine/Nardil®

Phenol

Phenoxybenzamine/Dibenzyline®

Phentermine/Ionamin®

Phentolamine/Regitine®

Phenylephrine/Neo-Synephrine®

Phosphorated carbohydrate solution/Emetrol[c]

Physostigmine

Phytonadione/AquaMephyton®, Mephyton®

Pilocarpine/Salagen®

Pimozide/Orap®

Pindolol/Visken®

Pioglitazone/Actos®

Perflutren/Definity®

Pneumococcal conjugate vaccine (7-valent)/Prevnar®

Pneumococcal polysaccharide vaccine/ Pneumovax 23®

Polidocanol/Asclera®

Poliovirus vaccine (inactivated)/IPOL®

Polyethylene glycol 3350/Miralax®, MoviPrep®

Polyethylene glycol-electrolyte solution/Colyte®, Golytely®, Nulytely®

Porfimer/Photofrin®

Posaconazole/Noxafil®

Potassium iodide/SSKI®

Pralatrexate/Folotyn®

Pramlintide/Symlin®—Caution, no data in hemodialysis

Prasugrel/Effient™

Pravastatin/Pravachol®—Caution, with history of significant renal dysfunction, starting dose is 10 mg daily

Praziquantel/Biltricide®

Prazosin/Minipress®

Prednisolone/Orapred®, Prelone®

Prednisone/Deltasone®

Prilocaine/Citanest®

Primaquine

Procaine/Novocain®

Procarbazine/Matulane®

Prochlorperazine/Compazine®

Progesterone/Prometrium®

Promethazine/Phenergan®

Propafenone/Rythmol®

Propantheline/Pro-Banthine®

Propofol/Diprivan®

Propranolol/Inderal®

Propylthiouracil

Protamine

Protriptyline/Vivactil®

Pseudoephedrine/Sudafed®

Psyllium/Metamucil®

Pyrantel pamoate/Combantrin™

Pyrazinamide

Pyrethrins and piperonyl butoxide/ Rid®

Pyridoxine

Pyrimethamine/Daraprim®

Quazepam/Doral®

Quetiapine/Seroquel®

Quinupristin and dalfopristin/ Synercid®

Rabeprazole/AcipHex®

Rabies immune globulin/HyperRab®

Raloxifene/Evista®

Raltegravir/Isentress®

Ramelteon/Rozerem®

Ranibizumab/Lucentis®

Rasagiline/Azilect®—Caution, no data in severe renal impairment

Rasburicase/Elitek®

Regadenoson/Lexiscan®

Remifentanil/Ultiva®—Caution, in patients >65 years, decrease starting dose by 50 %

Reteplase/Retavase®

Rh$_0$(D) immune globulin/RhoGam®

Ribavirin (inhaled)/Virazole®

Rilpivirine/Endurant™

Riboflavin

Rifapentine/Priftin®

Rifaximin/Xifaxan™

Rilpivirine/Edurant™

Riluzole/Rilutek®

RimabotulinumtoxinB/Myobloc®

Risperidone injection/Risperdal® Consta®

Ritonavir/Norvir®

Rituximab/Rituxan®—Caution, minimal data in renal impairment

Rivastigmine/Exelon®

Rizatriptan/Maxalt®

Rocuronium/Zemuron®

Roflumilast/Daliresp™

Romidepsin/Istodax®

Romiplostim/Nplate™

Ropinirole/Requip®

Ropvivacaine/Naropin®

Rosiglitazone/Avandia®

Rufinamide/Banzel™

Sacrosidase/Sucraid®

Saquinavir/Invirase®

Sargramostim/Leukine®

Scopolamine/Transderm Scōp®

Secobarbital/Seconal®

Selegiline/Eldepryl®

Selenium (homeopathic)/Male Libido™

Sertraline/Zoloft®

Sevelamer/Renagel®

Sevoflurane/Ultane®

Sildenafil/Revatio®, Viagra®—Caution, if CrCL < 30 mL/min, consider starting dose at Viagra 25 mg

Simethicone/Mylicon®

Simvastatin/Zocor®

Sipuleucel-T/Provenge®

Sirolimus/Rapamune®

Sodium bicarbonate

Sodium bicarbonate/Alka Seltzer® Heartburn and Acid Indigestion Relief

Sodium citrate and citric acid/Bicitra®

Sodium oxybate/Xyrem®

Sodium polystyrene sulfonate/ Kayexalate®

Sodium tetradecyl sulfate/Sotradecol®

Somatropin/Humatrope®

Sorbitol

Succimer/Chemet®—Caution in renal impairment

Succinylcholine/Anectine®

Sucralfate/Carafate®

Sufentanil/Sufenta®

Sulfadiazine

Sulfasalazine/Azulfidine®—Caution, 37 % cleared renally

Sulindac/Clinoril®—Caution, not recommended in advanced renal disease

Sumatriptan/Imitrex®

Tacrine/Cognex®

Tacrolimus/Prograf®—Caution, careful monitoring indicated in renal dysfunction

Tamoxifen/Nolvadex®

Telaprevir/Incivek™

Telmisartan/Micardis®

Temazepam/Restoril™

Temozolomide/Temodar®—Caution in severely impaired renal function (CrCL < 36 mL/min); no data in hemodialysis

Temsirolimus/Torisel®

Tenecteplase/TNKase®

Teniposide/Vumon®

Terazosin/Hytrin®

Teriparatide/Forteo®

Tesamorelin/Egrifta™—Caution, safety not established in renal impairment

Testosterone/Delatestryl®, Depo-Testosterone®

Tetanus immune globulin/ HyperTet™

Tetrabenazine/Xenazine®

Tetracaine/Pontocaine®

Thalidomide/Thalomid®

Theophylline/Elixophyllin®, Uniphyl®

Thiabendazole/Mintezol®—Caution in renal impairment

Thiamine

Thioguanine/Tabloid®

Thioridazine/Mellaril®

Thiotepa—Caution, use in low dosage, monitor carefully

Thiothixene/Navane®

Thyroid/Armour Thyroid®

Thyrotropin alfa/Thyrogen®

Tiagabine/Gabitril®

Ticagrelor/Brilinta™

Ticlopidine/Ticlid®

Tigecycline/Tygacil®

Timolol/Blocadren®

Tinidazole/Tindamax®

Tipranavir/Aptivus®

Tocilizumab/Actemra®

Tolazamide/Tolinase®

Tolbutamide/Orinase®

Tolcapone/Tasmar®—Caution in severe renal impairment (CrCL < 25 mL/min)

Tolvaptan/Samsca™

Toremifene/Fareston®

Torsemide/Demadex®

Tranylcypromine/Parnate®

Trastuzumab/Herceptin®

Trazodone/Desyrel®

Treprostinil/Remodulin®

Tretinoin/Vesanoid®—Caution, no data in renal impairment

Triamcinolone/Kenalog®, Aristospan®

Triazolam/Halcion®

Trientine/Syprine®

Trifluoperazine/Stelazine®

Trihexyphenidyl/Artane®

Trimethobenzamide/Tigan®

Trimipramine/Surmontil®

Triprolidine and pseudoephedrine/ Actifed®
Triptorelin/Trelstar®—Caution, rate of elimination is diminished in renal impairment
Typhoid Vaccine/Vivotif®
Urofollitropin/Bravelle®
Ursodiol/Actigall®, Urso®
Ustekinumab/Stelara®—Caution, minimal data in renal impairment
Valproic acid/Depacon®, Depakene®
Valsartan/Diovan®
Vancomycin (oral)/Vancocin®
Vardenafil/Levitra®

Varicella virus vaccine/Varivax®
Varicella-zoster immune globulin/ VariZIG™
Vasopressin/Pitressin®
Vecuronium/Norcuron®
Vemurafenib/Zelboraf™
Verapamil/Calan®, Isoptin®—Caution in renal impairment
Verteporfin/Visudyne®
Vilazodone/Viibryd™
Vinblastine/Velban®
Vincristine/Oncovin®
Vinorelbine/Navelbine®
Vismodegib/Erivedge™

Vitamin A/Aquasol A®
Vitamin E/Aquasol E®
Vorinostat/Zolinza®
Warfarin/Coumadin®
Yohimbine/Yocon®
Zafirlukast/Accolate®
Zaleplon/Sonata®
Zanamivir/Relenza®
Zileuton/Zyflo®
Zinc sulfate/Zincate®
Ziprasidone/Geodon®
Zolmitriptan/Zomig®
Zolpidem/Ambien®, Intermezzo®
Zoster vaccine/Zostavax®

A

L.K. Golightly et al. (eds.), *Renal Pharmacotherapy*,
DOI 10.1007/978-1-4614-5800-5_1, © Springer Science+Business Media New York 2013

<u>Acamprosate</u> - Selected References

Brasser SM, McCaul ME, Houtsmuller EJ. Alcohol effects during acamprosate treatment: a dose-response study in humans. Alcohol Clin Exp Res. 2004;28:1074–83.

Campral® tablet, delayed release [package insert]. St Louis: Forrest Pharmaceuticals Inc; 2010.

Hammarberg A, Beck O, Eksborg S, et al. Acamprosate determinations in plasma and cerebrospinal fluid after multiple dosing measured by liquid chromatography-mass spectroscopy: a pharmacokinetic study in healthy volunteers. Ther Drug Monit. 2010;32:489–96.

Johnson BA, O'Malley SS, Ciraulo DA, et al. Dose-ranging kinetics and behavioral pharmacology of naltrexone and acamprosate, both alone and combined, in alcohol-dependent subjects. J Clin Psychopharmacol. 2003;23:281–93.

Mason BJ, Goodman AM, Dixon RM, et al. A pharmacokinetic and pharmacodynamic drug interaction study of acamprosate and naltrexone. Neuropsychopharmacology. 2002;27:596–606.

Namkoong K, Lee B-O, Lee P-G, Choi M-J, Lee E. Acamprosate in Korean alcohol-dependent patients: a multi-centre, randomized, double-blind, placebo-controlled study. Alcohol Alcohol. 2003;38:135–41.

Rhee Y-S, Park S, Lee T-W, et al. Investigation of the relationship between in vitro and in vivo release behaviors of acamprosate from enteric-coated tablets. Arch Pharm Res. 2008;31:798–804.

Saivin S, Hulot T, Chabac S, Potgieter A, Durbin P, Houin G. Clinical pharmacokinetics of acamprosate. Clin Pharmacokinet. 1998;35:331–45.

Scott LJ, Figgitt DP, Keam SJ, Waugh J. Acamprosate: a review of its use in maintenance of abstinence in patients with alcohol dependence. CNS Drugs. 2005;19:445–64.

Umhau JC, Momenan R, Schwandt ML, et al. Effect of acamprosate on magnetic resonance spectroscopy measures of central glutamate in detoxified alcohol-dependent individuals: a randomized controlled experimental medicine study. Arch Gen Psychiatry. 2010;67:1069–77.

Dosage Adjustment of Medications Eliminated by the Kidneys

<u>Acamprosate</u>/Campral®	{Alcohol deterrent; putative glutamate/GABA receptor modifier}

Usual initial dose:	666 mg orally
Usual maintenance dose:	666 mg (two 333 mg tablets) orally three times daily
Typical maximum dose:	1,998 mg/day
Proportion eliminated unchanged:	~90 %

Adjustment for Kidney Disease

FDA-approved product labeling:	*CrCL >50 mL/min*	*666 mg orally three times daily*
	CrCL 30–50 mL/min	*333 mg orally three times daily*
	CrCL <30 mL/min	*Contraindicated*
Alternative adjustment:	*Data not available*	

Dosage Adjustment of Medications Eliminated by the Kidneys

Acarbose - Selected References

Abe M, Okada K, Soma M. Antidiabetic agents in patients with chronic kidney disease and end-stage renal disease on dialysis: metabolism and clinical practice. Curr Drug Metab. 2011;12:57–69.

Aronoff GA, Bennett WM, Berns JS, et al. Drug prescribing in renal failure: dosing guidelines for adults and children. 5th ed. Philadelphia: American College of Physicians; 2007.

Balfour JA, McTavish D. Acarbose: an update of its pharmacology and therapeutic use in diabetes mellitus. Drugs. 1993;46:1025–54.

Harrower AD. Pharmacokinetics of antihyperglycaemic agents in patients with renal insufficiency. Clin Pharmacokinet. 1996;31:111–9.

McIntyre CW, Owen PJ. Prescribing drugs in kidney disease. In: Brenner BM, editor. Brenner & Rector's the kidney. 8th ed. Philadelphia: Saunders Elsevier; 2008. p. 1930–55.

Olyaei AJ, Bennett WM. Pharmacologic approach to renal insufficiency. In: Dale DC, Federman DD, Antman K, editors. ACP medicine, WebMD June 2007 Update. Hamilton: BC Decker; 2007; NEPHROLOGY IX: Appendix A1–25.

Olyaei AJ, Bennett WM. Drug dosing in elderly patients with chronic kidney disease. Clin Geriatr Med. 2009;25:459–527.

Olyaei AJ, DeMattos AM, Bennett WM. Use of drugs in patients with renal failure. In: Schrier RW, editor. Diseases of the kidney and urinary tract. 8th ed. Philadelphia: Lippincott Williams & Wilkins; 2007. p. 2765–807.

Precose® tablet [package insert]. Wayne: Bayer HealthCare Pharmaceuticals Inc; 2008.

Salvatore T, Giugliamo D. Pharmacokinetic-pharmacodynamic relationships of acarbose. Clin Pharmacokinet. 1996;30: 94–106.

Dosage Adjustment of Medications Eliminated by the Kidneys

<u>Acarbose</u>/Precose®	{Antidiabetic; α-glucosidase inhibitor}	
Usual initial dose:	25 mg orally one to three times daily with meals	
Usual maintenance dose:	50–100 mg orally three times daily with meals	
Typical maximum dose:	50 mg orally three times daily (weight ≤60 kg); 100 mg orally three times daily (weight >60 kg)	
Proportion eliminated unchanged:	35 %	

Adjustment for Kidney Disease

FDA-approved product labeling:	*SCr >2.0 mg/dL*	*Clinical trials in diabetic patients with significant renal dysfunction (SCr >2.0 mg/dL) have not been conducted; therefore, treatment of these patients with (acarbose) is not recommended.*
Alternative adjustment:	*GFR >50 mL/min*	*50 mg orally three times daily with meals*
	GFR 10–50 mL/min	*Data not available. Preferably avoid unless no suitable alternative exists; if indeed necessary, begin with low doses and monitor carefully.*
	GFR <10 mL/min	*Data not available. Preferably avoid unless no suitable alternative exists; if indeed necessary, begin with low doses and monitor carefully.*
	Hemodialysis	*Data not available. Avoid unless no suitable alternative exists; if indeed necessary, begin with low doses and monitor carefully.*
	CAPD	*Data not available. Preferably avoid unless no suitable alternative exists; if indeed necessary, begin with low doses and monitor carefully.*
	CRRT	*Not applicable; preferably avoid unless no suitable alternative exists.*

Dosage Adjustment of Medications Eliminated by the Kidneys

Acebutolol - Selected References

Acebutolol hydrochloride capsule [package insert]. Morgantown: Mylan Pharmaceuticals Inc; 2006.

Aronoff GA, Bennett WM, Berns JS, et al. Drug prescribing in renal failure: dosing guidelines for adults and children. 5th ed. Philadelphia: American College of Physicians; 2007.

Bailey DG. Fruit juice inhibition of uptake transport: a new type of food-drug interaction. Br J Clin Pharmacol. 2010; 70:645–55.

Baker JG, Hall IP, Hill SJ. Agonist actions of "β-blockers" provide evidence for two agonist activation sites or conformations of the human β1-adrenoceptor. Mol Pharmacol. 2003;63:1312–21.

Begg E, Munn S, Bailey RR. Acebutolol in the treatment of patients with hypertension and renal functional impairment. N Z Med J. 1979;89:293–5.

Cuthbert MF, Collins RF. Plasma levels and β-adrenoceptor blockade with acebutolol, practolol and propranolol in man. Br J Clin Pharmacol. 1975;2:49–55.

Daly MJ, Flook JJ, Levy GP. The selectivity of β-adrenoceptor antagonists on cardiovascular and bronchodilator responses to isoprenaline in the anaesthetized dog. Br J Pharmacol. 1975;53:173–81.

Gabriel R. Acebutolol in the management of hypertension in patients with renal disease. Br J Clin Pract. 1979;33:259–62.

Gulaid A, James IM, Kaye CM, et al. Lack of correlation between acetylator status and the production of the acetyl metabolite of acebutolol in man [letter]. Br J Clin Pharmacol. 1978;5:261–2.

Kaye CM, Dufton JF. Preliminary observations on the elimination of acebutolol in severe chronic renal failure [letter]. Br J Clin Pharmacol. 1976;3:198–9.

Kirch W, Köhler H, Berggren G, Braun W. The influence of renal function on plasma levels and urinary excretion of acebutolol and its main N-acetyl metabolite. Clin Nephrol. 1982;18:88–94.

Lilja JJ, Raaska K, Neuvonen PJ. Effects of grapefruit juice on the pharmacokinetics of acebutolol. Br J Clin Pharmacol. 2005:60:659–63.

Martin MA, Phillips FC, Tucker GT, Smith AJ. Acebutolol in hypertension: relationships between drug concentration and effects. Eur J Clin Pharmacol. 1978;14:383–90.

McIntyre CW, Owen PJ. Prescribing drugs in kidney disease. In: Brenner BM, editor. Brenner & Rector's the kidney. 8th ed. Philadelphia: Saunders Elsevier; 2008. p. 1930–55.

Meffin PJ, Winkle RA, Peters FA, Harrison DC, Harapat SR, Yee Y-G. Dose-dependent acebutolol disposition after oral administration. Clin Pharmacol Ther. 1978;24:542–7.

Munn S, Bailey RR, Begg E, Ebert R, Ferry DG. Plasma and urine concentrations of acebutolol and its acetyl metabolite in patients with renal impairment. N Z Med J. 1980;91:289–91.

Olyaei AJ, Bennett WM. Pharmacologic approach to renal insufficiency. In: Dale DC, Federman DD, Antman K, editors. ACP medicine, WebMD June 2007 Update. Hamilton: BC Decker; 2007; NEPHROLOGY IX: Appendix A1–25.

Olyaei AJ, Bennett WM. Drug dosing in elderly patients with chronic kidney disease. Clin Geriatr Med. 2009;25:459–27.

Olyaei AJ, DeMattos AM, Bennett WM. Use of drugs in patients with renal failure. In: Schrier RW, editor. Diseases of the kidney and urinary tract. 8th ed. Philadelphia: Lippincott Williams & Wilkins; 2007. p. 2765–807.

Roux A, Aubert P, Buedon J, Flouvat B. Pharmacokinetics of acebutolol in patients with all grades of renal failure. Eur J Clin Pharmacol. 1980;17:339–48.

Salpeter SR, Ormiston TM, Salpeter EE, Wood-Baker R. Cardioselective beta-blockers for reversible airway disease (review). Cochrane Database Syst Rev. 2002;(4):CD002992. doi:10.1002/14651858.CD002992.

Singh BN, Thoden WR, Wahl J. Acebutolol: a review of its pharmacology, pharmacokinetics, clinical uses, and adverse effects. Pharmacotherapy. 1986;6:45–63.

Smith RS, Warren DJ, Renwick AG, George CF. Acebutolol pharmacokinetics in renal failure. Br J Clin Pharmacol. 1983;16:253–8.

Winkle RA, Meffin PJ, Ricks WB, Harrison DC. Acebutolol metabolite plasma concentration during chronic oral therapy. Br J Clin Pharmacol. 1977;4:519–22.

Dosage Adjustment of Medications Eliminated by the Kidneys

<u>Acebutolol</u>/Sectral®	**{Antihypertensive; antianginal; β-adrenergic receptor blocker}**
Usual initial dose:	200 mg orally twice daily
Usual maintenance dose:	400–800 mg/day orally
Typical maximum dose:	1,200 mg/day
Proportion eliminated unchanged:	55 % (acebutolol 18 %, primary active metabolite >90 %)

Adjustment for Kidney Disease

FDA-approved product labeling:	*CrCL <50 mL/min*	*100 mg orally twice daily (50 % decrease)*
	CrCL <25 mL/min	*100 mg orally once daily (75 % decrease)*
Alternative adjustment:	*GFR >50 mL/min*	*200 mg orally twice daily; titrate.*
	GFR 10–50 mL/min	*100 mg orally twice daily; titrate (50 % decrease).*
	GFR <10 mL/min	*100 mg orally once daily; titrate (75 % decrease).*
	Hemodialysis	*100 mg orally once daily; titrate; administer after hemodialysis on dialysis days.*
	CAPD	*Data not available. Preferably avoid unless no suitable alternative exists; if indeed necessary, begin with low doses and monitor carefully.*
	CRRT	*100 mg enterally twice daily; titrate.*

Dosage Adjustment of Medications Eliminated by the Kidneys

Acetaminophen - Selected References

Aronoff GA, Bennett WM, Berns JS, et al. Drug prescribing in renal failure: dosing guidelines for adults and children. 5th ed. Philadelphia: American College of Physicians; 2007.

Carpenter HM, Mudge GH. Acetaminophen nephrotoxicity: studies on renal acetylation and deacetylation. J Pharmacol Exp Ther. 1981;218:161–7.

Davenport A, Finn R. Paracetamol (acetaminophen) poisoning resulting in acute renal failure without hepatic coma. Nephron. 1988;50:55–6.

de Maat MM, Tijssen TA, Brüggemann RJ, Ponssen HH. Paracetamol for intravenous use in medium- and intensive-care patients: pharmacokinetics and tolerance. Eur J Clin Pharmacol. 2010:66:713–9.

Duggan ST, Scott LJ. Intravenous paracetamol (acetaminophen). Drugs. 2009;69:101–13.

Duggin GG, Mudge GH. Analgesic nephropathy: renal distribution of acetaminophen and its conjugates. J Pharmacol Exp Ther. 1976;199:1–9.

FeverAll® suppository [package insert]. Morristown: Actavis US; 2011.

Forrest JAH, Clements JA, Prescott LF. Clinical pharmacokinetics of paracetamol. Clin Pharmacokinet. 1982;7:93–107.

Holmér Pettersson P, Öwall A, Jakobsson J. Early bioavailability of paracetamol after oral or intravenous administration. Acta Anaesthesiol Scand. 2004;48:867–70.

Jahr JS, Lee VK. Intravenous acetaminophen. Anesthesiol Clin. 2010;28:619–45.

Levy G. Comparative pharmacokinetics of aspirin and acetaminophen. Arch Intern Med. 1981;141:279–81.

Liukas A, Kuusiemi K, Aantaa R, et al. Pharmacokinetics of intravenous paracetamol in elderly patients. Clin Pharmacokinet. 2011;60:121–9.

Lowenthal DT, Øie S, van Stone JC, Briggs WA, Levy G. Pharmacokinetics of acetaminophen elimination by anephric patients. J Pharmacol Exp Ther. 1976;196:570–8.

Marbury TC, Wang LH, Lee CS. Hemodialysis of acetaminophen in uremic patients. Int J Artif Organs. 1980;3:263–6.

Martin U, Temple RM, Winney RJ, Prescott LF. The disposition of paracetamol and its conjugates during multiple dosing in patients with end-stage renal failure maintained on haemodialysis. Eur J Clin Pharmacol. 1993;45:141–5.

Mattammal MB, Zenser TV, Brown WW, Herman CA, Davis BB. Mechanism of inhibition of renal prostaglandin production by acetaminophen. J Pharmacol Exp Ther. 1979;210:405–9.

Ofirmev™ injection [package insert]. San Diego: Cadence Pharmaceuticals Inc; 2010.

Øie S, Lowenthal DT, Briggs WA, Levy G. Effect of hemodialysis on acetaminophen elimination by anephric patients. Clin Pharmacol Ther. 1975;18:680–6.

Perneger TV, Whelton PK, Klag MJ. Risk of kidney failure associated with the use of acetaminophen, aspirin, and nonsteroidal antiinflammatory drugs. N Engl J Med. 1994;331:1675–9.

Plotz PH, Kimberly RP. Acute effects of aspirin and acetaminophen on renal function. Arch Intern Med. 1981;141:343–8.

Prescott LF. Kinetics and metabolism of paracetamol and phenacetin. Br J Clin Pharmacol. 1980;10:S291–8.

Prescott LF, Speirs GC, Critchley JAJH, Temple RM, Winney RJ. Paracetamol disposition and metabolite kinetics in patients with chronic renal failure. Eur J Clin Pharmacol. 1989;36:291–7.

Rawlins MD, Henderson DB, Hijab AR. Pharmacokinetics of paracetamol (acetaminophen) after intravenous and oral administration. Eur J Clin Pharmacol. 1977;11:283–6.

Sandler DP, Smith JC, Weinbert CR, et al. Analgesic use and chronic renal disease. N Engl J Med. 1989;320:1238–43.

Schreiner GE, McAnally JF, Winchester JF. Clinical analgesic nephropathy. Arch Intern Med. 1981;141:349–57.

Segasothy M, Suleiman AB, Puvaneswary M, Rohana A. Paracetamol: a cause for analgesic nephropathy and end-stage renal disease. Nephron. 1988;50:50–4.

Segasothy M, Tong BKC, Kamal A, Murad Z, Suleiman AB. Analgesic nephropathy associated with paracetamol. Aust N Z J Med. 1984;14:23–6.

Tylenol® Regular Strength Tablet [package insert]. Fort Washington: McNeil Consumer Healthcare; 2011.

Dosage Adjustment of Medications Eliminated by the Kidneys

__Acetaminophen__/Tylenol®, Ofirmev™   {Antipyretic; analgesic}

Usual initial dose:	650 mg orally or rectally or 1,000 mg IV
Usual maintenance dose:	650 mg orally or rectally or 1,000 mg IV every 6 h (PRN)
Typical maximum dose:	4,000 mg/day (3,250 mg/day in persons with evidence of liver disease)
Proportion eliminated unchanged:	4 %

Adjustment for Kidney Disease

FDA-approved product labeling:	*Severe renal impairment*	*Longer dosing intervals and a reduced total daily dose of acetaminophen may be warranted.*
Alternative adjustment:	*GFR >50 mL/min*	*650 mg orally or rectally or 1,000 mg IV every 6 h (PRN)*
	GFR 10–50 mL/min	*650 mg orally or rectally or 1,000 mg IV every 6 h (PRN) (no change)*
	GFR <10 mL/min	*650 mg orally or rectally or 1,000 mg IV every 8 h (PRN)*
	Hemodialysis	*650 mg orally or rectally or 1,000 mg IV every 8 h (PRN)*
	CAPD	*650 mg orally or rectally or 1,000 mg IV every 8 h (PRN)*
	CRRT	*650 mg orally or rectally or 1,000 mg IV every 6 h (PRN)*

Dosage Adjustment of Medications Eliminated by the Kidneys

Acetazolamide - Selected References

Acetazolamide injection USP [package insert]. Big Flats: X-GEN Pharmaceuticals Inc; 2009.

Acetazolamide tablet USP [package insert]. Hawthorne: Taro Pharmaceuticals USA Inc; 2005.

Alm A, Berggren L, Hartvig P, Roosdorp M. Monitoring acetazolamide treatment. Acta Ophthalmol (Copenh). 1982;60: 24–34.

Aronoff GA, Bennett WM, Berns JS, et al. Drug prescribing in renal failure: dosing guidelines for adults and children. 5th ed. Philadelphia: American College of Physicians; 2007.

Chapron DJ, Gomolin IH, Sweeney KR. Acetazolamide blood concentrations are excessive in the elderly: propensity for acidosis and relationship to renal function. J Clin Pharmacol. 1989;29:348–53.

Diamox® Sequels extended-release capsules [package insert]. Pomona: Duramed Pharmaceuticals Inc; 2008.

Kunka RL, Mattocks AM. Relationship for pharmacokinetics to pharmacological response for acetazolamide. J Pharm Sci. 1979;68:347–9.

McIntyre CW, Owen PJ. Prescribing drugs in kidney disease. In: Brenner BM, editor. Brenner & Rector's the kidney. 8th ed. Philadelphia: Saunders Elsevier; 2008. p. 1930–55.

Olyaei AJ, Bennett WM. Pharmacologic approach to renal insufficiency. In: Dale DC, Federman DD, Antman K, editors. ACP medicine, WebMD June 2007 update. Hamilton: BC Decker; 2007; NEPHROLOGY IX: Appendix A1–25.

Olyaei AJ, Bennett WM. Drug dosing in elderly patients with chronic kidney disease. Clin Geriatr Med. 2009;25:459–527.

Olyaei AJ, DeMattos AM, Bennett WM. Use of drugs in patients with renal failure. In: Schrier RW, editor. Diseases of the kidney and urinary tract. 8th ed. Philadelphia: Lippincott Williams & Wilkins; 2007. p. 2765–807.

Roy LF, Dufresne LR, Legault L, Long H, Morin C. Acetazolamide in hemodialysis patients: a rational use after ocular surgery. Am J Kidney Dis. 1992;20:650–2.

Schwenk MH, St Peter WL, Meese MG, Singhal PC. Acetazolamide toxicity and pharmacokinetics in patients receiving hemodialysis. Pharmacotherapy. 1995;15:522–7.

Tawil R, Moxley RT III, Griggs RC. Acetazolamide-induced nephrolithiasis: implications for treatment of neuromuscular disorders. Neurology. 1993;43:1105–6.

Yano I, Takayama A, Takano M, et al. Pharmacokinetics and pharmacodynamics of acetazolamide in patients with transient intraocular pressure elevation. Eur J Clin Pharmacol. 1998:54:63–8.

Dosage Adjustment of Medications Eliminated by the Kidneys

<u>Acetazolamide</u>/Diamox®   {Diuretic; antiepileptic; carbonic anhydrase inhibitor}

Usual initial dose:	250–500 mg orally or IV
Usual maintenance dose:	250–500 mg (approx 5 mg/kg) orally or IV every 6–12 h
Typical maximum dose:	1,000 mg/day
Proportion eliminated unchanged:	95 %

Adjustment for Kidney Disease

FDA-approved product labeling:	*Marked kidney disease or dysfunction*	*Contraindicated*
Alternative adjustment:	*GFR >50 mL/min*	*250 mg orally or IV every 6 h*
	GFR 10–50 mL/min	*125 mg orally or IV every 12 h*
	GFR <10 mL/min	*Data not available. Preferably avoid unless no suitable alternative exists; if indeed necessary, begin with low doses and monitor carefully.*
	Hemodialysis	*Minimal data available. Preferably avoid or use in reduced doses of 62.5–125 mg orally or IV every 24 h with careful clinical and serum level monitoring.**
	CAPD	*Data not available. Preferably avoid unless no suitable alternative exists; if indeed necessary, begin with low doses and monitor carefully.*
	CRRT	*250 mg orally or IV every 12 h*

*Therapeutic Drug Monitoring

Therapeutic Plasma Levels: *Mid-interval to trough concentration: 4–10 mg/L*

Dosage Adjustment of Medications Eliminated by the Kidneys

Acetohydroxamic Acid - Selected References

Aronoff GA, Bennett WM, Berns JS, et al. Drug prescribing in renal failure: dosing guidelines for adults and children. 5th ed. Philadelphia: American College of Physicians; 2007.

Burr RG, Nuseibeh I. The effect of acetohydroxamic acid on urinary saturation in stone-forming spinal cord patients. Br J Urol. 1983;55:162–5.

Feldman S, Putcha L, Griffith DP. Pharmacokinetics of acetohydroxamic acid: preliminary investigations. Invest Urol. 1978;15:498–501.

Griffith DP, Musher DM. Acetohydroxamic acid: potential use in urinary infection caused by urea-splitting bacteria. Urology. 1975;5:299–302.

Griffith DP, Gibson JR, Clinton CW, Musher DM. Acetohydroxamic acid: clinical studies of a urease inhibitor in patients with staghorn renal calculi. J Urol. 1978;119:9–15.

Griffith DP, Gleeson MJ, Lee H, Longuet R, Deman E, Earle N. Randomized, double-blind trial of Lithostat™ (acetohydroxamic acid) in the palliative treatment of infection-induced urinary calculi. Eur Urol. 1991;20:243–7.

Griffith DP, Khonsari F, Skurnick JH, James KE. A randomized trial of acetohydroxamic acid for the treatment and prevention of infection-induced urinary stones in spinal cord injury patients. J Urol. 1988;140:318-–24.

Lamm DL, Johnson SA, Friedlander AM, Gittes RF. Medical therapy of experimental infection stones. Urology. 1977;10:418–21.

Lithostat® tablet [package insert]. San Antonio: Mission Pharmacal Co; 2011.

Martelli A, Bull P, Cortecchia V. Acetohydroxamic acid therapy in infected renal stones. Urology. 1981;17:320–2.

McIntyre CW, Owen PJ. Prescribing drugs in kidney disease. In: Brenner BM, editor. Brenner & Rector's the kidney. 8th ed. Philadelphia: Saunders Elsevier; 2008. p. 1930–55.

Musher DM, Saenz C, Griffith DP. Interaction between acetohydroxamic acid and 12 antibiotics against 14 gram-negative pathogenic bacteria. Antimicrob Agents Chemother. 1974;5:106–10.

Putcha L, Griffith DP, Feldman S. Pharmacokinetics of acetohydroxamic acid in patients with staghorn renal calculi. Eur J Clin Pharmacol. 1985;28:439–45.

Rodman JS, Williams JJ, Jones RL. Hypercoagulability produced by treatment with acetohydroxamic acid. Clin Pharmacol Ther. 1987;42:346–50.

Rodman JS, Williams JJ, Peterson CM. Partial dissolution of struvite calculus with oral acetohydroxamic acid. Urology. 1983;22:410–2.

Williams JJ, Rodman JS, Peterson CM. A randomized double-blind study of acetohydroxamic acid in struvite nephrolithiasis. N Engl J Med. 1984;311:760–4.

Dosage Adjustment of Medications Eliminated by the Kidneys

Acetohydroxamic Acid/Lithostat®	{Antibacterial for chronic urea-splitting urinary infection; urease inhibitor}
Usual initial dose:	12 mg/kg/day total (e.g., one tablet [250 mg] three to four times a day)
Usual maintenance dose:	10–15 mg/kg/day
Typical maximum dose:	1.5 g/day
Proportion eliminated unchanged:	19–48 %

Adjustment for Kidney Disease

FDA-approved product labeling:	*SCr ≥1.8–2.5 mg/dL*	*Maximum dose 500 mg orally twice daily*
	SCr >2.5 mg/dL	*Contraindicated*
Alternative adjustment:	*GFR >50 mL/min*	*10–15 mg/kg/day orally in three to four divided doses*
	GFR 10–50 mL/min	*10–15 mg/kg/day in orally three to four divided doses*
	GFR <10 mL/min	*Preferably avoid due to risks of drug and metabolite accumulation, bone marrow depression, hypercoagulability, hypercarbia, and electrolyte derangements.*
	Hemodialysis	*Preferably avoid due to risks of drug and metabolite accumulation, bone marrow depression, hypercoagulability, hypercarbia, and electrolyte derangements.*
	CAPD	*Preferably avoid due to risks of drug and metabolite accumulation, bone marrow depression, hypercoagulability, hypercarbia, and electrolyte derangements.*
	CRRT	*Not applicable; preferably avoid.*

Dosage Adjustment of Medications Eliminated by the Kidneys

Acitretin - Selected References

Bavinck JNB, Tieben LM, Van Der Woude FJ, et al. Prevention of skin cancer and reduction of keratotic skin lesions during acitretin therapy in renal transplant recipients: a double-blind, placebo-controlled study. J Clin Oncol. 1995;13:1933–8.

Brindley CJ. Overview of recent clinical pharmacokinetic studies with acitretin (Ro 10-1670, etretin). Dermatologica. 1989;178:79–87.

Carneiro RV, Sotto MN, Azevedo LS, Ianhez LE, Rivitti EA. Acitretin and skin cancer in kidney transplanted patients. Clinical and histological evaluation and immunohistochemical analysis of lymphocytes, natural killer cells and Langerhans' cells in sun exposed and sun protected skin. Clin Transplant. 2005;19:115–21.

Chen K, Craig JC, Shumack S. Oral retinoids for the prevention of skin cancers in solid organ transplant recipients: a systematic review of randomized controlled trials. Br J Dermatol. 2005;152:518–23.

de Sévaux RGL, Smit JV, de Jong EMGJ, van de Kerkhof PCM, Hoitsma AJ. Acitretin treatment of premalignant and malignant skin disorders in renal transplant recipients: clinical effects of a randomized trial comparing two doses of acitretin. J Am Acad Dermatol. 2003;49:407–12.

Dunn LK, Gaar LR, Yentzer BA, O'Neill JL, Feldman SR. Acitretin in dermatology: a review. J Drugs Dermatol. 2011;10:772–82.

European Best Practice Guideline Expert Group on Renal Transplantation. Long-term management of the transplant recipient. IV.6.2. Skin cancers: prevention and treatment. Nephrol Dial Transplant. 2002;17(Suppl 4):31–6.

George R, Weightman W, Russ GR, Bannister KM, Mathew TH. Acitretin for chemoprevention of non-melanoma skin cancers in renal transplant recipients. Australas J Dermatol. 2002;43:269–73.

Lambert WE, Meyer E, De Leenheer AP, De Bersaques J, Kint AH. Pharmacokinetics and drug interactions of etretinate and acitretin. J Am Acad Dermatol. 1992;27 (6 Pt 2):S19–22.

Lambert WE, Meyer E, De Leenheer AP, De Bersaques J, Kint AH. Pharmacokinetics of acitretin. Acta Derm Venereol Suppl (Stockh). 1994;186:122–3.

Larsen FG. Pharmacokinetics of etretinate and acitretin with special reference to treatment of psoriasis. Acta Derm Venereol Suppl (Stockh). 1994;190:1–33.

Larsen FG, Jakobsen P, Eriksen H, Grønhøj J, Kragballe K, Nielsen-Kudsk F. The pharmacokinetics of acitretin and its 13-cis-metabolite in psoriatic patients. J Clin Pharmacol. 1991;31:477-83.

Larsen FG, Jakobsen P, Larsen CG, Kragballe K, Nielsen-Kudsk F. Pharmacokinetics of etretin and etretinate during long-term treatment of psoriasis patients. Pharmacol Toxicol. 1988;62:159–65.

Larsen FG, Jakobsen P, Larsen CG, Nørgaard A, Kragballe K, Nielsen-Kudsk F. Single dose pharmacokinetics of etretin and etretinate in psoriatic patients. Pharmacol Toxicol. 1987;61:85-–8.

McKenna DB, Murphy GM. Skin cancer chemoprophylaxis in renal transplant recipients: 5 years of experience using low-dose acitretin. Br J Dermatol. 1999;140:656–60.

Pang M-L, Murase JE, Koo J. An updated review of acitretin—a systemic retinoid for the treatment of psoriasis. Expert Opin Drug Metab Toxicol. 2008;4:953–64.

Paul C, Gallini A, Maza A, et al. Evidence-based recommendations on conventional systemic treatments in psoriasis: systematic review and expert opinion of a panel of dermatologists. J Eur Acad Dermatol Venereol. 2011;25(Suppl 2):2–11.

Pilkington T, Brogden RN. Acitretin: a review of its pharmacology and therapeutic use. Drugs. 1992;43:597–627.

Rubio F, Jensen BK, Henderson L, Garland WA, Szuna A, Town C. Disposition of [^{14}C]acitretin in humans following oral administration. Drug Metab Dispos. 1994;22:211–5.

Soriatane® capsule [package insert]. Research Triangle Park: Stiefel Laboratories Inc; 2011.

Stuck AE, Brindley CJ, Busslinger A, Frey FJ. Pharmacokinetics of acitretin and its 13-cis metabolite in patients on haemodialysis. Br J Clin Pharmacol. 1989;27:301–4.

Vahlquist A. Etretinate pharmacokinetics in chronic renal failure: a preliminary study in psoriasis patients. Dermatologica. 1987;175:224–8.

Wiegand U-W, Chou RC. Pharmacokinetics of acitretin and etretinate. J Am Acad Dermatol. 1998;39 (3 Pt 3):S25–33.

Acitretin/Soriatane®   {Antipsoriatic; retinol (vitamin A) derivative}

Usual initial dose: 25 mg orally once daily with the main meal

Usual maintenance dose: 25–50 mg orally once daily with the main meal, depending on response
                                            and tolerance

Typical maximum dose: 100 mg/day

Proportion eliminated unchanged: Nil (approx 20 % as minimally active oxidative and glucuronide
                                            metabolites)

Adjustment for Kidney Disease

    FDA-approved product labeling: *CrCL >~30 mL/min*   *25–50 mg orally once daily with the main
                                                                                       meal*

                                          Severely impaired kidney   Contraindicated
                                                             function

    Alternative adjustment: *Data not available*

        *Note: Reasons for the above contraindication are not clear and this
categorization is apparently unsupported. Single and multiple dose
investigations in patients with ESRD either receiving or not receiving
hemodialysis revealed that total acitretin exposure was approximately 50 %
lower than in matched patients without renal impairment and comparative
elimination characteristics showed little or no change. Substantial clinical
experience in kidney transplant recipients shows successful use of acitretin
in usual or slightly reduced (0.2–0.4 mg/kg) daily dosages.*

Dosage Adjustment of Medications Eliminated by the Kidneys

Acyclovir (IV) - Selected References

Acyclovir injection [package insert]. Bedford: Bedford Laboratories; 2005.

Aronoff GA, Bennett WM, Berns JS, et al. Drug prescribing in renal failure: dosing guidelines for adults and children. 5th ed. Philadelphia: American College of Physicians; 2007.

Bean B, Braun C, Balfour HH Jr. Acyclovir therapy for acute herpes zoster. Lancet. 1982;2:118–21.

Boelaert J, Schurgers M, Daneels R, Van Landuyt HW, Weatherley BC. Multiple dose pharmacokinetics of intravenous acyclovir in patients on continuous ambulatory peritoneal dialysis. J Antimicrob Chemother. 1987;20:69–76.

Brigden D, Rosling AE, Woods NC. Renal function after acyclovir intravenous injection. Am J Med. 1982;73(Suppl 1A):182–5.

Burgess ED, Gill MJ. Intraperitoneal administration of acyclovir in patients receiving continuous ambulatory peritoneal dialysis. J Clin Pharmacol. 1990;30:994–6.

de Miranda, Good SS, Laskin OL, Krasny HC, Connor JD, Lietman PS. Disposition of intravenous radioactive acyclovir. Clin Pharmacol Ther. 1981;30:662–72.

Heintz BH, Matzke GR, Dager WF. Antimicrobial dosing concepts and recommendations for critically ill adult patients receiving continuous renal replacement therapy or intermittent hemodialysis. Pharmacotherapy. 2009;29:562–77.

Jones T, Alderman C. Acyclovir clearance by CAVHD. Intensive Care Med. 1991;17:125–6.

Krasny HC, Liao SHT, de Miranda P, Laskin OL, Whelton A, Lietman PS. Influence of hemodialysis on acyclovir pharmacokinetics in patients with chronic renal failure. Am J Med. 1982;73(Suppl 1A):202–4.

Laskin OL. Clinical pharmacokinetics of acyclovir. Clin Pharmacokinet. 1983;8:187–201.

Laskin OL, Longstreth JA, Whelton A, et al. Acyclovir kinetics in end-stage renal disease. Clin Pharmacol Ther. 1982;31:594–601.

Laskin OL, Longstreth JA, Whelton A, et al. Effect of renal failure on the pharmacokinetics of acyclovir. Am J Med. 1982;73(Suppl 1A):197–201.

Meyers JD, Wade JC, Mitchell CD, et al. Multicenter collaborative trial of intravenous acyclovir for treatment of mucocutaneous herpes simplex virus infection in the immunocompromised host. Am J Med. 1982;73(Suppl 1A):229–35.

Mitchell CD, Bean B, Gentry SR, Groth KE, Boen JR, Balfour HH Jr. Acyclovir therapy for mucocutaneous herpes simplex infections in immunocompromised patients. Lancet. 1982;1:1389–92.

Morse GD, Shelton MJ, O'Donnell AM. Comparative pharmacokinetics of antiviral nucleoside analogues. Clin Pharmacokinet. 1993;24:101–23.

Nunan TO, King M, Bull P, Banatvala JE, Jones NF, Hilton PJ. Parenteral acyclovir therapy for cytomegalovirus infection after renal transplantation. Clin Nephrol. 1984;22:28–31.

Peterslund NA, Seyer-Hansen K, Ipsen J, Esmann V, Schonheyder H, Juhl H. Acyclovir in herpes zoster. Lancet. 1981;2:827–30.

Saral R, Burns WH, Laskin OL, Santos GW, Lietman PS. Acyclovir prophylaxis of herpes simplex-virus infections: a randomized, double-blind, controlled trial in bone-marrow transplant recipients. N Engl J Med. 1981;305:83–7.

Shah GM, Winer RL, Krasny HC. Acyclovir pharmacokinetics in a patient on continuous ambulatory peritoneal dialysis. Am J Kidney Dis. 1986;7:507–10.

Trotman RL, Williamson JC, Shoemaker M, Salzer WL. Antibiotic dosing in critically ill adult patients receiving continuous renal replacement therapy. Clin Infect Dis. 2005;41:1159–66.

van der Meer JWM, Versteeg J. Acyclovir in severe herpes virus infections. Am J Med. 1982;73(Suppl 1A):271–4.

Wade JC, Hintz M, McGuffin RW, Springmeyer SC, Connor JD, Meyers JD. Treatment of cytomegalovirus pneumonia with high-dose acyclovir. Am J Med. 1982;73(Suppl 1A):249–56.

Wade JC, Newton B, McLaren C, Fluornoy N, Keeney RE, Meyers JD. Intravenous acyclovir to treat mucocutaneous herpes simplex virus infection after bone marrow transplantation. Ann Intern Med. 1982;96:265–9.

Whitley RJ, Gnann JW Jr. Acyclovir: a decade later. N Engl J Med. 1992;327:782–9.

Whitley RJ, Gnann JW Jr, Hinthorn D, et al. Disseminated herpes zoster in the immunocompromised host: a comparative trial of acyclovir and vidarabine. J Infect Dis. 1992;165:450–5.

Dosage Adjustment of Medications Eliminated by the Kidneys

Acyclovir/Zovirax® (IV)	**{Antiviral; nucleoside analog; viral DNA polymerase inhibitor}**
Usual initial dose:	10 mg/kg (ideal body weight or lean body mass)
Usual maintenance dose:	5 mg/kg IV every 8 h for 7 days (mucosal and cutaneous herpes simplex [HSV-1 and HSV-2] infections in immunocompromised patients);
	5 mg/kg IV every 8 h for 5 days (severe initial episodes of herpes genitalis);
	10 mg/kg IV every 8 h for 7–10 days (herpes simplex encephalitis);
	10 mg/kg IV every 8 h for 7 days (varicella zoster infections in immunocompromised patients)
Typical maximum dose:	20 mg/kg IV every 8 h
Proportion eliminated unchanged:	77–99 %

Adjustment for Kidney Disease

FDA-approved product labeling: *Acyclovir dosage adjustments in renal impairment*

CrCL (mL/min)	Percent of recommended dose (%)	Dosing interval (h)
>50	100	8
25–50	100	12
10–25	100	24
0–10	50	24

Alternative adjustment:		
GFR >50 mL/min	5–10 mg/kg IV every 8 h
GFR 10–50 mL/min	5–10 mg/kg IV every 12–24 h
GFR <10 mL/min	2.5–5 mg/kg IV every 24 h
Hemodialysis	2.5–5 mg/kg IV every 24 h, dose after hemodialysis on dialysis days
CAPD	2.5–5 mg/kg IV every 24 h
CVVH	2.5–7.5 mg/kg IV every 24 h
CVVHD or CVVHDF	5–7.5 mg/kg IV every 24 h

Dosage Adjustment of Medications Eliminated by the Kidneys

Acyclovir (Enteral) - Selected References

Aronoff GA, Bennett WM, Berns JS, et al. Drug prescribing in renal failure: dosing guidelines for adults and children. 5th ed. Philadelphia: American College of Physicians; 2007.

Blum MR, Liao SHT, de Miranda P. Overview of acyclovir pharmacokinetic disposition in adults and children. Am J Med. 1982;73(Suppl 1A):186–92.

Boelaert J, Schurgers M, Daneels R, Van Landuyt HW, Weatherley BC. Multiple dose pharmacokinetics of intravenous acyclovir in patients on continuous ambulatory peritoneal dialysis. J Antimicrob Chemother. 1987;20:69–76.

Burgess ED, Gill MJ. Intraperitoneal administration of acyclovir in patients receiving continuous ambulatory peritoneal dialysis. J Clin Pharmacol. 1990;30:994–6.

Cobo LM, Foulks GN, Liesegang T, et al. Oral acyclovir in the therapy of acute herpes zoster ophthalmicus: an interim report. Ophthalmology. 1985;92:1574–83.

Fletcher CV, Chinnock BJ, Chace B, Balfour HH Jr. Pharmacokinetics and safety of high-dose oral acyclovir for suppression of cytomegalovirus disease after renal transplantation. Clin Pharmacol Ther. 1988;44:158–63.

Fletcher CV, Englund JA, Edelman CK, Gross CR, Dunn DL, Balfour HH Jr. Pharmacologic basis for high-dose oral acyclovir prophylaxis of cytomegalovirus disease in renal allograft recipients. Antimicrob Agents Chemother. 1991;35:938–43.

Heintz BH, Matzke GR, Dager WF. Antimicrobial dosing concepts and recommendations for critically ill adult patients receiving continuous renal replacement therapy or intermittent hemodialysis. Pharmacotherapy. 2009;29:562–77.

Huff JC, Bean B, Balfour HH Jr, et al. Therapy of Herpes zoster with oral acyclovir. Am J Med. 1988;85(Suppl 2A):84–9.

Jacobson MA, Berger TG, Fikrig S, et al. Acyclovir-resistant Varicella zoster virus infection after chronic oral acyclovir therapy in patients with the acquired immunodeficiency syndrome (AIDS). Ann Intern Med. 1990;112:187–91.

Jones T, Alderman C. Acyclovir clearance by CAVHD. Intensive Care Med. 1991;17:125–6.

Krasny HC, Liao SHT, de Miranda P, Laskin OL, Whelton A, Lietman PS. Influence of hemodialysis on acyclovir pharmacokinetics in patients with chronic renal failure. Am J Med. 1982;73(Suppl 1A):202–4.

Laskin OL. Clinical pharmacokinetics of acyclovir. Clin Pharmacokinet. 1983;8:187–201.

Laskin OL, Longstreth JA, Whelton A, et al. Effect of renal failure on the pharmacokinetics of acyclovir. Am J Med. 1982;73(Suppl 1A):197–201.

Leflore S, Anderson PL, Fletcher CV. A risk-benefit evaluation of aciclovir for the treatment and prophylaxis of herpes simplex virus infections. Drug Saf. 2000;23:131–42.

Mertz GJ, Eron L, Kaufman R, et al. Prolonged continuous versus intermittent oral acyclovir treatment in normal adults with frequently recurring genital herpes simplex virus infection. Am J Med. 1988;85(Suppl 2A):14–9.

Peterslund NA, Esmann V, Ipsen J, Dencker Christensen K, Petersen M. Oral and intravenous acyclovir are equally effective n herpes zoster. J Antimicrob Chemother. 1984;14:185–9.

Shah GM, Winer RL, Krasny HC. Acyclovir pharmacokinetics in a patient on continuous ambulatory peritoneal dialysis. Am J Kidney Dis. 1986;7:507–10.

Straus SE, Smith HA, Brickman C, de Miranda P, McLaren C, Keeney RE. Acyclovir for chronic mucocutaneous herpes simplex virus infection in immunosuppressed patients. Ann Intern Med. 1982;96:270–7.

Straus SE, Takiff HE, Seidlin M, et al. Suppression of frequently occurring genital herpes: a placebo-controlled double-blind trial of oral acyclovir. N Engl J Med. 1984;310:154–50.

Swan SK, Bennett WM. Oral acyclovir and neurotoxicity [letter]. Ann Intern Med. 1988;111:188–9.

Trotman RL, Williamson JC, Shoemaker M, Salzer WL. Antibiotic dosing in critically ill adult patients receiving continuous renal replacement therapy. Clin Infect Dis. 2005;41:1159–66.

Van Dyke RB, Connor JD, Wyborny D, Hintz M, Keeney RE. Pharmacokinetics of orally administered acyclovir in patients with herpes progenitalis. Am J Med. 1982;73(Suppl 1A):172–5.

Whitley RJ, Gnann JW Jr. Acyclovir: a decade later. N Engl J Med. 1992;327:782–9.

Wood MJ, Ogan PH, McKendrick MW, Care CD, McGill JI, Webb EM. Efficacy of oral acyclovir treatment of acute Herpes zoster. Am J Med. 1988;85(Suppl 2A):79–83.

Zovirax® tablet, capsule, suspension [package insert]. Research Triangle Park: GlaxoSmithKline; 2007.

Dosage Adjustment of Medications Eliminated by the Kidneys

Acyclovir/Zovirax® (Enteral)	{Antiviral; nucleoside analog}

Usual initial dose: 200–800 mg enterally

Usual maintenance dose: 800 mg enterally every 4 h, five times daily (acute treatment of herpes zoster); 200 mg orally every 4 h, five times daily (treatment of initial genital herpes); 400 mg orally two times daily for up to 12 months (chronic suppressive therapy for recurrent disease); 200 mg orally every 4 h, five times daily for 5 days (intermittent therapy, at the earliest sign or symptom [prodrome] of recurrence); 800 mg orally four times daily for 5 days (chickenpox)

Typical maximum dose: 800 mg five times daily (enteral)

Proportion eliminated unchanged: 50–90 %

Adjustment for Kidney Disease

FDA-approved product labeling: *Acyclovir dosage modification for renal impairment (enteral)*

Normal dosage regimen	CrCL (mL/min/ 1.73 m²)	Adjusted dosage regimen	
		Dose	Dosing interval
200 mg every 4 h	>10	200 mg	Every 4 h, 5× daily
	0–10	200 mg	Every 12 h
400 mg every 12 h	>10	400 mg	Every 12 h
	0–10	200 mg	Every 12 h
800 mg every 4 h	>25	800 mg	Every 4 h, 5× daily
	10–25	800 mg	Every 8 h
	0–10	800 mg	Every 12 h

Alternative adjustment:

GFR >50 mL/min	*200–800 mg orally or enterally five times daily*
GFR 10–50 mL/min	*200–800 mg orally or enterally every 8 h*
GFR <10 mL/min	*200–800 mg orally or enterally every 12 h*
Hemodialysis	*200–800 mg orally or enterally every 12 h; administer after hemodialysis on dialysis days*
CAPD	*200–800 mg orally or enterally every 12 h*
CRRT	*Not applicable (consider IV acyclovir)*

Dosage Adjustment of Medications Eliminated by the Kidneys

Adefovir - Selected References

Aronoff GA, Bennett WM, Berns JS, et al. Drug prescribing in renal failure: dosing guidelines for adults and children. 5th ed. Philadelphia: American College of Physicians; 2007.

Cundy KC. Clinical pharmacokinetics of the antiviral nucleotide analogues cidofovir and adefovir. Clin Pharmacokinet. 1999;36:127–43.

Cundy KC, Barditch-Crovo P, Walker RE, Collier AC, et al. Clinical pharmacokinetics of adefovir in human immunodeficiency virus type 1-infected patients. Antimicrob Agents Chemother. 1995;39:2401–5.

Fontaine H, Vallet-Pichard A, Chaix M-L, et al. Efficacy and safety of adefovir dipivoxil in kidney recipients, hemodialysis patients, and patients with renal insufficiency. Transplantation. 2005;80:1086–92.

Gupta SK, Eustace JA, Winston JA, et al. Guidelines for the management of chronic kidney disease in HIV-infected patients: recommendations of the HIV Medicine Section of the Infectious Diseases Society of America. Clin Infect Dis. 2005;40:1559–85.

Hepsera® tablet [package insert]. Foster City: Gilead Sciences Inc; 2009.

Olyaei AJ, Bennett WM. Drug dosing in elderly patients with chronic kidney disease. Clin Geriatr Med. 2009;25:459–527.

Ray AS, Vela JE, Olson L, Fridland A. Effective metabolism and long intracellular half life of the anti-hepatitis B agent adefovir in hepatic cells. Biochem Pharmacol. 2004;68:1825–31.

Shiffman ML, Pol S, Rostaing L, et al. Efficacy and pharmacokinetics of adefovir dipivoxil liquid suspension in patients with chronic hepatitis B and renal impairment. J Clin Pharmacol. 2010. Epub ahead of print. doi:10.1177/009127001381385.

Sokol EM, Kelly D, Wirth S, Mizerski J, Dhawan A, Frederick D. The pharmacokinetics and safety of adefovir dipivoxil in children and adolescents with chronic hepatitis B virus infection. J Clin Pharmacol. 2008;48:512–7.

Sun DS, Wang H-S, Ni M-Y, Wang B-J, Guo R-C. Pharmacokinetics, safety and tolerance of single- and multiple-dose adefovir dipivoxil in healthy Chinese subjects. Br J Clin Pharmacol. 2006;63:15–23.

Dosage Adjustment of Medications Eliminated by the Kidneys

<u>Adefovir</u>/Hepsera™   {Antiviral; anti-hepatitis B nucleotide analog}

Usual initial dose:	10 mg orally once daily
Usual maintenance dose:	10 mg orally once daily
Typical maximum dose:	10 mg orally once daily
Proportion eliminated unchanged:	>90 %

Adjustment for Kidney Disease

FDA-approved product labeling: *Adefovir dosing interval adjustment in adults with impaired renal function*

	CrCL (mL/min)[a]			
	≥50	*30–49*	*10–29*	*Hemodialysis*
Recommended dosage and dosing interval	10 mg orally every 24 h	10 mg orally every 48 h	10 mg orally every 72 h	10 mg orally every 7 days following dialysis

[a]CrCL calculated by Cockroft-Gault method using lean or ideal body weight

Alternative adjustment:

GFR >50 mL/min	*10 mg orally every 24 h*
GFR 20–50 mL/min	*10 mg orally every 48 h*
GFR <20 mL/min	*10 mg orally every 72 h*
Intermittent hemodialysis	*10 mg orally once weekly after dialysis*
CAPD	*Data not available. Preferably avoid or, if indeed necessary, administer 10 mg orally every 72 h and monitor carefully.*
CRRT	*Data not available. Preferably avoid or, if indeed necessary, administer 10 mg enterally every 48–72 h and monitor carefully.*

Dosage Adjustment of Medications Eliminated by the Kidneys

<u>Alendronate</u> - Selected References

Black DM, Cummings SR, Karpf DB, et al. Randomised trial of effect of alendronate on risk of fracture in women with existing vertebral fractures. Lancet. 1996;348:1535–41.

Dansereau RJ, Crail DJ, Perkins AC. In vitro disintegration and dissolution studies of once-weekly copies of alendronate sodium tablets (70 mg) and in vivo implications. Curr Med Res Opin. 2008;24:1137–45.

Fosamax® tablet and solution [package insert]. Whitehouse Station: Merck Sharp & Dohme Corp; 2011.

Gertz BJ, Holland SD Kline WF, et al. Studies of oral bioavailability of alendronate. Clin Pharmacol Ther. 1995;58:288–98.

Jamal SA, Bauer DC, Ensrud KE, et al. Alendronate treatment in women with normal to severely impaired renal function: an analysis of the Fracture Intervention Trial. J Bone Miner Res. 2007;22:503–7.

Koc M, Tuglular S, Arikan H, Ozener C, Akoglu E. Alendronate increases bone mineral density in long-term renal transplant recipients. Transplant Proc. 2002;34:2111–3.

Lamprecht G. In vitro determination of the release of alendronic acid from alendronate tablets of different brands during deglutition. J Pharm Sci. 2009;98:3575–81.

Lin JH, Chen I-W, Deluna FA. Nonlinear kinetics of alendronate: plasma protein binding and bone uptake. Drug Metab Dispos. 1994;22:400–5.

Ott SM, Drueke T, Elder G, et al. Renal function and bisphosphonate therapy [letter]. J Bone Miner Res. 2008;23:453–4.

Porras AG, Holland SD, Gertz BJ. Pharmacokinetics of alendronate. Clin Pharmacokinet. 1999;36:315–28.

Ringe JD, Möller G. Differences in persistence, safety and efficacy of generic and original branded once weekly bisphosphonates in patients with postmenopausal osteoporosis: 1-year results of a retrospective patient chart analysis. Rheumatol Int. 2009;30:213–21.

Strample W, Emkey R, Civitelli R. Safety considerations with bisphosphonates for the treatment of osteoporosis. Drug Saf. 2007;30:756–63.

Yun M-H, Woo J-S, Kown K-I. Bioequivalence and pharmacokinetics of 70 mg alendronate sodium tablets by measuring alendronate in plasma. Arch Pharm Res. 2006;29:328–32.

Zazgornik J, Grafinger P, Bisenbach G, Hubmann R, Fridrik M. Acute renal failure and alendronate [letter]. Nephrol Dial Transplant. 1997;12:2797–8.

Dosage Adjustment of Medications Eliminated by the Kidneys

<u>Alendronate</u>/Fosamax®   {Anti-osteoporotic; bisphosphonate}

Usual initial dose:	10 mg orally once daily or 35–70 mg orally once weekly
Usual maintenance dose:	10 mg orally once daily or 35–70 mg orally once weekly
Typical maximum dose:	70 mg/week
Proportion eliminated unchanged:	40–60 % of an assimilated dose; ~100 % of drug in plasma

Adjustment for Kidney Disease

FDA-approved product labeling:	*CrCL >60 mL/min*	*No adjustment needed: 10 mg orally once daily or 35–70 mg orally once weekly*
	CrCL 35–60 mL/min	*No adjustment needed: 10 mg orally once daily or 35–70 mg orally once weekly*
	CrCL <35 mL/min	*Not recommended due to lack of experience*
Alternative adjustment:	*eCrCL ≥60 mL/min*	*10 mg orally once daily or 35–70 mg orally once weekly*
	eCrCL 35–59 mL/min	*10 mg orally once daily (no adjustment needed)*
	eCrCL <35 mL/min	*10 mg orally once daily (no adjustment needed); only minimal clinical experience supports safety.*

Dosage Adjustment of Medications Eliminated by the Kidneys

Alfuzosin - Selected References

Chau LH, Tai DCK, Fung BTC, Li JCM, Fan CW, Li MKW. Medical expulsive therapy using alfuzosin for patient presenting with ureteral stone less than 10 mm: a prospective randomized trial. Int J Urol. 2011;18:510–4.

Cisternino A, Zeccolini G, Calpista A, et al. Obstructive primary bladder neck disease: evaluation of the efficacy and safety of α_1-blockers. Urol Int. 2006;76:150–3.

Guay RP. Extended-release alfuzosin hydrochloride: a new alpha-adrenergic receptor antagonist for symptomatic benign prostatic hyperplasia. Am J Geriatr Pharmacother. 2004;2:14–23.

Karadağ E, Öner S, Budak YU, Atahan Ö. Randomized crossover comparison of tamsulosin and alfuzosin in patients with urinary disturbances caused by benign prostatic hyperplasia. Int Urol Nephrol. 2011;43:949–54.

Lamb AD, Vowler SL, Johnston R, Dunn N, Wiseman OJ. Meta-analysis showing the beneficial effect of α-blockers on ureteric stent discomfort. BJU Int. 2011;108:1894–902.

Marbury TC, Blum RA, Rauch C, Pinquier J-L. Pharmacokinetics and safety of a single oral dose of once-daily alfuzosin, 10 mg, in male subjects with mild to severe renal impairment. J Clin Pharmacol. 2002;42:1311–7.

McKeage K, Plosker GL. Alfuzosin: a review of the therapeutic use of the prolonged-release formulation given once daily in the management of benign prostatic hyperplasia. Drugs. 2002;62:633–53.

Mottet N, Bressolle F, Delmas V, Robert M, Costa P. Prostatic tissual distribution of alfuzosin in patients with benign prostatic hyperplasia following repeated oral administration. Eur Urol. 2003;44:101–3.

Öztürk Mĺ, Kalkan S, Koca O, et al. Efficacy of alfuzosin and sildenafil combination in male patients with lower urinary tract symptoms. Andrologia. 2011. Epub ahead of print. doi:10.1111/j.1439-0272.2011.01268.x.

Uroxatral® tablet, extended-release [package insert]. Bridgewater: Sanofi-Aventis US LLC; 2009.

Dosage Adjustment of Medications Eliminated by the Kidneys

Alfuzosin/Uroxatral®   {α_1-Adrenergic receptor blocker; ℞ for benign prostatic hyperplasia}

Usual initial dose:	10 mg orally
Usual maintenance dose:	10 mg orally once daily with food/after a meal at the same time each day
Typical maximum dose:	10 mg/day
Proportion eliminated unchanged:	24 % (11 % as unchanged drug)

Adjustment for Kidney Disease

FDA-approved product labeling:	*CrCL >30 mL/min*	*10 mg orally once daily after a meal*
	CrCL ≤30 mL/min	*Safety not determined—Drug exposure (maximum blood levels and area under the plasma concentration time curve) are increased by 50 % as compared to patients with normal renal function.*
Alternative adjustment:	*eCrCL ≥60 mL/min*	*10 mg orally once daily after a meal*
	eCrCL 30–59 mL/min	*10 mg orally once daily after a meal*
	eCrCL <30 mL/min	*5 mg orally once daily after a meal*

Dosage Adjustment of Medications Eliminated by the Kidneys

Aliskiren - Selected References

Ali AK. Pharmacovigilance analysis of adverse event reports for aliskiren hemifumarate, a first-in-class direct renin inhibitor. Ther Clin Risk Manag. 2011;7:337–44.

Azizi M, Ménard J. Renin inhibitors and cardiovascular and renal protection: an endless quest? Cardiovasc Drugs Ther. 2010. Epub ahead of print. doi:10.1007/s10557-012-6380-6.

Berle T. Renal protection by inhibition of the renin-angiotensin aldosterone system. J Renin Angiotensin Aldosterone Syst. 2009;10:1–8.

Duggan ST, Chwieduk M, Curran MP. Aliskiren: a review of its use as monotherapy and as combination therapy in the management of hypertension. Drugs. 2010;70:2011–49.

FDA MedWatch Drug Safety Communication. Aliskiren-containing medications: new warning and contraindication. Available at http://www.fda.gov/Safety/MedWatch/SafetyInformation/SafetyAlertsforHumanMedicalProducts/ucm301120.htm?source=govdelivery. Accessed 20 Apr 2012.

Harel Z, Gilbert C, Wald R, et al. The effect of combination treatment with aliskiren and blockers of the renin-angiotensin system on hyperkalaemia and acute kidney injury: systematic review and meta-analysis. BMJ. 2012;344:e42. doi:10.1136/bmj.e42.

Jackson CE, MacDonald MR, Petrie MC, et al. Associations of albuminuria in patients with chronic heart failure: findings in the Aliskiren Observation of Heart Failure Treatment study. Eur J Heart Fail. 2011;13:746–54.

Moriyama T, Tsurut Y, Kojima C, et al. Beneficial effect of aliskiren combined with olmesartan in reducing urinary protein excretion in patients with chronic kidney disease. Int Urol Nephrol. 2011. Epub ahead of print. doi:10.1007/s11255-011-9991-0.

Nakamura T, Sato E, Amaha M, Kawagoe Y, Maeda S, Yamagishi S. Addition of aliskiren to angiotensin II receptor blockers ameliorates renal tubular injury and reduces intima media thickness of carotid artery in patients with diabetic nephropathy. Int J Cardiol. 2012;155:294–6.

Nakamura T, Sato E, Amaha M, Kawagoe Y, Maeda S, Yamagishi S. Addition of aliskiren to olmesartan ameliorates tubular injury in chronic kidney disease patients partly by reducing proteinuria. J Renin Angiotensin Aldosterone Syst. 2012;13:122–7.

Novartis International AG. Media release: Novartis announces termination of ALTITUDE study with Rasilez®/Tekturna® in high-risk patients with diabetes and renal impairment. Available at http://www.novartis.com/downloads/newsroom/rasilez-tekturna-information-center/20111220-rasilez-tekturna.pdf. Accessed 20 Apr 2012.

Parving H-H, Persson F Lewis JB, Lewis EJ, Hollenberg NK, AVOID Study Investigators. Aliskiren combined with losartan in type 2 diabetes and nephropathy. N Engl J Med. 2008;358:2433–46.

Persson F, Lewis JB, Lewis EJ, Rossing P, Hollenberg NK, Parving H-H. Aliskiren in combination with losartan reduces albuminuria independent of baseline blood pressure in patients with type 2 diabetes and nephropathy. Clin J Am Soc Nephrol. 2011;6:1025–31.

Persson F, Rossing P, Reinhard H, et al. Renal effects of aliskiren compared with and in combination with irbesartan in patients with type 2 diabetes, hypertension, and albuminuria. Diabetes Care. 2009;32:1873–9.

Siamopoulos KC, Kalaitzidis RG. Inhibition of the renin-angiotensin system and chronic kidney disease. Int Urol Nephrol. 2008;40:1015–25.

Tekturna® tablet [package insert]. East Hanover: Novartis Pharmaceuticals Corp; 2012.

Vaidyanathan S, Bigler H, Jarugula V, et al. Pharmacokinetics of the oral direct renin inhibitor aliskiren alone and in combination with irbesartan in renal impairment. Clin Pharmacokinet. 2007;46:661–75.

Vaidyanathan S, Jarugula V, Dieterich HA, Howard D, Dole WP. Clinical pharmacokinetics and pharmacodynamics of aliskiren. Clin Pharmacokinet. 2008;47:515–31.

Venzin RM, Cohen CD, Maggiorini M, Wüthrich RP. Aliskiren-associated acute renal failure with hyperkalemia. Clin Nephrol. 2009;71:326–8.

White WB, Bresalier R, Laplan AP, et al. Safety and tolerability of the direct renin inhibitor aliskiren in combination with angiotensin receptor blockers and thiazide diuretics: a pooled analysis of clinical experience of 12,942 patients. J Clin Hypertens (Greenwich). 2011;13:506–16.

Zhao C, Vaidyanathan S, Yeh C-M, Maboudian M, Dieterich HA. Aliskiren exhibits similar pharmacokinetics in healthy volunteers and patients with type 2 diabetes mellitus. Clin Pharmacokinet. 2006;45:1125–34.

Dosage Adjustment of Medications Eliminated by the Kidneys

Aliskiren/Tekturna®   {**Antihypertensive; direct renin inhibitor**}

Usual initial dose:	150 mg orally
Usual maintenance dose:	150–300 mg orally once daily
Typical maximum dose:	300 mg/day
Proportion eliminated unchanged:	25 %

Adjustment for Kidney Disease

FDA-approved product labeling:	*Renal impairment (GFR <60 mL/min)*	*Avoid. Safety and effectiveness not established (patients with CrCL <30 mL/min were excluded from controlled trials); monitor renal function—Patients with renal artery stenosis, heart failure, volume depletion, and those receiving an angiotensin-converting enzyme (ACE) inhibitor or angiotensin receptor blocker (ARB) may be at particular risk for developing acute renal failure. Contraindicated in patients with diabetes who are receiving ARBs or ACE inhibitors because of the increased risk of renal impairment, hyperkalemia, and hypotension*
Alternative adjustment:	*eCrCL 31–59 mL/min*	*Preferably avoid. If indeed necessary, 150–300 mg orally once daily (no adjustment necessary); monitor carefully—Be aware of contraindications and markedly increased risk of acute kidney injury, hyperkalemia, and hypotension in patients receiving ARBs and/or ACE inhibitors.*
	eCrCL ≤30 mL/min	*Preferably avoid. If indeed necessary, 150–300 mg orally once daily (no adjustment necessary); monitor carefully—Be aware of contraindications and markedly increased risk of acute kidney injury, hyperkalemia, and hypotension in patients receiving ARBs and/or ACE inhibitors.*
	Hemodialysis	*Preferably avoid. Minimal data available; if indeed necessary, initiate therapy with 150 mg orally once daily with careful clinical and biochemical monitoring.*
	CRRT	*Preferably avoid. No published data available; if indeed necessary, initiate with 150 mg enterally once daily with careful monitoring.*

Dosage Adjustment of Medications Eliminated by the Kidneys

Allopurinol - Selected References

Aloprim® injection [package insert]; Lake Forest: Bioniche Pharma USA LLC; 2008.

Alsarraf D, Reese L. Management of acute renal failure due to marked hyperuricemia. Can Med Assoc J. 1972;106:352–4.

Appelbaum SJ, Mayersohn M, Dorr RT, Perrier D. Allopurinol kinetics and bioavailability: intravenous, oral and rectal administration. Cancer Chemother Pharmacol. 1982;8:93–8.

Aronoff GA, Bennett WM, Berns JS, et al. Drug prescribing in renal failure: dosing guidelines for adults and children. 5th ed. Philadelphia: American College of Physicians; 2007.

Day RO, Graham GG, Hicks M, McLachlan AJ, Stocker SL, Williams KM. Clinical pharmacokinetics and pharmacodynamics of allopurinol and oxypurinol. Clin Pharmacokinet. 2007;46:623–44.

Elion GB, Benezra FM, Beardmore TD. Studies with allopurinol in patients with impaired renal function. Adv Exp Biol Med. 1980;122A:263–7.

Elion GB, Yü T-F, Gutman AB, Hitchings GH. Renal clearance of oxypurinol, the chief metabolite of allopurinol. Am J Med. 1968;45:69-77.

Fagugli RM, Gentile G, Ferrara, Brugnano R. Acute renal and hepatic failure associated with allopurinol treatment. Clin Nephrol. 2008;70:523–6.

Favel MA, Ernst ME. Management of gout in the older adult. Am J Geriatr Pharmacother. 2011;9:271–85.

Goldfinger S, Klinenberg JR, Seegmiller JE. The renal excretion of oxypurines. J Clin Invest. 1965;44:623–8.

Hanlon JT, Aspinall SL, Semla TP, et al. Consensus guidelines for oral dosing of primarily renally cleared medications in older adults. J Am Geriatr Soc. 2009;57:335–40.

Haririan A, Metireddy M, Cangro C, et al. Association of serum uric acid with graft survival after kidney transplantation: a time-varying analysis. Am J Transplant. 2011;11:4943–50.

Kanbay M, Huddam B, Azak A, et al. A randomized study of allopurinol on endothelial function and estimated glomerular filtration rate in asymptomatic hyperuricemic subjects with normal renal function. Clin J Am Soc Nephrol. 2011;6:1887–94.

Kao MP, Ang DS, Gandy SJ, et al. Allopurinol benefits left ventricular mass and endothelial dysfunction in chronic kidney disease. J Am Soc Nephrol. 2011;22:1382–9.

McIntyre CW, Owen PJ. Prescribing drugs in kidney disease. In: Brenner BM, editor. Brenner & Rector's the kidney. 8th ed. Philadelphia: Saunders Elsevier; 2008. p. 1930–55.

Meléndez-Ramírez G, Pérez-Méndez O, López-Osorio D, Kurí-Alfaro J, Espinola-Zavaleta N. Effect of allopurinol on the endothelial function in patients with hyperuricemia. Endocr Res. 2011. Epub ahead of print. doi:10.3109/0735800.2011.566235.

Murrell GAC, Rapeport WG. Clinical pharmacokinetics of allopurinol. Clin Pharmacokinet. 1986;11:343–53.

Olyaei AJ, Bennett WM. Pharmacologic approach to renal insufficiency. In: Dale DC, Federman DD, Antman K, editors. ACP medicine, WebMD June 2007 update. Hamilton: BC Decker; 2007; NEPHROLOGY IX: Appendix A1–25.

Olyaei AJ, Bennett WM. Drug dosing in elderly patients with chronic kidney disease. Clin Geriatr Med. 2009;25:459–527.

Olyaei AJ, DeMattos AM, Bennett WM. Use of drugs in patients with renal failure. In: Schrier RW, editor. Diseases of the kidney and urinary tract. 8th ed. Philadelphia: Lippincott Williams & Wilkins; 2007. p. 2765–807.

Rundles RW. Allopurinol in gouty nephropathy and renal dialysis. Ann Rheum Dis. 1966;25(6 Suppl):694–6.

Siu Y-P, Leung K-T, Tong MK-H, Kwan TH. Use of allopurinol in slowing the progression of renal disease through its ability to lower serum uric acid level. Am J Kidney Dis. 2005;47:51–9.

Turnheim K, Drivanek P, Oberbauer R. Pharmacokinetics and pharmacodynamics of allopurinol in elderly and young subjects. Br J Clin Pharmacol. 1999;48:501–9.

Zyloprim® tablet [package insert]. San Diego CA: Prometheus Laboratories Inc; 2003.

Dosage Adjustment of Medications Eliminated by the Kidneys

Allopurinol/Zyloprim®, Aloprim®	{Anti-gout; xanthine oxidase inhibitor}

Usual initial dose:	200 mg/m² orally or IV
Usual maintenance dose:	200–400 mg/m²/day orally or IV
Typical maximum dose:	600 mg/day
Proportion eliminated unchanged:	10 % (plus 80 % of each dose as pharmacologically active primary metabolite, oxypurinol)

Adjustment for Kidney Disease

FDA-approved product labeling:	*CrCL 10–20 mL/min*	*200 mg orally or IV once daily*
	CrCL 3–10 mL/min	*100 mg orally or IV once daily*
	CrCL <3 mL/min	*100 mg/day orally or IV at extended intervals*
Alternative adjustment:	*GFR >50 mL/min*	*200 mg orally or IV once daily*
	GFR 10–50 mL/min	*150 mg orally or IV once daily*
	GFR <10 mL/min	*100 mg orally or IV once daily or 150 mg orally every 48 h*
	Hemodialysis	*100 mg orally or IV once daily or 150 mg orally every 48 h; administer supplemental half dose (50 %) after dialysis*
	CAPD	*Data not available*
	CRRT	*150 mg enterally or IV once daily*

Dosage Adjustment of Medications Eliminated by the Kidneys

Almotriptan - Selected References

Axert® tablet [package insert]. Titusville: Ortho-McNeil Neurologics; 2009.

Baldwin JR, Fleishaker JC, Azie NE, Carel BJ. A comparison of the pharmacokinetics and tolerability of the anti-migraine compound almotriptan in healthy adolescents and adults. Cephalgia. 2004;24:28–92.

Bou J, Domènech T, Puig J, et al. Pharmacological characterization of almotriptan: an indolic 5-HT receptor agonist for the treatment of migraine. Eur J Pharmacol. 2000;410:33–41.

Gras J, Llenas J, Jansat JM, Jáuregui J, Cabarrocas X, Palacios JM. Almotriptan, a new anti-migraine agent: a review. CNS Drug Rev. 2002;8:217–34.

Gras J, Llupià J, Llenas J, Palacios JM. Safety profile of almotriptan, a new antimigraine agent. Arzneimittelforschung. 2001;51:726–32.

Jansat JM, Costa J, Salvà P, Fernandez FJ, Martinez-Tobed A. Absolute bioavailability, pharmacokinetics, and urinary excretion of the novel antimigraine agent almotriptan in healthy male volunteers. J Clin Pharmacol. 2002;42:1303–10.

Keam SJ, Goa KL, Figgitt DP. Almotriptan: a review of its use in migraine. Drugs. 2002;62:387–414.

McEnroe JD, Fleishaker JC. Clinical pharmacokinetics of almotriptan, a serotonin 5-HT$_{1B/1D}$ receptor agonist for the treatment of migraine. Clin Pharmacokinet. 2005;44:237–46.

Dosage Adjustment of Medications Eliminated by the Kidneys

Almotriptan/Axert®   {**Anti-migraine; serotonin 5-HT$_3$ receptor antagonist**}

Usual initial dose:	12.5 mg orally
Usual maintenance dose:	6.25–12.5 mg orally; may be repeated once in 2 h if necessary
Typical maximum dose:	25 mg/day
Proportion eliminated unchanged:	45 %

Adjustment for Kidney Disease

FDA-approved product labeling:	*Severe renal impairment*	*6.25 mg orally; maximum daily dose should not exceed 12.5 mg over a 24-h period.*
Alternative adjustment:	*Data not available*	

Dosage Adjustment of Medications Eliminated by the Kidneys

Amantadine - Selected References

Aoki FY, Sitar DS. Clinical pharmacokinetics of amantadine hydrochloride. Clin Pharmacokinet. 1988;14:35–51.

Aronoff GA, Bennett WM, Berns JS, et al. Drug prescribing in renal failure: dosing guidelines for adults and children. 5th ed. Philadelphia: American College of Physicians; 2007.

Borison Rl. Amantadine-induced psychosis in a geriatric patient with renal disease. Am J Psychiatry. 1979;136:111–2.

Bridges CB, Fukuda K, Uyeki TM, Cox NJ, Singleton JA. Prevention and control of influenza: recommendations of the Advisory Committee on Immunization Practices (ACIP). MMWR Recomm Rep. 2002;51 (RR-3):1–31.

Deleu D, Northway MG, Hanssens Y. Clinical pharmacokinetic and pharmacodynamic properties of drugs used in the treatment of Parkinson's disease. Clin Pharmacokinet. 2002;41:261–309.

Giacino JT, Whyte J, Bagiella E, et al. Placebo-controlled trial of amantadine for severe traumatic brain injury. N Engl J Med. 2012;366:819–26.

Gilbert B, Robbins P, Livornese LL Jr. Use of antibacterial agents in renal failure. Med Clin North Am. 2011;95:677–702.

Gill J, Malyuk R, Djurdjev O, Levin A. Use of GFR equations to adjust drug doses in an elderly multi-ethnic group: a cautionary tale. Nephrol Dial Transplant. 2007;22:2894–9.

Hanlon JT, Aspinall SL, Semla TP, et al. Consensus guidelines for oral dosing of primarily renally cleared medications in older adults. J Am Geriatr Soc. 2009;57:335–40.

Ing TS, Daugirdas JT, Soung LS, et al. Toxic effects of amantadine in patients with renal failure. Can Med Assoc J. 1979; 120:695–8.

Ing TS, Mahurkar SD, Dunea G, Hayashi JA, Klawans HL, Markey WS. Removal of amantadine hydrochloride by dialysis in patients with renal insufficiency. Can Med Assoc J. 1976;115:515.

Kim E, Ko HH, Yoshida EM. Treatment issues surrounding hepatitis C in renal transplantation: a review. Ann Hepatol. 2011;10:5–14.

Kuang D, Verbine A, Ronco C. Pharmacokinetics and antimicrobial dosing adjustment in critically ill patients during continuous renal replacement therapy. Clin Nephrol. 2007;67:267–84.

Macchio GJ, Ito V, Sahgal V. Amantadine-induced coma. Arch Phys Med Rehabil. 1993:74:1119–20.

McIntyre CW, Owen PJ. Prescribing drugs in kidney disease. In: Brenner BM, editor. Brenner & Rector's the kidney. 8th ed. Philadelphia: Saunders Elsevier; 2008. p. 1930–55.

Miller KS, Miller JM. Toxic effects of amantadine in patients with renal failure [letter]. Chest. 1994;105:1630.

Nakai K, Takeda K, Kimura H, Miura S, Maeda A. Obstructive acute renal failure related to amantadine intoxication. Am J Emerg Med. 2009;27:371.e5–371.e7.

Nakata M, Ito S, Shirai W, Hattori T. Severe reversible neurological complications following amantadine treatment in three elderly patients with renal insufficiency. Eur Neurol. 2006;56:59–61.

Olyaei AJ, Bennett WM. Drug dosing in elderly patients with chronic kidney disease. Clin Geriatr Med. 2009;25:459–527.

Olyaei AJ, DeMattos AM, Bennett WM. Use of drugs in patients with renal failure. In: Schrier RW, editor. Diseases of the kidney and urinary tract. 8th ed. Philadelphia: Lippincott Williams & Wilkins; 2007. p. 2765–807.

Soung L-S, Ing TS, Daugirdas JT, et al. Amantadine hydrochloride pharmacokinetics in hemodialysis patients. Ann Intern Med. 1980;93:46–9.

Symmetrel® tablet and syrup [package insert]. Chadds Ford: Endo Pharmaceuticals Inc; 2009.

Wu MJ, Ing TS, Soung LS, Daugirdas JT, Hang JE, Gandhi VC. Amantadine hydrochloride pharmacokinetics in patients with impaired renal function. Clin Nephrol. 1982;17:19–23.

Dosage Adjustment of Medications Eliminated by the Kidneys

Amantadine/Symmetrel®   {Antiviral; anti-Parkinsonian; viral M2 protein transmembrane blocker; dopaminergic}

Usual initial dose: 100 mg orally

Usual maintenance dose: 100 mg orally twice daily

Typical maximum dose: 400 mg/day

Proportion eliminated unchanged: 90 %

Adjustment for Kidney Disease

FDA-approved product labeling: *Amantadine dosage in renal function impairment*

CrCL (mL/min)	Dosage
30–50	200 mg orally first day followed by 100 mg orally each day thereafter
15–29	200 mg orally first day followed by 100 mg on alternate days
<15	200 mg orally every 7 days

Hemodialysis: 200 mg orally every 7 days

Alternative adjustment:

GFR >50 mL/min	100 mg orally every 12 h (1.4 mg/kg/day)
GFR 10–50 mL/min	100 mg orally every 24–48 h
GFR <10 mL/min	100 mg orally every 7 days
Hemodialysis	200 mg orally every 7 days (no supplemental dose after dialysis)
CRRT	100–200 mg orally every 48–60 h

Dosage Adjustment of Medications Eliminated by the Kidneys

Amikacin - Selected References

Amikacin sulfate injection USP [package insert]. Lake Forest: Hospira Inc; 2004.

Armstrong DK, Hodgman T, Visconti JA, Reilley TE, Garner WL, Dasta JF. Hemodialysis of amikacin in critically ill patients. Crit Care Med. 1988;16:517–20.

Bauer LA, Blouin RA, Griffen WO JR, Record KE, Bell RM. Amikacin pharmacokinetics in morbidly obese patients. Am J Hosp Pharm. 1980;37:519–22.

Beaucaire G, Leroy O, Beusdart C, Karp P, Chidiac C, Caillaux M. Clinical and bacteriological efficacy, and practical aspects of amikacin given once daily for severe infections. J Antimicrob Chemother. 1991; 27(Suppl C):91–103.

Bogard KN, Peterson NT, Plumb TJ, Erwin MW, Fuller PW, Olsen KM. Antibiotic dosing during sustained low-efficiency dialysis: special considerations in adult critically ill patients. Crit Care Med. 2011;39:560–70.

Byl B, Baran D, Jacobs F, Herschuelz A, Thys J-P. Serum pharmacokinetics and sputum penetration of amikacin 30 mg/kg once daily and ceftazidime 200 mg/kg/day as a continuous infusion in cystic fibrosis patients [letter]. J Antimicrob Chemother. 2001;48:325–6.

Choi G, Gomersall CD, Tiaan Q, Joynt GM, Freebairn R, Lipman J. Principles of antibacterial dosing in continuous renal replacement therapy. Crit Care Med. 2009;37:2268–82.

Conil JM, Georges B, Breden A, et al. Increased amikacin dosage requirements in burn patients receiving a once-daily regimen. Int J Antimicrob Agents. 2006;28:226–30.

Giamarellou H, Yiallouros K, Petrikkos G, et al. Comparative kinetics and efficacy of amikacin administered once or twice daily in the treatment of systemic gram-negative infections. J Antimicrob Chemother. 1991;27(Suppl C):73–9.

Hatala R, Dinh T, Cook DJ. Once-daily aminoglycoside dosing in immunocompetent adults: a meta-analysis. Ann Intern Med. 1996;124:717–25.

Heintz BH, Matzke GR, Dager WF. Antimicrobial dosing concepts and recommendations for critically ill adult patients receiving continuous renal replacement therapy or intermittent hemodialysis. Pharmacotherapy. 2009;29:562–77.

Höffler D, Knoeppe P, Demers HG. Pharmacokinetics of amikacin for treatment of urinary tract infection in patients with reduced renal function. J Infect Dis. 1976;134(Suppl):S369–73.

McHenry MC, Wagner JG, Hall PM, Vidt DG, Gavan TL. Pharmacokinetics of amikacin in patients with impaired renal function. J Infect Dis. 1976;134(Suppl):S343–8.

Pijck J, Hallynck T, Soep H, Baert I, Daneels R, Boelaert J. Pharmacokinetics of amikacin in patients with renal insufficiency: relation of half-life and creatinine clearance. J Infect Dis. 1976;134(Suppl):S331–41.

Regeur L, Colding H, Jensen H, Kampmann JP. Pharmacokinetics of amikacin during hemodialysis and peritoneal dialysis. Antimicrob Agents Chemother. 1977;11:214–8.

Sarrubi FA Jr, Hull JH. Amikacin serum concentrations: prediction of levels and dosage guidelines. Ann Intern Med. 1978;89:612–8.

Smeltzer BD, Schwartzman MS, Bertino JS Jr. Amikacin pharmacokinetics during continuous ambulatory peritoneal dialysis. Antimicrob Agents Chemother. 1988;32:236–40.

Taccone FS, de Backer D, Laterre P-F, et al. Pharmacokinetics of a loading dose of amikacin in septic patients undergoing continuous renal replacement therapy. Int J Antimicrob Agents. 2011;37:531–5.

Taccone FS, Laterre P-F, Spapen H, et al. Revisiting the loading dose of amikacin for patients with severe sepsis and septic shock. Crit Care. 2010;14:R53. Epub ahead of print. doi:10.1186/cc8945.

Tian Q, Gomersall CD, Ip M, Tan PE, Joynt GM, Choi GYS. Adsorption of amikacin, significant mechanism of elimination by hemofiltration. Antimicrob Agents Chemother. 2008;52:1009–13.

Trotman RL, Williamson JC, Shoemaker M, Salzer WL. Antibiotic dosing in critically ill adult patients receiving continuous renal replacement therapy. Clin Infect Dis. 2005;41:1159–66.

Zaki M, Goetz MB. A meta-analysis of the relative efficacy and toxicity of single daily dosing versus multiple daily dosing of aminoglycosides. Clin Infect Dis. 1997;24:796–809.

Dosage Adjustment of Medications Eliminated by the Kidneys

Amikacin/Amikin®   {**Antibacterial; aminoglycoside**}

Usual initial dose: 7.5 mg/kg

Usual maintenance dose: 15 mg/kg/day IV once daily or divided into two or three equal doses (monitor[a], adjust)

Typical maximum dose: 20 (to 30) mg/kg/day not to exceed 1.5 g/day

Proportion eliminated unchanged: 95 %

Adjustment for Kidney Disease

    FDA-approved product labeling: *7.5 mg/kg every (nine times SCr in mg/dL) h*

    Alternative adjustment: *eCrCL >80 mL/min*   *7.5–20 mg/kg (up to 25–30 mg/kg in burn and cystic fibrosis patients) IV loading dose over 1 h followed by 7.5 mg/kg IV over 1 h every 12 h or 15–20 mg/kg IV over 1 h every 24 h[a]*

        eCrCL 30–80 mL/min   *5–7.5 mg/kg every 24 h[a]*

        eCrCL 10–30 mL/min   *5–7.5 mg/kg every 48 h[a]*

        eCrCL <10 mL/min   *3.75 mg/kg every 48–72 h[a]*

        Hemodialysis   *3.75 mg/kg after dialysis[a]*

        CAPD   *7.5 mg/kg IV followed by amikacin instilled in peritoneal dialysate at a (peak) concentration desired in plasma, usually 15–20 mg/L[a]*

        CVVH   *15 mg/kg followed by 7.5 mg/kg every 24–48 h according to plasma concentrations[a]*

        CVVHD   *15–25 mg/kg followed by 7.5 mg/kg every 24–48 h according to plasma concentrations[a]*

        CVVHDF   *15–25 mg/kg followed by 7.5 mg/kg every 24–48 h according to plasma concentrations[a]*

[a]Therapeutic drug monitoring

    Therapeutic plasma levels: *Peak*   *20–30 mg/L (conventional, multiple daily dosing)*

        Trough   *<10 mg/L; patients on extended-interval dosing generally should be re-dosed when levels fall below 5 mg/L.*

Dosage Adjustment of Medications Eliminated by the Kidneys

Amiloride - Selected References

Aronoff GA, Bennett WM, Berns JS, et al. Drug prescribing in renal failure: dosing guidelines for adults and children. 5th ed. Philadelphia: American College of Physicians; 2007.

George CF. Amiloride handling in renal failure. Br J Clin Pharmacol. 1980;9:94–5.

McIntyre CW, Owen PJ. Prescribing drugs in kidney disease. In: Brenner BM, editor. Brenner & Rector's the kidney. 8th ed. Philadelphia: Saunders Elsevier; 2008. p. 1930–55.

Midamor® tablet [package insert]. Minneapolis: Paddock Laboratories Inc; 2008.

Olyaei AJ, Bennett WM. Pharmacologic approach to renal insufficiency. In: Dale DC, Federman DD, Antman K, editors. ACP medicine, WebMD June 2007 update. Hamilton: BC Decker; 2007; NEPHROLOGY IX: Appendix A1–25.

Olyaei AJ, Bennett WM. Drug dosing in elderly patients with chronic kidney disease. Clin Geriatr Med. 2009;25:459–527.

Olyaei AJ, DeMattos AM, Bennett WM. Use of drugs in patients with renal failure. In: Schrier RW, editor. Diseases of the kidney and urinary tract. 8th ed. Philadelphia: Lippincott Williams & Wilkins; 2007. p. 2765–807.

Schwartz A, Seller R, Onesti G, Kim K, Swartz C, Brest AN. Pharmacodynamic effects of a new potassium-sparing diuretic, amiloride. J Clin Pharmacol. 1969;9:217–23.

Vidt DG. Mechanism of action, pharmacokinetics, adverse effects, and therapeutics of amiloride hydrochloride, a new potassium-sparing diuretic. Pharmacotherapy. 1981;1:179–87.

Dosage Adjustment of Medications Eliminated by the Kidneys

<u>Amiloride</u>/Midamor®	{Diuretic; potassium-sparing agent}
Usual initial dose:	5 mg orally daily
Usual maintenance dose:	5–10 mg orally once daily
Typical maximum dose:	20 mg/day
Proportion eliminated unchanged:	~50 %

Adjustment for Kidney Disease

FDA-approved product labeling:	*SCr >1.5 mg/dL or BUN >30 mg/dL*	*Use only with careful, frequent, and continuing monitoring of serum electrolytes, creatinine, and BUN levels.*
	Anuria, acute or chronic renal insufficiency and evidence of diabetic nephropathy	*Contraindicated*
Alternative adjustment:	*GFR >50 mL/min*	*5 mg orally once daily*
	GFR 10–50 mL/min	*2.5 mg orally once daily or 5 mg orally every 48 h*
	GFR <10 mL/min	*Preferably avoid due to risk for hyperkalemia and cardiac irregularities.*
	Hemodialysis	*Preferably avoid due to risk for hyperkalemia and cardiac irregularities.*
	CAPD	*Preferably avoid due to risk for hyperkalemia and cardiac irregularities.*
	CRRT	*Not applicable; preferably avoid due to risk for hyperkalemia and cardiac irregularities.*

_p_-Aminosalicylic Acid - Selected References

Abramowicz M, Zuccotti G, Pflomm J-M, et al. Handbook of antimicrobial therapy. 19th ed. New Rochelle: The Medical Letter; 2011.

Aronoff GA, Bennett WM, Berns JS, et al. Drug prescribing in renal failure: dosing guidelines for adults and children. 5th ed. Philadelphia: American College of Physicians; 2007.

Held H, Fried F. Elimination of para-aminosalicylic acid in patients with liver disease and renal insufficiency. Chemotherapy. 1977;23:405–15.

Holdiness MR. Clinical pharmacokinetics of the antituberculosis drugs. Clin Pharmacokinet. 1984;9:511–44.

Hong L, Jiang W, Pan H, Jiang Y, Zeng S, Zheng W. Brain regional pharmacokinetics of _p_-aminosalicylic acid an its N-acetylated metabolite: effectiveness in chelating brain manganese. Drug Metab Dispos. 2011;39:1904–9.

Hong L, Jiang W, Zheng W, Zeng S. HPLC analysis of para-aminosalicylic acid and its metabolite in plasma, cerebrospinal fluid and brain tissues. J Pharm Biomed Anal. 2011;54:1101–9.

Malone RS, Fish DN, Spiegel DM, Childs JM, Peloquin CA. The effect of hemodialysis on cycloserine, ethionamide, para-aminosalicylate, and clofazimine. Chest. 1999;116:984–90.

Paser® delayed release granules [package insert]. Princeton: Jacobus Pharmaceutical Co Inc; 1996.

Peloquin CA, Berning SE, Huitt GA, Childs JM, Singleton MD, James GT. Once-daily and twice-daily dosing of p-aminosalicylic acid granules. Am J Respir Crit Care Med. 1999;159:932–4.

Peloquin CA, Zhu M, Adam RD, Singleton MD, Nix DE. Pharmacokinetics of _para_-aminosalicylic acid granules under four dosing conditions. Ann Pharmacother. 2001;35:1332–8.

Pentikäinen PJ, Wan SH, Azarnoff DL. Bioavailability of aminosalicylic acid and its various salts in humans. IV: comparison of four brands of the sodium salt. J Pharm Sci. 1974;63:1431–4.

Reid J, Marciniuk D, Peloquin CA, Hoeppner V. Pharmacokinetics of antituberculosis medications delivered via percutaneous gastrojejunostomy tube. Chest. 2002;121:281–4.

Dosage Adjustment of Medications Eliminated by the Kidneys

<u>*p*-Aminosalicylic Acid</u>/Paser®, PAS   {Antitubercular; folic acid synthesis inhibitor}

Usual initial dose:	50 mg/kg orally
Usual maintenance dose:	4 g orally three times daily or 150 mg/kg/day orally in two to three equally divided doses
Typical maximum dose:	300 mg/kg/day
Proportion eliminated unchanged:	35 %

Adjustment for Kidney Disease

FDA-approved product labeling:	*Severe renal disease*	*Contraindicated*
Alternative adjustment:	*GFR >50 mL/min*	*50 mg/kg (approximately 4 g [1 granule packet]) orally every 8 h*
	GFR 10–50 mL/min	*25–35 mg/kg orally every 8 h (25–50 % decrease)*
	GFR <10 mL/min	*25 mg/kg orally every 8 h (50 % decrease)*
	Hemodialysis	*25 mg/kg orally every 8 h; dose after dialysis (50 % decrease)*
	CAPD	*25 mg/kg orally every 8 h (50 % decrease)*
	CRRT	*25–35 mg/kg orally every 8 h (25–50 % decrease)*

Ammonium Chloride - Selected References

Ammonium chloride injection concentrate (5 mEq/mL) [package insert]. Lake Forest: Hospira Inc; 2009.

Bear R, Goldstein M, Phillipson E, et al. Effect of metabolic alkalosis on respiratory function in patients with chronic obstructive lung disease. Can Med Assoc J. 1977;117:900–3.

Brenes LG, Sanchez MI. Impaired urinary ammonium excretion in patients with isolated proximal renal tubular acidosis. J Am Soc Nephrol. 1993;4:1073–8.

Brest AN, Moyer JH. Clinical pharmacology of diuretic drugs. Am J Cardiol. 1966;17:626–30.

Jarrell MA, Greer M, Maren TH. The effect of acidosis in hypokalemic periodic paralysis. Arch Neurol. 1976;33:791–3.

Levene DL, Knight A. Ammonium chloride poisoning in chronic renal disease. Can Med Assoc J. 1974;111:335–8.

Martin MJ, Matzke GR. Treating severe metabolic alkalosis. Clin Pharm. 1982;1:42–8.

Mashford ML, Robertson MB. Spironolactone and ammonium and potassium chloride [letter]. Br Med J. 1972;4:298–9.

Mégarbane B, Bruneel F, Bédos JP, Régnier B. Ammonium chloride poisoning; a misunderstood cause of metabolic acidosis with normal anion gap [letter]. Intensive Care Med. 2000;26:1869.

Reynolds TM, Burgess N, Matanhelia S, Brain A, Penney MD. The frusemide test: simple screening test for renal acidification defect in urolithiasis. Br J Urol. 1993;72:153–6.

Simpson DP. Control of hydrogen ion homeostasis and renal acidosis. Medicine (Baltimore). 1971;50:503–41.

Stein TP, Leskiw MJ, Wallace HW. Metabolism of parenterally administered ammonia. J Surg Res. 1976;21:17–20.

Warren SE, Swerdlin ARH, Steinberg SM. Treatment of alkalosis with ammonium chloride: a case report. Clin Pharmacol Ther. 1979;25:624–7.

Ammonium Chloride

{Systemic acidifier; electrolyte replenisher}

Usual initial dose:	100–200 mEq IV in 500–1,000 mL 0.9 % sodium chloride IV over 3 h (not to exceed 5 mL/h)
Usual maintenance dose:	As required by repeated sodium bicarbonate determinations
Typical maximum dose:	200 mEq/day
Proportion eliminated unchanged:	Nil

Adjustment for Kidney Disease

FDA-approved product labeling:	*Severe renal function impairment*	*Contraindicated*
Alternative adjustment:	*Data not available*	

Dosage Adjustment of Medications Eliminated by the Kidneys

Amoxicillin - Selected References

Abramowicz M, Zuccotti G, Pflomm J-M, et al. Handbook of antimicrobial therapy. 19th ed. New Rochelle: The Medical Letter; 2011.

Amoxicillin powder for suspension [package insert]. Jacksonville: Ranbaxy Laboratories Inc; 2008.

Arancibia A, Drouquett MT, Fuentes G, et al. Pharmacokinetics of amoxicillin in subjects with normal and impaired renal function. Int J Clin Pharmacol Ther Toxicol. 1982;20:447–53.

Arancibia A, Guttmann J, González G, González C. Absorption and disposition kinetics of amoxicillin in normal human subjects. Antimicrob Agents Chemother. 1980;17:199–202.

Aronoff GA, Bennett WM, Berns JS, et al. Drug prescribing in renal failure: dosing guidelines for adults and children. 5th ed. Philadelphia: American College of Physicians; 2007.

Garbutt JM, Banister C, Spitznagel E, Piccirillo JF. Amoxicillin for acute rhinosinusitis: a randomized controlled trial. JAMA. 2012;307:685–92.

Humbert G, Spyker DA, Fillastre JP, Leroy A. Pharmacokinetics of amoxicillin: dosage nomogram for patients with impaired renal function. Antimicrob Agents Chemother. 1979;15:28–33.

Kucers A, Bennett NMcK, Kemp RJ. The use of antibiotics: a comprehensive review with clinical emphasis. 4th ed. Philadelphia: JB Lippincott Co;1987:172–95.

Lawson DH, Henderson AK. Amoxycillin: pharmacokinetic studies in normal subjects, patients with pernicious anaemia and those with renal failure. Postgrad Med J. 1974;50:500–3.

McIntyre CW, Owen PJ. Prescribing drugs in kidney disease. In: Brenner BM, editor. Brenner & Rector's the kidney. 8th ed. Philadelphia: Saunders Elsevier; 2008. p. 1930–55.

Meyer B, Guttmann C, Dittrich E, Schmaldienst S, Thalhammer R. Intermittent administration of betalactam-antibiotics for treatment of severe infection in hemodialysis patients. Eur J Med Res. 2005;10:140–4.

Moxatag® tablet extended release [package insert]. San Diego: Victory Pharma Inc; 2008.

Olyaei AJ, Bennett WM. Pharmacologic approach to renal insufficiency. In: Dale DC, Federman DD, Antman K, editors. ACP medicine, WebMD June 2007 update. Hamilton: BC Decker; 2007; NEPHROLOGY IX: Appendix A1–25.

Olyaei AJ, Bennett WM. Drug dosing in elderly patients with chronic kidney disease. Clin Geriatr Med. 2009;25:459–527.

Olyaei AJ, DeMattos AM, Bennett WM. Use of drugs in patients with renal failure. In: Schrier RW, editor. Diseases of the kidney and urinary tract. 8th ed. Philadelphia: Lippincott Williams & Wilkins; 2007. p. 2765–807.

Sjövall J, Alván G, Westerlund D. Dose-dependent absorption of amoxycillin and bacampicillin. Clin Pharmacol Ther. 1985;38:2141–50.

Sjövall J, Westerlund D, Alván G. Renal excretion of intravenously infused amoxycillin and ampicillin. Br J Clin Pharmacol. 1985;19:191–201.

Spyker DA, Rugloski RJ, Vann RL, O'Brien WM. Pharmacokinetics of amoxicillin: dose dependence after intravenous, oral, and intramuscular administration. Antimicrob Agents Chemother. 1977;11:132–41.

Zarowny D, Ogilvie R, Tamblyn D, MacLeod C, Ruedy J. Pharmacokinetics of amoxicillin. Clin Pharmacol Ther. 1974; 16:1045–51.

Dosage Adjustment of Medications Eliminated by the Kidneys

Amoxicillin/Amoxil®, Moxatag™	{Antibacterial; aminopenicillin}
Usual initial dose:	500 mg orally
Usual maintenance dose:	250–500 mg orally every 8–12 h
Typical maximum dose:	3,000 mg single dose or 2,000 mg/day
Proportion eliminated unchanged:	60–80 %

Adjustment for Kidney Disease

FDA-approved product labeling:	*CrCL 10–30 mL/min*	*250–500 mg orally or enterally every 12 h*
	CrCL <10 mL/min	*250–500 mg orally or enterally every 24 h*
	Hemodialysis	*250–500 mg orally or enterally every 24 h + additional dose both during and after dialysis*
Alternative adjustment:	*GFR >50 mL/min*	*250–500 mg orally or enterally every 8 h*
	GFR 10–50 mL/min	*250–500 mg orally or enterally every 8–12 h*
	GFR <10 mL/min	*250–500 mg orally or enterally every 12–24 h*
	Hemodialysis	*250–500 mg orally or enterally every 12–24 h*
	CAPD	*250 mg orally or enterally every 8 h*
	CRRT	*Not applicable (consider IV ampicillin)*

Dosage Adjustment of Medications Eliminated by the Kidneys

Amoxicillin and Clavulanate - Selected References

Abramowicz M, Zuccotti G, Pflomm J-M, et al. Handbook of antimicrobial therapy. 19th ed. New Rochelle: The Medical Letter; 2011.

Amsden GW. Tables of antimicrobial agent pharmacology. In: Mandell GL, Bennett JE, Dolin R, editors. Mandell, Douglas, and Bennett's principles and practice of infectious diseases, vol. 1. 6th ed. Philadelphia: Elsevier; 2005. p. 634–700.

Aronoff GA, Bennett WM, Berns JS, et al. Drug prescribing in renal failure: dosing guidelines for adults and children. 5th ed. Philadelphia: American College of Physicians; 2007.

Augmentin® tablet, chewable tablet, and powder for suspension [package insert]. Research Triangle Park: GlaxoSmithKline; 2005.

Borrows R, Chusney G, Loucaidou M, et al. The magnitude and time course of changes in mycophenolic acid 12-hour pre-dose levels during antibiotic therapy in mycophenolate mofetil-based renal transplantation. Ther Drug Monit. 2007;29:122–6.

Brumfitt W, Hamilton-Miller JMT. Comparative study of cephradine and amoxicillin-clavulanate in treatment of recurrent urinary tract infections. Antimicrob Agents Chemother. 1990;34:1803–5.

Evans CM, Purohit S, Colbert JW, et al. Amoxycillin-clavulanic acid (Augmentin) antibiotic prophylaxis against wound infections in renal failure patients. J Antimicrob Chemother. 1988;22:363–9.

Ferslew KE, Daigneault EA, Aten EM, Roseman JM. Pharmacokinetics and urinary excretion of clavulanic acid after oral administration of amoxicillin and potassium clavulanate. J Clin Pharmacol. 1984;24:452–6.

Horber FF, Frey FJ, Descoeudres C, Murray Beubl FC. Differential effect of impaired renal function on the kinetics of clavulanic acid and amoxicillin. Antimicrob Agents Chemother. 1986;29:614–9.

Lim KB, Thirumoorthy T, Lee CT, Sng EH, Tan T. Three regimens of procaine penicillin G, Augmentin, and probenecid compared for treating acute gonorrhoea in men. Genitourin Med. 1986;62:82–5.

Ratna P, Mathew BS, Anapandian VM, et al. Pharmacokinetic drug interaction of mycophenolate with co-amoxiclav in renal transplant patients [letter]. Transplantation. 2011;91:e36–8. doi:10.1097/TP.0b013e31820a6a79.

Slaughter RL, Kohli R, Brass C. Effects of hemodialysis on the pharmacokinetics of amoxicillin/clavulanic acid combination. Ther Drug Monit. 1984;6:424–7.

Wald ER, Chiponis D, Ledesma-Medina J. Comparative effectiveness of amoxicillin and amoxicillin-clavulanate potassium in acute paranasal sinus infections in children: a double-blind, placebo-controlled trial. Pediatrics. 1986;77:795–800.

Watson ID, Stewart MJ, Platt DJ. Clinical pharmacokinetics of enzyme inhibitors in antimicrobial chemotherapy. Clin Pharmacokinet. 1988;15:133–64.

Weber DJ, Tolkoff-Rubin NE, Rubin RH. Amoxicillin and potassium clavulanate: an antibiotic combination. Mechanism of action, pharmacokinetics, antimicrobial spectrum, clinical efficacy and adverse effects. Pharmacotherapy. 1984;4:122–36.

Woodruff G, Berry V, Kernutt I, Mizen L. Penetration of amoxycillin, ticarcillin and clavulanic acid into lymph after intravenous infusion in rabbits to simulate human serum pharmacokinetics. J Antimicrob Chemother. 1990;26:695–704.

Dosage Adjustment of Medications Eliminated by the Kidneys

<u>Amoxicillin and Clavulanate</u>/Augmentin®   {Antibacterial; aminopenicillin/β-lactamase inhibitor}

Usual initial dose:	500 mg orally
Usual maintenance dose:	250–500 mg orally or enterally every 8 h or 500–875 mg orally every 12 h
Typical maximum dose:	1,750 mg/day
Proportion eliminated unchanged:	60–80 %/25–40 %

Adjustment for Kidney Disease

FDA-approved product labeling:

CrCL >30 mL/min	*250–500 mg orally or enterally every 8–12 h*
CrCL 10–30 mL/min	*250–500 mg orally or enterally every 12 h*
CrCL <10 mL/min	*250–500 mg orally or enterally every 24 h*
Hemodialysis	*250–500 mg orally or enterally every 24 h; administer an additional dose both during and at the end of dialysis.*
CAPD	*No data*
CRRT	*No data*

Alternative adjustment:

eCrCL >80 mL/min	*250–500 mg orally or enterally every 8–12 h*
eCrCL 51–80 mL/min	*250–500 mg orally or enterally every 8–12 h*
eCrCL 10–50 mL/min	*250–500 mg orally or enterally every 12 h*
eCrCL <10 mL/min	*250–500 mg orally or enterally every 24 h*
Hemodialysis	*250–500 mg orally or enterally every 24 h; give 250–500 mg enterally after dialysis*
CAPD	*250 mg orally or enterally every 12 h*
CRRT	*Not applicable (consider IV ampicillin/ sulbactam)*

Dosage Adjustment of Medications Eliminated by the Kidneys

Ampicillin (Enteral) - Selected References

Ampicillin trihydrate capsule [package insert]. Fort Lee: DAVA Pharmaceuticals Inc; 2011.

Ampicillin trihydrate suspension [package insert]. Fort Lee: DAVA Pharmaceuticals Inc; 2010.

Aronoff GA, Bennett WM, Berns JS, et al. Drug prescribing in renal failure: dosing guidelines for adults and children. 5th ed. Philadelphia: American College of Physicians; 2007.

Buck AC, Cohen SL. Absorption of antibiotics during peritoneal dialysis in patients with renal failure. J Clin Pathol. 1968;21:88–92.

Heintz BH, Matzke GR, Dager WF. Antimicrobial dosing concepts and recommendations for critically ill adult patients receiving continuous renal replacement therapy or intermittent hemodialysis. Pharmacotherapy. 2009;29:562–77.

Hori R, Okumura K, Kamiya A, Nihira H, Nakano H. Ampicillin and cephalexin in renal insufficiency. Clin Pharmacol Ther. 1983;34:792–8.

Kucers A, Bennett NMcK, Kemp RJ. The use of antibiotics: a comprehensive review with clinical emphasis. 4th ed. Philadelphia: JB Lippincott Co; 1987. p. 133–71.

Lee HA, Hill LF. The use of ampicillin in renal disease. Br J Clin Pract. 1968;22:354–7.

Olyaei AJ, Bennett WM. Pharmacologic approach to renal insufficiency. In: Dale DC, Federman DD, Antman K, editors. ACP medicine, WebMD June 2007 update. Hamilton: BC Decker; 2007; NEPHROLOGY IX: Appendix A1–25.

Olyaei AJ, Bennett WM. Drug dosing in elderly patients with chronic kidney disease. Clin Geriatr Med. 2009;25:459–527.

Olyaei AJ, DeMattos AM, Bennett WM. Use of drugs in patients with renal failure. In: Schrier RW, editor. Diseases of the kidney and urinary tract. 8th ed. Philadelphia: Lippincott Williams & Wilkins; 2007. p. 2765–807.

Ruedy J. The effects of peritoneal dialysis on the physiological disposition of oxacillin, ampicillin and tetracycline in patients with renal disease. Can Med Assoc J. 1966;94:257–61.

Sjövall J, Westerlund D, Alván G. Renal excretion of intravenously infused amoxicillin and ampicillin. Br J Clin Pharmacol. 1985;19:191–201.

Dosage Adjustment of Medications Eliminated by the Kidneys

<u>**Ampicillin (Enteral)**</u>/**Polycillin®**   {Antibacterial; aminopenicillin}

Usual initial dose:	250–1,000 mg or 3.5 g once only enterally
Usual maintenance dose:	250–500 mg enterally every 6 h (≥1 h prior to or ≥2 h after meals)
Typical maximum dose:	3,000 mg/day
Proportion eliminated unchanged:	60 %

Adjustment for Kidney Disease

FDA-approved product labeling:	*CrCL >50 mL/min*	*250–500 mg orally or enterally every 6 h*
	CrCL 10–50 mL/min	*250–500 mg orally enterally every 6–12 h*
	CrCL <10 mL/min	*250–500 mg orally or enterally every 12–16 h*
	Hemodialysis	*250–500 mg orally or enterally every12–24 h; give supplemental dose after dialysis*
	CAPD	*250 mg orally or enterally every 12 h*
Alternative adjustment:	*GFR >50 mL/min*	*250–500 mg enterally every 6 h*
	GFR 10–50 mL/min	*250–500 mg enterally every 8 h*
	GFR <10 mL/min	*250–500 mg enterally every 12 h*
	Hemodialysis	*250–500 mg enterally every 12 h; administer after hemodialysis on dialysis days.*
	CRRT	*Not applicable (consider IV ampicillin)*

Dosage Adjustment of Medications Eliminated by the Kidneys

Ampicillin (IV) - Selected References

Abramowicz M, Zuccotti G, Pflomm J-M, et al. Handbook of antimicrobial therapy. 19th ed. New Rochelle: The Medical Letter; 2011.

Ampicillin sodium injection [package insert]. New York: Pfizer Laboratories Division of Pfizer Inc; 2010.

Aronoff GA, Bennett WM, Berns JS, et al. Drug prescribing in renal failure: dosing guidelines for adults and children. 5th ed. Philadelphia: American College of Physicians; 2007.

Buck AC, Cohen SL. Absorption of antibiotics during peritoneal dialysis in patients with renal failure. J Clin Pathol. 1968;21:88–92.

Bulger RJ, Bennett JV. Intraperitoneal administration of broad-spectrum antibiotics in patients with renal failure. JAMA. 1965:194:1198–202.

Gilbert B, Robbins P, Livornese LL Jr. Use of antibacterial agents in renal failure. Med Clin North Am. 2011;95:677–702.

Gouveia EL, Reis JN, Flannery B, et al. Clinical outcome of pneumococcal meningitis during the emergence of penicillin-resistant *Streptococcus pneumoniae*: an observational study. BMC Infect Dis. 2011;11:323. doi:10.1186/1471-2334-11-323.

Heintz BH, Matzke GR, Dager WF. Antimicrobial dosing concepts and recommendations for critically ill adult patients receiving continuous renal replacement therapy or intermittent hemodialysis. Pharmacotherapy. 2009;29:562–77.

Kucers A, Bennett NMcK, Kemp RJ. The use of antibiotics: a comprehensive review with clinical emphasis. 4th ed. Philadelphia: JB Lippincott Co;1987:133–71.

Lee HA, Hill LF. The use of ampicillin in renal disease. Br J Clin Pract. 1968;22:354–7.

McIntyre CW, Owen PJ. Prescribing drugs in kidney disease. In: Brenner BM, editor. Brenner & Rector's the kidney. 8th ed. Philadelphia: Saunders Elsevier; 2008. p. 1930–55.

Olyaei AJ, Bennett WM. Pharmacologic approach to renal insufficiency. In: Dale DC, Federman DD, Antman K, editors. ACP medicine, WebMD June 2007 update. Hamilton: BC Decker; 2007; NEPHROLOGY IX: Appendix A1–25.

Olyaei AJ, Bennett WM. Drug dosing in elderly patients with chronic kidney disease. Clin Geriatr Med. 2009;25:459–527.

Olyaei AJ, DeMattos AM, Bennett WM. Use of drugs in patients with renal failure. In: Schrier RW, editor. Diseases of the kidney and urinary tract. 8th ed. Philadelphia: Lippincott Williams & Wilkins; 2007. p. 2765–807.

Ruedy J. The effects of peritoneal dialysis on the physiological disposition of oxacillin, ampicillin and tetracycline in patients with renal disease. Can Med Assoc J. 1966;94:257–61.

Sjövall J, Westerlund D, Alván G. Renal excretion of intravenously infused amoxicillin and ampicillin. Br J Clin Pharmacol. 1985;19:191–201.

Dosage Adjustment of Medications Eliminated by the Kidneys

<u>**Ampicillin (IV)**</u>**/Polycillin®**   {Antibacterial; aminopenicillin}

Usual initial dose:	2 g IV
Usual maintenance dose:	1–2 g IV every 6 h
Typical maximum dose:	50 mg/kg/dose (~3 g/dose) or 250 mg/kg/day (~12 g/day)
Proportion eliminated unchanged:	60 %

Adjustment for Kidney Disease

FDA-approved product labeling:	*CrCL >50 mL/min*	*1–2 g IV every 4–6 h or 12 g/day continuous IV infusion*
	CrCL 10–50 mL/min	*1–2 g IV every 6–12 h*
Alternative adjustment:	*GFR >50 mL/min*	*1–2 g IV every 6 h*
	GFR 10–50 mL/min	*1–2 g IV every 8 h*
	GFR <10 mL/min	*500–1,500 mg IV every 12 h*
	Hemodialysis	*1 g IV every 12 h; administer after hemodialysis on dialysis days.*
	CAPD	*250 mg IV every 12 h*
	CVVH	*1–2 g IV every 8–12 h*
	CVVHD	*1–2 g IV every 8 h*
	CVVHDF	*1–2 g IV every 6–8 h*

Dosage Adjustment of Medications Eliminated by the Kidneys

Ampicillin and Sulbactam - Selected References

Abramowicz M, Zuccotti G, Pflomm J-M, et al., editors. Handbook of antimicrobial therapy. 19th ed. New Rochelle: The Medical Letter; 2011.

Blackwell BG, Leggett JE II, Johnson CA, Zimmerman SW Craig WA II. Ampicillin and sulbactam pharmacokinetics and pharmacodynamics in continuous ambulatory peritoneal dialysis (CAPD). Perit Dial Int. 1990;10:221–6.

Blum RA, Kohli RK, Harrison NJ, Schentag JJ. Pharmacokinetics of ampicillin (2.0 grams) and sulbactam (1.0 gram) coadministered to subjects with normal an abnormal renal function and with end-stage renal disease on hemodialysis. Antimicrob Agents Chemother. 1989;33:1470–6.

Foulds G, Stankewich JP, Marshall DC, et al. Pharmacokinetics of sulbactam in humans. Antimicrob Agents Chemother. 1983;23:692–9.

Hardin TC, Butler SC, Ross S, Wakeford JH, Jorgensen JH. Comparison of ampicillin-sulbactam and ticarcillin-clavulanic acid in patients with chronic renal failure: effects of differential pharmacokinetics on serum bactericidal activity. Pharmacotherapy. 1994;14:147–52.

Heintz BH, Matzke GR, Dager WF. Antimicrobial dosing concepts and recommendations for critically ill adult patients receiving continuous renal replacement therapy or intermittent hemodialysis. Pharmacotherapy. 2009;29:562–77.

Kielstein JT, Lorenzen J, Kaever V, et al. Risk of underdosing of ampicillin/sulbactam in patients undergoing extended daily dialysis: a single case. Nephrol Dial Transplant. 2009;25:2283–5.

Kuang D, Verbine A, Ronco C. Pharmacokinetics and antimicrobial dosing adjustment in critically ill patients during continuous renal replacement therapy. Clin Nephrol. 2007;67:267–84.

Oliveira MS, Prado GVB, Costa SF, Grinbaum RS, Levin AS. Ampicillin/sulbactam compared with polymyxins for the treatment of infections caused by carbapenem-resistant *Acinetobacter* spp. J Antimicrob Chemother. 2008;61:1369–75.

Rho JP, Jones A, Woo M, et al. Single-dose pharmacokinetics of intravenous ampicillin plus sulbactam in healthy elderly and young adult subjects. J Antimicrob Chemother. 1989;24:573–80.

Ripa S, Ferrante L, Prenna M. Pharmacokinetics of sulbactam/ampicillin in humans after intravenous and intramuscular injection. Chemotherapy. 1990;36:185–92.

Skoulas G, Bayer AS, Pogliano J, et al. Ampicillin enhances daptomycin- and cationic host defense peptide-mediated killing of ampicillin- and vancomycin-resistant *Enterococcus faecium*. Antimicrob Agents Chemother. 2011. Epub ahead of print. doi:10.1128/AAC.05551-11.

Trotman RL, Williamson JC, Shoemaker M, Salzer WL. Antibiotic dosing in critically ill adult patients receiving continuous renal replacement therapy. Clin Infect Dis. 2005;41:1159–66.

Unasyn® injection [package insert]. New York: Roerig Division of Pfizer Inc; 2010.

Watson ID, Stewart MJ, Platt DJ. Clinical pharmacokinetics of enzyme inhibitors in antimicrobial chemotherapy. Clin Pharmacokinet. 1988;15:133–64.

Wright N, Wise R. The elimination of sulbactam alone and combined with ampicillin in patients with renal dysfunction. J Antimicrob Chemother. 1983;11:583–7.

Dosage Adjustment of Medications Eliminated by the Kidneys

<u>Ampicillin and Sulbactam</u>/Unasyn® {Antibacterial; aminopenicillin/β-lactamase inhibitor}

Usual initial dose:	1.5–3 g IV
Usual maintenance dose:	1.5–3 g IV every 6 h
Typical maximum dose:	3 g IV
Proportion eliminated unchanged:	35 %

Adjustment for Kidney Disease

FDA-approved product labeling: *Ampicillin and sulbactam for injection dosage guide for patients with renal impairment*

CrCL (mL/min)	Ampicillin/sulbactam half-life (h)	Recommended ampicillin/ sulbactam for injection dosage
≥30	1	1.5–3 g IV q 6–q 8 h
15–29	5	1.5–3 IV g q 12 h
5–14	9	1.5–3 g IV q 24 h

Alternative adjustment:

GFR >50 mL/min	1.5–3 g IV every 6 h
GFR 10–50 mL/min	1.5–3 g IV every 12 h
GFR <10 mL/min	1.5–3 g IV every 24 h
Hemodialysis	3 g IV every 24 h; administer after hemodialysis on dialysis days.
Sustained low-efficiency dialysis	3 g IV every 12 h on dialysis days
CAPD	3 g IV every 12 h
CVVH	3 g IV every 12 h
CVVHD or CVVHDF	3 g IV every 8 h

Anakinra - Selected References

Balakrishnan VS, Jaber BL, Natov SN, et al. Interleukin-2 receptor antagonist synthesis by peripheral blood mononuclear cells in hemodialysis patients. Kidney Int. 1998;54:2106–12.

Donati D, Degiannis D, Mazzola E, et al. Interleukin-1 receptors and receptor antagonist in haemodialysis. Nephrol Dial Transplant. 1997;12:111–8.

Ghani BA, Zainudin S, Ctkong N, et al. Serum IL-6 and IL-1-ra with sequential organ failure assessment scores n septic patients receiving high-volume haemofiltration and continuous venovenous haemofiltration. Nephrology. 2006;11:386–93.

Kineret® injection [package insert]. Thousand Oaks: Amgen Inc; 2010.

Schiff MH, DiVittorio G, Tesser J, et al. The safety of anakinra in high-risk patients with rheumatoid arthritis: six-month observations of patients with comorbid conditions. Arthritis Rheum. 2004;50:1752–60.

Schindler R, Lonnemann G, Schäffer K, et al. The effect of ultrafiltered dialysate on the cellular content of interleukin-1 receptor antagonist in patients on chronic hemodialysis. Nephron. 1994;68:229–33.

Yang B-B, Baughman S, Sullivan JT. Pharmacokinetics of anakinra in subjects with different levels of renal function. Clin Pharmacol Ther. 2003;74:85–94.

Dosage Adjustment of Medications Eliminated by the Kidneys

Anakinra/Kineret®   **{Antirheumatic; human interleukin 1 receptor antagonist}**

Usual initial dose: 100 mg subcutaneously

Usual maintenance dose: 100 mg subcutaneously once daily

Typical maximum dose: 100 mg/day

Proportion eliminated unchanged: Unknown; plasma clearance decreased by 75 % in end-stage renal disease

Adjustment for Kidney Disease

FDA-approved product labeling:	*CrCL >30 mL/min*	*100 mg subcutaneously once daily*
	CrCL ≤30 mL/min	*100 mg subcutaneously every 48 h*
Alternative adjustment:	*GFR >50 mL/min*	*100 mg subcutaneously once daily*
	GFR 10–50 mL/min	*100 mg subcutaneously every 48 h*
	GFR <10 mL/min	*100 mg subcutaneously every 48 h*
	Hemodialysis	*100 mg subcutaneously every 48 h*
	CAPD	*100 mg subcutaneously every 48 h*
	CRRT	*Data not available*

Apomorphine - Selected References

Apokyn® injection [package insert]. Brisbane: Tercica Inc, a subsidiary of the Ipsen Group; 2010.

Corboy DL, Wagner ML, Sage JI. Apomorphine for motor fluctuations and freezing in Parkinson's disease. Ann Pharmacother. 1995;29:282–8.

Eeleu D, Northway MG, Hanssens Y. Clinical pharmacokinetics and pharmacodynamics of drugs used in the treatment of Parkinson's disease. Clin Pharmacokinet. 2002;41:261–309.

Gancher St Bennett W, English J. Studies of renal function in animals chronically treated with apomorphine. Res Commun Chem Pathol Pharmacol. 1989;66:163–6.

Dosage Adjustment of Medications Eliminated by the Kidneys

<u>**Apomorphine**</u>/**Apokyn**®   **{Anti-Parkinsonian; acetylcholinesterase inhibitor}**

Usual initial dose: 2 mg subcutaneously (test dose)

Usual maintenance dose: 3–6 mg subcutaneously three times daily

Typical maximum dose: 20 mg/day

Proportion eliminated unchanged: Unknown

Adjustment for Kidney Disease

    FDA-approved product labeling: *Mild to moderate renal impairment*   *1 mg subcutaneously three times daily (test dose and initial maintenance dose)*

                                                    Severe renal impairment   *Studies in subjects with severe renal impairment have not been conducted.*

    Alternative adjustment: *Data not available*

Arsenic Trioxide - Selected References

Au W-Y, Cheung GT, Yuen TW, Kumana CR, Kwong Y-L. Successful treatment of relapsed acute promyelocytic leukemia in a patient receiving continuous ambulatory peritoneal dialysis with oral arsenic trioxide [letter]. Arch Intern Med. 2005;165:1067–8.

Au W-Y, Kwong YL. Arsenic trioxide: safety issues and their management. Acta Pharmacol Sin. 2008;29:296–304.

Blythe D, Joyce DA. Clearance of arsenic by haemodialysis after poisoning with arsenic trioxide [letter]. Intensive Care Med. 2001;27:334.

Fujisawa S, Ohno R, Shigeno K, et al. Pharmacokinetics of arsenic species in Japanese patients with relapsed or refractory acute promyelocytic leukemia treated with arsenic trioxide. Cancer Chemother Pharmacol. 2007;59:485–93.

Mathews V, George B, Chendamarai E, et al. Single-agent arsenic trioxide in the treatment of newly diagnosed acute promyelocytic leukemia: long-term follow-up data. J Clin Oncol. 2010;28:3866–71.

Sasaki A, Oshima Y, Fujimura A. An approach to elucidate potential mechanism of renal toxicity of arsenic trioxide. Exp Hematol. 2007;35:252–67.

Shen Y, Shen Z-X, Yan H, et al. Studies on the clinical efficacy and pharmacokinetics of low-dose arsenic trioxide in the treatment of relapsed acute promyelocytic leukemia: a comparison with conventional dosage. Leukemia. 2001;15:735–41.

Shen Z-X, Chen G-Q, Ni J-H, et al. Use of arsenic trioxide (As2O3) in the treatment of acute promyelocytic leukemia (APL): II. Clinical efficacy and pharmacokinetics in relapsed patients. Blood. 1997;89:3354–60.

Soignet SL, Frankel SR, Douer D, et al. United States multicenter study of arsenic trioxide in relapsed acute promyelocytic leukemia. J Clin Oncol. 2001;19:3852–60.

Sweeney CJ, Takimoto C, Wood L, et al. A pharmacokinetic and safety study of intravenous arsenic trioxide in adult cancer patients with renal impairment. Cancer Chemother Pharmacol. 2010;66:345–56.

Trisenox® injection [package insert]. Frazer: Cephalon Inc; 2010.

Yamamoto Y, Sasaki M, Oshimi K, Sugimoto K. Arsenic trioxide in a hemodialytic patient with acute promyelocytic leukemia. Acta Haematol. 2009;52–3.

Yoon HS, Park TS, Jeong KH. Arsenic trioxide for the treatment of a relapsed acute promyelocytic leukemia with renal failure [letter]. Pediatr Blood Cancer. 2011;57:1085.

Dosage Adjustment of Medications Eliminated by the Kidneys

<u>Arsenic Trioxide</u>/Trisenox®	{Antineoplastic; fusion protein inhibitor; ℞ for acute promyelocytic leukemia}	
Usual initial dose:	0.15 mg/kg IV over 2 h	
Usual maintenance dose:	Induction—0.15 mg/kg IV over 2 h daily until bone marrow remission; total induction dose should not exceed 60 doses.	
	Consolidation—Beginning 3–6 weeks after completion of induction therapy, 0.15 mg/kg IV over 2 h daily for 25 doses over a period up to 5 weeks .	
Typical maximum dose:	0.15 mg/kg/day	
Proportion eliminated unchanged:	20 % increasing to 60 % with repeated doses	

Adjustment for Kidney Disease

FDA-approved product labeling:	*Severe renal impairment*	*Exposure of arsenic trioxide may be higher.*
	CrCL < 30 mL/min	*Monitor closely for toxicity (e.g., QT interval prolongation, seizures, muscle weakness, confusion); a dose reduction may be warranted (toxicity with signs of overdose should be treated with chelation therapy).*
Alternative adjustment:	*CrCL > 80 mL/min*	*Induction—0.15 mg/kg IV over 2 h daily until bone marrow remission; total induction dose should not exceed 60 doses.*
		Consolidation—Beginning 3–6 weeks after completion of induction therapy, 0.15 mg/kg IV over 2 h daily for 25 doses over a period up to 5 weeks.
	CrCL 50– 80 mL/min	*Total arsenic exposure appears to be unchanged as compared to patients without renal impairment, but distribution volume of arsenic is contracted; although too few data are available to suggest exact dosages, consider dose reduction to 0.08 mg/kg IV daily.*
	CrCL 30– 49 mL/min	*As compared to patients without renal impairment, distribution volume of arsenic is contracted, total exposure is increased, and the percentage of arsenic dose excreted in urine is decreased; although too few data are available to suggest exact dosages, consider dose reduction to 0.15 mg/kg IV twice weekly.*
	CrCL < 30 mL/min	*As compared to patients without renal impairment, distribution volume of arsenic is contracted, total exposure is increased, and the percentage of arsenic dose excreted in urine is substantially decreased; although too few data are available to suggest exact dosages, consider dose reduction to 0.15 mg/kg IV twice weekly.*
	Hemodialysis	*Very small numbers of patients have been treated with 0.15 mg/kg IV two to three times weekly with monitoring of plasma arsenic levels; hemodialytic clearance of arsenic has been calculated as approximately 5 mL/min.*
	CAPD	*Presently, data not available for use of IV arsenic trioxide*
	CRRT	*Data not available*

Dosage Adjustment of Medications Eliminated by the Kidneys

Aspirin - Selected References

Aronoff GA, Bennett WM, Berns JS, et al. Drug prescribing in renal failure: dosing guidelines for adults and children. 5th ed. Philadelphia: American College of Physicians; 2007.

Bayer® Advanced Aspirin Extra Strength tablet [package insert]. Morristown; Bayer HealthCare LLC; 2010.

Berg KJ. Acute effects of acetylsalicylic acid in patients with chronic renal insufficiency. Eur J Clin Pharmacol. 1977;11:111–6.

Berg KJ. Acute effects of acetylsalicylic acid on renal function in normal man. Eur J Clin Pharmacol. 1977;11:117–23.

Burch JW, Stanford N, Majerus PW. Inhibition of platelet prostaglandin synthetase by oral aspirin. J Clin Invest. 1978;61:314–9.

Campbell EJM, MacLaurin RE. Acute renal failure in salicylate poisoning. Br Med J. 1958;1:503–5.

Cerletti C, Marchi S, Lauri D, et al. Pharmacokinetics of enteric-coated aspirin and inhibition of platelet thromboxane A_2 and vascular prostacyclin generation in humans. Clin Pharmacol Ther. 1987;42:175–80.

Chen Y-T, Yang W-C, Lin C-C g Y-Y, Chen J-Y, Li S-Y. Comparison of peptic ulcer disease risk between peritoneal and hemodialysis patients. Am J Nephrol. 2010;32:212–8.

Collins R, Peto R, Hennekens C, et al. Aspirin in the primary and secondary prevention of vascular disease: collaborative meta-analysis of individual participant data from randomised trials. Lancet. 2009;373:1849–60.

Cuny G, Royer RJ, Mur JM, et al. Pharmacokinetics of salicylates in the elderly. Gerontology. 1979;25:49–55.

Doherty CC, McGeown MG. Aspirin and renal function [letter]. Lancet. 1977;1:1056–7.

Gault MH, Rudwal TC, Engles WD, Dossetor JB. Syndrome associated with the abuse of analgesics. Ann Intern Med. 1968;68:906–25.

Greenblatt DJ, Abernethy DR, Divoll M, Ochs HR, Shader RI. Antipyretic analgesic drugs as models for studies of drug disposition in old age. Am J Med. 1983;75(Suppl 5A):127–40.

Kearon C, Hirsh J. Optimal dose for starting and maintaining low-dose aspirin. Arch Intern Med. 1993;153:700–2.

Kelton JG, Hirsh J, Carter CJ, Buchanan MR. Thrombogenic effect of high-dose aspirin in rabbits: relationship to inhibition of vessel wall synthesis of prostaglandin I_2-like activity. J Clin Invest. 1978;62:892–5.

Levy G. Clinical pharmacokinetics of aspirin. Pediatrics. 1978;62(5 Pt 2 Suppl):867–72.

Mason WD, Winer N. Kinetics of aspirin, salicylic acid, and salicyluric acid following oral administration of aspirin as a tablet and two buffered solutions. J Pharm Sci. 1981;70:262–5.

McIntyre CW, Owen PJ. Prescribing drugs in kidney disease. In: Brenner BM, editor. Brenner & Rector's the kidney. 8th ed. Philadelphia: Saunders Elsevier; 2008. p. 1930–55.

Olyaei AJ, Bennett WM. Pharmacologic approach to renal insufficiency. In: Dale DC, Federman DD, Antman K, editors. ACP medicine, WebMD June 2007 update. Hamilton: BC Decker; 2007; NEPHROLOGY IX: Appendix A1–25.

Olyaei AJ, Bennett WM. Drug dosing in elderly patients with chronic kidney disease. Clin Geriatr Med. 2009;25:459–527.

Olyaei AJ, DeMattos AM, Bennett WM. Use of drugs in patients with renal failure. In: Schrier RW, editor. Diseases of the kidney and urinary tract. 8th ed. Philadelphia: Lippincott Williams & Wilkins; 2007. p. 2765–807.

Plotz PH, Kimberly RP. Acute effects of aspirin and acetaminophen on renal function. Arch Intern Med. 1981;141:343–8.

Saito Y, Soejima H, Morimoto T, et al. Low-dose aspirin therapy in patients with type 2 diabetes and reduced glomerular filtration rate. Diabetes Care. 2011;34:280–5.

Schreiner GE, McAnally JF, Winchester JF. Clinical analgesic nephropathy. Arch Intern Med. 1981;141:349–57.

Shea-Donohue T, Steel L, Montcalm-Mazzili E, Dubois A. Aspirin-induced changes in gastric function: role of endogenous prostaglandins and mucosal damage. Gastroenterology. 1990;98:284–92.

Dosage Adjustment of Medications Eliminated by the Kidneys

Aspirin/Bayer Aspirin®, Ecotrin®	{**Anti-inflammatory; analgesic; platelet aggregation inhibitor**}
Usual initial dose:	325–650 mg orally or rectally
Usual maintenance dose:	81–325 mg orally once daily (antiplatelet) or 300–650 mg orally or rectally every 4 h as necessary (analgesic/antipyretic)
Typical maximum dose:	4,000 mg/day
Proportion eliminated unchanged:	2–80 %

Adjustment for Kidney Disease

FDA-approved product labeling:	*CrCL ≥50 mL/min*	*81–325 mg orally once daily (antiplatelet) or 300–650 mg orally or rectally every 4 h as necessary (analgesic/antipyretic)*
	Kidney problems	*Ask a doctor before use.*
Alternative adjustment:	*GFR >50 mL/min*	*81–325 mg orally once daily (antiplatelet) or 650 mg orally or rectally every 4 h as necessary (analgesic/antipyretic)*
	GFR 10–50 mL/min	*81–162 mg orally once daily (antiplatelet) or 650 mg orally or rectally every 6 h as necessary (analgesic/antipyretic)*
	GFR <10 mL/min	*Data not available. Preferably avoid unless no suitable alternative exists; if indeed necessary, begin with low doses (e.g., 81 mg/day) and monitor carefully.*
	Hemodialysis	*81–162 mg orally or rectally after hemodialysis on dialysis days*
	CAPD	*Minimal data available. Preferably avoid unless no suitable alternative exists; if indeed necessary, begin with low doses (e.g., 81 mg/day) and monitor carefully.*
	CRRT	*81–162 mg orally once daily (antiplatelet) or 650 mg enterally or rectally every 6 h as necessary (analgesic/antipyretic)*

Dosage Adjustment of Medications Eliminated by the Kidneys

Atazanavir - Selected References

Aronoff GA, Bennett WM, Berns JS, et al. Drug prescribing in renal failure: dosing guidelines for adults and children. 5th ed. Philadelphia: American College of Physicians; 2007.

Boffito M, Kurowski M, Kruse G, et al. Atazanavir enhances saquinavir hard-gel concentrations in a ritonavir-boosted once-daily regimen. AIDS. 2004;18:1291–7.

Cleijsen RMM, van de Ende ME, Kroon FP, et al. Therapeutic drug monitoring of the HIV protease inhibitor atazanavir in clinical practice. J Antimicrob Chemother. 2007;60:897–900.

Colombe S, Buclin T, Cavassini M, et al. Population pharmacokinetics of atazanavir in patients with human immunodeficiency virus infection. Antimicrob Agents Chemother. 2006;50:3801–8.

Drusano GL, Bilello JA, Preston SL, et al. Hollow-fiber evaluation of a new human immunodeficiency virus type 1 protease inhibitor, BMS-232632, for determination of the linked pharmacodynamic variable. J Infect Dis. 2001;1126–9.

Izzedine H, Launay-Vacher V, Peytavin G, Valantin MA, Deray G. Atazanavir: a novel inhibitor of HIV-protease in haemodialysis [letter]. Nephrol Dial Transplant. 2005;20:852–3.

Le Tiec C, Barrail A, Goujard C, Taburet A-M. Clinical pharmacokinetics and summary of efficacy and tolerability of atazanavir. Clin Pharmacokinet. 2005;44:1035–50.

Reyataz® capsule [package insert]. Princeton: Bristol-Myers Squibb Co; 2011.

Solas C, Gagnieu M-C, Ravaux I, et al. Population pharmacokinetics of atazanavir in human immunodeficiency virus-infected patients. Ther Drug Monit. 2008;30:670–3.

Dosage Adjustment of Medications Eliminated by the Kidneys

Atazanavir/Reyataz® {Antiretroviral; protease inhibitor}

Usual initial dose: 300 mg orally with ritonavir 100 mg or 400 mg orally (without ritonavir) with food once daily

Usual maintenance dose: 300 mg orally with ritonavir 100 mg or 400 mg orally (without ritonavir) with food once daily

Typical maximum dose: 400 mg/day

Proportion eliminated unchanged: 7 %

Adjustment for Kidney Disease

FDA-approved product labeling:	*Renal impairment, including patients with severe renal impairment not managed with hemodialysis*	*400 mg orally every 24 h (no dose adjustment necessary)*
	Treatment-naïve patients with ESRD managed with hemodialysis	*300 mg orally once daily with ritonavir 100 mg orally once daily*
	HIV-treatment-experienced patients with ESRD managed with hemodialysis	*Do not administer; avoid.*
Alternative adjustment:	*GFR >50 mL/min*	*400 mg orally every 24 h*
	GFR 10–50 mL/min	*Data not available*
	GFR <10 mL/min	*Data not available*
	Hemodialysis	*400 mg orally every 24 h (no dose adjustment necessary—only very limited data available)*
	CAPD	*Data not available*
	CRRT	*Data not available*

Atenolol - Selected References

Aronoff GA, Bennett WM, Berns JS, et al. Drug prescribing in renal failure: dosing guidelines for adults and children. 5th ed. Philadelphia: American College of Physicians; 2007.

Boyd RA, Chin SK, Don-Pedro O, Williams RL, Giacomini KM. The pharmacokinetics of the enantiomers of atenolol. Clin Pharmacol Ther. 1989;45:403–10.

Brown HC, Carruthers SG Johnston GD, et al. Clinical pharmacological observations on atenolol, a beta-adrenoceptor blocker. Clin Pharmacol Ther. 1976;20:524–34.

Fitzgerald JD, Ruffin R, Smedstad KG, Roberts R, McAinsch J. Studies on the pharmacokinetics of atenolol in man. Eur J Clin Pharmacol. 1978;13:81–9.

Flouvat B, Decourt S, Aubert P, et al. Pharmacokinetics of atenolol in patients with terminal renal failure and influence of haemodialysis. Br J Clin Pharmacol. 1980;9:379–85.

McAinsh J. Clinical pharmacokinetics of atenolol. Postgrad Med J. 1977;53(Suppl):74–8.

McAinsh J, Holmes BF, Smith S, Hood D, Warren D. Atenolol kinetics in renal failure. Clin Pharmacol Ther. 1980;28:302–9.

McIntyre CW, Owen PJ. Prescribing drugs in kidney disease. In: Brenner BM, editor. Brenner & Rector's the kidney. 8th ed. Philadelphia: Saunders Elsevier; 2008. p. 1930–55.

Olyaei AJ, Bennett WM. Pharmacologic approach to renal insufficiency. In: Dale DC, Federman DD, Antman K, editors. ACP medicine, WebMD June 2007 update. Hamilton: BC Decker; 2007; NEPHROLOGY IX: Appendix A1–25.

Olyaei AJ, Bennett WM. Drug dosing in elderly patients with chronic kidney disease. Clin Geriatr Med. 2009;25:459–527.

Olyaei AJ, DeMattos AM, Bennett WM. Use of drugs in patients with renal failure. In: Schrier RW, editor. Diseases of the kidney and urinary tract. 8th ed. Philadelphia: Lippincott Williams & Wilkins; 2007. p. 2765–807.

Rubin PC, Scott PJ, McLean K, Pearson A, Ross D, Reid JL. Atenolol disposition in young and elderly subjects. Br J Clin Pharmacol. 1982;13:235–7.

Salahudeen AK, Wilkinson R, McAinsh J, Bateman DN. Atenolol pharmacokinetics in patients on continuous ambulatory peritoneal dialysis. Br J Clin Pharmacol. 1984;18:457–60.

Sassard J, Pozet N, McAinsh J, Legheand J, Zech P. Pharmacokinetics of atenolol in patients with renal impairment. Eur J Clin Pharmacol. 1977;12:175–80.

Tenormin® injection [package insert]. Wilmington: AstraZeneca Pharmaceuticals LP; 2004.

Tenormin® tablet [package insert]. Wilmington: AstraZeneca Pharmaceuticals LP; 2008.

Dosage Adjustment of Medications Eliminated by the Kidneys

Atenolol/Tenormin® {**Antihypertensive; antianginal; β-adrenergic receptor blocker**}

Usual initial dose: 25–50 mg orally or 5 mg IV followed by 5 mg IV 10 min later

Usual maintenance dose: 50–100 mg orally once daily

Typical maximum dose: 2 mg/kg/day up to 100 mg daily

Proportion eliminated unchanged: 95 %

Adjustment for Kidney Disease

FDA-approved product labeling: *Atenolol dosage adjustment in renal impairment*

CrCL (mL/min)	Atenolol elimination half-life (h)	Maximum dosage
15–35	16–27	50 mg orally daily
<15	>27	25 mg orally daily

Hemodialysis: 25–50 mg orally after each dialysis

Alternative adjustment:

GFR >50 mL/min	*50–100 mg orally daily*
GFR 10–50 mL/min	*25–50 mg orally every 24 h (~75 % of usual dose)*
GFR <10 mL/min	*25 mg orally every 24 h (~50 % of usual dose)*
Hemodialysis	*25–50 mg orally every 24 h; dose after hemodialysis on dialysis days*
CAPD	*25 mg orally every 24 h (~50 % of usual dose)*
CRRT	*25–50 mg orally every 24 h; titrate.*

Atovaquone and Proguanil - Selected References

Gillotin C, Mamet JP, Veronese L. Lack of a pharmacokinetic interaction between atovaquone and proguanil. Eur J Clin Pharmacol. 1999;55:311–5.

Hussein Z, Eaves CJ, Hutchinson DB, Canfield CJ. Population pharmacokinetics of proguanil in patients with acute *P. falciparum* malaria after combined therapy with atovaquone. Br J Clin Pharmacol. 1996;42:589–97.

Hussein Z, Eaves CJ, Hutchinson DB, Canfield CJ. Population pharmacokinetics of atovaquone in patients with acute malaria caused by *Plasmodium falciparum*. Clin Pharmacol Ther. 1997;64:518–30.

Malarone® tablet [package insert]. Research Triangle Park: GlaxoSmithKline; 2010.

Sabchareon A, Attanath P, Phanuaksook P, et al. Efficacy and pharmacokinetics of atovaquone and proguanil in children with multidrug-resistant *Plasmodium falciparum* malaria. Trans R Soc Trop Med Hyg. 1998;92:201–6.

Thapar MM, Ashton M, Lindegårdh N, et al. Time-dependent pharmacokinetics and drug metabolism of atovaquone plus proguanil (Malarone) when taken as chemoprophylaxis. Eur J Clin Pharmacol. 2002;58:19–27.

Dosage Adjustment of Medications Eliminated by the Kidneys

<u>**Atovaquone and Proguanil**</u>/Malarone®	{**Antimalarial; ubiquinone-mediated mitochondrial electron transport and dihydrofolate reductase inhibitor**}

Usual initial dose: Malaria treatment—1,000 mg/400 mg (four tablets) orally once daily for three consecutive days

Malaria prevention—250 mg/100 mg (one tablet) orally once daily beginning 1–2 days prior to entering malaria-endemic area

Usual maintenance dose: Malaria prevention—250 mg/100 mg (one tablet) daily, continuing for 7 days after leaving malaria-endemic area

Typical maximum dose: 1,000 mg/400 mg (four tablets)

Proportion eliminated unchanged: 40–60 % (proguanil)

Adjustment for Kidney Disease

FDA-approved product labeling: *CrCL ≥30 mL/min*   *Malaria treatment—1,000 mg/400 mg (four tablets) orally once daily for three consecutive days*

Malaria prevention—250 mg/100 mg (one tablet) orally once daily

CrCL <30 mL/min   *Malaria treatment—Use with caution only if the benefits of the 3-day regimen outweigh the potential risks associated with increased drug exposure.*

Malaria prophylaxis—contraindicated

Alternative adjustment: *Data not available*

Auranofin - Selected References

Aronoff GA, Bennett WM, Berns JS, et al. Drug prescribing in renal failure: dosing guidelines for adults and children. 5th ed. Philadelphia: American College of Physicians; 2007.

Blocka K. Auranofin versus injectable gold: comparison of pharmacokinetic properties. Am J Med. 1983;75(Suppl 6A): 114–22.

Blocka K, Furst DE, Landaw E, Dromgoole S, Blomberg A, Paulus HE. Single dose pharmacokinetics of auranofin in rheumatoid arthritis. J Rheumatol Suppl. 1982;8:110–9.

Blocka KLN, Paulus HE, Furst DE. Clinical pharmacokinetics of oral and injectable gold compounds. Clin Pharmacokinet. 1986;11:133–43.

Blodget RC Jr. Auranofin: experience to date. Am J Med. 1983;75(Suppl 6A):86–9.

Blodgett RC Jr, Heuer MA, Pietrusko RG. Auranofin: a unique oral chrysotherapeutic agent. Semin Arthritis Rheum. 1984;13:255–73.

Furst DE. Mechanism of action, pharmacology, clinical efficacy and side effects of auranofin, an orally administered organic gold compound for the treatment of rheumatic arthritis. Pharmacotherapy. 1983;3:284–98.

Jarner D, Nielsen AM. Auranofin (SK+F 39162) induced enterocolitis in rheumatoid arthritis: a case report. Scand J Rheumatol. 1983;12:254–6.

Kvien TK, Høyeraal HM, Sandstad B, Kass E. Auranofin therapy in juvenile rheumatoid arthritis: a 48-week phase II study. Scand J Rheumatol Suppl. 1986;63:79–84.

Luthra HS, Bunch TW, O'Duffy JD, Dillon AM, Lakhanpal S, O'Fallon WM. Double-blind study comparing auranofin and d-penicillamine in rheumatoid arthritis. Scand J Rheumatol Suppl. 1986;63:55–8.

McIntyre CW, Owen PJ. Prescribing drugs in kidney disease. In: Brenner BM, editor. Brenner & Rector's the kidney. 8th ed. Philadelphia: Saunders Elsevier; 2008. p. 1930–55.

Olyaei AJ, Bennett WM. Pharmacologic approach to renal insufficiency. In: Dale DC, Federman DD, Antman K, editors. ACP medicine, WebMD June 2007 update. Hamilton: BC Decker; 2007; NEPHROLOGY IX: Appendix A1–25.

Olyaei AJ, Bennett WM. Drug dosing in elderly patients with chronic kidney disease. Clin Geriatr Med. 2009;25:459–527.

Olyaei AJ, DeMattos AM, Bennett WM. Use of drugs in patients with renal failure. In: Schrier RW, editor. Diseases of the kidney and urinary tract. 8th ed. Philadelphia: Lippincott Williams & Wilkins; 2007. p. 2765–807.

Ridaura® capsule [package insert]. San Diego: Prometheus Laboratories Inc; 2007.

Walz DT, DiMartino MJ, Griswold DE, Intoccia AP, Flanagan TL. Biologic actions and pharmacokinetic studies of auranofin. Am J Med. 1983;75(Suppl 6A):90–108.

Walz DT, DiMartino MJ, Griswold DE. The pharmacological profile of auranofin, an orally active gold compound. Scand J Rheumatol Suppl. 1983;51:16–25.

Ward JR, Williams HJ, Boyce E, Egger MJ, Reading JC, Samuelson CO Jr. Comparison of auranofin, gold sodium thiomalate, and placebo in the treatment of rheumatoid arthritis: subsets of responses. Am J Med. 1983;75(Suppl 6A):133–7.

Wenger ME, Alexander S, Bland JH, Blechman WJ. Auranofin versus placebo in the treatment of rheumatoid arthritis. Am J Med. 1983;75(Suppl 6A):123–7.

Dosage Adjustment of Medications Eliminated by the Kidneys

__Auranofin__/Ridaura®	{Antirheumatic; gold macrophage phagocytosis and lysosomal enzyme inhibitor}

Usual initial dose:	3 mg orally
Usual maintenance dose:	3 mg orally twice daily or 6 mg orally once daily
Typical maximum dose:	9 mg/day
Proportion eliminated unchanged:	60 %

Adjustment for Kidney Disease

> **FDA-approved product labeling:** *The potential benefits of using (auranofin) in patients with progressive renal disease should be weighed against (1) the potential risks of gold toxicity on organ systems previously compromised or with decreased reserve and (2) the difficulty in quickly detecting and correctly attributing the toxic effect.*

> **Alternative adjustment:**

GFR >50 mL/min	*3 mg orally every 24 h (50 % decrease)*
GFR 10–50 mL/min	*Preferably avoid due to risk for acute kidney injury and proteinuria and/or hematological toxicity.*
GFR <10 mL/min	*Preferably avoid due to risk for acute kidney injury and proteinuria and/or hematological toxicity.*
Hemodialysis	*Preferably avoid due to risk for acute kidney injury and proteinuria and/or hematological toxicity.*
CAPD	*Preferably avoid due to risk for acute kidney injury and proteinuria and/or hematological toxicity.*
CRRT	*Preferably avoid due to risk for acute kidney injury and proteinuria and/or hematological toxicity.*

Dosage Adjustment of Medications Eliminated by the Kidneys

Azacitidine - Selected References

Buckstein R, Yee K, Wells RA. 5-Azacitidine in myelodysplastic syndromes: a clinical practice guideline. Cancer Treat Rev. 2011;37:160–7.

Campelo MD, Delgado RG, Molias ACG, Sanchez JF. Azacitidine for the treatment of myelodysplastic syndromes in the elderly. Adv Ther. 2011;28(Suppl 2):10–5.

Edlin R, Connock M, Tubeuf S, et al. Azacitidine for the treatment of myelodysplastic syndrome, chronic myelomonocytic leukaemia and acute myeloid leukaemia. Health Technol Assess. 2010;14(Suppl 1):69–74.

Garcia-Manero G, Stoltz ML, Ward MR, Kantarjian H, Sharma S. A pilot pharmacokinetic study of oral azacitidine. Leukemia. 2008;22:1680–4.

Israili AH, Vogler WR, Mingioli ES, Pirkis JL, Smithwick RW, Goldstein JH. The disposition and pharmacokinetics in humans of 5-azacytidine administered intravenously or by continuous infusion. Cancer Res. 1976;36;1453–61.

Marcucci G, Silverman L Eller M, Lintz L, Beach CL. Bioavailability of azacitidine subcutaneous versus intravenous in patients with the myelodysplastic syndromes. J Clin Pharmacol. 2005;45:597–602.

Scott BL, Deeg HJ. Myelodysplastic syndromes. Annu Rev Med. 2010;61:145–58.

Sullivan M, Hahn K, Kolesar JM. Azacitidine: a novel agent for myelodysplastic syndromes. Am J Health Syst Pharm. 2005;62:1567–73.

Trostel WM, Weiss AJ, Stambaugh JE, Laucius JF, Manthel RW. Absorption, distribution, and excretion of 5-azacytidine (NSC-102816) in man. Cancer Chemother Rep. 1972;56:405–11.

Vidaza® injection [package insert]. Summit: Celgene Corp; 2008.

Dosage Adjustment of Medications Eliminated by the Kidneys

__Azacitidine__/Vidaza®	__{Antineoplastic; DNA demethylation agent, ℞ for myelodysplastic syndromes}__

__Usual initial dose:__	75 mg/m² IV or subcutaneously
__Usual maintenance dose:__	75 mg/m² subcutaneously daily for seven consecutive days every 4 weeks for a minimum of four cycles
__Typical maximum dose:__	100 mg/m²/day (if no beneficial effect is seen after. two lower-dose treatment cycles and if no toxicity other than nausea and vomiting has occurred)
__Proportion eliminated unchanged:__	85 %

Adjustment for Kidney Disease

FDA-approved product labeling:	*Impaired renal function*	*Imparts greater risk of toxic reactions; if unexplained elevations of SCr or BUN occur, the next cycle should be delayed until values return to normal or baseline and the dose should be reduced to 50 % on the next treatment course.*
Alternative adjustment:	*Data not available*	

Azathioprine - Selected References

Aronoff GA, Bennett WM, Berns JS, et al. Drug prescribing in renal failure: dosing guidelines for adults and children. 5th ed. Philadelphia: American College of Physicians; 2007.

Azathioprine sodium injection [package insert]. Bedford: Bedford Laboratories Inc; 2011.

Chan GLC, Canafax DM, Johnson CA. The therapeutic use of azathioprine in renal transplantation. Pharmacotherapy. 1987;7:165–77.

Imuran® tablet [package insert]. San Diego: Prometheus Laboratories Inc; 2009.

McIntyre CW, Owen PJ. Prescribing drugs in kidney disease. In: Brenner BM, editor. Brenner & Rector's the kidney. 8th ed. Philadelphia: Saunders Elsevier; 2008. p. 1930–55.

Odlind B, Grefberg N, Hartvig P, Lindström B, Lönnerholm G. Pharmacokinetics of azathioprine and 6-mercaptopurine: methodological aspects and preliminary results in uremic patients. Scand J Urol Nephrol Suppl. 1981;64:213–9.

Olyaei AJ, Bennett WM. Pharmacologic approach to renal insufficiency. In: Dale DC, Federman DD, Antman K, editors. ACP medicine, WebMD June 2007 update. Hamilton: BC Decker; 2007; NEPHROLOGY IX: Appendix A1–25.

Olyaei AJ, Bennett WM. Drug dosing in elderly patients with chronic kidney disease. Clin Geriatr Med. 2009;25:459–527.

Olyaei AJ, DeMattos AM, Bennett WM. Use of drugs in patients with renal failure. In: Schrier RW, editor. Diseases of the kidney and urinary tract. 8th ed. Philadelphia: Lippincott Williams & Wilkins; 2007. p. 2765–807.

Schusziarra V, Ziekursch V, Schlamp R, Siemensen HC. Pharmacokinetics of azathioprine under haemodialysis. Int J Clin Pharmacol Biopharm. 1976;14:298–302.

Yatscoff RW, Aspeslet LJ, Gallant HL. Pharmacodynamic monitoring of immunosuppressive drugs. Clin Chem. 1998;44: 428–32.

Dosage Adjustment of Medications Eliminated by the Kidneys

<u>Azathioprine</u>/Imuran®   {**Immunosuppressive; antirheumatic; T cell effect suppressor**}

Usual initial dose: 3–5 mg/kg orally or IV daily

Usual maintenance dose: 1–3 mg/kg orally or IV once daily

Typical maximum dose: 5 mg/kg/day

Proportion eliminated unchanged: <2 %

Adjustment for Kidney Disease

FDA-approved product labeling: *Relatively oliguric patients, especially those with tubular necrosis in the immediate postcadaveric transplant period, may have delayed clearance of azathioprine or its metabolites, may be particularly sensitive to this drug, and are usually given lower doses.*

Alternative adjustment: | | |
|---|---|
| *GFR >50 mL/min* | *1.5–2.5 mg/kg orally or IV every 24 h* |
| *GFR 10–50 mL/min* | *1.125–1.875 mg/kg orally or IV every 24 h (~25 % decrease)* |
| *GFR <10 mL/min* | *0.75–1.25 mg/kg orally or IV every 24 h (~50 % decrease)* |
| *Hemodialysis* | *0.75–1.25 mg/kg orally or IV every 24 h (~50 % decrease); supplement 0.25 mg/kg after hemodialysis on dialysis days.* |
| *CAPD* | *Data not available* |
| *CRRT* | *1.125–1.875 mg/kg orally or IV every 24 h (~25 % decrease)* |

Dosage Adjustment of Medications Eliminated by the Kidneys

Aztreonam - Selected References

Aronoff GA, Bennett WM, Berns JS, et al. Drug prescribing in renal failure: dosing guidelines for adults and children. 5th ed. Philadelphia: American College of Physicians; 2007.

Azactam® injection [package insert]. South San Francisco: Elan Pharmaceuticals Inc; 2009.

Brown J, Altmann P, Cunningham, Shaw E, Marsh F. Pharmacokinetics of once-daily intra-peritoneal aztreonam and vancomycin in the treatment of CAPD peritonitis. J Antimicrob Chemother. 1990;25:141–7.

Cheng IKP, Chan C-Y, Wong WT. A randomised prospective comparison of oral ofloxacin and intraperitoneal vancomycin plus aztreonam in the treatment of bacterial peritonitis complicating continuous ambulatory peritoneal dialysis (CAPD). Perit Dial Int. 1991;11:27–30.

Creasey WA, Platt TB, Frantz M, Sugerman AA. Pharmacokinetics of aztreonam in elderly male volunteers. Br J Clin Pharmacol. 1985;19:233–7.

Fillastre JP, Leroy A, Baudoin C, et al. Pharmacokinetics of aztreonam in patients with chronic renal failure. Clin Pharmacokinet. 1985;10:91–100.

Friedrich LV, White RL, Kays MB, Brundage DM, Yarbrough D III. Aztreonam pharmacokinetics in burn patients. Antimicrob Agents Chemother. 1991;35:57–61.

Gerig JS, Bolton ND, Swabb EA, Scheld WM, Bolton WK. Effect of hemodialysis and peritoneal dialysis on aztreonam pharmacokinetics. Kidney Int. 1984;26:308–18.

Gilbert B, Robbins P, Livornese LL Jr. Use of antibacterial agents in renal failure. Med Clin North Am. 2011;95:677–702.

Heintz BH, Matzke GR, Dager WE. Antimicrobial dosing concepts and recommendations for critically ill adult patients receiving continuous renal replacement therapy or intermittent hemodialysis. Pharmacotherapy. 2009;29:562–77.

Janicke DM, Cafarell RF, Parker SW, Apicella MA, Jusko WJ. Pharmacokinetics of aztreonam in patients with gram-negative infections. Antimicrob Agents Chemother. 1985;27:16–20.

Kuang D, Verbine A, Ronco C. Pharmacokinetics and antimicrobial dosing adjustment in critically ill patients during continuous renal replacement therapy. Clin Nephrol. 2007;67:267–84.

Mattie H. Clinical pharmacokinetics of aztreonam: an update. Clin Pharmacokinet. 1984;26:99–106.

McIntyre CW, Owen PJ. Prescribing drugs in kidney disease. In: Brenner BM, editor. Brenner & Rector's the kidney. 8th ed. Philadelphia: Saunders Elsevier; 2008. p. 1930–55.

Mihindu JCL, Scheld WM, Bolton ND, Spyker DA, Swabb EA, Bolton WK. Pharmacokinetics of aztreonam in patients with various degrees of renal dysfunction. Antimicrob Agents Chemother. 1983;24:252–61.

Nikolaidis PK, Dombros N, Alexiou P, Balaskas E, Tourkantonis A. Pharmacokinetics of aztreonam administered IP in continuous ambulatory peritoneal dialysis (CAPD) patients. Perit Dial Int. 1989;9:57–9.

Scully BE, Swabb EA, Neu HC. Pharmacology of aztreonam after intravenous infusion. Antimicrob Agents Chemother. 1983;24:18–22.

Sion ML, Pyrpasopoulos M, Nicolaidis P, Papagianni C, Tsurutsoglu G. Efficacy and safety of aztreonam in the treatment of patients with renal failure. Rev Infect Dis. 1991;13(Suppl 7):S652–4.

Swabb EA, Sugerman AA. A review of single- and multiple-dose pharmacokinetics of the monobactam azthreonam (SQ 26,776) in healthy subjects. Antimicrob Agents Chemother. 1983;23:125–132.

Swabb EA, Sugerman AA, McKinstry DN. Multiple-dose pharmacokinetics of the monobactam, aztreonam (SQ 26,776) in healthy subjects. Chemotherapy. 1983;29:313–21.

Trotman RL, Williamson JC, Shoemaker M, Salzer WL. Antibiotic dosing in critically ill adult patients receiving continuous renal replacement therapy. Clin Infect Dis. 2005;41:1159–66.

Watson AJS, Stout RL, Whelton A. The intrarenal distribution of aztreonam in healthy and diseased kidneys: clinical therapeutic implications. J Infect Dis. 1984;150:631–5.

Wiggins KJ, Johnson DW, Craig JC, Strippoli GFM. Treatment of peritoneal dialysis-associated peritonitis: a systematic review of randomized controlled trials. Am J Kidney Dis. 2007;50:967–88.

Wise R, Dyas A, Hegarty A, Andrews JM. Pharmacokinetics and tissue penetration of azthreonam. Antimicrob Agents Chemother. 1982;22:969–71.

Dosage Adjustment of Medications Eliminated by the Kidneys

<u>Aztreonam</u>/Azactam®   {**Antibacterial; monobactam**}

Usual initial dose: 1–2 g IV

Usual maintenance dose: 1–2 g IV every 6–12 h

Typical maximum dose: 8 g/day

Proportion eliminated unchanged: 75 %

Adjustment for Kidney Disease

FDA-approved product labeling:	*CrCL 10–30 mL/min*	*500–1,000 mg IV every 6–12 h*
	CrCL <10 mL/min	*250–500 mg IV every 6–12 h*
	Hemodialysis	*250–500 mg IV every 6–12 h plus 125–250 mg after dialysis*
	CAPD	*250–500 mg IV every 6–12 h*
Alternative adjustment:	*GFR >50 mL/min*	*500–2,000 mg IV every 8–12 h*
	GFR 10–50 mL/min	*500–1,000 mg IV every 8–12 h*
	GFR <10 mL/min	*500 mg IV every 8 h*
	Hemodialysis	*1,000 mg IV every 12 h*
	CAPD	*500 mg IV every 8 h or add to dialysate qs 1,000 mg/L ×1 then 250 mg/L*
	CVVH	*1,000–2,000 mg IV every 12 h*
	CVVHD or CVVHDF	*2,000 mg IV every 12 h*

B

L.K. Golightly et al. (eds.), *Renal Pharmacotherapy*,
DOI 10.1007/978-1-4614-5800-5_2, © Springer Science+Business Media New York 2013

Dosage Adjustment of Medications Eliminated by the Kidneys

Bacitracin - Selected References

BACiiM® injection [package insert]. Northport: X-Gen Pharmaceuticals Inc; 2003.

Battistella M, Bhola C, Lok CE. Long-term follow-up of the Hemodialysis Infection Prevention with Polysporin Ointment (HIPPO) study: a quality improvement report. Am J Kidney Dis. 2011;57:432–41.

Chapnick EK, Gradon JD, Kreiswirth B, et al. Comparative killing kinetics of methicillin-resistant *Staphylococcus aureus* by bacitracin or mupirocin. Infect Control Hosp Epidemiol. 1996;17:178–80.

Davis JE, Siemsen AW, Anderson RW. Uremia, deafness, and paralysis due to irrigating antibiotic solutions. Arch Intern Med. 1970;125:135–9.

Eagle H, Newman EV, Greif R, Burkholder TM, Goodman SC. The blood levels and renal clearance in rabbits and man of an antibiotic derived from *B subtilis* (bacitracin). J Clin Invest. 1947;26:919–28.

Ericsson CD, Duke JH Jr, Pickering LK, Hussain Qadri AM. Systemic absorption of bacitracin after peritoneal lavage. Am J Surg. 1979;137:65–7.

Genkins G, Uhr JW, Bryer MS. Bacitracin nephropathy: report of a case of acute renal failure and death. J Am Med Assoc. 1954;155:894–7.

Jackson EA, McLeod DC. Pharmacokinetics and dosing of antimicrobial agents in renal impairment, part II. Am J Hosp Pharm. 1974;31:137–48.

Kunin CM. Nephrotoxicity of antibiotics. JAMA. 1967;202:204–8.

Lok CE, Stanley KE, Hux JE, Richardson R, Tobe SW, Conly J. Hemodialysis infection prevention with Polysporin ointment. J Am Soc Nephrol. 2003;14:169–79.

McCann M, Moore ZEH. Interventions for preventing infectious complications in haemodialysis patients with central venous catheters (review). Cochrane Database Syst Rev. 2010;(1):CD006894. doi:10.1002/14651858.CD006894.pub

Prince MEP, Lemkert RJ. Analysis of intranasal distribution of ointment. J Otolaryngol. 1997;26:657–60.

Smith LW, Schultz FH Jr, Ott WL, Payne HG. A comparative study of the renal damage produced in mice by various lots of bacitracin. J Clin Invest. 1949;28:1018–21.

Weinstein MR, Dedier H, Brunton J, Campbell I, Conly JM. Lack of efficacy of oral bacitracin plus doxycycline for the eradication of stool colonization with vancomycin-resistant *Enterococcus faecium*. Clin Infect Dis. 1999;29:361–6.

Zintel HA, Ma RA, Ellis H. The absorption, distribution, excretion and toxicity of bacitracin in man. Am J Med Sci. 1949;218:439–45.

Dosage Adjustment of Medications Eliminated by the Kidneys

<u>**Bacitracin**</u>/BACiiM™	{**Antibacterial; polypeptide complex derived from *Bacillus subtilis*}**

Usual initial dose	50,000 units IM
Usual maintenance dose	50,000 units IM every 6 h
Typical maximum dose	200,000 units/day
Proportion eliminated unchanged	87 %

Adjustment for Kidney Disease

FDA-approved product labeling: *To reduce the development of drug-resistant bacteria and maintain the effectiveness of bacitracin and other antibacterial drugs, bacitracin should be used only to treat or prevent infections that are proven or strongly suspected to be caused by bacteria.*

Warning—nephrotoxicity: Bacitracin in parenteral (intramuscular) therapy may cause renal failure due to tubular and glomerular necrosis. Its use should be restricted to infants with staphylococcal pneumonia and empyema when due to organisms shown to be susceptible to bacitracin. It should be used only where adequate laboratory facilities are available and when constant supervision of the patient is possible.

Renal function should be carefully determined prior to and daily during therapy. The recommended daily dose should not be exceeded and fluid intake and urinary output maintained at proper levels to avoid kidney toxicity. If renal toxicity occurs, the drug should be discontinued. The concurrent use of other nephrotoxic drugs, particularly streptomycin, kanamycin, polymyxin B, polymyxin E (colistin), neomycin, and viomycin, should be avoided.

Alternative adjustment: *eGFR < 60 mL/min*   *Avoid peritoneal lavage and IM/IV administration due to risk of drug accumulation and nephrotoxicity.*

Dosage Adjustment of Medications Eliminated by the Kidneys

Benazepril - Selected References

Aronoff GA, Bennett WM, Berns JS, et al. Drug prescribing in renal failure: dosing guidelines for adults and children. 5th ed. Philadelphia: American College of Physicians; 2007.

Balfour JA, Goa K. Benazepril: a review of its pharmacodynamic and pharmacokinetic properties, and therapeutic efficacy in hypertension and congestive heart failure. Drugs. 1991;42:511–39.

De Cesaris R, Ranieri G, Andriani A, et al. Effects of benazepril and nicardipine on microalbuminuria in normotensive and hypertensive patients with diabetes. Clin Pharmacol Ther. 1996;60:472–8.

Dessi-Fulgheri P, Motolese M, Di Noto G, et al. Blunting of atrial natriuretic factor response to volume expansion by benazepril in hypertensive patients. J Hypertens. 1989;7(Suppl 6):S300–1.

Fujita N, Hartiala J, O'Sullivan M, et al. Assessment of left ventricular diastolic function in dilated cardiomyopathy with cine magnetic resonance imaging: effect of an angiotensin converting enzyme inhibitor, benazepril. Am Heart J. 1993;125:171–8.

Gengo FM, Brady E. The pharmacokinetics of benazepril relative to other ACE inhibitors. Clin Cardiol. 1991;14 (Suppl 4):44–50.

Harrigan JR, Lees KR, Meredith PA. Age and the physiologically realistic characterization of benazepril pharmacokinetics [abstract]. Br J Clin Pharmacol. 1990;29:589P.

Kaiser G, Ackerman R, Sioufi A. Pharmacokinetics of a new angiotensin-converting enzyme inhibitor, benazepril hydrochloride, in special populations. Clin Pharmacol Ther. 1989;117:746–50.

Kaiser G, Ackerman R, Dieterle W, et al. Pharmacokinetics and pharmacodynamics of the ace inhibitor benazepril hydrochloride in the elderly. Eur J Clin Pharmacol. 1990;38:379–85.

Kuroda K, Fukuda Y, Nadao K, Inukai T. Antihypertensive mechanism of action of the novel angiotensin converting enzyme inhibitor benazepril. Arzneimittelforschung. 1990;40:968–73.

Lotensin® tablet [package insert]. East Hanover: Novartis Pharmaceuticals Corp; 2009.

Macdonald N-J, Sioufi A, Howie CA, Wade JR, Elliott HL. The effects of age on the pharmacokinetics of single oral doses of benazepril and enalapril. Br J Clin Pharmacol. 1993;36:205–9.

Maschio G, Alberti D, Janin G, et al. Effect of the angiotensin-converting-enzyme inhibitor benazepril on the progression of chronic renal insufficiency. N Engl J Med. 1996;334:939–45.

McIntyre CW, Owen PJ. Prescribing drugs in kidney disease. In: Brenner BM, editor. Brenner & Rector's the kidney. 8th ed. Philadelphia: Saunders/Elsevier; 2008. p. 1930–55.

Noormohamed FH, Fuller GN, Lant AF. Effect of salt balance on the renal and hemodynamic actions of benazepril in normal men. J Clin Pharmacol. 1989;29:928–37.

Olyaei AJ, Bennett WM. Pharmacologic approach to renal insufficiency. In: Dale DC, Federman DD, Antman K, editors. ACP medicine, WebMD June 2007 update. Hamilton: BC Decker; 2007. NEPHROLOGY IX: Appendix A1–25.

Olyaei AJ, Bennett WM. Drug dosing in elderly patients with chronic kidney disease. Clin Geriatr Med. 2009;25:459–527.

Olyaei AJ, DeMattos AM, Bennett WM. Use of drugs in patients with renal failure. In: Schrier RW, editor. Diseases of the kidney and urinary tract. 8th ed. Philadelphia: Lippincott Williams & Wilkins; 2007. p. 2765–807.

Reams GP, Lau A, Bauer JH. Effect of benazepril monotherapy in subjects with hypertension associated with renal dysfunction. J Clin Pharmacol. 1989;29:609–14.

Shionoiri H, Ueda S, Minamisawa K, et al. Pharmacokinetics and pharmacodynamics of benazepril in hypertensive patients with normal and impaired renal function. J Cardiovasc Pharmacol. 1992;20:348–56.

Waldmeier F, Kaiser G, Ackermann R, et al. The disposition of [¹⁴C]-labelled benazepril HCl in normal adult volunteers after single and repeated oral doses. Xenobiotica. 1991;21:251–61.

Yamamoto S, Takemori E, Hasegawa Y, et al. General pharmacology of the novel angiotensin converting enzyme inhibitor benazepril hydrochloride. Arzneimittelforschung. 1991;41:913–23.

Dosage Adjustment of Medications Eliminated by the Kidneys

<u>Benazepril</u>/Lotensin®   {Antihypertensive; vasodilator; angiotensin-converting enzyme (ACE)/ renin inhibitor}

Usual initial dose	10 mg orally daily
Usual maintenance dose	20–40 mg/day orally as either a single dose or two equally divided doses
Typical maximum dose	40 mg/day
Proportion eliminated unchanged	18 % (as active benazeprilat)

Adjustment for Kidney Disease

FDA-approved product labeling:	*CrCL < 30 mL/min*	*Initial dose is 5 mg once daily, increasing as necessary to maximum 40 mg/day*
Alternative adjustment:	*GFR > 50 mL/min*	*20–40 mg orally daily (100 % of usual dose)*
	GFR 10–50 mL/min	*15–30 mg orally daily (75 % of usual dose)*
	GFR < 10 mL/min	*5–20 mg orally daily (25–50 % of usual dose)*
	Hemodialysis	*5–20 mg orally daily (25–50 % of usual dose)*
	CAPD	*5–20 mg orally daily (25–50 % of usual dose)*
	CRRT	*15–30 mg orally daily (75 % of usual dose)*

Dosage Adjustment of Medications Eliminated by the Kidneys

Bendamustine - Selected References

Chovan JP, Li F, Yu E, Ring SC. Metabolic profile of [^{14}C]bendamustine in rat urine and bile: preliminary structural identification of metabolites. Drug Metab Dispos. 2007;35:1744–53.

Garnock-Jones KP. Bendamustine: a review of its use in the management of indolent non-Hodgkin's lymphoma and mantle cell lymphoma. Drugs. 2010;70:1703–18.

Knauf WU, Lissichkov T, Aldaoud A, et al. Phase III randomized study of bendamustine compared with chlorambucil in previously untreated patients with chronic lymphocytic leukemia. J Clin Oncol. 2009;27:4378–84.

Ogura M, Uchida T, Taniwaki M, et al. Phase I and pharmacokinetic study of bendamustine hydrochloride in relapsed or refractory indolent B-cell non-Hodgkin lymphoma and mantle cell lymphoma. Cancer Sci. 2010;101:2054–8.

Treanda® injection [package insert]. Frazer: Cephalon Inc; 2010.

von Minckwitz G, Chernozemsky I, Sirakova L, et al. Bendamustine prolongs progression-free survival in metastatic breast cancer (MBC): a phase III prospective, randomized, multicenter trial of bendamustine hydrochloride, methotrexate and 5-fluorouracil (BMF) versus cyclophosphamide, methotrexate and 5-fluorouracil (CMF) as first-line treatment of MBC. Anticancer Drugs. 2005;16:871–7.

Dosage Adjustment of Medications Eliminated by the Kidneys

<u>Bendamustine</u>/Treanda®   {Antineoplastic; alkylating agent, mechlorethamine derivative}

Usual initial dose   100 mg/m² IV

Usual maintenance dose   100 mg/m² administered IV over 30 min on days 1 and 2 of a 28-day cycle, up to 6 cycles

Typical maximum dose   100 mg/m²

Proportion eliminated unchanged   ~10 %

Adjustment for Kidney Disease

FDA-approved product labeling:	*CrCL > 40 mL/min*	*100 mg/m² administered IV over 30 min on days 1 and 2 of a 28-day cycle, up to 6 cycles*
	CrCL ≤ 40 mL/min	*Avoid; safety not established*
Alternative adjustment:	*Data not available*	

Bismuth Subsalicylate - Selected References

Akpolat I, Kahrman H, Arik N, Akpolat T, Kandemir B, Cengiz K. Acute renal failure due to overdose of colloidal bismuth [letter]. Nephrol Dial Transplant. 1996;11:1890–1.

Burr RE, Gotto AMK, Beaver DL. Isolation and analysis of renal bismuth inclusions. Toxicol Appl Pharmacol. 1965;7:588–91.

Cengiz N, Uslu Y, Gök F, Anarat A. Acute renal failure after overdose of colloidal bismuth subcitrate. Pediatr Nephrol. 2005;20:1355–8.

Czerwinski AW, Ginn HE. Bismuth nephrotoxicity. Am J Med. 1964;37:969–75.

Gryboski JD, Gotoff SP. Bismuth nephrotoxicity: report of a case. N Engl J Med. 1961;265:1289–91.

Hespe W, Staal HJM, Hall DWR. Bismuth absorption from the colloidal subcitrate [letter]. Lancet. 1988;2:1258.

Hruz P, Mayr M, Löw R, Drewe J, Huber G. Fanconi's syndrome, acute renal failure, and tonsil ulcerations after colloidal bismuth subcitrate intoxication. Am J Kidney Dis. 2002;39:e18. doi:10.1053/ajkd.2002.31429.

Hudson M, Mowat NAG. Reversible toxicity in poisoning with colloidal bismuth subcitrate. Br Med J. 1989;299:159.

James JA. Acute renal failure due to a bismuth preparation. Calif Med. 1968;109:317–9.

Jungreis AC, Schaumburg HH. Encephalopathy from abuse of bismuth subsalicylate (Pepto-Bismol). Neurology. 1993;43:1265.

Leussink BT, Slikkerveer A, Krauwinkel WJJ, et al. Bismuth biokinetics and kidney histopathology after bismuth overdose in rats. Arch Toxicol. 2000;74:349–55.

Mayer L, Baehr G. Bismuth poisoning: a clinical and pathological report. Surg Gynecol Obstet. 1912;15:309–22.

Mendelowitz PC, Hoffman RS, Weber S. Bismuth absorption and myoclonic encephalopathy during bismuth subsalicylate therapy. Ann Intern Med. 1990;112:140–1.

Peptic Relief Liquid [package insert]. Duluth: Rugby Laboratories Inc; 2007.

Playford RJ, Matthews CH, Campbell MJ, et al. Bismuth induced encephalopathy caused by tri potassium dicitrato bismuthate in a patient with chronic renal failure. Gut. 1990;31:359–60.

Slikkerveer A, de Wolff FA. Pharmacokinetics and toxicity of bismuth compounds. Med Toxicol Adverse Drug Exp. 1989;4:303–23.

Taylor EG, Klenerman P. Acute renal failure after colloidal bismuth subcitrate overdose [letter]. Lancet. 1990;335:670–1.

Urizar R, Vernier RI. Bismuth nephropathy. JAMA. 1966;198:187–9.

Weil J, Bell GD, Powell K. Disposition of bismuth and renal function [letter]. Aliment Pharmacol Ther. 1992;6:395–7.

Bismuth Subsalicylate/Pepto-Bismol®   {Antidiarrheal; antiflatulent}

Usual initial dose	30 mL (524 mg) orally every 30–60 min PRN upset stomach, indigestion, simple diarrhea, and nausea
Usual maintenance dose	N/A
Typical maximum dose	240 mL/day
Proportion eliminated unchanged	Unknown

Adjustment for Kidney Disease

FDA-approved product labeling:	*Data not available*	
Alternative adjustment:	*GFR < 50 mL/min*	*Preferably avoid due to risk for bismuth and/or salicylic acid accumulation and heavy metal or salicylate toxicity.*
	Hemodialysis	*Preferably avoid due to risk for bismuth and/or salicylic acid accumulation and heavy metal or salicylate toxicity.*
	CAPD	*Preferably avoid due to risk for bismuth and/or salicylic acid accumulation and heavy metal or salicylate toxicity.*
	CRRT	*Preferably avoid due to risk for bismuth and/or salicylic acid accumulation and heavy metal or salicylate toxicity.*

Dosage Adjustment of Medications Eliminated by the Kidneys

Bisoprolol - Selected References

Aronoff GA, Bennett WM, Berns JS, et al. Drug prescribing in renal failure: dosing guidelines for adults and children. 5th ed. Philadelphia: American College of Physicians; 2007.

Benetos A, Adamopoulos C, Argyriadis P, Bean K, Consoli S, Safar M. Clinical results with bisoprolol 2.5 mg/hydrochlorothiazide 6.25 mg combination in systolic hypertension in the elderly. J Hypertens. 2002;20(Suppl 1):S21–5.

Castagno D, Jhund PS, McMurray JJV, et al. Improved survival with bisoprolol in patients with heart failure and renal impairment: an analysis of the cardiac insufficiency bisoprolol study II (CIBIS-II) trial. Eur J Heart Fail. 2010;12:607–16.

Damman K, Voors AA, Hillege HL, et al. Congestion in chronic systolic heart failure is related to renal dysfunction and increased mortality. Eur J Heart Fail. 2010;12:974–82.

Dobre D, van Veldhuisen DJ, Goulder MA, Krum H, Willenheimer R. Clinical effects of initial 6 months of monotherapy with bisoprolol versus enalapril in the treatment of patients with mild to moderate chronic heart failure: data from the CIBIS II Trial. Cardiovasc Drugs Ther. 2008;22:399–405.

Dunkelgrun M, Boersma E, Schouten O, et al. Bisoprolol and fluvastatin for the reduction of perioperative cardiac mortality and myocardial infarction in intermediate-risk patients undergoing noncardiovascular surgery: a randomized controlled trial (DECREASE-IV). Ann Surg. 2009;249:921–6.

Dutta A, Lanc R, Begg E, et al. Dose proportionality of bisoprolol enantiomers in humans after oral administration of the racemate. J Clin Pharmacol. 1994;34:829–36.

Haeusler G, Schliep H-J, Schelling P, et al. High β_1 selectivity and favourable pharmacokinetics as the outstanding properties of bisoprolol. J Cardiovasc Pharmacol. 1986;8(Suppl 11):S2–15.

Jovanović, Ćušić S, Rančić D, Srnić D, Perković-Vukčević N. A pharmacokinetic comparison of tablets containing bisoprolol with the innovator formulation in healthy volunteers. J Clin Pharmacol. 2006;46:1217–22.

Le Coz F, Sauleman P, Poirier JM, et al. Oral pharmacokinetics of bisoprolol in resting and exercising healthy volunteers. J Cardiovasc Pharmacol. 1991;18:28–34.

Leeman M, van de Borne P, Collart F, et al. bisoprolol and atenolol in essential hypertension: effects on systemic and renal hemodynamics and on ambulatory blood pressure. J Cardiovasc Pharmacol. 1993;22:785–91.

Leopold G. Balanced pharmacokinetics and metabolism of bisoprolol. J Cardiovasc Pharmacol. 1986;8(Suppl 11):S16–20.

Lewis R, Maclean D, Ioannides C, Johnston A, McDevitt DG. A comparison of bisoprolol and atenolol in the treatment of mild to moderate hypertension. Br J Clin Pharmacol. 1988;26:53–9.

McIntyre CW, Owen PJ. Prescribing drugs in kidney disease. In: Brenner BM, editor. Brenner & Rector's the kidney. 8th ed. Philadelphia: Saunders/Elsevier; 2008. p. 1930–55.

Zebeta® tablet [package insert]. Pomona: Duramed Pharmaceuticals Division of Barr Pharmaceuticals Inc; 2010.

Dosage Adjustment of Medications Eliminated by the Kidneys

<u>Bisoprolol</u>/Zebeta®   {**Antihypertensive; antianginal; β-adrenergic receptor blocker**}

Usual initial dose	5 mg orally once daily
Usual maintenance dose	10–20 mg orally once daily
Typical maximum dose	20 mg/day
Proportion eliminated unchanged	50 %

Adjustment for Kidney Disease

FDA-approved product labeling:	*CrCL < 40 mL/min*	*The initial daily dose should be 2.5 mg orally and caution should be used in dose titration*
Alternative adjustment:	*GFR > 50 mL/min*	*5 mg orally every 24 h*
	GFR 10–50 mL/min	*2.5–5 mg orally every 24 h (~25 % decrease)*
	GFR < 10 mL/min	*2.5 mg orally every 24 h (50 % decrease)*
	Hemodialysis	*2.5 mg orally every 24 h (50 % decrease), dose after hemodialysis on dialysis days*
	CAPD	*2.5 mg orally every 24 h (50 % decrease)*
	CRRT	*2.5 mg orally every 24 h (50 % decrease)*

Dosage Adjustment of Medications Eliminated by the Kidneys

Bivalirudin - Selected References

Angiomax® injection [package insert]. Parsippany: The Medicines Co; 2010.

Curran MP. Bivalirudin in patients with ST-segment elevation myocardial infarction. Drugs. 2010;70:909–18.

Dangas GC, Mehran R, Nikolsky E, et al. Effect of switching antithrombin agent for primary angioplasty in acute myocardial infarction: The HORIZONS-SWITCH analysis. J Am Coll Cardiol. 2011;57:2309–16.

Garcia DA, Baglin TP, Weitz JI, Samama MM. Parenteral anticoagulants: antithrombotic therapy and prevention of thrombosis, 9th ed: American College of Chest Physicians Evidence-Based Clinical Practice Guidelines. Chest. 2012;141(2 Suppl):e24–43S. doi:10.1378/chest.11-2291.

Kiser TH, Fish DN. Evaluation of bivalirudin treatment for heparin-induced thrombocytopenia in critically ill patients with hepatic and/or renal dysfunction. Pharmacotherapy. 2006;26:452–60.

Kiser TH, Burch JC, Klem PD, Hassell KL. Safety, efficacy, and dosing requirements of bivalirudin in patients with heparin-induced thrombocytopenia. Pharmacotherapy. 2008;28:1115–24.

Kiser TH, MacLaren R, Fish DN, Hassell KL, Teitelbaum I. Bivalirudin versus unfractionated heparin for prevention of hemofilter occlusion during continuous renal replacement therapy. Pharmacotherapy. 2010;30:1117–26.

Kiser TH, Mann AM, Trujillo TC, Hassell KL. Evaluation of empiric versus nomogram-based thrombin inhibitor management in patients with suspected heparin-induced thrombocytopenia. Am J Hematol. 2011;86:267–72.

Kumar D, Dangas G, Mehran R, et al. Comparison of bivalirudin versus bivalirudin plus glycoprotein IIb/IIIa inhibitor in patients with acute coronary syndromes having percutaneous intervention for narrowed saphenous vein aorto-coronary grafts (the ACUITY Trial Investigators). Am J Cardiol. 2010;106:941–5.

Mueller SW, MacLaren R, Fish DN, Kiser TH. Prefilter bivalirudin for preventing hemofilter occlusion in continuous renal replacement therapy. Ann Pharmacother. 2009;43:1360–5.

Robson R, White H, Aylward P, Frampton C. Bivalirudin pharmacokinetics and pharmacodynamics: effect of renal function, dose, and gender. Clin Pharmacol Ther. 2002;71:433–9.

Runyan CL, Cabral KP, Riker RR, et al. Correlation of bivalirudin dose with creatinine clearance during treatment of heparin-induced thrombocytopenia. Pharmacotherapy. 2011;31:850–6.

Skrupky LP, Smith JR, Deal EN, et al. Comparison of bivalirudin and argatroban for the management of heparin-induced thrombocytopenia. Pharmacotherapy. 2010;30:1229–38.

Stone GW, McLaurin BT, Cox DA, et al. Bivalirudin for patients with acute coronary syndromes. N Engl J Med. 2006;355:2203–16.

Stone GW, Witzenbichler B, Guagliumi G, et al. Bivalirudin during primary PCI in acute myocardial infarction. N Engl J Med. 2008;358:2218–30.

Stone GW, Witzenbichler B, Guagliumi G, et al. Heparin plus a glycoprotein IIb/IIIa inhibitor versus bivalirudin monotherapy and paclitaxel-eluting stents versus bare-metal stents in acute myocardial infarctions (HORIZONS-AMI): final 3-year results from a multicentre, randomised controlled trial. Lancet. 2011;377:2193–204.

Tsu LV, Dager WE. Comparison of bivalirudin dosing strategies using total, adjusted, and ideal body weights in obese patients with heparin-induced thrombocytopenia. Pharmacotherapy. 2012;32:20–6.

Weitz JI, Crowther M. Direct thrombin inhibitors. Thromb Res. 2002;106:V275–83.

Weitz JI, Hudoba M, Massel D, Maraganore J, Hirsch J. Clot-bound thrombin is protected from inhibition by heparin-antithrombin III but is susceptible to inactivation by antithrombin III-independent inhibitors. J Clin Invest. 1990;86:385–91.

White HD, Ohman EM, Lincoff AM, et al. Safety and efficacy of bivalirudin with and without glycoprotein IIb/IIIa inhibitors in patients with acute coronary syndromes undergoing percutaneous coronary intervention: 1-year results from the ACUITY (Acute Catheterization and Urgent Intervention Triage strategy) Trial. J Am Coll Cardiol. 2008;52:807–14.

Witzenbichler B, Mehran R, Guagliumi G, et al. Impact of diabetes mellitus on the safety and effectiveness of bivalirudin in patients with acute myocardial infarction undergoing primary angioplasty: analysis from the HORIZONS-AMI (Harmonizing Outcomes with RevasculariZatiON and Stents in Acute Myocardial Infarction) trial. JACC Cardiovasc Interv. 2011;4:760–8.

Dosage Adjustment of Medications Eliminated by the Kidneys

<u>Bivalirudin</u>/Angiomax®   {Antithrombotic; direct thrombin inhibitor}

Usual initial dose   0.75 mg/kg IV

Usual maintenance dose   Continuous IV infusion of 1.75 mg/kg/h for the duration of the percutaneous coronary intervention procedure

Typical maximum dose   As required to attain aPTT 1.5–2.5 times baseline or control value

Proportion eliminated unchanged 20 %

Adjustment for Kidney Disease

    FDA-approved product labeling: *For anticoagulation in patients undergoing percutaneous coronary intervention*

CrCL ≥ 60 mL/min	*0.75 mg/kg* *IV followed by infusion of 1.75 mg/kg/h*
CrCL 30–59 mL/min	*0.75 mg/kg* *IV followed by infusion of 1.75 mg/kg/h*
CrCL < 30 mL/min	*0.75 mg/kg* *IV followed by infusion of 1.00 mg/kg/h*
Hemodialysis	*0.75 mg/kg* *IV followed by infusion of 0.25 mg/kg/h*

    Alternative adjustment: *For anticoagulation in patients with venous thromboembolism*

eCrCL ≥ 60 mL/min	*Continuous IV infusion of 0.15 mg/kg/h* *(no initial bolus)*
eCrCL 44–60 mL/min	*Continuous IV infusion of 0.075 mg/kg/h* *(no initial bolus)*
eCrCL 30–43 mL/min	*Continuous IV infusion of 0.05 mg/kg/h* *(no initial bolus)*
eCrCL < 30 mL/min	*Continuous IV infusion of 0.025 mg/kg/h* *(no initial bolus)*
CRRT	*Continuous IV (prefilter) infusion of 0.02 mg/kg/h* *(no initial bolus)*

Note: dosage usually should be based on total body weight in normal body weight and obese patients

Dosage Adjustment of Medications Eliminated by the Kidneys

<u>Bleomycin</u> - Selected References

Aronoff GA, Bennett WM, Berns JS, et al. Drug prescribing in renal failure: dosing guidelines for adults and children. 5th ed. Philadelphia: American College of Physicians; 2007.

Bleomycin injection USP [package insert]. Bedford: Bedford Laboratories; 2006

Crooke ST, Luft F, Broughton A, Strong J, Casson K, Einhorn L. Bleomycin serum pharmacokinetics as determined by a radioimmunoassay and a microbiologic assay in a patient with compromised renal function. Cancer. 1977;39:1430–4.

Krakoff IH, Cvitkovic E, Currie V, Yeh S, LaMonte C. Clinical pharmacologic and therapeutic studies of bleomycin given by continuous infusion. Cancer. 1977;40:2027–37.

Kramer WG, Feldman S, Broughton A, Strong JE, Hall SW, Holoye PY. The pharmacokinetics of bleomycin in man. J Clin Pharmacol. 1978;18:346–52.

Lewis BM, Izbicki R. Routine pulmonary tests during bleomycin therapy: tests may be ineffective and potentially misleading. JAMA. 1980;243:347–51.

McIntyre CW, Owen PJ. Prescribing drugs in kidney disease. In: Brenner BM, editor. Brenner & Rector's the kidney. 8th ed. Philadelphia: Saunders/Elsevier; 2008. p. 1930–55.

Oken MM, Crooke ST, Elson MK, Strong JE, Shafer RB. Pharmacokinetics of bleomycin after im administration in man. Cancer Treat Rep. 1981;68:485–9.

Umezawa H. Chemistry and mechanism of action of bleomycin. Fed Proc. 1974;33:2296–302.

Yagoda A, Mukherji B, Young C, et al. Bleomycin, an antitumor antibiotic: clinical experience in 274 patients. Ann Intern Med. 1972;77:861–70.

Yee GC, Crom WR, Champion JE, Brodeur GM, Evans WE. Cisplatin-induced changes in bleomycin elimination. Cancer Treat Rep. 1983;67:587–9.

Dosage Adjustment of Medications Eliminated by the Kidneys

<u>Bleomycin</u>/Blenoxane®	**{Antineoplastic; DNA, RNA, and protein synthesis inhibitor}**

Usual initial dose
0.25–0.50 units/kg (10–20 units/m^2) given IV, IM, or subcutaneously weekly or twice weekly; because of the possibility of an anaphylactoid reaction, lymphoma patients should be given 2 units or less for the first two doses.

Usual maintenance dose
0.25–0.50 units/kg (10–20 units/m^2) given IV, IM, or subcutaneously weekly or twice weekly. After a 50 % response, a maintenance dose of 1 unit daily or 5 units weekly intravenously or intramuscularly should be given.

Typical maximum dose
400 units (total dose)

Proportion eliminated unchanged
65 %

Adjustment for Kidney Disease

FDA-approved product labeling:
Bleomycin clearance may be reduced in patients with impaired renal function. Bleomycin should be used with extreme caution in patients with significant renal impairment.

Alternative adjustment:

GFR > 50 mL/min	*10–20 units/m^2 IV, IM, or subcutaneously weekly or twice weekly*
GFR 10–50 mL/min	*7.5–15 units/m^2 IV, IM, or subcutaneously weekly or twice weekly (25 % decrease)*
GFR < 10 mL/min	*5–10 units/m^2 IV, IM, or subcutaneously weekly or twice weekly (50 % decrease)*
Hemodialysis	*Minimal data available, effective dose unclear*
CAPD	*Data not available*
CRRT	*7.5–15 units/m^2 IV, IM, or subcutaneously weekly or twice weekly (25 % decrease)*

Buspirone - Selected References

Aronoff GA, Bennett WM, Berns JS, et al. Drug prescribing in renal failure: dosing guidelines for adults and children. 5th ed. Philadelphia: American College of Physicians; 2007.

BuSpar® tablet [package insert]. Princeton: Bristol-Myers Squibb Co; 2010.

Gammans RE, Mayol FR, Labudde JA. Metabolism and disposition of buspirone. Am J Med. 1986;80(Suppl 3B):41–51.

Gammans RE, Westrick ML, Shea JP, Mayol RF, LaBudde JA. Pharmacokinetics of buspirone in elderly subjects. J Clin Pharmacol. 1989;29:72–8.

Jann MW. Buspirone: an update on a unique anxiolytic agent. Pharmacotherapy. 1988;8:100–16.

McIntyre CW, Owen PJ. Prescribing drugs in kidney disease. In: Brenner BM, editor. Brenner & Rector's the kidney. 8th ed. Philadelphia: Saunders/Elsevier; 2008. p. 1930–55.

Olyaei AJ, Bennett WM. Pharmacologic approach to renal insufficiency. In: Dale DC, Federman DD, Antman K, editors. ACP medicine, WebMD June 2007 update. Hamilton: BC Decker; 2007. NEPHROLOGY IX: Appendix A1–25.

Olyaei AJ, Bennett WM. Drug dosing in elderly patients with chronic kidney disease. Clin Geriatr Med. 2009;25:459–527.

Olyaei AJ, DeMattos AM, Bennett WM. Use of drugs in patients with renal failure. In: Schrier RW, editor. Diseases of the kidney and urinary tract. 8th ed. Philadelphia: Lippincott Williams & Wilkins; 2007. p. 2765–807.

Sethy VH, Francis JW. Pharmacokinetics of buspirone as determined by ex vivo (3H)-DPAT binding. Life Sci. 1988;42:1045–8.

Dosage Adjustment of Medications Eliminated by the Kidneys

Buspirone/BuSpar® {Anxiolytic; serotonin 5-HT$_{1A}$ and D$_2$ dopamine receptor modifier}

Usual initial dose	7.5 mg orally twice daily
Usual maintenance dose	10–15 mg orally twice daily
Typical maximum dose	60 mg/day
Proportion eliminated unchanged	Minimal

Adjustment for Kidney Disease

FDA-approved product labeling:	*Severe renal impairment*	*Not recommended; after multiple-dose administration of buspirone to renally impaired (CrCL = 10–70 mL/min/1.73 m²) patients, steady state AUC of buspirone increased 4-fold compared with healthy (CrCL ≥ 80 mL/min/1.73 m²) subjects.*
Alternative adjustment:	*GFR > 50 mL/min*	*10–15 mg orally twice daily*
	GFR 10–50 mL/min	*5–10 mg orally twice daily (~25 % decrease)*
	GFR < 10 mL/min	*2.5–7.5 mg orally twice daily (~50 % decrease)*
	Hemodialysis	*2.5–7.5 mg orally twice daily*
	CAPD	*2.5–7.5 mg orally twice daily*
	CRRT	*5–10 mg enterally twice daily*

Butorphanol - Selected References

Aronoff GA, Bennett WM, Berns JS, et al. Drug prescribing in renal failure: dosing guidelines for adults and children. 5th ed. Philadelphia: American College of Physicians; 2007.

Bullingham RES, McQuay HJ, Moore RA. Clinical pharmacokinetics of narcotic agonist–antagonist drugs. Clin Pharmacokinet. 1983;8:332–43.

Davis GA, Rudy AC, Archer SM, Wermeling DP. Bioavailability of intranasal butorphanol administered from a single-dose sprayer. Am J Health Syst Pharm. 2005;62:48–53.

Gaver RC, Vasilev M, Wong H, Monkovic I, Swigor JE, van Harken DR, Smyth RD. Disposition of parenteral butorphanol in man. Drug Metab Dispos. 1980;8:230–5.

Gillis JC, Benfield P, Goa K. Transnasal butorphanol: a review of its pharmacodynamic and pharmacokinetic properties, and therapeutic potential in acute pain management. Drugs. 1995:50:157–75.

Groenendaal D, Freijer J, Rosier A, et al. Pharmacokinetic/pharmacodynamic modeling of the EEG effects of opioids: the role of complex biophase distribution kinetics. Eur J Pharm Sci. 2008;34:149–63.

Henry H II, Nordan J, Tomlin EM. Comparison of butorphanol tartrate and meperidine in moderate to severe renal colic. Urology. 1987;29:339–45.

Shyu WC, Pittman KA, Robinson DA, Barbhaiya RH. Multiple-dose phase I study of transnasal butorphanol. Clin Pharmacol Ther. 1993a;54:34–41.

Shyu WC, Pittman KA, Robinson DA, Barbhaiya RH. The absolute bioavailability of transnasal butorphanol in patients experiencing rhinitis. Eur J Clin Pharmacol. 1993a;45:559–62.

Shyu WC, Morgenthien EA, Barbhaiya RH. Pharmacokinetics of butorphanol nasal spray in patients with renal impairment. Br J Clin Pharmacol. 1996;41:397–402.

Stadol® injection and spray [package insert]. Dayton: Apothecon/Geneva Pharmaceuticals Inc; 2002.

Vachharajani NN, Shyu WC, Greene DS, Barbhaiya BH. The pharmacokinetics of butorphanol and its metabolites at steady state following nasal administration in humans. Biopharm Drug Dispos. 1997;18:191–202.

Wu-Pong S, Schnoll S, Weaver M. Butorphanol pharmacokinetics in a CRPS patient. J Pain Symptom Manage. 1999;17:1–2.

Dosage Adjustment of Medications Eliminated by the Kidneys

Butorphanol/Stadol®	{Analgesic; opioid μ-receptor partial agonist}	
Usual initial dose	1 mg IV or IM or 1 mg (1 spray in 1 nostril) intranasally	
Usual maintenance dose	1–2 mg IV or IM every 4 h as necessary or 1–2 mg (1 spray in 1 or 2 nostrils) intranasally every 4 h PRN	
Typical maximum dose	4 mg/dose	
Proportion eliminated unchanged	4 %	

Adjustment for Kidney Disease

FDA-approved product labeling:	*CrCL < 30 mL/min*	*0.5–1 mg IV or IM every 6 h as necessary (50 % decrease) or 1 mg (1 spray in 1 nostril) followed, if needed, by 1 mg (1 spray in 1 nostril) in 90–120 min; repeat doses should be determined by response but given at intervals of no less than 6 h*
Alternative adjustment:	*GFR > 50 mL/min*	*0.5–1 mg IV or IM every 6 h PRN*
	GFR 10–50 mL/min	*0.375–0.75 mg IV or IM every 6 h PRN (25 % decrease)*
	GFR < 10 mL/min	*0.25–0.5 mg IV or IM every 6 h PRN (50 % decrease)*
	Hemodialysis	*Data not available*
	CAPD	*Data not available*
	CRRT	*0.375–0.75 mg IV or IM every 6 h PRN (25 % decrease)*

C

L.K. Golightly et al. (eds.), *Renal Pharmacotherapy*,
DOI 10.1007/978-1-4614-5800-5_3, © Springer Science+Business Media New York 2013

Dosage Adjustment of Medications Eliminated by the Kidneys

Capecitabine - Selected References

Beigner B, Verweij J, Dirix L, et al. Effect of food on the pharmacokinetics of capecitabine and its metabolites following oral administration in cancer patients. Clin Cancer Res. 1998;4:941–8.

Cassidy J, Twelves C, Cameron D, et al. Bioequivalence of two tablet formulations of capecitabine and exploration of age, gender, body surface area, and creatinine clearance as factors influencing system exposure in cancer patients. Cancer Chemother Pharmacol. 1999;44:453–60.

Desmoulin F, Gilard V, Malet-Martino M, Martino R. Metabolism of capecitabine, an oral fluorouracil prodrug: 19F NMR studies in animal models and human urine. Drug Metab Dispos. 2002;30:1221–9.

Dooley M, Goa KL. Capecitabine. Drugs. 1999;58:69–76.

Gieschke R, Burger H-U, Reigner BG, Blesch KS, Steimer J-L. Population pharmacokinetics and concentration-effect relationships of capecitabine metabolites in colorectal cancer patients. Br J Clin Pharmacol. 2003;55:252–63.

Gieschke R, Reigner B, Blesch KS, Steimer J-L. Population pharmacokinetic analysis of the major metabolites of capecitabine. J Pharmacokinet Pharmacodyn. 2002;29:25–47.

Mackean M, Planting A, Twelves C, et al. Phase I and pharmacologic study of intermittent twice-daily oral therapy with capecitabine in patients with advanced and/or metastatic cancer. J Clin Oncol. 1998;16:2977–85.

McIntyre CW, Owen PJ. Prescribing drugs in kidney disease. In: Brenner BM, editor. Brenner & Rector's the kidney. 8th ed. Philadelphia: Saunders Elsevier; 2008. p. 1930–55.

Poole C, Gardiner J, Twelves C, et al. Effect of renal impairment on the pharmacokinetics and tolerability of capecitabine (Xeloda) in cancer patients. Cancer Chemother Pharmacol. 2002;49:225–34.

Pronk LC, Vasey P, Sparreboom A, et al. A phase I and pharmacokinetic study of the combination of capecitabine and docetaxel in patients with advanced solid tumors. Br J Cancer. 2000;83:22–9.

Royce ME, Hoff PM, Padzur R. Novel chemotherapy agents for colorectal cancer: oral fluoropyrimidines, oxaliplatin, and raltitrexed. Curr Oncol Rep. 1999;1:161–7.

Skirvin JA, Lichtman SM. Pharmacokinetic considerations of oral chemotherapy in elderly patients with cancer. Drugs Aging. 2002;19:25–42.

Tsukamoto Y, Kato Y, Ura M, et al. A physiologically based pharmacokinetic analysis of capecitabine, a triple prodrug of 5-FU, in humans: the mechanism for tumor-selective accumulation of 5-FU. Pharm Res. 2001;18:1190–202.

Tsukamoto Y, Kato Y, Ura M, et al. Investigation of 5-FU disposition after oral administration of capecitabine, a triple-prodrug of 5-FU, using a physiologically based pharmacokinetic model in a human cancer xenograft model: comparison of the simulated 5-FU exposures in the tumour tissue between human and xenograft model. Biopharm Drug Dispos. 2001;22:1–14.

Twelves C, Glynne-Jones R, Cassidy J, et al. Effect of hepatic dysfunction due to liver metastases on the pharmacokinetics of capecitabine and its metabolites. Clin Cancer Res. 1999;5:1696–702.

Villalona-Calero MA, Blum JL, Jones SE, et al. A phase I and pharmacologic study of capecitabine and paclitaxel in breast cancer patients. Ann Oncol. 2001;12:605–14.

Villalona-Calero MA, Weiss GR, Burris HA, et al. Phase I and pharmacokinetic study of the oral fluoropyrimidine capecitabine in combination with paclitaxel in patients with advanced solid malignancies. J Clin Oncol. 1999;17:1915–25.

Xeloda® tablet [package insert]. South San Francisco: Genentech USA Inc; 2011.

Dosage Adjustment of Medications Eliminated by the Kidneys

<u>Capecitabine</u>/Xeloda®   {Antineoplastic; antimetabolite, 5-fluorouracil prodrug}

Usual initial dose:	1,250 mg/m^2 orally twice daily
Usual maintenance dose:	1,250 mg/m^2 orally twice daily for 2 weeks in 3-week cycles
Typical maximum dose:	2,500 mg/m^2/day
Proportion eliminated unchanged:	86 % (as parent drug and active metabolites)

Adjustment for Kidney Disease

FDA-approved product labeling:	*CrCL >50 mL/min*	*1,250 mg/m^2 orally twice daily for 2 weeks in 3-week cycles*
	CrCL 30–50 mL/min	*950 mg/m^2 orally twice daily*
	CrCL <30 mL/min	*Contraindicated*
Alternative adjustment:	*Data not available*	

Note: Hematological and other considerations may suggest further dosage adjustments.

Capreomycin - Selected References

Aronoff GA, Bennett WM, Berns JS, et al. Drug prescribing in renal failure: dosing guidelines for adults and children. 5th ed. Philadelphia: American College of Physicians; 2007.

Black HR, Griffith RS, Peabody GAM. Absorption, excretion and metabolism of capreomycin in normal and diseased states. Ann NY Acad Sci. 1966;135:974–82.

Capastat® sulfate injection [package insert]. Indianapolis: Eli Lilly Co. 2008.

Darr M, Hamburger S, Ellerbeck E. Acid-base and electrolyte abnormalities due to capreomycin. South Med J. 1982;75:627–8.

Garfield JW, Jones JM, Cohen NL, Daly JF, McClement JH. The auditory, vestibular and renal effects of capreomycin in humans. Ann NY Acad Sci. 1966;135:1039–46.

Holdiness MR. Clinical pharmacokinetics of the antituberculosis drugs. Clin Pharmacokinet. 1984;9:511–44.

Jassal M, Bishai WR. Extensively drug-resistant tuberculosis. Lancet Infect Dis. 2009;9:19–30.

Lee SH, Shin J, Choi JM, et al. The impurities of capreomycin make a difference in the safety and pharmacokinetic profiles [letter]. Int J Antimicrob Agents. 2003;22:81–3.

Lehmann CR, Garrett LE, Winn RE, et al. Capreomycin kinetics in renal impairment and clearance by hemodialysis. Am Rev Respir Dis. 1988;138:1312–3.

Miller JD, Popplewell AG, Landwehr A, Greene ME. Toxicology studies in patients on prolonged therapy with capreomycin. Ann NY Acad Sci. 1966;135:1047–56.

Peloquin CA. Pharmacology of antimycobacterial drugs. Med Clin North Am. 1993;77:1253–62.

Steiner RW, Omachi AS. A Bartter's-like syndrome from capreomycin, and a similar gentamicin tubulopathy. Am J Kidney Dis. 1986;7:245–9.

Yue WY, Cohen SS. Toxic nephritis with acute renal insufficiency caused by administration of capreomycin: case report with necropsy findings. Dis Chest. 1966;49:549–51.

Zietse R, Zoutendijk R, Hoorn EJ. Fluid, electrolyte and acid-base disorders associated with antibiotic therapy. Nat Rev Nephrol. 2009;5:193–202.

Dosage Adjustment of Medications Eliminated by the Kidneys

Capreomycin/Capastat®	{Antitubercular; polypeptide antibiotic}

Usual initial dose: 1,000 mg IV or IM

Usual maintenance dose: 1,000 mg IV or IM once daily (not to exceed 20 mg/kg/day) for 60–120 days followed by 1,000 mg IV or IM 2–3 times/week

Typical maximum dose: 20 mg/kg/day

Proportion eliminated unchanged: 50 %

Adjustment for Kidney Disease

FDA-approved product labeling: *Estimated dosages to attain mean steady-state serum capreomycin concentration of 10 mcg/mL (based on CrCL)*

CrCL (mL/min)	Capreomycin clearance ($L/g/h \times 10^{-2}$)	Half-life (h)	Dose (mg/kg) for the following dosing intervals		
			24 h	48 h	72 h
0	0.54	55.5	1.29	2.58	3.87
10	1.01	29.4	2.43	4.87	7.3
20	1.49	20	3.58	7.16	10.7
30	1.97	15.1	4.72	9.45	14.2
40	2.45	12.2	5.87	11.7	–
50	2.92	10.2	7.01	14	–
60	3.4	8.8	8.16	–	–
80	4.35	6.8	10.4	–	–
100	5.31	5.6	12.7	–	–
110	5.78	5.2	13.9	–	–

Alternative adjustment:

GFR >50 mL/min	*1 g IV every 24 h*
GFR 10–50 mL/min	*1 g IV every 24–48 h*
GFR <10 mL/min	*1 g IV every 48 h*
Hemodialysis	*1 g IV after hemodialysis on dialysis days only*
CAPD	*Data not available*
CRRT	*5 mg/kg IV every 24 h*

Captopril - Selected References

Aronoff GA, Bennett WM, Berns JS, et al. Drug prescribing in renal failure: dosing guidelines for adults and children. 5th ed. Philadelphia: American College of Physicians; 2007.

Capoten® tablet [package insert]. Spring Valley: Par Pharmaceutical Companies Inc; 2007.

Cody RJ, Covit A, Schaer G, Williams G. Captopril pharmacokinetics and the acute hemodynamic and hormonal response in patients with severe chronic congestive heart failure. Am Heart J. 1982;104:180–3.

Deray G. Captopril pharmacokinetics [letter]. Br J Clin Pharmacol. 1985;20:20–1.

Duchin KL, Pierides AM, Heald A, Singhvi SM, Rommel AJ. Elimination kinetics of captopril in patients with renal failure. Kidney Int. 1984;25:942–7.

Duchin KL, Singhvi SM, Willard DA, Migdalof BH, McKinstry DN. Captopril kinetics. Clin Pharmacol Ther. 1982;31:452–8.

Fujimura A, Kajiyama H, Ebihara A, Washita K, Nomura Y. Kawahara Y. Pharmacokinetics and pharmacodynamics of captopril in patients undergoing continuous ambulatory peritoneal dialysis. Nephron. 1986;44:324–8.

Giudicelli JF, Chaignon M, Richer C, Giroux B, Guedon J. Influence of chronic renal failure on captopril pharmacokinetics and clinical and biological effects in hypertensive patients. Br J Clin Pharmacol. 1984;18:749–58.

Migdalof BH, Antonaccio MJ, McKinstry DN, et al. Captopril: pharmacology, metabolism, and disposition. Drug Metab Rev. 1984;15:841–69.

Olyaei AJ, Bennett WM. Drug dosing in elderly patients with chronic kidney disease. Clin Geriatr Med. 2009;25:459–527.

Olyaei AJ, Bennett WM. Pharmacologic approach to renal insufficiency. In: Dale DC, Federman DD, Antman K, editors. ACP medicine, WebMD June 2007 update. Hamilton: BC Decker; 2007; NEPHROLOGY IX: Appendix A1–25.

Olyaei AJ, DeMattos AM, Bennett WM. Use of drugs in patients with renal failure. In: Schrier RW, editor. Diseases of the kidney and urinary tract. 8th ed. Philadelphia: Lippincott Williams & Wilkins; 2007. p. 2765–807.

Richer C, Giroux B, Plouin PF, Maarek B, Giudicelli JF. Captopril: pharmacokinetics, antihypertensive and biological effects in hypertensive patients. Br J Clin Pharmacol. 1984;17:243–50.

Singhvi AM, McKinstry DN, Shaw JM, Willard DA, Migdalof BH. Effect of food on the bioavailability of captopril in healthy subjects. J Clin Pharmacol. 1982;22:135–40.

Dosage Adjustment of Medications Eliminated by the Kidneys

<u>Captopril</u>/Capoten®   {**Antihypertensive, vasodilator, angiotensin-converting enzyme (ACE)/ renin inhibitor**}

Usual initial dose:	6.25–12.5 mg orally three times daily
Usual maintenance dose:	25–50 mg orally three times daily
Typical maximum dose:	450 mg/day
Proportion eliminated unchanged:	30 %

Adjustment for Kidney Disease

FDA-approved product labeling: *For patients with significant renal impairment, initial daily dosage of captopril should be reduced, and smaller increments utilized for titration.*

Alternative adjustment:		
	GFR >50 mL/min	*25–50 mg orally every 8–12 h*
	GFR 10–50 mL/min	*18.75–37.5 mg orally every 12 h (~25 % decrease)*
	GFR <10 mL/min	*12.5–25 mg orally every 24 h (~50 % decrease)*
	Hemodialysis	*12.5–25 mg orally every 24 h (~50 % decrease); dose after hemodialysis on dialysis days*
	CAPD	*18.75–37.5 mg orally (~25 % decrease) every 12–18 h*
	CRRT	*18.75–37.5 mg enterally every 12 h (~25 % decrease)*

Dosage Adjustment of Medications Eliminated by the Kidneys

Carboplatin - Selected References

Ando Y, Minami H, Saka H, Ando M, Sakai S, Shimokata K. Adjustment of creatinine clearance improves accuracy of Calvert's formula for carboplatin dosing. Br J Cancer. 1997;76:1067–71.

Aronoff GA, Bennett WM, Berns JS, et al. Drug prescribing in renal failure: dosing guidelines for adults and children. 5th ed. Philadelphia: American College of Physicians; 2007.

Calvert AH, Newell DR, Gumbrell LA, et al. Carboplatin dosage: prospective evaluation of a simple formula based on renal function. J Clin Oncol. 1989;7:1748–56.

Carboplatin injection [package insert]. Bedford: Bedford Laboratories; 2009.

Chatelut E, Rostaing L, Gualano V, et al. Pharmacokinetics of carboplatin in a patient suffering from advanced ovarian carcinoma with hemodialysis-dependent renal insufficiency. Nephron. 1994;66:157–61.

Daley-Yates PT, McBrien DCH. The renal fractional clearance of platinum antitumour compounds in relation to nephrotoxicity. Biochem Pharmacol. 1985;34:1423–8.

Egorin MJ Van Echo DA, Tipping SJ, et al. Pharmacokinetics and dosage reduction of cis-diammine(1, 1-cyclobutanedicarboxylato) platinum in patients with impaired renal function. Cancer Res. 1984;44:5432–8.

Ekhart C, de Jonge ME, Huitema ADR, Schellens JHM, Rodenhuis S, Beijnen JH. Flat dosing of carboplatin is justified in adult patients with normal renal function. Clin Cancer Res. 2006;12:6502–8.

Ekhart C, Rodenhuis S, Schellens JHM, Beijnen JH, Huitema ADR. Carboplatin dosing in overweight and obese patients with normal renal function, does weight matter? Cancer Chemother Pharmacol. 2009;64:115–22.

Elferink F, van der Vijgh WJ, Klein I, Vermorken JB, Gall HE, Pinedo HM. Pharmacokinetics of carboplatin after IV administration. Cancer Treat Rep. 1987;71:1231–7.

El-Yazigi A, Alfurayh O, Amer M. Pharmacokinetics of carboplatin in a patient with cervical cancer with ureteral obstruction before, during, and after hemodialysis. J Clin Pharmacol. 1995;35:1003–7.

English MW, Lowis SP, Peng B, et al. Pharmacokinetically guided dosing of carboplatin and etoposide during peritoneal dialysis and haemodialysis. Br J Cancer. 1996;73:775–80.

Harland SJ, Newell DR, Siddik ZH, Chadwick R, Calvert AH, Harap KR. Pharmacokinetics of cis-diammine-1, 1-cyclobutane dicarboxylate platinum(II) in patients with normal and impaired renal function. Cancer Res. 1984;44:1693–7.

Heijns JB, van der Burg MEL, van Gelder T, et al. Continuous ambulatory peritoneal dialysis: pharmacokinetics and clinical outcome of paclitaxel and carboplatin treatment. Cancer Chemother Pharmacol. 2008;62:841–7.

Murry DJ, Sandland JT, Stricklin LM, Rodman JH. Pharmacokinetics and acute renal effects of continuously infused carboplatin. Clin Pharmacol Ther. 1993;54:374–80.

Oguri S, Sakakibara T, Mase H, et al. Clinical pharmacokinetics of carboplatin. J Clin Pharmacol. 1988;28:208–15.

Oguri T, Shimokata T, Inada M, et al. Pharmacokinetic analysis of carboplatin in patients with cancer who are undergoing hemodialysis. Cancer Chemother Pharmacol. 2010;66:813–7.

Shord SS, Bressler LR, Radhakrishnan L, Chen, Villano JL. Evaluation of the modified diet in renal disease equation for calculation of carboplatin dose. Ann Pharmacother. 2009;43:235–41.

Sørensen BT, Strömgren A, Jakobsen P, Nielsen J, Andersen LS, Jakobsen A. Renal handing of carboplatin. Cancer Chemother Pharmacol. 1992;30:317–20.

Suzuki S, Koide M, Sakamoto S, Matsuo T. Pharmacokinetics of carboplatin and etoposide in a haemodialysis patient with Merkel-cell carcinoma. Nephrol Dial Transplant. 1997;12:137–40.

Takezawa K, Okamoto I, Fukuoka M, Nakagawa K. Pharmacokinetic analysis of carboplatin and etoposide in a small cell lung cancer patient undergoing hemodialysis. J Thorac Oncol. 2008;3:1073–5.

Tanizawa K, Fukunaga K, Okumura N, et al. Successful chemotherapy for small-cell lung cancer in an elderly patient undergoing continuous ambulatory peritoneal dialysis. Intern Med. 2010;49:1179–83.

Yanagawa H, Takisita Y, Bando H, Sumitani H, Okada S. Carboplatin-based chemotherapy in patients undergoing hemodialysis. Anticancer Res. 1996;16:533–5.

Dosage Adjustment of Medications Eliminated by the Kidneys

Carboplatin/Paraplatin®   {Antineoplastic; platinum coordination complex; DNA cross-link disruptor}

Usual initial dose: 300–360 mg/m^2 IV

Usual maintenance dose: 300–360 mg/m^2 IV every 4 weeks, or

Total dose (mg) = (target AUC [usually 4–6 mg/mL • min]) × (GFR [mL/min] + 25)

Typical maximum dose: 360 mg/m^2

Proportion eliminated unchanged: 50–75 %

Adjustment for Kidney Disease

FDA-approved product labeling: *Carboplatin dosage modifications in adults with renal function impairment*

Creatinine clearance (mL/min)	Carboplatin dose
41–59	250 mg/m^2 IV
16–40	200 mg/m^2 IV
≤15	Not recommended

Alternative adjustment:

GFR >50 mL/min	300 mg/m^2 IV
GFR 10–50 mL/min	150 mg/m^2 IV (50 % decrease)
GFR <10 mL/min	75 mg/m^2 IV (75 % decrease)
Hemodialysis	150 mg/m^2 IV (50 % decrease)
CAPD	75 mg/m^2 IV (75 % decrease)
CRRT	200 mg/m^2 IV

Note: Hematological and other considerations may suggest further dosage adjustments.

Dosage Adjustment of Medications Eliminated by the Kidneys

Carmustine - Selected References

Aronoff GA, Bennett WM, Berns JS, et al. Drug prescribing in renal failure: dosing guidelines for adults and children. 5th ed. Philadelphia: American College of Physicians; 2007.

BiCNU® injection [package insert]. Princeton: Bristol-Myers Squibb Co; 2010.

DeVita VT, Denham C, Davidson JD, Oliverio VT. The physiological disposition of the carcinostatic 1,3-bis (2-chlorethyl)-1-nitrosourea (BCNU) in man and animals. Clin Pharmacol Ther. 1967;8:566–77.

Flemming AB, Saltzman WM. Pharmacokinetics of the carmustine implant. Clin Pharmacokinet. 2002;41:403–19.

Hammond LA, Eckardt JR, Kuhn JG, et al. A randomized phase I and pharmacological trial of sequences of 1,3-bis(chloroethyl)-1-nitrosourea and temozolomide in patients with advanced solid neoplasms. Clin Cancer Res. 2004;10:1645–56.

Henner WD, Peters WP, Eder JP, Antman K, Schnipper L, Frei E III. Pharmacokinetics and immediate effects of high-dose carmustine in man. Cancer Treat Rep. 1986;70:877–80.

Jones RB, Matthes S, Shpall EJ, et al. Acute lung injury following treatment with high-dose cyclophosphamide, cisplatin, and carmustine: pharmacodynamic evaluation of carmustine. J Natl Cancer Inst. 1993;85:640–7.

Kintzel PE, Dorr RT. Anticancer drug renal toxicity and elimination: dosing guidelines for altered renal function. Cancer Treat Rev. 1995;21:33–64.

Levin VA, Hoffman W, Weinkam RJ. Pharmacokinetics of BCNU in man: a preliminary study of 20 patients. Cancer Treat Rep. 1978;62:1305–12.

Schacht RG, Feiner HD, Gallo GR, Lieberman A, Baldwin DS. Nephrotoxicity of nitrosoureas. Cancer. 1981;48:1328–34.

Dosage Adjustment of Medications Eliminated by the Kidneys

Carmustine/BiCNU®   {Antineoplastic; nitrosourea alkylating agent}

Usual initial dose:	150 mg/m² IV
Usual maintenance dose:	150–200 mg/m² IV every 6 weeks
Typical maximum dose:	200 mg/m² (up to 1,200 mg/m² IV in autologous stem cell transplantation)
Proportion eliminated unchanged:	65 % (as active metabolites and unchanged drug)

Adjustment for Kidney Disease

FDA-approved product labeling: *Risk of toxic reactions may be greater in patients with impaired renal function.*

Alternative adjustment:	*GFR 45–60 mL/min*	*110–150 mg/m² IV every 2 weeks (25 % reduction)*
	GFR 10–45 mL/min	*Preferably avoid due to increased risk for drug accumulation and resultant toxicity*
	GFR <10 mL/min	*Preferably avoid due to increased risk for drug accumulation and resultant toxicity*
	Hemodialysis	*Preferably avoid due to increased risk for drug accumulation and resultant toxicity*
	CAPD	*Preferably avoid due to increased risk for drug accumulation and resultant toxicity*
	CRRT	*Data not available*

Dosage Adjustment of Medications Eliminated by the Kidneys

Cefadroxil - Selected References

Amsden GW. Tables of antimicrobial agent pharmacology. In: Mandell GL, Bennett JE, Dolin R, editors. Mandell, Douglas, and Bennett's principles and practice of infectious diseases, vol 1. 6th ed. Philadelphia: Elsevier; 2005. p. 634–700.

Aronoff GA, Bennett WM, Berns JS, et al. Drug prescribing in renal failure: dosing guidelines for adults and children. 5th ed. Philadelphia: American College of Physicians; 2007.

Cutler R. Cefadroxil kinetics in patients with impaired renal function. J Int Med Res. 1980;8(Suppl 1):17–20.

Cutler RE, Blair AD, Kelly MR. Cefadroxil kinetics in patients with renal insufficiency. Clin Pharmacol Ther. 1979;25:14–21.

Duricef® capsule [package insert]. Rockaway: Warner Chilcott Co; 2007.

Garrigues TM, Martín U, Peris-Ribera JE, Prescott LF. Dose-dependent absorption and elimination of cefadroxil. Eur J Clin Pharmacol. 1991;41:179–83.

Granero L, Gimeno MJ, Torres-Molina F, Chesa-Jiménez J, Peris JE. Studies on the renal excretion mechanisms of cefadroxil. Drug Metab Dispos. 1994;22:447–50.

Hampel B, Lode H, Wagner J, Koeppe P. Pharmacokinetics of cefadroxil and cefaclor during an eight-day dosage period. Antimicrob Agents Chemother. 1982;22:1061–3.

Humbert G, Leroy A, Fillastre JP, Godin M. Pharmacokinetics of cefadroxil in normal subjects and in patients with renal insufficiency. Chemotherapy. 1979;25:189–95.

La Rosa F, Ripa S, Prenna M, Ghezzi A, Pfeffer M. Pharmacokinetics of cefadroxil after oral administration. Antimicrob Agents Chemother. 1982;21:320–2.

Leroy A, Humbert G, Godin M, Fillastre JP. Pharmacokinetics of cefadroxil in patients with impaired renal function. J Antimicrob Chemother. 1982;10(Suppl B):39–46.

Lode H, Stahlmann R, Koeppe P. Comparative pharmacokinetics of cephalexin, cefaclor, cefadroxil, and CGP 9000. Antimicrob Agents Chemother. 1979;16:1–6.

Mariño EL, Dominguez-Gil A. Influence of dose on the pharmacokinetics of cefadroxil. Eur J Clin Pharmacol. 1980;18:505–9.

Mariño EL, Dominguez-Gil A, Muriel C. Influence of dosage form and administration route on the pharmacokinetic parameters of cefadroxil. Int J Clin Pharmacol Ther Toxicol. 1982;20:73–7.

McIntyre CW, Owen PJ. Prescribing drugs in kidney disease. In: Brenner BM, editor. Brenner & Rector's the kidney. 8th ed. Philadelphia: Saunders Elsevier; 2008. p. 1930–55.

Olyaei AJ, Bennett WM. Drug dosing in elderly patients with chronic kidney disease. Clin Geriatr Med. 2009;25:459–527.

Olyaei AJ, Bennett WM. Pharmacologic approach to renal insufficiency. In: Dale DC, Federman DD, Antman K, editors. ACP medicine, WebMD June 2007 update. Hamilton: BC Decker; 2007; NEPHROLOGY IX: Appendix A1–25.

Olyaei AJ, DeMattos AM, Bennett WM. Use of drugs in patients with renal failure. In: Schrier RW, editor. Diseases of the kidney and urinary tract. 8th ed. Philadelphia: Lippincott Williams & Wilkins; 2007. p. 2765–807.

Pfeffer M, Jackson A, Ximenes J, Perche de Menezes J. Comparative human oral clinical pharmacology of cefadroxil, cephalexin, and cephradine. Antimicrob Agents Chemother. 1977;11:331–8.

Santella PJ, Henness D. A review of the bioavailability of cefadroxil. J Antimicrob Chemother. 1982;10(Suppl B):17–25.

Dosage Adjustment of Medications Eliminated by the Kidneys

<u>Cefadroxil</u>/Duricef®	{**Antibacterial; first-generation cephalosporin**}
Usual initial dose:	1 g orally
Usual maintenance dose:	1–2 g/day orally in single or divided doses (twice daily) for 10 days
Typical maximum dose:	2 g/day in single or divided (twice daily) doses
Proportion eliminated unchanged:	85 %

Adjustment for Kidney Disease

FDA-approved product labeling: *In patients with renal impairment, initial dose is 1 g of cefadroxil orally, and the maintenance dose (based on the creatinine clearance rate [mL/min]) is 500 mg orally at the time intervals listed below*

CrCL (mL/min)	Dosage interval (h)
0–10	*36*
10–25	*24*
25–50	*12*
>50	*12*

Alternative adjustment:

GFR >50 mL/min	*1,000 mg orally every 12 h*
GFR 10–50 mL/min	*500–1,000 mg orally every 12–24 h*
GFR <10 mL/min	*1,000 mg orally every 48 h*
Hemodialysis	*1,000 mg orally every 72 h, after hemodialysis on dialysis days*
CAPD	*500 mg orally every 24 h*
CRRT	*Not applicable (consider an IV cephalosporin)*

Dosage Adjustment of Medications Eliminated by the Kidneys

Cefazolin - Selected References

Ahern JW, Possidente CJ, Hood V, Alston WK. Cefazolin dosing protocol for patients receiving long-term hemodialysis. Am J Health Syst Pharm. 2003;60:178–81.

Amsden GW. Tables of antimicrobial agent pharmacology. In: Mandell GL, Bennett JE, Dolin R, editors. Mandell, Douglas, and Bennett's principles and practice of infectious diseases, vol 1. 6th ed. Philadelphia: Elsevier; 2005. p. 634–700.

Ancef® injection [package insert]. Research Triangle Park: GlaxoSmithKline; 2005.

Aronoff GA, Bennett WM, Berns JS, et al. Drug prescribing in renal failure: dosing guidelines for adults and children. 5th ed. Philadelphia: American College of Physicians; 2007.

Brogard JM, Pinget M, Brandt C, Lavillaureix J. Pharmacokinetics of cefazolin in patients with renal failure; special reference to hemodialysis. J Clin Pharmacol. 1977;17:225–30.

Bunke CM, Aronoff GR, Brier ME, Sloan RS, Luft FC. Cefazolin and cephalexin kinetics in continuous ambulatory peritoneal dialysis. Clin Pharmacol Ther. 1983;33:66–72.

Bunke CM, Aronoff GR, Luft FC. Pharmacokinetics of common antibiotics used in continuous ambulatory peritoneal dialysis. Am J Kidney Dis. 1983;3:114–7.

Craig WA, Welling PG, Jackson TC, Kunin CM. Pharmacology of cefazolin and other cephalosporins in patients with renal insufficiency. J Infect Dis. 1973;128(Suppl):S347–53.

Fogel MA, Nussbaum PB, Feintzeig ID, Hunt WA, Gavin JP, Kim RC. Cefazolin in chronic hemodialysis patients: a safe, effective alternative to vancomycin. Am J Kidney Dis. 1998;32:401–9.

Gold JA, McKee JJ, Ziv DS. Experience with cefazolin: an overall summary of pharmacologic and clinical trials in man. J Infect Dis. 1973;128(Suppl):S415–21.

Heintz BH, Matzke GR, Dager WF. Antimicrobial dosing concepts and recommendations for critically ill adult patients receiving continuous renal replacement therapy or intermittent hemodialysis. Pharmacotherapy. 2009;29:562–77.

Johnson CA, Zimmerman SW, Rogge M. The pharmacokinetics of antibiotics used to treat peritoneal dialysis-associated peritonitis. Am J Kidney Dis. 1984;4:3–17.

Kaye D, Wenger N, Agarwal B. Pharmacology of intraperitoneal cefazolin in patients undergoing peritoneal dialysis. Antimicrob Agents Chemother. 1978;14:318–21.

Kefzol®, sterile cefazolin sodium USP [package insert]. Indianapolis: Eli Lilly Co; 1990.

Kirby WMM, Regamy C. Pharmacokinetics of cefazolin compared with four other cephalosporins. J Infect Dis. 1973;128(Suppl):S341–6.

Levison MF, Levison SP, Ries K, Kaye D. Pharmacology of cefazolin in patients with normal and abnormal renal function. J Infect Dis. 1973;128(Suppl):S354–7.

Madhavan T, Yaremchuk K, Levin N, et al. Effects of renal failure and dialysis on cefazolin pharmacokinetics. Antimicrob Agents Chemother. 1975;8:63–6.

Marx MA, Frye RF, Matzke GR, Golper TA. Cefazolin as empiric therapy in hemodialysis-related infections: efficacy and blood concentrations. Am J Kidney Dis. 1998;32:410–4.

McIntyre CW, Owen PJ. Prescribing drugs in kidney disease. In: Brenner BM, editor. Brenner & Rector's the kidney. 8th ed. Philadelphia: Saunders Elsevier; 2008. p. 1930–55.

Olyaei AJ, Bennett WM. Drug dosing in elderly patients with chronic kidney disease. Clin Geriatr Med. 2009;25:459–527.

Olyaei AJ, DeMattos AM, Bennett WM. Use of drugs in patients with renal failure. In: Schrier RW, editor. Diseases of the kidney and urinary tract. 8th ed. Philadelphia: Lippincott Williams & Wilkins; 2007. p. 2765–807.

Paton TW, Manuel MA, Walker SE. Pharmacokinetics of tobramycin and cefazolin in patients undergoing continuous ambulatory peritoneal dialysis [abstract]. Clin Pharmacol Ther. 1982;31:259–60.

Sowinski KM, Mueller B, Grabe DW, et al. Cefazolin dialytic clearance by high-efficiency and high-flux hemodialyzers. Am J Kidney Dis. 2001;37:766–76.

Trotman RL, Williamson JC, Shoemaker M, Salzer WL. Antibiotic dosing in critically ill adult patients receiving continuous renal replacement therapy. Clin Infect Dis. 2005;41:1159–66.

Wiggins KJ, Johnson DW, Craig JC, Strippoli GFM. Treatment of peritoneal dialysis-associated peritonitis: a systematic review of randomized controlled trials. Am J Kidney Dis. 2007;50:967–88.

Dosage Adjustment of Medications Eliminated by the Kidneys

Cefazolin/Ancef®   {Antibacterial; first-generation cephalosporin}

Usual initial dose: 1–2 g IV

Usual maintenance dose: 1–2 g IV every 8 h

Typical maximum dose: 6 g/day IV

Proportion eliminated unchanged: 96 %

Adjustment for Kidney Disease

FDA-approved product labeling:	*CrCL ≥55 mL/min or SCr ≤1.5 mg/dL*	*500 mg–2 g IV every 8 h*
	CrCL 35–54 mL/min or SCr 1.6–3.0 mg/dL	*500 mg–2 g IV every 12 h*
	CrCL 11–34 mL/min or SCr 3.1–4.5 mg/dL	*250–1,000 mg IV every 12 h*
	CrCL ≤10 mL/min or SCr ≥4.6 mg/dL	*250–1,000 mg IV every 18–24 h*
Alternative adjustment:	*GFR >50 mL/min*	*500–2,000 mg IV every 8 h*
	GFR 10–50 mL/min	*250–1,000 mg IV every 12 h*
	GFR <10 mL/min	*250–1,000 mg IV every 24 h*
	Hemodialysis	*20 mg/kg (1,000–2,000 mg) IV after each dialysis*
	CAPD	*500 mg IV every 12 h or add 1,000 mg/2 L dialysate 4 × daily*
	CVVH	*1–2 g IV every 12 h*
	CVVHD or CVVHDF	*2 g IV every 12 h*

Cefdinir - Selected References

Aronoff GA, Bennett WM, Berns JS, et al. Drug prescribing in renal failure: dosing guidelines for adults and children. 5th ed. Philadelphia: American College of Physicians; 2007.

Guay DRP. Cefdinir: an expanded-spectrum oral cephalosporin. Ann Pharmacother. 2000;34:1469–77.

Hishida A, Ohishi K, Nagashima S, Kanamuru M, Obara M, Kitada A. Pharmacokinetic study of an oral cephalosporin, cefdinir, in hemodialysis patients. Antimicrob Agents Chemother. 1998;42:1718–24.

Kimura Y, Kawamura M, Owada M, Fujiwara T, Maesawa C, Hiramori K. Successful steroid therapy for cefdinir-induced acute tubulointerstitial nephritis with progressive renal failure. Intern Med. 2001;40:114–7.

Omnicef® capsule and suspension [package insert]. North Chicago: Abbott Laboratories; 2005.

Paris MM, Devcich KJ. Overview of cefdinir: pharmacokinetics, safety, and efficacy in the treatment of uncomplicated skin and skin structure infections. Cutis. 2004;73:14–8.

Perry CM, Scott LJ. Cefdinir: a review of its use in the management of mild-to-moderate bacterial infections. Drugs. 2004;64:1433–64.

Tomino Y, Fukui M, Hamada C, Inoue S, Osada S. Pharmacokinetics of cefdinir and its transfer to dialysate in patients with chronic renal failure undergoing continuous ambulatory peritoneal dialysis. Arzneimittelforschung. 1998;48:862–7.

Dosage Adjustment of Medications Eliminated by the Kidneys

<u>Cefdinir</u>/Omnicef®   {**Antibacterial; third-generation cephalosporin**}

Usual initial dose:	600 mg orally
Usual maintenance dose:	300 mg orally every 12 h or 600 mg orally every 24 h
Typical maximum dose:	600 mg/day
Proportion eliminated unchanged:	15 %

Adjustment for Kidney Disease

FDA-approved product labeling:	*CrCL <30 mL/min*	*300 mg orally once daily*
	Hemodialysis	*300 mg or 7 mg/kg dose every other day. At the conclusion of each hemodialysis session, 300 mg (or 7 mg/kg) should be given.*
Alternative adjustment:	*GFR >50 mL/min*	*300 mg orally every 12 h*
	GFR 10–50 mL/min	*300 mg orally every 24 h*
	GFR <10 mL/min	*300 mg orally every 48 h*
	Hemodialysis	*300 mg orally every 48 h, after hemodialysis on dialysis days*
	CAPD	*300 mg orally every 48 h*
	CRRT	*Not applicable (consider an IV cephalosporin)*

Cefditoren - Selected References

Amsden GW. Tables of antimicrobial agent pharmacology. In: Mandell GL, Bennett JE, Dolin R, editors. Mandell, Douglas, and Bennett's principles and practice of infectious diseases, vol 1. 6th ed. Philadelphia: Elsevier; 2005. p. 634–700.

Aronoff GA, Bennett WM, Berns JS, et al. Drug prescribing in renal failure: dosing guidelines for adults and children. 5th ed. Philadelphia: American College of Physicians; 2007.

Granizo JJ, Sádaba B, Honorato J, et al. Monte Carlo simulation describing the pharmacodynamic profile of cefditoren in plasma from healthy volunteers [letter]. Int J Antimicrob Agents. 2008;31:396–8.

Guay DRP. Review of cefditoren, an advanced-generation, broad-spectrum oral cephalosporin. Clin Ther. 2001;23:1924–7.

Li J-T, Hou F, Lu H, Li T, Li H. Phase I clinical trial of cefditoren pivoxil (ME 1207): pharmacokinetics in healthy volunteers. Drugs Exp Clin Res. 1997;23:145–50.

Miyazaki S, Miyazaki Y, Tsuji A, Nishida M, Goto S. In vitro antibacterial activity of ME1207, a new oral cephalosporin. Antimicrob Agents Chemother. 1991;35:1691–4.

Sábada B, Azanza JR, Quetglas EG, et al. Pharmacokinetic/pharmacodynamic serum and urine profile of cefditoren following single-dose and multiple twice- and thrice-daily regimens in healthy volunteers: a phase I study. Rev Esp Quimioter. 2007;20:51–60.

Spectracef® tablet film coated [package insert]. Cary: Cornerstone Therapeutics Inc; 2009.

Tamura A, Okamoto R, Yoshida T, et al. In vitro and in vivo antibacterial activities of ME1207, a new oral cephalosporin. Antimicrob Agents Chemother. 1988;32:1421–6.

Wellington K, Curran MP. Cefditoren pivoxil: a review of its use in the treatment of bacterial infections. Drugs. 2004;64:2597–18.

Dosage Adjustment of Medications Eliminated by the Kidneys

<u>**Cefditoren**</u>/**Spectracef®**   {**Antibacterial; second-generation cephalosporin**}

Usual initial dose: 400 mg orally

Usual maintenance dose: 200–400 mg orally every 12 h for 10 days

Typical maximum dose: 400 mg

Proportion eliminated unchanged: >90 %

Adjustment for Kidney Disease

FDA-approved product labeling: *CrCL 50–80 mL/min* — *200–400 mg orally every 12 h with meals*

CrCL 30–49 mL/min — *200 mg orally every 12 h with meals*

CrCL <30 mL/min — *200 mg orally every 24 h with meals (Note: the appropriate dose in patients with end-stage renal disease has not been determined.)*

Alternative adjustment: *GFR >50 mL/min* — *200–400 mg orally every 12 h with meals*

GFR 10–50 mL/min — *200 mg orally every 12 h with meals*

GFR <10 mL/min — *200 mg orally every 24 h with meals*

Hemodialysis — *200 mg orally every 24 h with meals; administer after hemodialysis on dialysis days.*

CAPD — *300 mg orally every 48 h with meals*

CRRT — *Not applicable (consider an IV cephalosporin)*

Dosage Adjustment of Medications Eliminated by the Kidneys

Cefepime - Selected References

Allaochiche B, Breilh D, Jaumain H, Gillard B, Renard S, Saux M-C. Pharmacokinetics of cefepime during continuous venovenous hemodiafiltration. Antimicrob Agents Chemother. 1997;41:2424–7.

Aronoff GA, Bennett WM, Berns JS, et al. Drug prescribing in renal failure: dosing guidelines for adults and children. 5th ed. Philadelphia: American College of Physicians; 2007.

Bächer K, Schaeffer M, Lode H, Nord CE, Bormer K, Koeppe P. Multiple dose pharmacokinetics, safety, and effects on faecal microflora of cefepime in healthy volunteers. J Antimicrob Chemother. 1992;32:365–75.

Barbey F, Bubnon D, Wauters J-P. Severe neurotoxicity of cefepime in uremic patients [letter]. Ann Intern Med. 2001;135:1011.

Barbhaiya RH, Forgue ST, Gleason CR, Knupp CA, Pittman KA, Weidler DJ, Martin RR. Safety, tolerance, and pharmacokinetic evaluation of cefepime after administration of single intravenous doses. Antimicrob Agents Chemother. 1990;34:1118–22.

Barbhaiya RH, Knupp CA, Forgue ST, et al. Disposition of the cephalosporin cefepime in normal and renally impaired subjects. Drug Metab Dispos. 1991;19:68–73.

Barbjaoua RH, Knupp CA, Forgue ST, Matzke GR, Guay DRP, Pittman K. Pharmacokinetics of cefepime in subjects with renal insufficiency. Clin Pharmacol Ther. 1990;48:268–76.

Chatellier D Jourdain M, Mangalaboyi J, et al. Cefepime-induced neurotoxicity: an underestimated complication of antibio-therapy in patients with acute renal failure. Intensive Care Med. 2002;28:214–7.

Cheatham SC, Shea KM, Healy DP, et al. Steady-state pharmacokinetics and pharmacodynamics of cefepime administered by prolonged infusion in hospitalised patients. Int J Antimicrob Agents. 2011;37:46–50.

Cronqvist J, Nilsson-Ehle I, Ōqvist B, Norrby SR. Pharmacokinetics of cefepime dihydrochloride arginine in subjects with renal impairment. Antimicrob Agents Chemother. 1992;36:2676–80.

Elwell RJ, Frye RF, Bailie GR. Pharmacokinetics of intraperitoneal cefepime in automated peritoneal dialysis. Perit Dial Int. 2005;25:380–6.

Ferrara N, Abete P, Giodanano M, et al. Neurotoxicity induced by cefepime in a very old hemodialysis patient. Clin Nephrol. 2003;59:388–90.

Heintz BH, Matzke GR, Dager WF. Antimicrobial dosing concepts and recommendations for critically ill adult patients receiving continuous renal replacement therapy or intermittent hemodialysis. Pharmacotherapy. 2009;29:562–77.

Icasio AM, Ariano RE, Zelenitsky SA, et al. Population pharmacokinetics of high-dose, prolonged-infusion cefepime in adult critically ill patients with ventilator-associated pneumonia. Antimicrob Agents Chemother. 2009;53:1476–81.

Isla A, Gascóm AR, Maynar J, Arzuaga A, Toral D, Pedraz JL. Cefepime and continuous renal replacement therapy (CRRT): in vitro permeability of two CRRT membranes and pharmacokinetics in four critically ill patients. Clin Ther. 2005;27:599–608.

Lipman J, Wallis SC, Rickard C. Low plasma cefepime levels in critically ill septic patients: pharmacokinetic modeling indicates improved troughs with revised dosing. Antimicrob Agents Chemother. 1999;43:2559–61.

Malone RS, Fish DN, Abraham E, Teitelbaum I. Pharmacokinetics of cefepime during continuous renal replacement therapy in critically ill patients. Antimicrob Agents Chemother. 2001;45:3148–55.

Maxipime® injection [package insert]. Princeton: Bristol-Myers Squibb Co; 2010.

Moriyama B, Henning SA, Neuhauser MN, Danner RL, Walsh TJ. Continuous-infusion β-lactam antibiotics during continuous venovenous hemofiltration for the treatment of resistant gram-negative bacteria. Ann Pharmacother. 2009;43:1324–7.

Schmaldienst S, Traunmiler F, Burgmann H, et al. Multiple-dose pharmacokinetics of cefepime in long-term hemodialysis with high-flux membranes. Eur J Clin Pharmacol. 2000;56:61–4.

Sonck J, Lureys G, Verbeelen D. The neurotoxicity and safety of treatment with cefepime in patients with renal failure. Nephrol Dial Transplant. 2008;23:966–70.

Tam VH, McKinnon PS, Akins RL, Drusano GL, Rybak MJ. Pharmacokinetics and pharmacodynamics of cefepime in patients with various degrees of renal function. Antimicrob Agents Chemother. 2003;47:1853–61.

Wong KM, Chan WK. Chan YH, Li CS. Cefepime-related neurotoxicity in a haemodialysis patient. Nephrol Dial Transplant. 1999;14:2266–6.

Dosage Adjustment of Medications Eliminated by the Kidneys

Cefepime/Maxipime® {Antibacterial; fourth-generation cephalosporin}

Usual initial dose: 2 g IV

Usual maintenance dose: 500 mg–2 g IV every 8–12 h or 1 g IV every 8 h infused over 4 h

Typical maximum dose: 2 g IV

Proportion eliminated unchanged: 85 %

Adjustment for Kidney Disease

FDA-approved product labeling: *Cefepime dosing for adults with renal function impairment*

CrCL (mL/min)	Recommended maintenance schedule, dependent upon severity of infection			
>60 (normal)	500 mg q 12 h	1 g q 12 h	2 g q 12 h	2 g q 8 h
30–60	500 mg q 24 h	1 g q 24 h	2 g q 24 h	2 g q 12 h
11–29	500 mg q 24 h	500 mg q 24 h	1 g q 24 h	2 g q 24 h
<11	250 mg q 24 h	250 mg q 24 h	500 mg q 24 h	1 g q 24 h
CAPD	500 mg q 48 h	1 g q 48 h	2 g q 48 h	2 g q 48 h
Hemodialysis	1 g on day 1, then 500 mg q 24 h thereafter			1 g q 24 h

On hemodialysis days, cefepime should be administered following dialysis. Whenever possible, cefepime should be administered at the same time each day

Alternative adjustment:

GFR >50 mL/min	1 g IV every 4 h or 1 g IV over 4 h every 8 h or 1–2 g IV every 8–12 h
GFR 10–50 mL/min	1–2 g IV every 12–24 h
GFR <10 mL/min	500–1,000 mg IV every 24 h
Hemodialysis	1 g IV every 24 h; dose after hemodialysis on dialysis days
CAPD	500–1,000 mg IV every 24 h
CVVH	1–2 g IV every 12 h
CVVHD or CVVHDF	1–2 g IV every 12 h (consider 2 g IV every 8 h for gram-negative pathogens with MIC ≥4 mg/L)

Dosage Adjustment of Medications Eliminated by the Kidneys

Cefixime - Selected References

Aronoff GA, Bennett WM, Berns JS, et al. Drug prescribing in renal failure: dosing guidelines for adults and children. 5th ed. Philadelphia: American College of Physicians; 2007.

Dhib M, Moulin B, Leroy A, et al. Relationship between renal function and disposition of oral cefixime. Eur J Clin Pharmacol. 1991;41:579–83.

Faulkner RD, Bohaychuk W, Desjardins FE, et al. Pharmacokinetics of cefixime after once-a-day and twice-a-day dosing to steady state. J Clin Pharmacol. 1987;27:807–12.

Faulkner RD, Bohaychuk W, Lanc RA, et al. Pharmacokinetics of cefixime in the young and elderly. J Antimicrob Chemother. 1988;21:787–94.

Faulkner RD, Fernandez P, Lawrence G, et al. Absolute bioavailability of cefixime in man. J Clin Pharmacol. 1988;28:700–6.

Guay DRP, Meatherall RC, Harding GK, Brown GR. Pharmacokinetics of cefixime (CL 284,635; FK 027) in healthy subjects and patients with renal insufficiency. Antimicrob Agents Chemother. 1986;30:485–90.

McIntyre CW, Owen PJ. Prescribing drugs in kidney disease. In: Brenner BM, editor. Brenner & Rector's the kidney. 8th ed. Philadelphia: Saunders Elsevier; 2008. p. 1930–55.

Olyaei AJ, Bennett WM. Drug dosing in elderly patients with chronic kidney disease. Clin Geriatr Med. 2009;25:459–527.

Olyaei AJ, Bennett WM. Pharmacologic approach to renal insufficiency. In: Dale DC, Federman DD, Antman K, editors. ACP medicine, WebMD June 2007 update. Hamilton: BC Decker; 2007; NEPHROLOGY IX: Appendix A1–25.

Olyaei AJ, DeMattos AM, Bennett WM. Use of drugs in patients with renal failure. In: Schrier RW, editor. Diseases of the kidney and urinary tract. 8th ed. Philadelphia: Lippincott Williams & Wilkins; 2007. p. 2765–807.

Suprax® suspension [package insert]. Baltimore: Lupin Pharmaceuticals Inc; 2005.

Dosage Adjustment of Medications Eliminated by the Kidneys

<u>Cefixime</u>/Suprax®   {**Antibacterial; third-generation cephalosporin**}

Usual initial dose:	400 mg orally
Usual maintenance dose:	400 mg/day orally
Typical maximum dose:	400 mg
Proportion eliminated unchanged:	85 %

Adjustment for Kidney Disease

FDA-approved product labeling:

Cefixime dosage in renal function impairment

CrCL (mL/min)	Dosage
>60	Standard (400 mg/day orally)
21–60 or hemodialysis[a]	75 % of standard (300 mg/day orally)
<20 or continuous ambulatory peritoneal dialysis[a]	50 % of standard (200 mg/day orally)

[a]*Neither hemodialysis nor peritoneal dialysis removes significant amounts of drug from the body*

Alternative adjustment:

GFR >50 mL/min	*400 mg orally once daily*
GFR 10–50 mL/min	*400 mg orally once daily*
GFR <10 mL/min	*200 mg orally once daily (50 % decrease)*
Hemodialysis	*300 mg orally once daily, after hemodialysis on dialysis days*
CAPD	*200 mg orally once daily*
CRRT	*Not recommended (consider an IV cephalosporin)*

Dosage Adjustment of Medications Eliminated by the Kidneys

Cefotaxime - Selected References

Andrassy K. Pharmacokinetics of cefotaxime in dialysis patients. Diagn Microbiol Infect Dis. 1995;22:85–7.

Aronoff GA, Bennett WM, Berns JS, et al. Drug prescribing in renal failure: dosing guidelines for adults and children. 5th ed. Philadelphia: American College of Physicians; 2007.

Bergquist S-O, Eriksson I, Eriksson S, et al. Retrospective analysis of the efficacy of cefotaxime sodium dosed twice daily: the Swedish experience. Diagn Microbiol Infect Dis. 1995;22:163–6.

Burke JP, Pestotnik SL, Classen DC, Lloyd JF. A retrospective analysis of twice-daily cefotaxime compared to conventional therapy for the treatment of infections in a USA hospital. Diagn Microbiol Infect Dis. 1995;22:167–9.

Claforan® injection [package insert]. Bridgewater: Sanofi-Aventis US LLC; 2009.

Fillastre JP, Leroy A, Humbert G, Godin M. Pharmacokinetics of cefotaxime in subjects with normal and impaired renal function. J Antimicrob Chemother. 1980;6(Suppl A):103–11.

Heintz BH, Matzke GR, Dager WF. Antimicrobial dosing concepts and recommendations for critically ill adult patients receiving continuous renal replacement therapy or intermittent hemodialysis. Pharmacotherapy. 2009;29:562–77.

Imada A, Itagaki N, Hasegawa H, Horiuchi A. Comparative study of the pharmacokinetics of various β-lactams after intravenous and intraperitoneal administration in patients undergoing continuous ambulatory peritoneal dialysis. Drugs. 1988;35(Suppl 2):82–7.

Karimi A, Seeger K, Stolke D, Knothe H. Cefotaxime concentration in cerebrospinal fluid. J Antimicrob Chemother. 1980;6(Suppl A):119–20.

Kosmidis J, Stathakis C, Mantopoulos K, Pouriezi T, Papathanassiou B, Daikos GK. Clinical pharmacology of cefotaxime including penetration into bile, sputum, bone and cerebrospinal fluid. J Antimicrob Chemother. 1980;6(Suppl A):147–51.

Kuang D, Verbine A, Ronco C. Pharmacokinetics and antimicrobial dosing adjustment in critically ill patients during continuous renal replacement therapy. Clin Nephrol. 2007;67:267–84.

LeFrock JL, Prince RA, Leff RD. Mechanism of action, antimicrobial activity, pharmacology, adverse effects, and clinical efficacy of cefotaxime. Pharmacotherapy. 1982;2:174–84.

McIntyre CW, Owen PJ. Prescribing drugs in kidney disease. In: Brenner BM, editor. Brenner & Rector's the kidney. 8th ed. Philadelphia: Saunders Elsevier; 2008. p. 1930–55.

Nix DE, Schentag JJ. Role of pharmacokinetics and pharmacodynamics in the design of dosage schedules for 12-h cefotaxime alone and in combination with other antibiotics. Diagn Microbiol Infect Dis. 1995;22:71–6.

Olyaei AJ, Bennett WM. Drug dosing in elderly patients with chronic kidney disease. Clin Geriatr Med. 2009;25:459–527.

Olyaei AJ, Bennett WM. Pharmacologic approach to renal insufficiency. In: Dale DC, Federman DD, Antman K, editors. ACP medicine, WebMD June 2007 update. Hamilton: BC Decker; 2007; NEPHROLOGY IX: Appendix A1–25.

Olyaei AJ, DeMattos AM, Bennett WM. Use of drugs in patients with renal failure. In: Schrier RW, editor. Diseases of the kidney and urinary tract. 8th ed. Philadelphia: Lippincott Williams & Wilkins; 2007. p. 2765–807.

Patel KA, Nicolau DP, Nightingale CH, Quintilani R. Pharmacokinetics of cefotaxime in healthy volunteers and patients. Diagn Microbiol Infect Dis. 1995;22:49–55.

Shah PM, Stille W. Cefotaxime versus ceftriaxone for the treatment of nosocomial pneumonia: results of a multicenter study. Diagn Microbiol Infect Dis. 1995;22:171–2.

Simmons BP, Gelfand MS, Grogan J, Craft B. Cefotaxime twice daily versus ceftriaxone once daily: a randomized controlled study in patients with serious infections. Diagn Microbiol Infect Dis. 1995;22:155–7.

Trotman RL, Williamson JC, Shoemaker M, Salzer WL. Antibiotic dosing in critically ill adult patients receiving continuous renal replacement therapy. Clin Infect Dis. 2005;41:1159–66.

Young JPW, Husson JM, Bruch K, Blomer RJ, Savopoulos C. The evaluation of efficacy and safety of cefotaxime: a review of 2500 cases. J Antimicrob Chemother. 1980;6(Suppl A):293–300.

Dosage Adjustment of Medications Eliminated by the Kidneys

Cefotaxime/Claforan®	{Antibacterial; third-generation cephalosporin}
Usual initial dose:	1–2 g IV
Usual maintenance dose:	1–2 g IV every 8 h
Typical maximum dose:	12 g/day IV
Proportion eliminated unchanged:	60 %

Adjustment for Kidney Disease

FDA-approved product labeling:	*CrCL ≥20 mL/min*	*1–2 g IV every 6–8 h*
	CrCL <20 mL/min	*0.5–1 g IV every 8 h (50 % decrease)*
Alternative adjustment:	*GFR >50 mL/min*	*1–2 g IV every 8–12 h*
	GFR 10–50 mL/min	*1–2 g IV every 12 h*
	GFR <10 mL/min	*1–2 g IV every 24 h*
	Hemodialysis	*1–2 g IV every 24 h; administer after hemodialysis on dialysis days.*
	CAPD	*0.5–1 g every 24 h*
	CVVH	*1–2 g IV every 8–12 h*
	CVVHD	*1–2 g IV every 8 h*
	CVVHDF	*1–2 g IV every 6–8 h*

Dosage Adjustment of Medications Eliminated by the Kidneys

Cefotetan - Selected References

Aronoff GA, Bennett WM, Berns JS, et al. Drug prescribing in renal failure: dosing guidelines for adults and children. 5th ed. Philadelphia: American College of Physicians; 2007.

Cefotan® injection [package insert]. Wilmington: AstraZeneca Pharmaceuticals LP; 2004

Fraschini F, Scaglione F, Mezzetti M, et al. Pharmacokinetic profile of cefotetan in different clinical conditions. Drugs Exp Clin Res. 1988;14:547–53.

Geckler RW, Eng RHK, Fabian TC, et al. A multicenter comparative study of cefotetan once daily and cefoxitin thrice daily for the treatment of infections of the skin and superficial soft tissue. Am J Med. 1988;155(Suppl 5A):91–5.

Gribble MJ, Mandell LA, Bergeron M, et al. Cefotetan: a second-generation cephalosporin active against anaerobic bacteria. Can Med Assoc J. 1994;151:537–42.

Martin C, Thomachot L, Albanese J. Clinical pharmacokinetics of cefotetan. Clin Pharmacokinet. 1994;26:248–58.

McIntyre CW, Owen PJ. Prescribing drugs in kidney disease. In: Brenner BM, editor. Brenner & Rector's the kidney. 8th ed. Philadelphia: Saunders Elsevier; 2008. p. 1930–55.

Nakagawa K, Koyama M, Tachibana A, Komiya M, Kikuchi Y, Yano K. Pharmacokinetics of cefotetan (YM09330) in humans. Antimicrob Agents Chemother. 1982;22:935–41.

Ohkawa M, Hirano S, Tokunaga S, et al. Pharmacokinetics of cefotetan in normal subjects and patients with impaired renal function. Antimicrob Agents Chemother. 1983;23:31–5.

Olyaei AJ, Bennett WM. Drug dosing in elderly patients with chronic kidney disease. Clin Geriatr Med. 2009;25:459–527.

Olyaei AJ, Bennett WM. Pharmacologic approach to renal insufficiency. In: Dale DC, Federman DD, Antman K, editors. ACP medicine, WebMD June 2007 update. Hamilton: BC Decker; 2007; NEPHROLOGY IX: Appendix A1–25.

Olyaei AJ, DeMattos AM, Bennett WM. Use of drugs in patients with renal failure. In: Schrier RW, editor. Diseases of the kidney and urinary tract. 8th ed. Philadelphia: Lippincott Williams & Wilkins; 2007. p. 2765–807.

Orr JW Jr, Sisson PF, Barrett JM, Ellington JR, Jennings RH, Taylor DL. Pharmacokinetics and tissue dynamics of 1 g cefotetan prophylaxis in abdominal or vaginal surgery. Am J Obstet Gynecol. 1988;158:742–3.

Smith BR, LeFrock JL, Thyrum PT, et al. Cefotetan pharmacokinetics in volunteers with various degrees of renal function. Antimicrob Agents Chemother. 1986;29:887–93.

Wright N, Wise R, Hegarty T. Cefotetan elimination in patients with varying degrees of renal dysfunction. J Antimicrob Chemother. 1983;11(Suppl A):213–6.

Yates RA, Cockshott ID, Houghton HL, Wardleworth A, Adam H, Donnelly RJ. Pharmacokinetics and dynamics of single intramuscular doses of cefotetan in normal Caucasian volunteers. J Antimicrob Chemother. 1983;11(Suppl A):207–12.

Dosage Adjustment of Medications Eliminated by the Kidneys

Cefotetan/Cefotan®   {**Antibacterial; second-generation cephalosporin**}

Usual initial dose: 2 g IV

Usual maintenance dose: 1–2 g IV every 12 h

Typical maximum dose: 6 g/day

Proportion eliminated unchanged: 75 %

Adjustment for Kidney Disease

FDA-approved product labeling: *Cefotetan dosage in patients with renal function impairment*

CrCL (mL/min)	Dose	Frequency
>30	Usual recommended dosage	Every 12 h
10–30	Usual recommended dosage	Every 24 h
<10	Usual recommended dosage	Every 48 h

Alternative adjustment:

GFR >50 mL/min	1–2 g IV every 12 h
GFR 10–50 mL/min	1–2 g IV every 24 h
GFR <10 mL/min	1–2 g IV every 48 h or 0.5 g IV every 24 h
Hemodialysis	1 g IV after hemodialysis on dialysis days only
CAPD	1 g IV daily
CRRT	1–2 g IV every 24 h

Dosage Adjustment of Medications Eliminated by the Kidneys

Cefoxitin - Selected References

Andriole VT. Pharmacokinetics of cephalosporins in patients with normal or reduced renal function. J Infect Dis. 1978;137(Suppl):S88–99.

Aronoff GA, Bennett WM, Berns JS, et al. Drug prescribing in renal failure: dosing guidelines for adults and children. 5th ed. Philadelphia: American College of Physicians; 2007.

Brumfitt W, Kosmidis J, Hamilton-Miller JMT, Gilchrist JNG. Cefoxitin and cephalothin: antimicrobial activity, human pharmacokinetics, and toxicology. Antimicrob Agents Chemother. 1974;6:290–9.

Garcia MJ, Dominguez-Gil A, Tabernero JM, Diaz Molina M. Pharmacokinetics of cefoxitin during haemofiltration. Eur J Clin Pharmacol. 1983;25:395–8.

Garcia MJ, Dominguez-Gil A, Tabernero JM, Sanchez Tomero JA. Pharmacokinetics of cefoxitin in patients with normal or impaired renal function. Eur J Clin Pharmacol. 1979;16:119–24.

Garcia MJ, Garcia A, Nieto MJ, Dominguez-Gil A, Alonso G, Mellado L. Disposition of cefoxitin in the elderly. Int J Clin Pharmacol Ther Toxicol. 1980;18:503–9.

Goodwin CS, Raftery EB, Goldberg AD, Skeggs H, Till AE, Martin CM. Effects of rate of infusion and probenecid on serum levels, renal excretion, and tolerance of intravenous doses of cefoxitin in humans: comparison with cephalothin. Antimicrob Agents Chemother. 1974;6:338–46.

Humbert G, Fillastre JP, Leroy A, Godin M, Van Winzum C. Pharmacokinetics of cefoxitin in normal subjects and in patients with renal insufficiency. Rev Infect Dis. 1979;1:118–26.

Kuang D, Verbine A, Ronco C. Pharmacokinetics and antimicrobial dosing adjustment in critically ill patients during continuous renal replacement therapy. Clin Nephrol. 2007;67:267–84.

McCue JD. Cefoxitin resistance in community-acquired gram-negative bacillary bacteremia: associated clinical factors. Arch Intern Med. 1985;145:834–6.

McIntyre CW, Owen PJ. Prescribing drugs in kidney disease. In: Brenner BM, editor. Brenner & Rector's the kidney. 8th ed. Philadelphia: Saunders Elsevier; 2008. p. 1930–55.

Mefoxin® injection [package insert]. Whitehouse Station: Merck & Co Inc; 2006.

Neu HC. Cefoxitin: an overview of clinical studies in the United States. Rev Infect Dis. 1979;1:233–9.

Olyaei AJ, Bennett WM. Drug dosing in elderly patients with chronic kidney disease. Clin Geriatr Med. 2009;25:459–527.

Olyaei AJ, Bennett WM. Pharmacologic approach to renal insufficiency. In: Dale DC, Federman DD, Antman K, editors. ACP medicine, WebMD June 2007 update. Hamilton: BC Decker; 2007; NEPHROLOGY IX: Appendix A1–25.

Olyaei AJ, DeMattos AM, Bennett WM. Use of drugs in patients with renal failure. In: Schrier RW, editor. Diseases of the kidney and urinary tract. 8th ed. Philadelphia: Lippincott Williams & Wilkins; 2007. p. 2765–807.

Sutter VL, Oberhammer I, Kwok Y-Y. Finegold SM. Susceptibility of anaerobes to cefoxitin and cephalothin. J Antimicrob Chemother. 1978;4(Suppl B):41–6.

Dosage Adjustment of Medications Eliminated by the Kidneys

<u>Cefoxitin</u>/Mefoxin® {**Antibacterial; second-generation cephalosporin**}

Usual initial dose:	1–2 g IV
Usual maintenance dose:	1–2 g IV every 6–8 h
Typical maximum dose:	2 g IV every 4 h or 3 g IV every 6 h
Proportion eliminated unchanged:	80 %

Adjustment for Kidney Disease

FDA-approved product labeling:

Maintenance cefoxitin dosage in adults with renal impairment

Renal function	CrCL (mL/min)	Dose (g)	Frequency
Mild impairment	30–50	1–2	Every 8–12 h
Moderate impairment	10–29	1–2	Every 12–24 h
Severe impairment	5–9	0.5–1	Every 12–24 h
Essentially anephric	<5	0.5–1	Every 24–48 h

Alternative adjustment:

GFR >50 mL/min	1–2 g IV every 6 h
GFR 10–50 mL/min	1–2 g IV every 8–12 h
GFR <10 mL/min	1–2 g IV every 12 h
Hemodialysis	As tabulated above plus 1–2 g IV after hemodialysis on dialysis days
CAPD	1 g IV every 24 h
CVVH	1–2 g IV every 12–18 h
CVVHD	1–2 g IV every 12 h
CVVHDF	1–2 g IV every 12 h

Dosage Adjustment of Medications Eliminated by the Kidneys

Cefpodoxime - Selected References

Backhouse C, Wade A, Williamson P, Tremblay D, Lenfant B. Multiple dose pharmacokinetics of cefpodoxime in young adult and elderly patients. J Antimicrob Chemother. 1990; 26(Suppl E):29–34.

Borin MT, Ferry JJ, Forbes KK, Hughes GS. Pharmacokinetics of cefpodoxime proxetil in healthy young and elderly volunteers. J Clin Pharmacol. 1994;34:774–81.

Borin MT, Hughes GS, Kelloway JS, Shapiro BE, Halstenson CE. Disposition of cefpodoxime proxetil in hemodialysis patients. J Clin Pharmacol. 1992;32:1038–44.

Borin MT, Hughes GS, Spillers CR, Patel RK. Pharmacokinetics of cefpodoxime in plasma and skin blister fluid following oral dosing of cefpodoxime proxetil. Antimicrob Agents Chemother. 1990;34:1094–9.

Dumont R, Guetat F, Andrews JM, Sultan E, Lenfant B. Concentrations of cefpodoxime in plasma and pleural fluid after a single oral dose of cefpodoxime proxetil. J Antimicrob Chemother. 1990;26(Suppl E):41–6.

Höffler D, Koeppe P, Corcilium M, Przyklink A. Cefpodoxime proxetil in patients with endstage renal failure on hemodialysis. Infection. 1990;18:157–62.

Johnson CA, Ateshkadi A, Zimmerman SW, et al. Pharmacokinetics and ex vivo susceptibility of cefpodoxime proxetil in patients receiving continuous ambulatory peritoneal dialysis. Antimicrob Agents Chemother. 1993;37:2650–55.

McIntyre CW, Owen PJ. Prescribing drugs in kidney disease. In: Brenner BM, editor. Brenner & Rector's the kidney. 8th ed. Philadelphia: Saunders Elsevier; 2008. p. 1930–55.

Olyaei AJ, Bennett WM. Pharmacologic approach to renal insufficiency. In: Dale DC, Federman DD, Antman K, editors. ACP medicine, WebMD June 2007 update. Hamilton: BC Decker; 2007; NEPHROLOGY IX: Appendix A1–25.

Olyaei AJ, Bennett WM. Drug dosing in elderly patients with chronic kidney disease. Clin Geriatr Med. 2009;25:459–527.

Olyaei AJ, DeMattos AM, Bennett WM. Use of drugs in patients with renal failure. In: Schrier RW, editor. Diseases of the kidney and urinary tract. 8th ed. Philadelphia: Lippincott Williams & Wilkins; 2007. p. 2765–807.

Phillips H, Van Hook CJ, Butler T, Todd WM. A comparison of cefpodoxime proxetil and cefaclor in the treatment of acute exacerbation of COPD in adults. Chest. 1993;104:1387–92.

Schatz BS, Karavokiros KT, Taeubel MA, Itokazu GS. Comparison of cefprozil, cefpodoxime proxetil, loracarbef, cefixime, and ceftibuten. Ann Pharmacother. 1996;30:258–68.

St Peter JV, Borin MT, Hughes GS, Kelloway JS, Shapiro BE, Halstenson CE. Disposition of cefpodoxime proxetil in healthy volunteers and patients with impaired renal function. Antimicrob Agents Chemother. 1992;36:126–31.

Vantin® tablet and suspension [package insert]. New York: Pharmacia & Upjohn Co division of Pfizer Inc; 2007.

Dosage Adjustment of Medications Eliminated by the Kidneys

<u>Cefpodoxime</u>/Vantin®　　　　　　{**Antibacterial; third-generation cephalosporin**}

Usual initial dose:	200 mg orally
Usual maintenance dose:	200 mg orally every 12 h
Typical maximum dose:	400 mg/day
Proportion eliminated unchanged:	50 %

Adjustment for Kidney Disease

FDA-approved product labeling:	*CrCL <30 mL/min*	*200 mg orally every 24 h*
	Hemodialysis	*200 mg orally 3 times/week after hemodialysis*
Alternative adjustment:	*GFR >50 mL/min*	*200 mg orally every 12 h*
	GFR 10–50 mL/min	*200 mg orally every 12 h*
	GFR <10 mL/min	*100 mg orally every 12 h*
	Hemodialysis	*100–200 mg orally every 12 h, dose after dialysis*
	CAPD	*100–200 mg orally every 12 h*
	CRRT	*Not applicable (consider an IV cephalosporin)*

Dosage Adjustment of Medications Eliminated by the Kidneys

Cefprozil - Selected References

Aronoff GA, Bennett WM, Berns JS, et al. Drug prescribing in renal failure: dosing guidelines for adults and children. 5th ed. Philadelphia: American College of Physicians; 2007.

Barbhaiya RH, Gleason CR, Shyu WC, Wilber RB, Martin RR, Pittman KA. Phase I study of single-dose BMY-28100, a new oral cephalosporin. Antimicrob Agents Chemother. 1990;34:202–5.

Barbhaiya RH, Shukla UA, Gleason CR, Shyu WC, Pittman KA. Comparison of the effects of food on the pharmacokinetics of cefprozil and cefaclor. Antimicrob Agents Chemother. 1990;34:1210–3.

Barriere SL. Pharmacology and pharmacokinetics of cefprozil. Clin Infect Dis. 1992;14(Suppl 2):S184–8.

Cefprozil tablet film coated and suspension [package insert]. Princeton: Sandoz Inc; 2008.

McIntyre CW, Owen PJ. Prescribing drugs in kidney disease. In: Brenner BM, editor. Brenner & Rector's the kidney. 8th ed. Philadelphia: Saunders Elsevier; 2008. p. 1930–55.

Nye K, O'Neill P, Andrews JM, Wise R. Pharmacokinetics and tissue penetration of cefprozil. J Antimicrob Chemother. 1990;25:831–5.

Shyu WC, Haddad J, Reilly J, et al. Penetration of cefprozil into middle ear fluid of patients with otitis media. Antimicrob Agents Chemother. 1994;38:2210–2.

Shyu WC, Pittman KA, Wilber RB, Matzke GR, Barbhaiya RH. Pharmacokinetics of cefprozil in healthy subjects and patients with renal impairment. J Clin Pharmacol. 1991;31:362–71.

Shyu WC, Shah VR, Campbell DA, Wilber RB, Pittman KA, Barbhaiya RH. Oral absolute bioavailability and intravenous dose-proportionality of cefprozil in humans. J Clin Pharmacol. 1992;32:798–302.

Shyu WC, Wilber RB, Pittman KA, Barbhaiya RH. Effect of antacid on the bioavailability of cefprozil. Antimicrob Agents Chemother. 1992;36:962–5.

Smith PF, Tsuji B, Booker BM, et al. Pharmacodynamics of cefprozil against Haemophilus influenzae in an in vitro pharmacodynamic model. Diagn Microbiol Infect Dis. 2006;56:379–86.

Tomatsu K, Ando S, Masuyoshi S, et al. In vitro and in vivo evaluations of BMY-28100, a new oral cephalosporin. J Antibiot (Tokyo). 1987;40:1175–83.

Wiseman LR, Benfield P. Cefprozil: a review of its antibacterial activity, pharmacokinetic properties, and therapeutic potential. Drugs. 1993;45:295–317.

Dosage Adjustment of Medications Eliminated by the Kidneys

<u>Cefprozil</u>/Cefzil®	{Antibacterial; second-generation cephalosporin}
Usual initial dose:	500 mg orally
Usual maintenance dose:	250–500 mg orally every 12–24 h
Typical maximum dose:	1,000 mg/day
Proportion eliminated unchanged:	65 %

Adjustment for Kidney Disease

FDA-approved product labeling: *Cefprozil dosing in renal impairment*

CrCL (mL/min)	Dosage	Dosing interval
30–120	*250–500 mg orally*	*Every 12–24 h*
0–29	*125–250 mg orally*	*Every 12–24 h*

Hemodialysis: 250–500 mg orally after completion of hemodialysis

Alternative adjustment:

GFR >50 mL/min	*250–500 mg orally every 24 h*
GFR 10–50 mL/min	*125–250 mg orally every 24 h*
GFR <10 mL/min	*125–250 mg orally every 24 h*
Hemodialysis	*125–250 mg orally every 24 h; administer supplemental 250 mg orally after hemodialysis on dialysis days.*
CAPD	*125–250 mg orally every 24 h*
CRRT	*Not applicable (consider an IV cephalosporin)*

Dosage Adjustment of Medications Eliminated by the Kidneys

Ceftaroline - Selected References

Biek D, Critchley IA, Riccobene TA, Thye DA. Ceftaroline fosamil: a novel broad-spectrum cephalosporin with expanded anti-gram-positive activity. J Antimicrob Chemother. 2010;65(Suppl 4):iv9–16.

Cédric J, Amador G, Caillon J, et al. Efficacy of the new cephalosporin ceftaroline in the treatment of experimental methicillin-resistant *Staphylococcus aureus* acute osteomyelitis. J Antimicrob Chemother. 2010;65:1749–52.

Corey GR, Wilcox M, Talbot GH, et al. Integrated analysis of CANVAS 1 and 2: phase 3, multicenter, randomized, double-blind studies to evaluate the safety and efficacy of ceftaroline versus vancomycin plus aztreonam in complicated skin and skin-structure infection. Clin Infect Dis. 2010;51:641–50.

Drusano G. Pharmacodynamics of ceftaroline fosamil for complicated skin and skin-structure infection: rationale for improved anti-methicillin-resistant Staphylococcus aureus activity. J Antimicrob Chemother. 2010;65(Suppl 4):iv33–9.

File TM Jr, Low DE, Eckburg PB, et al. FOCUS 1: a randomized, double-blinded, multicentre, phase III trial of the efficacy and safety of ceftaroline fosamil versus ceftriaxone in community-acquired pneumonia. J Antimicrob Chemother. 2010;65(Suppl 4):iv19–32.

Kaushik D, Rathi S, Jain A. Ceftaroline: a comprehensive update. Int J Antimicrob Agents. 2011;37:389–95.

Low DE, File TM Jr, Eckburg PB, et al. FOCUS 2: a randomized, double-blinded, multicentre, phase III trial of the efficacy and safety of ceftaroline fosamil versus ceftriaxone in community-acquired pneumonia. J Antimicrob Chemother. 2010;65(Suppl 4):iv33–44.

Rank DR, Friedland HD, Laudano JB. Integrated safety summary of FOCUS 1 and FOCUS 2 trials: phase III randomized, double-blind studies evaluating ceftaroline fosamil for the treatment of patients with community-acquired pneumonia. J Antimicrob Chemother. 2010;65(Suppl 4):iv53–9.

Saravolatz LD, Stein GE, Johnson LB. Ceftaroline: a novel cephalosporin with activity against methicillin-resistant Staphylococcus aureus. Clin Infect Dis. 2011;52:1156–63.

Steed ME, Rybak MJ. Ceftaroline: a new cephalosporin with activity against resistant gram-positive pathogens. Pharmacotherapy. 2010;30:375–89.

Teflaro™ injection [package insert]. St Louis: Forest Pharmaceuticals Inc; 2010.

Wilcox MH, Corey GR, Talbot GH, et al. CANVAS 2: the second phase III, randomized, double-blind study evaluating ceftaroline fosamil for the treatment of patients with complicated skin and skin structure infections. J Antimicrob Chemother. 2010;65(Suppl 4):iv53–65.

Zhanel GG, Sniezek G, Schweizer F, et al. Ceftaroline: a novel broad-spectrum cephalosporin with activity against methicillin-resistant Staphylococcus aureus. Drugs. 2009;69:809–31.

Dosage Adjustment of Medications Eliminated by the Kidneys

Ceftaroline/Teflaro™   {**Antibacterial; third-generation cephalosporin**}

Usual initial dose: 600 mg IV over 1 h

Usual maintenance dose: 600 mg IV over 1 h every 12 h

Typical maximum dose: 1,200 mg/day

Proportion eliminated unchanged: 50 %

Adjustment for Kidney Disease

FDA-approved product labeling: *Ceftaroline injection dosage in renal impairment*

Estimated CrCL (mL/min)	Ceftaroline recommended dosage regimen
>50 mL/min	600 mg IV every 12 h
>30 to ≤50 mL/min	400 mg IV every 12 h
≥15 to ≤30 mL/min	300 mg IV every 12 h
ESRD including hemodialysis	200 mg IV every 12 h

Alternative adjustment: *Renal impairment*   *Presently (May 2012), data not available*

CRRT   *Presently (May 2012), data not available*

Dosage Adjustment of Medications Eliminated by the Kidneys

Ceftazidime - Selected References

Angus BJ, Smith MD, Suputtamongkol Y, et al. Pharmacokinetic-pharmacodynamic evaluation of ceftazidime continuous infusion vs intermittent bolus injection in septicaemic melioidosis. Br J Clin Pharmacol. 2000;49:184–91.

Aronoff GA, Bennett WM, Berns JS, et al. Drug prescribing in renal failure: dosing guidelines for adults and children. 5th ed. Philadelphia: American College of Physicians; 2007.

Berkhout J, Visser LG, van den Broek PJ, van de Klundert JAM, Mattie H. Clinical pharmacokinetics of cefamandole and ceftazidime by continuous intravenous infusion. Antimicrob Agents Chemother. 2003;47:1862–6.

Buijk SLCE, Gyssens IC, Mouton JW, Van Vliet A, Verbrugh HA, Bruining HA. Pharmacokinetics of ceftazidime in serum and peritoneal exudate during continuous versus intermittent administration to patients with severe intra-abdominal infections. J Antimicrob Chemother. 2002;49:121–8.

Dailly E, Brun A, Kergueris M-F, Victorri-Vignoli C, Milpied N, Jolliet P. A simple formula for individualising ceftazidime dosage administered by continuous infusion in patients with haematological malignancies. Int J Antimicrob Agents. 2006;27:553–6.

Fillastre JP, Humbert G, Olier B, Leguy F, Borsa F, Spenser GR. Pharmacokinetics of ceftazidime in renal failure [letter]. J Antimicrob Chemother. 1983;11:487–8.

Georges B, Conil, J-M, Seguin T, et al. Population pharmacokinetics of ceftazidime in intensive care unit patients: influence of glomerular filtration rate, mechanical ventilation, and reason for admission. Antimicrob Agents Chemother. 2009;53:4483–9.

Gravert C, Schulz E, Sack K. Ceftazidime in intensive care medicine and hemofiltration. J Antimicrob Chemother. 1983;12(Suppl A):177–80.

Heintz BH, Matzke GR, Dager WF. Antimicrobial dosing concepts and recommendations for critically ill adult patients receiving continuous renal replacement therapy or intermittent hemodialysis. Pharmacotherapy. 2009;29:562–77.

Highet VS, Forrest A, Ballow CH, Schentag JJ. Antibiotic dosing issues in lower respiratory tract infection: population-derived area under inhibitory curve is predictive of efficacy. J Antimicrob Chemother. 1999;43(Suppl A):55–63.

Höffler D, Koeppe P, Williams KJ. The pharmacokinetics of ceftazidime in normal and impaired renal function. J Antimicrob Chemother. 1983;12(Suppl A):241–45.

Kim K, Hwang Y-H, Ro H, et al. Pharmacokinetic profiles of intravenous ceftazidime administration in patients undergoing automated peritoneal dialysis. Antimicrob Agents Chemother. 2011;55:2523–7.

Mariat C, Venet C, Jehl F, et al. Continuous infusion of ceftazidime in critically ill patients undergoing continuous venovenous haemodiafiltration: pharmacokinetic evaluation and dose recommendation. Crit Care. 2006;10:R26. doi:10.1186/cc3993.

Matzke GR, Frye RF, Joy MS, Palevsky PM. Determinants of ceftazidime clearance by continuous venovenous hemofiltration and continuous venovenous hemodialysis. Antimicrob Agents Chemother. 2000;44:1639–44.

McKinnon PS, Paladino JA, Schentag JJ. Evaluation of area under the inhibitory curve (AUIC) and time above the minimum inhibitory concentration (T > MIC) as predictors of outcome for cefepime and ceftazidime n serious bacterial infections. Int J Antimicrob Agents. 2008;31:345–51.

Norrby SR, Burman LÅ, Linderholm H, Trollfors B. Ceftazidime: pharmacokinetics in patients and effect on the renal function. J Antimicrob Chemother. 1982;10:199–206.

Tazicef® injection [package insert]. Lake Forest: Hospira Worldwide Inc; 2004.

Tourkantonis A, Nicolaidis P. Pharmacokinetics of ceftazidime in patients undergoing peritoneal dialysis. J Antimicrob Chemother. 1983;12(Suppl A):263–7.

Trotman RL, Williamson JC, Shoemaker M, Salzer WL. Antibiotic dosing in critically ill adult patients receiving continuous renal replacement therapy. Clin Infect Dis. 2005;41:1159–66.

Warns H, Lode H, Harnoss CM, Kemmerich B, Koeppe P, Wagner J. Multiple dose pharmacokinetics and therapeutic results with ceftazidime. J Antimicrob Chemother. 1983;12(Suppl A):235–40.

Welage LS, Schultz RW, Schentag JJ. Pharmacokinetics of ceftazidime in patients with renal insufficiency. Antimicrob Agents Chemother. 1984;25:201–4.

Dosage Adjustment of Medications Eliminated by the Kidneys

Ceftazidime/Fortaz®, Tazicef®	{**Antibacterial; third-generation cephalosporin**}
Usual initial dose:	2 g IV
Usual maintenance dose:	1–2 g IV every 8 h or 6 g/24 h continuous IV infusion
Typical maximum dose:	6 g/day
Proportion eliminated unchanged:	85 %

Adjustment for Kidney Disease

FDA-approved product labeling: *Ceftazidime dosage in renal impairment*

CrCL (mL/min)	*Dose (g)*	*Frequency of dosing*
31–50	*1–1.5*	*Every 12 h*
16–30	*1–1.5*	*Every 24 h*
6–15	*0.5–0.75*	*Every 24 h*
<5	*0.5–0.75*	*Every 48 h*

Hemodialysis: 1 g IV followed by 1 g IV after each hemodialysis
CAPD: 1 g IV followed by 500 mg IV every 24 h

Alternative adjustment:

GFR >50 mL/min	*1–2 g IV every 8 h or 6g/24 h continuous IV infusion*
GFR 10–50 mL/min	*1–2 g IV every 12–24 h or 0.6–1.2 mg/kg/min continuous IV infusion*
GFR <10 mL/min	*0.5–1 g IV every 24 h or 0.3 mg/kg/min continuous IV infusion*
Hemodialysis	*0.5–1 g IV every 24 h; administer after hemodialysis on dialysis days or give supplemental 1 g IV after each dialysis.*
CAPD	*0.5 g IV every 24 h or 0.25 g/2 L dialysate*
Automated PD	*15 mg/kg IV every 24 h or 20 mg/kg intraperitoneally during long off-cycler dwell*
CVVH	*1–2 g IV every 12 h*
CVVHD	*2 g IV every 12 h*
CVVHDF	*2 g IV every 12 h (consider 2 g IV every 8 h for gram-negative pathogens with MIC ≥4 mg/L) or 3 g/24 h continuous IV infusion*

Ceftibuten - Selected References

Aronoff GA, Bennett WM, Berns JS, et al. Drug prescribing in renal failure: dosing guidelines for adults and children. 5th ed. Philadelphia: American College of Physicians; 2007.

Barr WH, Lin C-C, Radwanski E, Lim J, Symchowicz S, Affrime M. The pharmacokinetics of ceftibuten in humans. Diagn Microbiol Infect Dis. 1991;14:93–100.

Bressolle F, Galtier M, Kinowski JM, et al. Multiple-dose pharmacokinetics of ceftibuten after oral administration to healthy volunteers. J Pharm Sci. 1994;83:1236–40.

Cedax® capsule and powder for oral suspension [package insert]. Atlanta: Sciele Pharma Inc; 2009.

Kelloway JS, Awni WM, Lin CC, et al. Pharmacokinetics of ceftibuten-*cis* and its *trans* metabolite in healthy volunteers and in patients with chronic renal insufficiency. Antimicrob Agents Chemother. 1991;35:2267–74.

Lin C, Lim J, Radwanski E, Marco A, Affrime M. Pharmacokinetics and dose proportionality of ceftibuten in men. Antimicrob Agents Chemother. 1995;39:359–61.

Lin C, Radwanski E, Affrime M, Cayen MN. Multiple-dose pharmacokinetics of ceftibuten in healthy volunteers. Antimicrob Agents Chemother. 1995;39:356–8.

McIntyre CW, Owen PJ. Prescribing drugs in kidney disease. In: Brenner BM, editor. Brenner & Rector's the kidney. 8th ed. Philadelphia: Saunders Elsevier; 2008. p. 1930–55.

Onyeji CO, Nicolau DP, Nightingale CH, Quintillani R. Optimal times above MICs of ceftibuten and cefaclor in experimental intra-abdominal infections. Antimicrob Agents Chemother. 1994;38:1112–7.

Wise R, Nye K, O'Neill P, Wostenholme M, Andrews JM. Pharmacokinetics and tissue penetration of ceftibuten. Antimicrob Agents Chemother. 1990;34:1053–5.

Dosage Adjustment of Medications Eliminated by the Kidneys

<u>**Ceftibuten**</u>/Cedax® **{Antibacterial; third-generation cephalosporin}**

Usual initial dose: 400 mg orally

Usual maintenance dose: 400 mg orally once daily for 10 days

Typical maximum dose: 400 mg/day

Proportion eliminated unchanged: 65 %

Adjustment for Kidney Disease

FDA-approved product labeling: *Ceftibuten dosing in renal impairment*

CrCL (mL/min)	Recommended dosing schedule
>50	9 mg/kg or 400 mg every 24 h
30–49	4.5 mg/kg or 200 mg every 24 h
5–29	2.25 mg/kg or 100 mg every 24 h

Hemodialysis: 400 mg or 9 mg/kg (maximum 400 mg) orally after each hemodialysis

Alternative adjustment:

GFR >50 mL/min	*400 mg orally every 24 h*
GFR 10–50 mL/min	*200 mg orally every 24 h (50 % decrease)*
GFR <10 mL/min	*100 mg orally every 24 h (75 % decrease)*
Hemodialysis	*400 mg orally three times weekly or after each dialysis*
CAPD	*100 mg orally every 24 h*
CRRT	*Not applicable (consider an IV cephalosporin)*

Dosage Adjustment of Medications Eliminated by the Kidneys

Ceftizoxime - Selected References

Amsden GW. Tables of antimicrobial agent pharmacology. In: Mandell GL, Bennett JE, Dolin R, editors. Mandell, Douglas, and Bennett's principles and practice of infectious diseases, vol 1. 6th ed. Philadelphia: Elsevier; 2005. p. 634–700.

Burgess ED, Blair AD. Pharmacokinetics of ceftizoxime in patients undergoing continuous ambulatory peritoneal dialysis. Antimicrob Agents Chemother. 1983;24:237–9.

Cefizox® injection [package insert]. Deerfield: Fujisawa Healthcare Inc; 2007.

Cutler RE, Blair AD, Burgess ED, Parks D. Pharmacokinetics of ceftizoxime. J Antimicrob Chemother. 1982;10 (Suppl C):91–7.

Dubb J, Actor P, Pitkin D, et al. Ceftizoxime kinetics and renal handling. Clin Pharmacol Ther. 1982;31:516–21.

Gross ML, Somani P, Ribner BS, Raeader R, Freimer EH, Higgins JR Jr. Ceftizoxime elimination kinetics in continuous ambulatory peritoneal dialysis. Clin Pharmacol Ther. 1983;34:673–80.

Gundert-Remy U, Hildebrandt R, Stiehl A, Schlegel P. Pharmacokinetics of ceftizoxime. Eur J Clin Pharmacol. 1985;28:463–7.

Imada A, Itagaki N, Hasegawa H, Horiuchi A. Comparative study of the pharmacokinetics of various β-lactams after intravenous and intraperitoneal administration in patients undergoing continuous ambulatory peritoneal dialysis. Drugs. 1988;35(Suppl 2):82–7.

Johnson CA, Zimmerman SW, Bayer W, Craig WA. Pharmacokinetics of intravenous ceftizoxime in patients on continuous ambulatory peritoneal dialysis. Clin Nephrol. 1985;23:120–4.

Johnson CA, Zimmerman SW, Rogge M. The pharmacokinetics of antibiotics used to treat peritoneal dialysis-associated peritonitis. Am J Kidney Dis. 1984;4:3–17.

Kowalsky SF, Echols RM, Venezia AR, Andrews EA. Pharmacokinetics of ceftizoxime in subjects with various degrees of renal function. Antimicrob Agents Chemother. 1983;24:151–5.

McIntyre CW, Owen PJ. Prescribing drugs in kidney disease. In: Brenner BM, editor. Brenner & Rector's the kidney. 8th ed. Philadelphia: Saunders Elsevier; 2008. p. 1930–55.

Neuhauser MM, McKinnon PS, Hershberger E, Rybak MJ. Pharmacokinetics and pharmacodynamics of ceftizoxime in patients with dosages adjusted for renal function. Pharmacotherapy. 2000;20:554–61.

Ohkawa M, Okasho A, Sugata T, Kuroda K. Elimination kinetics of ceftizoxime in humans with and without renal insufficiency. Antimicrob Agents Chemother. 1982;22:308–11.

Peterson LR, Gerding DN, van Etta LL, Eckfeldt, Larson TA. Pharmacokinetics, protein binding, and extracellular distribution of ceftizoxime in normal subjects. Antimicrob Agents Chemother. 1982;22:878–81.

Quintillani R, Nightingale CH. Comparative pharmacokinetics of ceftizoxime and other third-generation cephalosporins in humans. J Antimicrob Chemother. 1982;10(Suppl C):99–104.

Sánchez-Navarro A, Colino C-I, Sánchez Recio MM. A retrospective analysis of pharmacokinetic-pharmacodynamic parameters as indicators of the clinical efficacy of ceftizoxime. Clin Pharmacokinet. 2001;40:125–34.

Dosage Adjustment of Medications Eliminated by the Kidneys

Ceftizoxime/Cefizox® {**Antibacterial; third-generation cephalosporin**}

Usual initial dose:	1,000–2,000 mg IV
Usual maintenance dose:	1,000–2,000 mg IV every 8–12 h
Typical maximum dose:	12,000 mg/day
Proportion eliminated unchanged:	57–93 %

Adjustment for Kidney Disease

FDA-approved product labeling: *Ceftizoxime dosing in renal impairment (severe/life-threatening infection)*

CrCL (mL/min)	Dosage (mg)	Dosing interval
50–79	750–1,500	Every 8 h
5–49	500–1,000	Every 12 h

Hemodialysis (CrCL <4 mL/min): 500–1,000 mg every 48 h or 500 mg every 24 h. In patients undergoing hemodialysis, no additional supplemental dosing is required following hemodialysis; however, dosing should be timed so that the patient receives the dose at the end of dialysis

Alternative adjustment:

GFR >50 mL/min	*1–2 g IV every 8–12 h*
GFR 10–50 mL/min	*1 g IV every 8–12 h*
GFR <10 mL/min	*500–1,000 mg IV every 24 h*
Hemodialysis	*500 mg IV every 24 h; administer after hemodialysis on dialysis days.*
CAPD	*1 g IV every 24 h or 3 g IV every 48 h*
CRRT	*500–1,000 mg IV every 12 h*

Dosage Adjustment of Medications Eliminated by the Kidneys

Cefuroxime Axetil - Selected References

Aronoff GA, Bennett WM, Berns JS, et al. Drug prescribing in renal failure: dosing guidelines for adults and children. 5th ed. Philadelphia: American College of Physicians; 2007.

Ceftin® tablet and oral suspension [package insert]. Research Triangle Park: GlaxoSmithKline, 2010.

Cox CE, Sherrill JM, Cocchetto DM. Evaluation of cefuroxime axetil, cefaclor, and cephalexin in the treatment of urinary tract infections in adults. Curr Ther Res. 1987;42:124–37.

Fong IW, Linton W, Simbul M, Hinton NA. Comparative clinical efficacy of single oral doses of cefuroxime axetil and amoxicillin in uncomplicated gonococcal infections. Antimicrob Agents Chemother. 1986;30:321–2.

Gottlieb A, Mills J. Cefuroxime axetil for treatment of uncomplicated gonorrhea. Antimicrob Agents Chemother. 1986;30:333–4.

Hebblethwaite EM, Brown GW, Cox DM. A comparison of the efficacy and safety of cefuroxime axetil and Augmentin in the treatment of upper respiratory infections. Drugs Exp Clin Res. 1987;13:91–4.

Iravani A, Richard GA. Single-dose cefuroxime axetil versus multiple-dose cefaclor in the treatment of acute urinary tract infections. Antimicrob Agents Chemother. 1989;33:1212–6.

Konishi K, Suzuki H, Hayashi M, Saruta T. Pharmacokinetics of cefuroxime axetil in patients with normal and impaired renal function. J Antimicrob Chemother. 1993;31:413–20.

Marx MA, Fant WK. Cefuroxime axetil. Drug Intell Clin Pharm. 1988;22:651–8.

McIntyre CW, Owen PJ. Prescribing drugs in kidney disease. In: Brenner BM, editor. Brenner & Rector's the kidney. 8th ed. Philadelphia: Saunders Elsevier; 2008. p. 1930–55.

Olyaei AJ, Bennett WM. Drug dosing in elderly patients with chronic kidney disease. Clin Geriatr Med. 2009;25:459–527.

Olyaei AJ, Bennett WM. Pharmacologic approach to renal insufficiency. In: Dale DC, Federman DD, Antman K, editors. ACP medicine, WebMD June 2007 update. Hamilton: BC Decker; 2007; NEPHROLOGY IX: Appendix A1–25.

Olyaei AJ, DeMattos AM, Bennett WM. Use of drugs in patients with renal failure. In: Schrier RW, editor. Diseases of the kidney and urinary tract. 8th ed. Philadelphia: Lippincott Williams & Wilkins; 2007. p. 2765–807.

Pistos C, Michalea S, Kalovidouris M, Kontopoulos G, Georgarakis M. Bioequivalence evaluation of 2 brands of cefuroxime axetil 250 mg tablets in healthy human volunteers. Int J Clin Pharmacol Ther. 2004;42:367–72.

Reichman RC, Nolte FS, Wolinsky SM, Greisberger CA, Trupei MA, Nitzkin J. Single-dose cefuroxime axetil in the treatment of uncomplicated gonorrhea: a controlled trial. Sex Transm Dis. 1985;12:184–7.

Ridgway E, Stewart K, Rai G, Kelsey MC, Bielawska C. The pharmacokinetics of cefuroxime axetil in the sick elderly patient. J Antimicrob Chemother. 1991;27:663–8.

Ruiz-Carretero P, Merino-Sanjuán M, Nácher A, Casabó VG. Pharmacokinetic models for the saturable absorption of cefuroxime axetil and saturable elimination of cefuroxime. Eur J Pharm Sci. 2004;21:217–23.

Schleupner CJ, Anthony WC, Tan J, et al. Blinded comparison of cefuroxime to cefaclor for lower respiratory tract infections. Arch Intern Med. 1988;148:343–8.

Sommers DK, van Wyk M, Williams PEO, Harding SM. Pharmacokinetics and tolerance of cefuroxime axetil in volunteers during repeated dosing. Antimicrob Agents Chemother. 1984;25:244–7.

Spencer RC, Griggs JV, Brown GW. A dose-ranging study of cefuroxime axetil in the treatment of lower respiratory tract infections in general practice. Drugs Exp Clin Res. 1987;13:101–3.

Williams PEO, Harding SM. The absolute bioavailability of oral cefuroxime axetil in male and female volunteers after fasting and after food. J Antimicrob Chemother. 1984;13:191–6.

Williams KJ, Hebblethwaite EM, Brown GW, Cox DM, Plested SJ. Cefuroxime axetil in the treatment of uncomplicated UTI: a comparison with cefaclor and Augmentin. Drugs Exp Clin Res. 1987;13:95–9.

Dosage Adjustment of Medications Eliminated by the Kidneys

Cefuroxime Axetil/Ceftin®   {**Antibacterial; second-generation cephalosporin**}

Usual initial dose:	500 mg orally
Usual maintenance dose:	250–500 mg orally twice daily with meals
Typical maximum dose:	1,000 mg/day
Proportion eliminated unchanged:	65 %

Adjustment for Kidney Disease

FDA-approved product labeling: *The safety and efficacy of cefuroxime axetil in patients with renal failure have not been established. Since cefuroxime is renally eliminated, its half-life will be prolonged in patients with renal failure.*

Alternative adjustment:

eCrCL >30 mL/min	*250–500 mg orally twice daily with meals*
eCrCL 10–29 mL/min	*250–500 mg orally every 24 h*
eCrCL <10 mL/min	*250–500 mg orally every 48 h*
Hemodialysis	*250–500 mg orally every 24 h; administer after hemodialysis on dialysis days.*
CAPD	*250–500 mg orally every 48 h*
CRRT	*Not applicable (consider an IV cephalosporin)*

Dosage Adjustment of Medications Eliminated by the Kidneys

Cefuroxime Sodium - Selected References

Aronoff GA, Bennett WM, Berns JS, et al. Drug prescribing in renal failure: dosing guidelines for adults and children. 5th ed. Philadelphia: American College of Physicians; 2007.

Broekhuysen J, Deger F, Douchamps J, et al. Pharmacokinetic study of cefuroxime in the elderly. Br J Clin Pharmacol. 1981;12:801–5.

Bundtzen RW, Toothaker RD, Nielson OS, Madsen PO, Welling PG, Craig WA. Pharmacokinetics of cefuroxime in normal and impaired renal function: comparison of high-pressure liquid chromatography and microbiological assays. Antimicrob Agents Chemother. 1981;19:443–9.

Cantu TG. Cefuroxime dosage in renal failure [letter]. Ann Intern Med. 1988;109:989–90.

Chan MK, Browning AK, Poole CJM, et al. Cefuroxime pharmacokinetics in continuous and intermittent peritoneal dialysis. Nephron. 1985;41:161–5.

Cockram CS, Richards P, Bax RP. The safety of cefuroxime and gentamicin in patients with reduced renal function. Curr Med Res Opin. 1980;6:398–403.

Crenshaw CA, Glanges E, Webber CE Jr, McReynolds DB. Single-dose cefuroxime versus multiple-dose cefamandole for prophylaxis in general surgical procedures. Hosp Formul. 1989;24(Suppl C):28–31.

Edwards MS, Baker CJ, Butler KM, Mason EO Jr, Laurent JP, Cheek WR. Penetration of cefuroxime into ventricular fluid in cerebrospinal fluid shunt infections. Antimicrob Agents Chemother. 1989;33:1108–10.

Foord RD. Cefuroxime: human pharmacokinetics. Antimicrob Agents Chemother. 1976;9:741–7.

Goddard JK, Janning SW, Gass JS, Wilson RE. Cefuroxime-induced renal failure. Pharmacotherapy. 1994;14:488–91.

Gold B, Rodriguez WJ. Cefuroxime: mechanisms of action, antimicrobial activity, pharmacokinetics, clinical applications, adverse reactions and therapeutic indications. Pharmacotherapy. 1983;3:82–100.

Gower PE, Dash CH. The pharmacokinetics of cefuroxime after intravenous injection. Eur J Clin Pharmacol. 1977;12:221–7.

Gower PE, Kennedy MRK, Dash CH. The effect of renal failure and dialysis on the pharmacokinetics of cefuroxime. Proc R Soc Med. 1977;70(Suppl 9):151–7.

Höffler D, Sassman M. Pharmacokinetic studies of cefuroxime dosage recommendations in patients with impaired renal function. Proc R Soc Med. 1977;70(Suppl 9):144–7.

Kosmidis J, Stathakis C, Anyfantis A, Daikos GK. Cefuroxime in renal insufficiency: therapeutic results and pharmacokinetics including effects of dialysis. Proc R Soc Med. 1977;70(Suppl 9):139–43.

Leong CL, Thiruventhiran T. Cefuroxime-induced acute renal failure [letter]. Nephron. 2000;84:185.

Local FK, Munro AJ, Kerr DNS, Sussman M. Pharmacokinetics and intraperitoneal cefuroxime in patients undergoing peritoneal dialysis. Clin Nephrol. 1981;16:40–3.

McIntosh ME, Smith WGJ, Junor RJR, Forrest G, Brodie MJ. Increased peritoneal permeability in patients with peritonitis undergoing continuous ambulatory peritoneal dialysis. Eur J Clin Pharmacol. 1985;28:187–91.

Slama TG, Sklar SJ, Misinski J, Fess SW. Randomized comparison of cefamandole, cefazolin, and cefuroxime prophylaxis in open-heart surgery. Hosp Formul. 1989;24(Suppl C):16–20.

van Dalen R, Vree TB, Hafkenscheid JCM, Gimbrère JSF. Determination of plasma and renal clearance of cefuroxime and its pharmacokinetics in renal insufficiency. J Antimicrob Chemother. 1979;5:281–92.

Verhagen CA, Mattie H, Van Strijen E. The renal clearance of cefuroxime and ceftazidime and the effect of probenecid on their tubular excretion. Br J Clin Pharmacol.1994;37:193–7.

Walstad RA, Nilsen OG, Berg KJ. Pharmacokinetics and clinical effects of cefuroxime in patients with severe renal insufficiency. Eur J Clin Pharmacol. 1983;24:391–8.

Weiss LG, Cars O, Danielson BG, Grahnen A, Wikström B. Pharmacokinetics of intravenous cefuroxime during intermittent and continuous arteriovenous hemofiltration. Clin Nephrol. 1988;30:282–6.

Zinacef® injection [package insert]. Research Triangle Park: GlaxoSmithKline; 2009.

Dosage Adjustment of Medications Eliminated by the Kidneys

Cefuroxime Sodium/Zinacef®   {Antibacterial; second-generation cephalosporin}

Usual initial dose: 750–1,500 mg IV

Usual maintenance dose: 750 mg to 1,500 mg IV every 8 h

Typical maximum dose: 9 g/day IV

Proportion eliminated unchanged: 90 %

Adjustment for Kidney Disease

FDA-approved product labeling: *Cefuroxime dosing in renal impairment*

CrCL (mL/min)	Recommended dosing schedule
>20	750–1,500 mg every 8 h
10–20	750 mg every 24 h
<10	750 mg every 24 h

Hemodialysis: 750 mg every 24 h; give after hemodialysis on dialysis days

Alternative adjustment:

GFR >50 mL/min	750–1,500 mg IV every 8 h
GFR 10–50 mL/min	750–1,500 mg IV every 8–12 h
GFR <10 mL/min	750 mg IV every 24 h
Hemodialysis	750 mg IV every 24 h; administer after hemodialysis on dialysis days.
CAPD	750 mg IV every 24 h
CRRT	1,500 mg IV once followed by 750 mg IV every 12 h

Celecoxib - Selected References

Ahmad SR, Kortepeter C, Brinker A, Chen M, Beitz J. Renal failure associated with the use of celecoxib and rofecoxib. Drug Saf. 2002;25:537–44.

Alper AB Jr, Meleg-Smith S, Krane K. Nephrotic syndrome and interstitial nephritis associated with celecoxib. Am J Kidney Dis. 2002;40:1086–90.

Celebrex® capsule [package insert]. New York: GD Searle LLC division of Pfizer Inc; 2011.

Cherney DZI, Miller JA, Scholery JW, et al. The effect of cyclooxygenase-2 inhibition on renal hemodynamic function in humans with type 1 diabetes. Diabetes. 2008;57:688–95.

Clifford TM, Pajoumand M, Johnston TD. Celecoxib-induced nephrotoxicity in a renal transplant recipient. Pharmacotherapy. 2005;25:773–7.

Davies NM, McLachlan AJ, Day RO, Williams KM. Clinical pharmacokinetics and pharmacodynamics of celecoxib, a selective cyclo-oxygenase-2 inhibitor. Clin Pharmacokinet. 2000;38:225–42.

Esteve J-B, Launay-Vacher V, Brocheriou I, Grimaldi A, Izzedine H. COX-2 inhibitors and acute interstitial nephritis: case report and review of the literature. Clin Nephrol. 2005;63:385–9.

Harirforoosh S, Aghazadeh-Habashi A, Jamali F. Extent of renal effect of cyclo-oxygenase-2-selective inhibitors is pharmacokinetic dependent. Clin Exp Pharmacol Physiol. 2006;33:917–24.

Hermann M, Shaw S, Kiss E, et al. Selective COX-2 inhibitors and renal injury in salt-sensitive hypertension. Hypertension. 2005;45:193–7.

Markowitz GS, Falkowitz DC, Isom R, et al. Membranous glomerulopathy and acute interstitial nephritis following treatment with celecoxib. Clin Nephrol. 2003;59:137–42.

Moore RA, Derry S, Makinson GT, McQuay HJ. Tolerability and adverse events in clinical trials of celecoxib in osteoarthritis and rheumatoid arthritis: systematic review and meta-analysis of information from company clinical trial reports. Arthritis Res Ther. 2005;7:R644–65.

Noroian G, Clive D. Cyclo-oxygenase-2 inhibitors and the kidney: a case for caution. Drug Saf. 2002;25:166–72.

Schneider V, Lévesque LE, Zhang B, Hutchinson T, Brophy JM. Association of selective and conventional nonsteroidal antiinflammatory drugs with acute renal failure: a population-based, nested case–control study. Am J Epidemiol. 2006;164:881–9.

Schwartz JI, Vandormael K, Malice MP, et al. Comparison of rofecoxib, celecoxib, and naproxen on renal function in elderly subjects receiving a normal-salt diet. Clin Pharmacol Ther. 2002;72:50–61.

Zhang J, Ding EL, Song Y. Adverse effects of cyclooxygenase 2 inhibitors on renal and arrhythmia events: meta-analysis of randomized trials. JAMA. 2006;296:1619–32.

Dosage Adjustment of Medications Eliminated by the Kidneys

<u>Celecoxib</u>/Celebrex®

{Anti-inflammatory; nonsteroidal anti-inflammatory drug; selective cyclooxygenase (COX)-2 inhibitor}

Usual initial dose: 200 mg orally

Usual maintenance dose: 100–200 mg orally once or twice daily

Typical maximum dose: 400 mg/day

Proportion eliminated unchanged: 3 % as unchanged drug, ~30 % as minimally active primary metabolite

Adjustment for Kidney Disease

FDA-approved product labeling: *Severe renal insufficiency*   *Use not recommended*

Alternative adjustment: *GFR <30 mL/min*   *Minimal data available. Preferably avoid due to risk for renal and/or gastrointestinal toxicity; if indeed necessary, begin with low doses and monitor carefully.*

Cephalexin - Selected References

Abramowicz M, Zuccotti G, Pflomm J-M, et al., editors. Handbook of antimicrobial therapy. 19th ed. New Rochelle: The Medical Letter; 2011.

Androle VT. Pharmacokinetics of cephalosporins in patients with normal and reduced renal function. J Infect Dis. 1978;137(Suppl):S88–99.

Aronoff GA, Bennett WM, Berns JS, et al. Drug prescribing in renal failure: dosing guidelines for adults and children. 5th ed. Philadelphia: American College of Physicians; 2007.

Brogard JM, Pinget M, Dorner M, Lavillaureix J. Determination of cefalexin pharmacokinetics and dosage adjustments in relation to renal function. J Clin Pharmacol. 1975;15:666–73.

Bunke CM, Aronoff GR, Brier ME, Sloan RS, Luft FC. Cefazolin and cephalexin kinetics in continuous ambulatory peritoneal dialysis. Clin Pharmacol Ther. 1983;33:66–72.

Bunke CM, Aronoff GR, Luft FC. Pharmacokinetics of common antibiotics used in continuous ambulatory peritoneal dialysis. Am J Kidney Dis. 1983;3:114–7.

Burt RAP. A review of the drug events reported by 12,917 patients treated with cephalexin. Postgrad Med J. 1983;59(Suppl):47–50.

Drew PJT, Casewell MW, Desai N, Houang ET, Simpson CN, Marsh FP. Cephalexin for the treatment of CAPD peritonitis. J Antimicrob Chemother. 1984;13:153–9.

Greene DS, Flanagan DR, Quintilani R, Nightingale CH. Pharmacokinetics of cephalexin: an evaluation of one- and two-compartment model pharmacokinetics. J Clin Pharmacol. 1976;16:257–64.

Hori R, Okumura K, Kamiya A, Nihira H, Nakano H. Ampicillin and cephalexin in renal insufficiency. Clin Pharmacol Ther. 1983;34:792–8.

Johnson CA, Zimmerman SW, Rogge M. The pharmacokinetics of antibiotics used to treat peritoneal dialysis-associated with peritonitis. Am J Kidney Dis. 1984;4:3–17.

Keflex® capsules [package insert]. Germantown: Advancis Pharmaceutical Corp; 2006.

Kirby WMM, Regamy C. Pharmacokinetics of cefazolin compared with four other cephalosporins. J Infect Dis. 1973;128(Suppl):S341–6.

Liu R, Tang AMY, Tan Yl, Limenta LMG, Lee EJD. Effects of sodium bicarbonate and ammonium chloride pre-treatment on PEPT2 (SLC15A2) mediated renal clearance of cephalexin in healthy subjects. Drug Metab Pharmacokinet. 2011;26:87–93.

Lode H, Stahlmann R, Koeppe P. Comparative pharmacokinetics of cephalexin, cefaclor, cefadroxil, and CGP 9000. Antimicrob Agents Chemother. 1979;16:1–6.

McIntyre CW, Owen PJ. Prescribing drugs in kidney disease. In: Brenner BM, editor. Brenner & Rector's the kidney. 8th ed. Philadelphia: Saunders Elsevier; 2008. p. 1930–55.

Olyaei AJ, Bennett WM. Drug dosing in elderly patients with chronic kidney disease. Clin Geriatr Med. 2009;25:459–527.

Olyaei AJ, Bennett WM. Pharmacologic approach to renal insufficiency. In: Dale DC, Federman DD, Antman K, editors. ACP medicine, WebMD June 2007 update. Hamilton: BC Decker; 2007; NEPHROLOGY IX: Appendix A1–25.

Olyaei AJ, DeMattos AM, Bennett WM. Use of drugs in patients with renal failure. In: Schrier RW, editor. Diseases of the kidney and urinary tract. 8th ed. Philadelphia: Lippincott Williams & Wilkins; 2007. p. 2765–807.

Pfeffer M, Jackson A, Ximenes J, Perche de Menezes J. Comparative human oral clinical pharmacology of cefadroxil, cephalexin, and cephradine. Antimicrob Agents Chemother. 1977;11:331–8.

Spyker DA, Thomas BL, Sande MA, Bolton WK. Pharmacokinetics of cefaclor and cephalexin: dosage nomograms for impaired renal function. Antimicrob Agents Chemother. 1978;14:172–7.

Sullivan JW Bueschen AJ, Schlegel JU. Nitrofurantoin, sulfamethoxazole and cephalexin urinary concentration in unequally functioning pyelonephritic kidneys. J Urol. 1975;114:343–7.

Dosage Adjustment of Medications Eliminated by the Kidneys

<u>Cephalexin</u>/Keflex® {**Antibacterial; first-generation cephalosporin**}

Usual initial dose:	500 mg orally
Usual maintenance dose:	1–4 g/day orally in divided doses
Typical maximum dose:	4 g/day
Proportion eliminated unchanged:	96 %

Adjustment for Kidney Disease

FDA-approved product labeling: *Administer with caution in the presence of markedly impaired renal function. Under such conditions, careful clinical observation and laboratory studies should be made because safe dosage may be lower than that usually recommended.*

Alternative adjustment:

GFR >50 mL/min	*250–500 mg orally every 6 h*
GFR 10–50 mL/min	*260–500 mg orally every 6–8 h*
GFR <10 mL/min	*250–500 mg orally every 12–24 h*
Hemodialysis	*250–500 mg orally every 12–24 h; administer supplemental dose after hemodialysis on dialysis days.*
CAPD	*250–500 mg orally every 12–24 h*
CRRT	*Not applicable (consider an IV cephalosporin)*

Cetirizine - Selected References

Aronoff GA, Bennett WM, Berns JS, et al. Drug prescribing in renal failure: dosing guidelines for adults and children. 5th ed. Philadelphia: American College of Physicians; 2007.

Awni WM, Yeh J, Halstenson CE, Opsahl JA, Matzke GR. Effect of haemodialysis on the pharmacokinetics of cetirizine. Eur J Clin Pharmacol. 1990;38:67–9.

Baltes E, Coupez R, Giezek H, Voss G, Meyerhoff C, Strolin Benedetti M. Absorption and disposition of levocetirizine, the eutomer of cetirizine, administered alone or as cetirizine to healthy volunteers. Fundam Clin Pharmacol. 2001;15:269–77.

Desager J-P, Horsmans Y. Pharmacokinetic-pharmacodynamic relationships of H_1-antihistamines. Clin Pharmacokinet. 1995;28:419–32.

Golightly LK, Greos LS. Second-generation antihistamines: actions and efficacy in the management of allergic disorders. Drugs. 2005;65:341–84.

Lefebvre RA, Rosseel MT, Bernheim J. Single-dose pharmacokinetics of cetirizine in young and elderly volunteers. Int J Clin Pharmacol Res. 1988;8:463–70.

Matzke GR, Yeh J, Awni WM, Halstenson CE, Chung M. Pharmacokinetics of cetirizine in the elderly and patients with renal insufficiency. Ann Allergy. 1987;59(6 Pt 2):25–30.

McIntyre CW, Owen PJ. Prescribing drugs in kidney disease. In: Brenner BM, editor. Brenner & Rector's the kidney. 8th ed. Philadelphia: Saunders Elsevier; 2008. p. 1930–55.

Noiri E, Ozawa H, Fujita T, Nakao A. Pharmacokinetics of cetirizine in chronic hemodialysis patients: multiple-dose study. Nephron. 2001;89:101–4.

Pagliara A, Test B, Carrupt P-A, et al. Molecular properties and pharmacokinetic behavior of cetirizine, a zwitterionic H_1-receptor antagonist. J Med Chem. 1998;41:853–63.

Srinivas NR. Stereoselective renal tubular secretion of cetirizine enantiomers: initial plasma and urine data analysis may hold the key [letter]. Fundam Clin Pharmacol. 2009;23:537–8.

Strolin Benedetti M, Plisnier M, Kaise J, et al. Absorption, distribution, metabolism and excretion of [^{14}C]levocetirizine, the R enantiomer of cetirizine, in healthy volunteers. Eur J Clin Pharmacol. 2001;57:571–82.

Strolin Benedetti M, Whomsley R, Mathy F-X, Jacques P, Espie P, Canning M. Stereoselective renal tubular secretion of levocetirizine and dextrocetirizine, the two enantiomers of the H_1-antihistamine cetirizine. Fundam Clin Pharmacol. 2008;22:19–23.

Tillement J-P, Testa B, Brée F. Compared pharmacological characteristics in humans of racemic cetirizine and levocetirizine, two histamine H^1-receptor antagonists. Biochem Pharmacol. 2003;66:1123–6.

Tsuruoka S, Ioka T, Wakaumi M, Sakamoto K, Ookami H, Fujimura A. Severe arrhythmia as a result of the interaction of cetirizine and pilsicainide in a patient with renal insufficiency: first case presentation showing competition for excretion via renal multidrug resistance protein 1 and organic cation transporter 2. Clin Pharmacol Ther. 2006;79:389–96.

Urien S, Tillement J-P, Ganem B, Kuch M-D. A pharmacokinetic-pharmacodynamic modeling of the antihistaminic (H_1) effects of cetirizine. Int J Clin Pharmacol Ther. 1999;37:499–502.

Wood SG, John BA, Chasseaud LF, Yeh J, Chung M. The metabolism and pharmacokinetics of ^{14}C-cetirizine in humans. Ann Allergy. 1987;59(6 Pt 2):31–4.

Zyrtec® [package insert]. New York: Pfizer Labs division of Pfizer Inc; 2006.

Dosage Adjustment of Medications Eliminated by the Kidneys

Cetirizine/Zyrtec® {Antihistamine; second-generation histamine H$_1$ blocker}

Usual initial dose: 10 mg orally

Usual maintenance dose: 5–10 mg orally once daily, depending on symptom severity

Typical maximum dose: 20 mg daily

Proportion eliminated unchanged: 70 %

Adjustment for Kidney Disease

FDA-approved product labeling: *Cetirizine dosing in renal impairment*

CrCL (mL/min)	Recommended dosing schedule
≥32	10 mg every 24 h
11–31	5 mg every 24 h
≤10	Not recommended

Alternative adjustment:

GFR >50 mL/min	5–10 mg orally once daily
GFR 10–50 mL/min	5 mg orally once daily
GFR <10 mL/min	5 mg orally once daily
Hemodialysis	5 mg orally three times weekly to 5 mg orally daily; no supplemental dose after dialysis
CAPD	5 mg orally once daily
CRRT	Data not available

Cetrorelix - Selected References

Cetrotide® injection [package insert]. Rockland: EMD Serono Inc; 2008.

Duijkers IJM, Klipping C, Willemsen WNP, Krone D, Schneider E, Niebch G, Hermann R. Single and multiple dose pharmacokinetics of the gonadotrophin-releasing hormone antagonist cetrorelix in healthy female volunteers. Hum Reprod. 1998;13:2392–8.

Erb K, Junge K, Pechstein B, Schneider E, Derendorf H, Hermann R. Novel formulations of cetrorelix in healthy men: pharmacodynamic effects and noncompartmental pharmacokinetics. J Clin Pharmacol. 2002;42:995–1001.

Erb K, Klipping C, Duijkers I, Pechstein B, Schueler A, Hermann R. Pharmacodynamic effects and plasma pharmacokinetics of single doses of cetrorelix acetate in healthy premenopausal women. Fertil Steril. 2001;75:316–23.

Nagaraja NV, Pechsterin B, Erb K, et al. Pharmacokinetic and pharmacodynamic modeling of cetrorelix, an LH-RH antagonist, after subcutaneous administration in healthy postmenopausal women. Clin Pharmacol Ther. 2000;68:617–25.

Dosage Adjustment of Medications Eliminated by the Kidneys

<u>**Cetrorelix**</u>/**Cetrotide**®   **{Gonadotropin-releasing hormone antagonist}**

Usual initial dose:	3 mg subcutaneously once or 0.25 mg subcutaneously daily
Usual maintenance dose:	3 mg subcutaneously once during early- to mid-follicular phase or 0.25 mg subcutaneously once daily until the day of hCG administration
Typical maximum dose:	~3.5 mg/cycle
Proportion eliminated unchanged:	7–14 %

Adjustment for Kidney Disease

     FDA-approved product labeling: *Severe renal impairment*   *Contraindicated*

     Alternative adjustment: *Data not available*

Chloral Hydrate - Selected References

Breimer DD. Clinical pharmacokinetics of hypnotics. Clin Pharmacokinet. 1977;2:93–109.

Buur T, Larsson R, Norlander B. Pharmacokinetics of chloral hydrate poisoning treated with hemodialysis and hemoperfusion. Acta Med Scand. 1988;223:269–74.

Garrett ER, Lambert HJ. Pharmacokinetics of trichloroethanol and metabolites and interconversions among variously referenced pharmacokinetic parameters. J Pharm Sci. 1973;62:550–72.

Gorecki DKJ, Hindmarsh KW, Hall CA, Mayers DJ. Determination of chloral hydrate metabolism in adult and neonate biological fluids after single-dose administration. J Chromatogr. 1990;528:333–41.

McIntyre CW, Owen PJ. Prescribing drugs in kidney disease. In: Brenner BM, editor. Brenner & Rector's the kidney. 8th ed. Philadelphia: Saunders Elsevier; 2008. p. 1930–55.

Müller G, Spassovski M, Henschler D. Metabolism of trichloroethylene in man. II. Pharmacokinetics of metabolites. Arch Toxicol. 1974;32:283–95.

Ni Y-C, Wong T-Y, Kadlubar FF, Fu PP. Hepatic metabolism of chloral hydrate to free radical(s) and induction of lipid peroxidation. Biochem Biophys Res Commun. 1994;204:937–43.

Somnote® capsule [package insert]. Boca Raton: Breckenridge Pharmaceutical Inc; 2007.

Chloral <u>Hydrate</u>/Somnote® {**Sedative hypnotic**}

Usual initial dose:	500–1,000 mg orally at bedtime or 30 min prior to procedure
Usual maintenance dose:	500–1,000 mg orally at bedtime
Typical maximum dose:	2 g/day
Proportion eliminated unchanged:	Minimal; active metabolite (trichloroethanol) primarily eliminated in urine

Adjustment for Kidney Disease

FDA-approved product labeling: *Marked renal impairment*   *Contraindicated*

Alternative adjustment: *Data not available*

Chlorambucil - Selected References

Alberts DS, Chang SY, Chen H-SG, Larcom BJ, Jones SE. Pharmacokinetics and metabolism of chlorambucil in man: a preliminary report. Cancer Treat Rev. 1979;6(Suppl):9–17.

Aronoff GA, Bennett WM, Berns JS, et al. Drug prescribing in renal failure: dosing guidelines for adults and children. 5th ed. Philadelphia: American College of Physicians; 2007.

Blank DW, Nanji AA, Schreiber DH, Sanders HD. Acute renal failure and seizures associated with chlorambucil overdose. J Toxicol Clin Toxicol. 1983;20:361–5.

Dathan JRE, Heyworth MF, MacIver AG. Nephrotic syndrome in chronic lymphocytic leukemia. Br Med J. 1974;3:655–7.

Ehrsson H, Wallin I, Nilsson S-O, Johansson B. Pharmacokinetics of chlorambucil in man after administration of the free drug and its prednisolone ester (prednimustine, Leo 1031). Eur J Clin Pharmacol. 1983;24:251–3.

Ehrsson H, Wallin I, Simonsson S, Hartvig P, Öberg G. Effect of food on pharmacokinetics of chlorambucil and its main metabolite, phenylacetic acid mustard. Eur J Clin Pharmacol. 1984;27:111–4.

Greig NH, Stahle PL, Shetty U. High-performance liquid chromatographic analysis of chlorambucil tert-butyl ester and its active metabolites chlorambucil and phenylacetic mustard in plasma and tissue. J Chromatogr. 1990;534:279–86.

Ho WKW, Robertson MR, Macdonald GJ, Charlesworth JA, Pussell BA. Association of acute leukaemia with chlorambucil after renal transplantation [letter]. Lancet. 1994;343:1298–9.

Leff P, Bardsley WG. Pharmacokinetics of chlorambucil in ovarian carcinoma using a new HPLC assay. Biochem Pharmacol. 1979;28:1289–92.

Leukeran® tablet [package insert]. Research Triangle Park: GlaxoSmithKline; 2006.

McIntyre CW, Owen PJ. Prescribing drugs in kidney disease. In: Brenner BM, editor. Brenner & Rector's the kidney. 8th ed. Philadelphia: Saunders Elsevier; 2008. p. 1930–55.

McLean A, Woods RL, Catovsky D, Farmer P. Pharmacokinetics and metabolism of chlorambucil in patients with malignant disease. Cancer Treatment Rev. 1979;6(Suppl):33–42.

Newell DR, Calvert AH, Harrap KR, McElwain TJ. Studies on the pharmacokinetics of chlorambucil and prednimustine in man. Br J Clin Pharmacol. 1983;15:253–8.

Ponticelli C, Zucchelli P, Passerini P, et al. Methylprednisolone plus chlorambucil as compared with methylprednisolone alone for the treatment of idiopathic membranous nephropathy. N Engl J Med. 1992;327:599–603.

Silvernnoinen R, Malminiemi K, Malminiemi O, Seppälä E, Vilpo J. Pharmacokinetics of chlorambucil in patients with chronic lymphocytic leukaemia: comparison of different days, cycles and doses. Pharmacol Toxicol. 2000;87:223–8.

Dosage Adjustment of Medications Eliminated by the Kidneys

<u>Chlorambucil</u>/Leukeran®   {Antineoplastic; nitrogen mustard alkylating agent}

Usual initial dose:	0.1–0.2 mg/kg orally once daily
Usual maintenance dose:	0.1 mg/kg orally once daily (~2–4 mg)
Typical maximum dose:	0.4 mg/kg/day
Proportion eliminated unchanged:	<1 % (~95 % of each dose appears in urine as cytotoxic metabolite)

Adjustment for Kidney Disease

FDA-approved product labeling: *Not available*

Alternative adjustment:

GFR >50 mL/min	*0.1 mg/kg orally every 24 h*
GFR 10–50 mL/min	*0.075 mg/kg orally every 24 h (25 % decrease)*
GFR <10 mL/min	*0.05 mg/kg orally every 24 h (50 % decrease)*
Hemodialysis	*0.05 mg/kg orally every 24 h (50 % decrease)*
CAPD	*0.05 mg/kg orally every 24 h (50 % decrease)*
CRRT	*Data not available*

Note: Hematological and other considerations may suggest further dosage adjustments.

Chlorothiazide - Selected References

Aronoff GA, Bennett WM, Berns JS, et al. Drug prescribing in renal failure: dosing guidelines for adults and children. 5th ed. Philadelphia: American College of Physicians; 2007.

Baer JE, Leidy HL, Brooks AV, Beyer KH. The physiological disposition of chlorothiazide (Diuril) in the dog. J Pharmacol Exp Ther. 1959;125:295–302.

Brettell HR, Aikawa JK, Gordon GS. Studies with chlorothiazide tagged with radioactive carbon (C^{14}) in human beings. Arch Intern Med. 1960;109:109–15.

Chlorothiazide sodium injection [package insert]. Schaumburg: APP Pharmaceuticals LLC; 2009.

Chlorothiazide tablet [package insert]. Eatontown: West-ward Pharmaceuticals Corp; 2005.

Corrigan OI, O'Driscoll KM. The effect of dosage on the bioavailability of chlorothiazide administered in solution. J Pharm Pharmacol. 1980;32:547–9.

Diuril® suspension [package insert]. Whitehouse Station: Merck & Co; 2006.

Gold H, Kwit NT, Messeloff CR, et al. Comparison of chlorothiazide and meralluride: new rapid method for quantitative evaluation of diuretics in bed-patients in congestive heart failure. JAMA. 1960;173:745–52.

Kiil F. Permutation trial of diuretics: chlorothiazide and hydroflumethiazide. Circulation. 1960;21:717–23.

Lavender AR, Pullman TN. The renal effects of chlorothiazide. J Pharmacol Exp Ther. 1961;134:281–5.

Lee J-J, Cook JA, Smith DE. Renal transport kinetics of chlorothiazide in the isolated perfused rat kidney. J Pharmacol Exp Ther. 1988;247:203–8.

Morgan TO, Adam WR, Hodgson N, Myers J. Duration of effect of different diuretics. Med J Aust. 1979;2:315–6.

Murphy J, Casey W, Lasagna L. The effect of dosage regimen on the diuretic efficacy of chlorothiazide in human subjects. J Pharmacol Exp Ther. 1961;134:286–90.

Rahn KH. Clinical pharmacology of diuretics. Clin Exp Hypertens A. 1983;5:157–66.

Shah VP, Knight P, Prasad VK, Cabana BE. Thiazides IV: comparison of dissolution with bioavailability of chlorothiazide tablets. J Pharm Sci. 1982;71:822–4.

Straughn AB, Melikian AP, Meyer MC. Bioavailability of chlorothiazide tablets in humans. J Pharm Sci. 1979;68:1099–102.

Thakker KM. Predicting the dose-dependent bioavailability of hydrocortisone and chlorothiazide in humans [letter]. J Pharm Sci. 1983;72:577–8.

Welling PG, Barbhaiya RH. Influence of food and fluid volume on chlorothiazide bioavailability: comparison of plasma and urinary excretion methods. J Pharm Sci. 1982;71:32–5.

Dosage Adjustment of Medications Eliminated by the Kidneys

<u>**Chlorothiazide**</u>/Diuril®   **{Diuretic; thiazide}**

Usual initial dose:	125–500 mg enterally or IV
Usual maintenance dose:	500–1,000 mg enterally or IV once or twice daily
Typical maximum dose:	2,000 mg/day
Proportion eliminated unchanged:	25 %

Adjustment for Kidney Disease

FDA-approved product labeling: *Use with caution in severe renal disease.*

Alternative adjustment:

GFR >50 mL/min	*500–1,000 mg enterally or IV every 12–24 h*
GFR 30–50 mL/min	*500–1,000 mg enterally or IV every 12–24 h*
GFR <30 mL/min	*Possibly ineffective; may be effective at low GFR in combination with loop diuretic*
GFR <10 mL/min	*Usually ineffective. Preferably avoid unless no suitable alternative exists; if indeed necessary, begin with low doses and monitor carefully.*
Hemodialysis	*Data not available*
CAPD	*Usually ineffective. Preferably avoid unless no suitable alternative exists; if indeed necessary, begin with low doses and monitor carefully.*
CRRT	*Not applicable*

Chlorpropamide - Selected References

Aronoff GA, Bennett WM, Berns JS, et al. Drug prescribing in renal failure: dosing guidelines for adults and children. 5th ed. Philadelphia: American College of Physicians; 2007.

Chlorpropamide tablet [package insert]. Pomona: Barr Laboratories Inc; 2007.

Hanlon JT, Aspinall SL, Semla TP, et al. Consensus guidelines for oral dosing of primarily renally cleared medications in older adults. J Am Geriatr Soc. 2009;57:335–40.

Harrower ADB. Pharmacokinetics of oral antihyperglycaemic agents in patients with renal insufficiency. Clin Pharmacokinet. 1996;31:111–9.

Hensen J, Haenelt M, Gross P. Water retention after oral chlorpropamide is associated with an increase in renal papillary arginine vasopressin receptors. Eur J Endocrinol. 1995;132:459–64.

Ludwig SM, McKenzie J, Faiman C. Chlorpropamide overdose in renal failure: management with charcoal hemoperfusion. Am J Kidney Dis. 1987;10:457–60.

McIntyre CW, Owen PJ. Prescribing drugs in kidney disease. In: Brenner BM, editor. Brenner & Rector's the kidney. 8th ed. Philadelphia: Saunders Elsevier; 2008. p. 1930–55.

Olyaei AJ, Bennett WM. Drug dosing in elderly patients with chronic kidney disease. Clin Geriatr Med. 2009;25:459–527.

Olyaei AJ, Bennett WM. Pharmacologic approach to renal insufficiency. In: Dale DC, Federman DD, Antman K, editors. ACP medicine, WebMD June 2007 update. Hamilton: BC Decker; 2007; NEPHROLOGY IX: Appendix A1–25.

Olyaei AJ, DeMattos AM, Bennett WM. Use of drugs in patients with renal failure. In: Schrier RW, editor. Diseases of the kidney and urinary tract. 8th ed. Philadelphia: Lippincott Williams & Wilkins; 2007. p. 2765–807.

Rothfield EL, Crews AS Jr, Ribo S, Bernstein A. Severe hypoglycemia: result of renal retention of chlorpropamide. Arch Intern Med. 1965;115:468–9.

Seltzer HS. Drug-induced hypoglycemia: a review of 1418 cases. Endocrinol Metab Clin North Am. 1989;18:163–83.

Dosage Adjustment of Medications Eliminated by the Kidneys

<u>Chlorpropamide</u>/Diabinese®   {Antidiabetic; sulfonylurea}

Usual initial dose:	100–250 mg
Usual maintenance dose:	50–250 mg orally once daily
Typical maximum dose:	500 mg orally once daily
Proportion eliminated unchanged:	85 %

Adjustment for Kidney Disease

FDA-approved product labeling:	*Renal insufficiency*	*May increase the risk of serious hypoglycemic reactions*
Alternative adjustment:	*GFR >50 mL/min*	*50–250 mg orally once daily*
	GFR 10–50 mL/min	*Avoid due to risk for severe, prolonged hypoglycemia.*
	GFR <10 mL/min	*Avoid due to risk for severe, prolonged hypoglycemia.*
	Hemodialysis	*Avoid due to risk for severe, prolonged hypoglycemia.*
	CAPD	*Avoid due to risk for severe, prolonged hypoglycemia.*
	CRRT	*Not applicable; avoid due to risk for severe, prolonged hypoglycemia.*

Dosage Adjustment of Medications Eliminated by the Kidneys

Chlorthalidone - Selected References

Aronoff GA, Bennett WM, Berns JS, et al. Drug prescribing in renal failure: dosing guidelines for adults and children. 5th ed. Philadelphia: American College of Physicians; 2007.

Collste P, Garle M, Rawlins MD, Sjöqvist F. Interindividual differences in chlorthalidone concentration in plasma and red cells of man after single and multiple doses. Eur J Clin Pharmacol. 1976;9:319–25.

Colussi D, Schoeller JP, Richard A, Sioufi A. Pharmacokinetics of chlorthalidone in the elderly after single and multiple doses [letter]. Br J Clin Pharmacol. 1983;16:755–6.

Friis T, Lintrup J, Nissen NI. Comparative studies on spironolactone (Aldactone) and chlorthalidone (Hygroton) in the treatment of arterial hypertension. Acta Med Scand. 1966;179:371–81.

McIntyre CW, Owen PJ. Prescribing drugs in kidney disease. In: Brenner BM, editor. Brenner & Rector's the kidney. 8th ed. Philadelphia: Saunders Elsevier; 2008. p. 1930–55.

Mulley BA, Parr GD, Rye RM. Pharmacokinetics of chlorthalidone: dependence of biological half life on blood carbonic anhydrase levels. Eur J Clin Pharmacol. 1980;17:203–7.

Olyaei AJ, Bennett WM. Drug dosing in elderly patients with chronic kidney disease. Clin Geriatr Med. 2009;25:459–527.

Olyaei AJ, Bennett WM. Pharmacologic approach to renal insufficiency. In: Dale DC, Federman DD, Antman K, editors. ACP medicine, WebMD June 2007 update. Hamilton: BC Decker; 2007; NEPHROLOGY IX: Appendix A1–25.

Olyaei AJ, DeMattos AM, Bennett WM. Use of drugs in patients with renal failure. In: Schrier RW, editor. Diseases of the kidney and urinary tract. 8th ed. Philadelphia: Lippincott Williams & Wilkins; 2007. p. 2765–807.

Sica DA. Chlorthalidone – a renaissance in use? Expert Opin Pharmacother. 2009;10:2037–9.

Thalitone® tablet [package insert]. Bristol: Monarch Pharmaceuticals Inc; 2008.

Wright JT Jr, Probstfield JL, Cushman WC, et al. ALLHAT findings revisited in the context of subsequent analyses, other trials, and meta-analyses. Arch Intern Med. 2009;169:832–42.

Dosage Adjustment of Medications Eliminated by the Kidneys

<u>Chlorthalidone</u>/Thalitone®, Hygroton®   {Diuretic; thiazide-like}

Usual initial dose:	25 mg orally
Usual maintenance dose:	25 mg orally once daily
Typical maximum dose:	100 mg orally once daily
Proportion eliminated unchanged:	95 %

Adjustment for Kidney Disease

  FDA-approved product labeling:

Severe renal disease	*Use with caution.*
Anuria	*Contraindicated*

  Alternative adjustment:

GFR >50 mL/min	*25 mg orally once daily*
GFR 10–50 mL/min	*25 mg orally once daily*
GFR <10 mL/min	*Usually ineffective; preferably avoid.*
Hemodialysis	*Usually ineffective; preferably avoid.*
CAPD	*Usually ineffective; preferably avoid.*
CRRT	*Not applicable; preferably avoid.*

Dosage Adjustment of Medications Eliminated by the Kidneys

Cidofovir - Selected References

Aronoff GA, Bennett WM, Berns JS, et al. Drug prescribing in renal failure: dosing guidelines for adults and children. 5th ed. Philadelphia: American College of Physicians; 2007.

Brody SR, Humphreys MH, Gambertoglio JG, et al. Pharmacokinetics of cidofovir n renal insufficiency and in continuous ambulatory peritoneal dialysis or high-flux dialysis. Clin Pharmacol Ther. 1999;65:21–8.

Cihlar T, Ho ES, Lin DC, Mulato AS. Human renal organic anion transporter 1 (hOAT1) and its role in the nephrotoxicity of antiviral nucleotide analogs. Nucleosides Nucleotides Nucleic Acids. 2001;20:641–8.

Cundy KC. Clinical pharmacokinetics of the antiviral nucleotide analogues cidofovir and adefovir. Clin Pharmacokinet. 1999;36:127–43.

Cundy KC, Petty BG, Flaherty J, et al. Clinical pharmacokinetics of cidofovir in human immunodeficiency virus-infected patients. Antimicrob Agents Chemother. 1995;39:1247–52.

Ganguly N, Clough LA, DuBois LK, et al. Low-dose cidofovir in the treatment of symptomatic BK virus infection in patients undergoing allogeneic hematopoietic stem cell transplantation: a retrospective analysis of an algorithmic approach. Transpl Infect Dis. 2010;12:406–11.

Ho ES, Lin DC, Mendel DB, Cihlar T. Cytotoxicity of antiviral nucleotides adefovir and cidofovir is induced by the expression of human renal organic anion transporter 1. J Am Soc Nephrol. 2000;11:383–93.

Kadambi PV, Josephson MA, Willims J, et al. Treatment of refractory BK virus-associated nephropathy with cidofovir. Am J Transplant. 2003;3:186–91.

Kay TD, Hogan PG, McLeod SE, Johnson DW. Severe irreversible proximal renal tubular acidosis and azotaemia secondary to cidofovir [letter]. Nephron. 2000;86:348–9.

Keller LS, Peh CA, Nolan J, Bannister KM, Clarkson AR, Faull RJ. BK transplant nephropathy successfully treated with cidofovir. Nephrol Dial Transplant. 2003;18:1013–4.

Ljungman P, Ribaud P, Eyrich M, et al. Cidofovir for adenovirus infections after allogeneic hematopoietic stem cell transplantation: a survey by the Infectious Diseases Working Party of the European Group for Blood and Marrow Transplantation. Bone Marrow Transplant. 2003;31:481–6.

Meier P, Dautheville-Guibal S, Ronco PM, Rossert J. Cidofovir-induced end-stage renal failure. Nephrol Dial Transplant. 2002;17:148–9.

Miller DS. Nucleoside phosphonate interactions with multiple organic anion transporters in renal proximal tubule. J Pharmacol Exp Ther. 2001;299:567–74.

Nagafuji K, Aoki K, Henzan H, et al. Cidofovir for treating adenoviral hemorrhagic cystitis in hematopoietic stem cell transplant recipients. Bone Marrow Transplant. 2004;34:909–14.

Ramos E, Vincenti F, Lu WX, et al. Retransplantation in patients with graft loss caused by polyoma virus nephropathy. Transplantation. 2004;77:131–3.

Saqiob R. Melton LB, Chandrakantan A, et al. Disseminated adenovirus infection in renal transplant recipients: the role of cidofovir and intravenous immunoglobulin. Transpl Infect Dis. 2010;12:77–83.

Savona MR, Newton D, Frame D, Levine JE, Mineishi S, Kaul. Low-dose cidofovir treatment of BK virus-associated hemorrhagic cystitis in recipients of hematopoietic stem cell transplant. Bone Marrow Transplant. 2007;39:783–7.

Trofe J, Hirsch HH, Ramos E. Polyomavirus-associated nephropathy: update of clinical management in kidney transplant patients. Transpl Infect Dis. 2006;8:76–85.

Vistide® injection [package insert]. Foster City: Gilead Sciences Inc; 2000.

Wachsman M, Pety BG, Cundy KC, et al. Pharmacokinetics, safety and bioavailability of HPMPC (cidofovir) in human immunodeficiency virus-infected patients. Antiviral Res. 1996;29:153–61.

Wolf DL, Rodríguez CA, Mucci M, Ingrosso A, Duncan BA, Nickens DJ. Pharmacokinetics and renal effects of cidofovir with a reduced dose of probenecid in HIV-infected patients with cytomegalovirus retinitis. J Clin Pharmacol. 2003;43:43–51.

Wu S-W, Chang H-R, Lian J-D. The effect of low-dose cidofovir on the long-term outcome of polyomavirus-associated nephropathy in renal transplant recipients. Nephrol Dial Transplant. 2009;24:1034–8.

Zedtwitz-Liebenstein K, Presterl E, Deviatko E, Graninger W. Acute renal failure in a lung transplant patient after therapy with cidofovir [letter]. Transpl Int. 2001;14:445–6.

Dosage Adjustment of Medications Eliminated by the Kidneys

<u>Cidofovir</u>/Vistide®　　　　　　{Antiviral; ℞ for cytomegalovirus infection}

Usual initial dose: 5 mg/kg IV

Usual maintenance dose: 5 mg/kg IV over 1 h once weekly for 2 weeks; maintenance 5 mg/kg IV every other week (with probenecid 2 g administered orally 3 h prior to the cidofovir infusion and again at 8 h after completion of the cidofovir infusion)

Typical maximum dose: 5 mg/kg IV

Proportion eliminated unchanged: 90 %

Adjustment for Kidney Disease

FDA-approved product labeling: *With acute increase in SCr of 0.3–0.5 mg/dL over baseline, decrease dose to 3 mg/kg IV weekly ×2; discontinue for an increase in SCr of ≥0.5 mg/dL above baseline or development of ≥3+ proteinuria (with probenecid).*

Contraindicated in patients with SCr ≥1.5 mg/dL, calculated CrCL <55 mL/ min, and/or urine protein >100 mg/dL (equivalent to ≥2+ proteinuria); contraindicated in patients receiving agents with nephrotoxic potential or within 7 days after use of such agents

Alternative adjustment:	*GFR >55 mL/min*	*5 mg/kg IV weekly ×2 then 5 mg/kg IV every other week or 0.5–1 mg/kg IV weekly or 0.25 mg/kg IV weekly until symptom resolution (with probenecid 2 g orally 1 h prior to the cidofovir infusion)*
	GFR 10–55 mL/min	*Preferably avoid unless no suitable alternative exists; if indeed necessary, 0.25–0.5 mg/kg IV every 2 weeks (with probenecid; minimal data available).*
	GFR <10 mL/min	*Preferably avoid unless no suitable alternative exists; if indeed necessary, 0.25–0.5 mg/kg IV every 2 weeks (with probenecid; minimal data available).*
	Hemodialysis	*Preferably avoid unless no suitable alternative exists; if indeed necessary, 0.25–0.5 mg/kg IV every 2 weeks (without probenecid; minimal data available).*
	CAPD	*Preferably avoid unless no suitable alternative exists; if indeed necessary, 0.25–0.5 mg/kg IV every 2 weeks (without probenecid; minimal data available).*
	CRRT	*Preferably avoid unless no suitable alternative exists; if indeed necessary, 2 mg/kg IV weekly (with probenecid).*

Dosage Adjustment of Medications Eliminated by the Kidneys

Cimetidine - Selected References

Aronoff GA, Bennett WM, Berns JS, et al. Drug prescribing in renal failure: dosing guidelines for adults and children. 5th ed. Philadelphia: American College of Physicians; 2007.

Cimetidine in 0.9 % sodium chloride injection [package insert]. Lake Forest: Hospira Inc; 2006.

Cimetidine tablet [package insert]. Morgantown: Mylan Pharmaceuticals Inc; 2005.

Finkelstein W, Isselbacher KJ. Drug therapy: cimetidine. N Engl J Med. 1978;299:992–6.

Freston JW. Cimetidine. I. Developments, pharmacology, and efficacy. Ann Intern Med. 1982;97:573–80.

Freston JW. Cimetidine. II. Adverse reactions and patterns of use. Ann Intern Med. 1982;97:728–34.

Grahnén A, von Bahr, Lindström B, Rosén A. Bioavailability and pharmacokinetics of cimetidine. Eur J Clin Pharmacol. 1979;16:335–40.

Hanlon JT, Aspinall SL, Semla TP, et al. Consensus guidelines for oral dosing of primarily renally cleared medications in older adults. J Am Geriatr Soc. 2009;57:335–40.

Hyneck ML, Murphy JF, Lischutz DE. Cimetidine clearance during intermittent and chronic peritoneal dialysis. Am J Hosp Pharm. 1981;38:1760–2.

Iberti TTJ, Paluch TA, Helmer L, Murgolo VA, Benjamin E. The hemodynamic effects of intravenous cimetidine in intensive care unit patients: a double-blind, prospective study. Anesthesiology. 1986;64:87–9.

Kay WA, Passero MA, Solomon RJ, Johnson LA. Cimetidine-induced interstitial nephritis with response to prednisone therapy. Arch Intern Med. 1983;143:811–2.

Ma KW, Brown DC, Masler DS, Selvis SE. Effects of renal failure on blood levels of cimetidine. Gastroenterology. 1978;74:473–7.

McIntyre CW, Owen PJ. Prescribing drugs in kidney disease. In: Brenner BM, editor. Brenner & Rector's the kidney. 8th ed. Philadelphia: Saunders Elsevier; 2008. p. 1930–55.

Ochs H, Gugler R, Guthoff T, Greenblatt DJ. Effect of cimetidine on digoxin kinetics and creatinine clearance. Am Heart J. 1984;107:170–2.

Olyaei AJ, Bennett WM. Drug dosing in elderly patients with chronic kidney disease. Clin Geriatr Med. 2009;25:459–527.

Olyaei AJ, Bennett WM. Pharmacologic approach to renal insufficiency. In: Dale DC, Federman DD, Antman K, editors. ACP medicine, WebMD June 2007 update. Hamilton: BC Decker; 2007; NEPHROLOGY IX: Appendix A1–25.

Olyaei AJ, DeMattos AM, Bennett WM. Use of drugs in patients with renal failure. In: Schrier RW, editor. Diseases of the kidney and urinary tract. 8th ed. Philadelphia: Lippincott Williams & Wilkins; 2007. p. 2765–807.

Somogyi A, Gugler R. Clinical pharmacokinetics of cimetidine. Clin Pharmacokinet. 1983;8:463–95.

Somogyi A, McLean A, Heinzow B. Cimetidine-procainamide pharmacokinetic interaction in man: evidence of competition for tubular secretion of basic drugs. Eur J Clin Pharmacol. 1983;25:339–45.

Tagamet® tablet, liquid, and injection [package insert]. Philadelphia: SmithKline Beecham Pharmaceuticals; 1991.

Vaziri KD, Ness RL, Barton CH. Hemodialysis clearance of cimetidine. Arch Intern Med. 1978;138:1685–6.

Webster J, Barber HE, Hawksworth GM, et al. Cimetidine: a clinical and pharmacokinetic study. Br J Clin Pharmacol. 1981;11:333–8.

Dosage Adjustment of Medications Eliminated by the Kidneys

<u>Cimetidine</u>/Tagamet®	{Antacid; histamine H_2 receptor antagonist}
Usual initial dose:	300 mg IV
Usual maintenance dose:	300 mg IV every 6–8 h or 400–800 mg orally twice daily or 800 mg orally at bedtime
Typical maximum dose:	2,400 mg/day
Proportion eliminated unchanged:	50–80 %

Adjustment for Kidney Disease

FDA-approved product labeling:	*Impaired renal function (CrCL <30 mL/min)*	*300 mg IV or orally every 12 h*
Alternative adjustment:	*GFR >50 mL/min*	*300 mg IV every 8 h or 400 mg orally twice daily*
	GFR 10–50 mL/min	*150 mg IV every 8 h or 200 mg orally twice daily*
	GFR <10 mL/min	*150 mg IV every 12 h or 200 mg orally once daily (avoid in older adults.)*
	Hemodialysis	*150 mg IV every 12 h or 200 mg orally once daily; administer after hemodialysis on dialysis days*
	CAPD	*150 mg IV every 12 h or 200 mg orally once daily*
	CRRT	*150 mg IV every 8 h or 200 mg enterally twice daily*

Dosage Adjustment of Medications Eliminated by the Kidneys

Ciprofloxacin - Selected References

Allon M, Lopez EJ, Min K-W. Acute renal failure due to ciprofloxacin. Arch Intern Med. 1990;150:2187–9.

Aronoff GA, Bennett WM, Berns JS, et al. Drug prescribing in renal failure: dosing guidelines for adults and children. 5th ed. Philadelphia: American College of Physicians; 2007.

Barrie JR, Mousdale S. Ciprofloxacin levels in a patient undergoing veno-venous haemodiafiltration. Intensive Care Med. 1992;18:437–8.

Bayer A, Gajewska A, Stephens M, Stark JM, Pathy J. Pharmacokinetics of ciprofloxacin in the elderly. Respiration. 1987;51:292–5.

Bergan T, Thorsteinsson SB, Rohwedder R, Scholl H. Elimination of ciprofloxacin and three major metabolites and consequences of reduced renal function. Chemotherapy. 1989;35:393–405.

Boelaert J, Valcke Y, Schurgers M, et al. The pharmacokinetics of ciprofloxacin in patients with impaired renal function. J Antimicrob Chemother. 1985;16:87–93.

Cipro® IV solution concentrate [package insert]. Wayne: Bayer HealthCare Pharmaceuticals Inc; 2011.

Cipro® tablet film coated [package insert]. Wayne: Bayer HealthCare Pharmaceuticals Inc; 2011.

Davies SP, Azadian BS, Kox WJ, Brown EA. Pharmacokinetics of ciprofloxacin and vancomycin in patients with acute renal failure treated by continuous haemodialysis. Nephrol Dial Transplant. 1992;7:848–54.

Dharmasena D, Roberts DE, Coles GA, Williams JD. Pharmacokinetics of intraperitoneal ciprofloxacin in patients with CAPD. J Antimicrob Chemother. 1989;23:253–9.

Drusano GL, Weir M, Forrest A, Plaisance K, Emm T, Standiford HC. Pharmacokinetics of intravenously administered ciprofloxacin in patients with various degrees of renal function. Antimicrob Agents Chemother. 1987;31:860–4.

Eliopoulos GM. New quinolones: pharmacology, pharmacokinetics, and dosing in patients with renal insufficiency. Rev Infect Dis. 1988;10(Suppl 1):S102–5.

Fleming LW, Moreland TA, Scott AC, Stewart WK, White LO. Ciprofloxacin in plasma and peritoneal dialysate after oral therapy in patients on continuous ambulatory peritoneal dialysis. J Antimicrob Chemother. 1987;19:493–503.

Fleming LW, Phillips G, Stewart WK, Scott AC. Oral ciprofloxacin in the treatment of peritonitis in patients on continuous ambulatory peritoneal dialysis. J Antimicrob Chemother. 1990;25:441–8.

Gasser TC, Ebert SC, Graversen PH, Madsen PO. Ciprofloxacin pharmacokinetics in patients with normal and impaired renal function. Antimicrob Agents Chemother. 1987;31:709–2.

Hayakawa M, Fujita I, Iseki K, Gando S. The administration of ciprofloxacin during continuous renal replacement therapy: pilot study. ASAIO J. 2009;55:243–5.

Heintz BH, Matzke GR, Dager WF. Antimicrobial dosing concepts and recommendations for critically ill adult patients receiving continuous renal replacement therapy or intermittent hemodialysis. Pharmacotherapy. 2009;29:562–77.

Hirata CAI, Guay DRP, Awni QM, Stein DJ, Peterson PK. Steady-state pharmacokinetics of intravenous and oral ciprofloxacin in elderly patients. Antimicrob Agents Chemother. 1989;33:1297–31.

Hootkins R, Fenves AZ, Stephens MK. Acute renal failure secondary to oral ciprofloxacin therapy: a presentation of three cases and a review of the literature. Clin Nephrol. 1989;32:75–8.

Kowalsky SF, Echols M, Schwarz MT, Bailie GR, McCormick E. Pharmacokinetics of ciprofloxacin in subjects with varying degrees of renal function and undergoing hemodialysis or CAPD. Clin Nephrol. 1993;39:53–8.

Lo WK, Rolston KVI, Rubenstein EB, Bodey GP. Ciprofloxacin-induced nephrotoxicity in patients with cancer. Arch Intern Med. 1993;153:1258–62.

Roberts DE, Williams JD. Ciprofloxacin in renal failure [editorial]. J Antimicrob Chemother. 1989;23:820–3.

Sedlacek M, Suriawinata AA, Schoolwerth A, Remillard BD. Ciprofloxacin crystal nephropathy—a 'new' cause of acute renal failure [letter]. Nephrol Dial Transplant. 2009;21:2339–40.

Singlas E, Taburet AM, Landru I, Albin H, Ryckelinck JP. Pharmacokinetics of ciprofloxacin tablets in renal failure: influence of haemodialysis. Eur J Clin Pharmacol. 1987;31:589–93.

Vance-Bryan K, Guay DRP, Rotschafer JC. Clinical pharmacokinetics of ciprofloxacin. Clin Pharmacokinet. 1990;19:434–61.

Wallis SC, Mullany DV, Lipman J, Rickard CM. Daley PJ. Pharmacokinetics of ciprofloxacin in ICU patients on continuous veno-venous haemodiafiltration. Intensive Care Med. 2001;27:665–72.

Dosage Adjustment of Medications Eliminated by the Kidneys

Ciprofloxacin/Cipro®	{Antibacterial; fluoroquinolone}
Usual initial dose:	500–750 mg orally or 400 mg IV
Usual maintenance dose:	250–750 mg orally every 12 h or 200–400 mg IV every 12 h or 400 mg IV every 8 h

Ciprofloxacin equivalent area under the curve (AUC) dosing regimens

Ciprofloxacin oral dosage	Equivalent ciprofloxacin IV dosage
250 mg tablet every 12 h	200 mg IV every 12 h
500 mg tablet every 12 h	400 mg IV every 12 h
750 mg tablet every 12 h	400 mg IV every 8 h

Typical maximum dose:	750 mg/dose orally or 400 mg/dose IV
Proportion eliminated unchanged:	50 %

Adjustment for Kidney Disease

FDA-approved product labeling: *Ciprofloxacin dosage adjustment in adults with renal function impairment*

CrCL (mL/min)	Dose
>50	250–750 mg orally every 12 h[a]
30–50	250–500 mg orally every 12 h[a]
5–29	250–500 mg orally every 18 h[a]
Hemodialysis or peritoneal dialysis	250–500 mg orally every 24 h (after hemodialysis on dialysis days)[a]

[a]See table above for equivalent ciprofloxacin IV dosages

Alternative adjustment:		
	GFR >50 mL/min	500–750 mg orally or 400 mg IV every 12 h
	GFR 10–50 mL/min	250–500 mg orally or 200 mg IV every 12 h
	GFR <10 mL/min	250 mg orally or 200 mg IV every 12 h
	Hemodialysis	250 mg orally or 200 mg IV every 12 h
	CAPD	250 mg orally or 200 mg IV every 12 h or addition to dialysate in a concentration of 25 mg/L
	CVVH	200–400 mg IV every 12 h
	CVVHD or CVVHDF	200–400 mg IV every 8 h

Dosage Adjustment of Medications Eliminated by the Kidneys

Cisplatin - Selected References

Anand AJ, Bashey B. Newer insights into cisplatin nephrotoxicity. Ann Pharmacother. 1993;27:1519–25.

Aronoff GA, Bennett WM, Berns JS, et al. Drug prescribing in renal failure: dosing guidelines for adults and children. 5th ed. Philadelphia: American College of Physicians; 2007.

Bennett WM, Pastore L, Houghton DC. Fatal bleomycin toxicity in cisplatin-induced acute renal failure. Cancer Treat Rep. 1980;64:921–4.

Blachley JD, Hill JB. Renal and electrolyte disturbances associated with cisplatin. Ann Intern Med. 1981;95:628–32.

Campbell AB, Kalman SM, Jacobs C. Plasma platinum levels: relationship to cisplatin dose and nephrotoxicity. Cancer Treat Rep. 1982;67:169–72.

Daley-Yates PT, McBrien DCH. The renal fractional clearance of platinum antitumour compounds in relation to nephrotoxicity. Biochem Pharmacol. 1985;34:1423–8.

Dobyan DC, Levi J, Jacobs C, Kosek J, Weiner MW. Mechanism of cis-platinum nephrotoxicity: II. Morphologic observations. J Pharmacol Exp Ther. 1980;213:551–6..

Fjeldborg P, Sørensen J, Helkjær PE. The long-term effect of cisplatin on renal function. Cancer. 1986;58:2214–7.

Frick GA, Ballentine R, Driever C. Kramer WG. Renal excretion kinetics of high-dose cis-dichlorodiammineplatinum(II) administered with hydration and mannitol diuresis. Cancer Treat Rep. 1978;63:13–6.

Gormley PE, Bull JM, LeRoy AF. Kinetics of cis-dichlorodiammineplatinum. Clin Pharmacol Ther. 1979;25:351–7.

Jacobs C, Kalman SM, Tretton M, Weiner MW. Renal handling of cis-diamminedichloroplatinum (II). Cancer Treat Rep. 1980;64:1223–6.

Kovacs CJ, Braunschweiger PG, Schenken LL, Burholt DR. Proliferative defects in renal and intestinal epithelium after cis-dichlorodiammine platinum (II). Br J Cancer. 1982;45:286–94.

Kröning R, Katz D, Lichtenstein AK, Nagami GT. Differential effects of cisplatin in proximal and distal renal tubule epithelial cell lines. Br J Cancer. 1999;79:293–9.

Lagrange JL, Médecin B, Etienne MC, et al. Cisplatin nephrotoxicity: a multivariate analysis of potential predisposing factors. Pharmacotherapy. 1997;17:1246–53.

Levi J, Jacobs C, Kalman SM, McTigue M, Weiner MW. Mechanism of cis-platinum nephrotoxicity: I. Effects of sulfhydryl groups in rat kidneys. J Pharmacol Exp Ther. 1980;213:545–50.

Loehrer PJ, Einhorn LH. Drugs five years later: cisplatin. Ann Intern Med. 1984;100:704–13.

Platinol® injection [package insert]. Princeton: Bristol-Myers Squibb Co; 2010.

Ribaud P, Gouveia J, Bonnay M, Mathe G. Clinical pharmacology and pharmacokinetics of cis-platinum and analogs. Cancer Treat Rep. 1981;65(Suppl 3):97–105.

Schilsky RL, Anderson T. Hypomagnesemia and renal magnesium wasting in patients receiving cisplatin. Ann Intern Med. 1979;90:929–31.

Stark JJ, Howell SB. Nephrotoxicity of cis-platinum (II) dichlorodiammine. Clin Pharmacol Ther. 1978;23:461–6.

van Barneveld PWC, Sleijfer DT, van der Mark TW, et al. Influence of platinum-induced renal toxicity on bleomycin-induced pulmonary toxicity in patients with disseminated testicular carcinoma. Oncology. 1984;41:4–7.

Dosage Adjustment of Medications Eliminated by the Kidneys

Cisplatin/Platinol®   {Antineoplastic; platinum coordination complex}

Usual initial dose:	75–100 mg/m² IV
Usual maintenance dose:	75–100 mg/m² IV every 3–4 weeks
Typical maximum dose:	120 mg/m² IV
Proportion eliminated unchanged:	30–40 %

Adjustment for Kidney Disease

FDA-approved product labeling:	*Preexisting renal impairment*	*Contraindicated*
Alternative adjustment:	*GFR >50 mL/min*	*75–100 mg/m² IV every 3–4 weeks (100 % of usual dose)*
	GFR 10–50 mL/min	*60–75 mg/m² every 3–4 weeks (25 % decrease)*
	GFR <10 mL/min	*37.5–50 mg/m² every 3–4 weeks (50 % decrease)*
	Hemodialysis	*37.5–50 mg/m² every 3–4 weeks (50 % decrease); administer supplemental dose after hemodialysis on dialysis days.*
	CAPD	*37.5–50 mg/m² every 3–4 weeks (50 % decrease)*
	CRRT	*60–75 mg/m² every 3–4 weeks (25 % decrease)*

Note: Hematological and other considerations may suggest further dosage adjustments.

Cladribine - Selected References

Aronoff GA, Bennett WM, Berns JS, et al. Drug prescribing in renal failure: dosing guidelines for adults and children. 5th ed. Philadelphia: American College of Physicians; 2007.

Baltz JK, Montello MJ. Cladribine for the treatment of hematologic malignancies. Clin Pharm. 1993;12:805–13.

Bryson HM, Sorkin EM. Cladribine: a review of its pharmacodynamic and pharmacokinetic properties and therapeutic potential in haematological malignancies. Drugs. 1993;46:872–94.

Crews KR, Wimmer PS, Hudson JQ, Howard SC, Bibeiro RC, Razzouk BI. Pharmacokinetics of 2-chlorodeoxyadenosine in a child undergoing hemofiltration and hemodialysis. J Pediatr Hematol Oncol. 2002;24:677–80.

Gandhi V, Estey E, Keating MJ, Chucrallah A, Plunkett W. Chlorodeoxyadenosine and arabinosylcytosine in patients with acute myelogenous leukemia: pharmacokinetic, pharmacodynamic, and molecular interactions. Blood. 1996;87:256–64.

Juliusson G, Heldal D, Hippe E, et al. Subcutaneous injections of 2-chlorodeoxyadenosine for symptomatic hairy cell leukemia. J Clin Oncol. 1995;13:989–95.

Kobayashi K, Vogelzang NJ, O'Brien SM, Vokes EE, Ratain MJ. A phase I study of intermittent infusion cladribine in patients with solid tumors. Cancer. 1994;74:168–73.

Leustatin® injection [package insert]. Raritan: Centocor Ortho Biotech Products LP; 2009.

Liliemark J. The clinical pharmacokinetics of cladribine. Clin Pharmacokinet. 1997;32:120–31.

Liliemark J, Albertioni F, Juliusson G, Eksborg S. A limited sampling strategy for estimation of the cladribine plasma area under the concentration versus time curve after intermittent iv infusion, sc injection, and oral administration. Cancer Chemother Pharmacol. 1996;38:536–40.

Saven A, Cheung WK, Smith I, et al. Pharmacokinetic study of oral and bolus intravenous 2-chlorodeoxyadenosine in patients with malignancy. J Clin Oncol. 1996;14:978–83.

Sonderegger T, Beticher DC, Cerny T, Lauterburg BH. Pharmacokinetics of 2-chloro-2'-deoxyadenosine administered subcutaneously or by continuous intravenous infusion. Cancer Chemother Pharmacol. 2000;46:40–2.

Weiss GR, Kuhn JG, Rizzo J, et al. A phase I pharmacokinetics study of 2-chlorodeoxyadenosine in patients with solid tumors. Cancer Chemother Pharmacol. 1995;35:397–402.

Dosage Adjustment of Medications Eliminated by the Kidneys

<u>Cladribine</u>/Leustatin®   {**Antineoplastic; pyrimidine analog antimetabolite**}

Usual initial dose: 0.09 mg/kg/day IV

Usual maintenance dose: 0.09 mg/kg/day continuous IV infusion for seven consecutive days

Typical maximum dose: 0.09 mg/kg/day IV

Proportion eliminated unchanged: 15 %

Adjustment for Kidney Disease

> **FDA-approved product labeling:** *Proceed carefully in patients with known or suspected renal insufficiency.*

> **Alternative adjustment:**

GFR >50 mL/min	*0.09 mg/kg/day continuous IV infusion*
GFR 10–50 mL/min	*0.0675 mg/kg/day continuous IV infusion*
GFR <10 mL/min	*0.045 mg/kg/day continuous IV infusion*
Hemodialysis	*Data not available*
CAPD	*0.045 mg/kg/day continuous IV infusion*
CRRT	*Limited data; preferably avoid unless no suitable alternative exists; if indeed necessary, begin with low doses and monitor carefully.*

> *Note: Hematological and other considerations may suggest further dosage adjustments.*

Dosage Adjustment of Medications Eliminated by the Kidneys

Clarithromycin - Selected References

Abramowicz M, Zuccotti G, Pflomm J-M, et al., editors. Handbook of antimicrobial therapy. 19th ed. New Rochelle: The Medical Letter; 2011.

Ammon S, Treiber G, Kees F, Klotz U. Influence of age on the steady state disposition of drugs commonly used for the eradication of *Helicobacter pylori*. Aliment Pharmacol Ther. 2000;14:759–66.

Aronoff GA, Bennett WM, Berns JS, et al. Drug prescribing in renal failure: dosing guidelines for adults and children. 5th ed. Philadelphia: American College of Physicians; 2007.

Biaxin® tablet and granules for suspension [package insert]. North Chicago: Abbott Laboratories Inc; 2008.

Chu S-Y, Deaton R, Cavanaugh J. Absolute bioavailability of clarithromycin after oral administration in humans. Antimicrob Agents Chemother. 1992;36:1147–50.

Chu S-Y, Sennello ST, Varga LL, Wilson DS, Sonders RC. Pharmacokinetics of clarithromycin, a new macrolide, after single ascending oral doses. Antimicrob Agents Chemother. 1992;36:2447–53.

Chu S-Y, Wilson DS, Deaton RL, Mackenthun AV, Eason CN, Cavanaugh JH. Single- and multiple-dose pharmacokinetics of clarithromycin, a new macrolide antimicrobial. J Clin Pharmacol. 1993;33:719–26.

Chu S-Y, Wilson DS, Guay DRP, Craft C. Clarithromycin pharmacokinetics in healthy young and elderly volunteers. J Clin Pharmacol. 1992;32:1045–9.

Davey PG. The pharmacokinetics of clarithromycin and its 14-OH metabolite. J Hosp Infect. 1991; 19(Suppl A):29–37.

Ferrari SL, Goffin E, Mourad M, Wallemacq P, Squifflet J-P, Pirson Y. The interaction between clarithromycin and cyclosporine in kidney transplant recipients [letter]. Transplantation. 1994;27:725–7.

Fish DN, Abraham E. Pharmacokinetics of clarithromycin suspension administered via nasogastric tube to seriously ill patients. Antimicrob Agents Chemother. 1999;43:1277–80.

Fraschini F, Scaglione F, Demartini G. Clarithromycin clinical pharmacokinetics. Clin Pharmacokinet. 1993;25:189–204.

McIntyre CW, Owen PJ. Prescribing drugs in kidney disease. In: Brenner BM, editor. Brenner & Rector's the kidney. 8th ed. Philadelphia: Saunders Elsevier; 2008. p. 1930–55.

Olyaei AJ, Bennett WM. Drug dosing in elderly patients with chronic kidney disease. Clin Geriatr Med. 2009;25:459–527.

Olyaei AJ, Bennett WM. Pharmacologic approach to renal insufficiency. In: Dale DC, Federman DD, Antman K, editors. ACP medicine, WebMD June 2007 update. Hamilton: BC Decker; 2007; NEPHROLOGY IX: Appendix A1–25.

Olyaei AJ, DeMattos AM, Bennett WM. Use of drugs in patients with renal failure. In: Schrier RW, editor. Diseases of the kidney and urinary tract. 8th ed. Philadelphia: Lippincott Williams & Wilkins; 2007. p. 2765–807.

Patel KB, Xuan D, Tessier PR, Russomanno JH, Quintilani R, Nightingale CH. Comparison of bronchopulmonary pharmacokinetics of clarithromycin and azithromycin. Antimicrob Agents Chemother. 1996;40:2375–9.

Peters DH, Clissold SP. Clarithromycin: a review of its antimicrobial activity, pharmacokinetic properties and therapeutic potential. Drugs. 1992;44:117–64.

Rodvold KA, Gotfried MH, Danziger LH, Servi RJ. Intrapulmonary steady-state concentrations of clarithromycin and azithromycin in healthy adult volunteers. Antimicrob Agents Chemother. 1997;41:1399–402.

Vance E, Watson-Bitar M, Gustavson L, Kazanjian P. Pharmacokinetics of clarithromycin and zidovudine in patients with AIDS. Antimicrob Agents Chemother. 1995;39:1355–60.

Dosage Adjustment of Medications Eliminated by the Kidneys

<u>Clarithromycin</u>/Biaxin®   **{Antibacterial, macrolide}**

Usual initial dose:	500 mg orally
Usual maintenance dose:	250–500 mg orally twice daily
Typical maximum dose:	1,500 mg/day
Proportion eliminated unchanged:	15 % (plus 7 % of absorbed dose as metabolite)

Adjustment for Kidney Disease

FDA-approved product labeling: *In the presence of severe renal impairment with or without coexisting hepatic impairment, decreased dosage or prolonged dosing intervals may be appropriate.*

Alternative adjustment:

GFR >50 mL/min	*250–500 mg orally every 12 h*
GFR 10–50 mL/min	*125–500 mg orally every 12 h*
GFR <10 mL/min	*125–250 mg orally every 12 h*
Hemodialysis	*Data not available*
CAPD	*Data not available*
CRRT	*125–500 mg enterally every 12 h*

Dosage Adjustment of Medications Eliminated by the Kidneys

<u>Clomipramine</u> - Selected References

Anafranil® capsule [package insert]. Hazelwood: Mallinckrodt Inc; 2009.

Aronoff GA, Bennett WM, Berns JS, et al. Drug prescribing in renal failure: dosing guidelines for adults and children. 5th ed. Philadelphia: American College of Physicians; 2007.

Balant-Gorgia AE, Gex-Fabry M, Balant LP. Clinical pharmacokinetics of clomipramine. Clin Pharmacokinet. 1991;20:447–62.

Dawling S, Braithwaite RA, McAuley R, Montgomery SA. Single oral dose pharmacokinetics of clomipramine in depressed patients. Postgrad Med J. 1980;56(Suppl 1):115–6.

de Cuyper HJA, van Praag HM, Mulder-Hajonides WREM, Westenberg HGM, de Zeeuw RA. Pharmacokinetics of clomipramine in depressive patients. Psychiatry Res. 1981;4:147–56.

Dubois J-P, Küng W, Theobald W, Wirz B. Measurement of clomipramine, n-desmethyl-clomipramine, imipramine, and dehydroimipramine in biological fluids by selective ion monitoring, and pharmacokinetics of clomipramine. Clin Chem. 1976;22:892–7.

Hullin RP. Variation in plasma concentrations of clomipramine and desmethyl-clomipramine during clomipramine therapy. Postgrad Med J. 1980;56(Suppl 1):117–9.

Kuss H-J, Jungkunz G. Nonlinear pharmacokinetics of chlorimipramine after infusion and oral administration in patients. Prog Neuropsychopharmacol Biol Psychiatry. 1986;10:739–48.

McIntyre CW, Owen PJ. Prescribing drugs in kidney disease. In: Brenner BM, editor. Brenner & Rector's the kidney. 8th ed. Philadelphia: Saunders Elsevier; 2008. p. 1930–55.

Moyes RB, Moyes JCA. Measurement of plasma antidepressant levels by high-performance liquid chromatography. Postgrad Med J. 1977;53(Suppl 4):117–23.

Olyaei AJ, Bennett WM. Drug dosing in elderly patients with chronic kidney disease. Clin Geriatr Med. 2009;25:459–527.

Olyaei AJ, Bennett WM. Pharmacologic approach to renal insufficiency. In: Dale DC, Federman DD, Antman K, editors. ACP medicine, WebMD June 2007 update. Hamilton: BC Decker; 2007; NEPHROLOGY IX: Appendix A1–25.

Olyaei AJ, DeMattos AM, Bennett WM. Use of drugs in patients with renal failure. In: Schrier RW, editor. Diseases of the kidney and urinary tract. 8th ed. Philadelphia: Lippincott Williams & Wilkins; 2007:2765–807.

Onishi A, Yamamoto H, Akimoto T, et al. Reversible acute renal failure associated with clomipramine-induced interstitial nephritis. Clin Exp Nephrol. 2007;11:241–3.

Dosage Adjustment of Medications Eliminated by the Kidneys

<u>**Clomipramine**</u>/**Anafranil®**   {**Antidepressant; tricyclic**}

Usual initial dose: 25 mg orally

Usual maintenance dose: 100 mg orally once daily

Typical maximum dose: 250 mg orally once daily

Proportion eliminated unchanged: 60 %

Adjustment for Kidney Disease

  FDA-approved product labeling: *Use with caution in patients with significantly impaired renal function.*

  Alternative adjustment: *GFR >50 mL/min*   *100 mg orally once daily*

                                       GFR 10–50 mL/min   *100 mg orally once daily*

                                       GFR <10 mL/min   *100 mg orally once daily*

                                       Hemodialysis   *100 mg orally once daily, supplemental dose after hemodialysis not required*

                                       CAPD   *100 mg orally once daily*

                                       CRRT   *Date not available. Preferably avoid unless no suitable alternative exists; if indeed necessary, begin with low doses and monitor carefully.*

Dosage Adjustment of Medications Eliminated by the Kidneys

Clozapine - Selected References

Balant-Gorgia AE, Balant L. Antipsychotic drugs: clinical pharmacokinetics of potential candidates for plasma concentration monitoring. Clin Pharmacokinet. 1987;13:65–90.

Baldessarini RJ, Frankenburg FR. Clozapine. N Engl J Med. 1991;324:746–54.

Choc MG, Hsuan F, Honigfeld G, et al. Single- vs multiple-dose pharmacokinetics of clozapine in psychiatric patients. Pharm Res. 1990;7:347–51.

Clozaril® tablet [package insert]. East Hanover: Novartis Pharmaceuticals Corp; 2010.

Elias TJ, Bannister KM, Clarkson AR, Faull D, Faull RJ. Clozapine-induced acute interstitial nephritis [letter]. Lancet. 1999;354:1180–1.

Fitton A, Heel RC. Clozapine: a review of its pharmacological properties and therapeutic use in schizophrenia. Drugs. 1990;40:722–47.

Haring C, Barnas C, Saria A, Humpel C, Fleischhacker WW. Dose-related plasma levels of clozapine [letters]. J Clin Psychopharmacol. 1989;9:71–2.

Haring C, Fleischhacker WW, Schett P, Humpel C, Barnas C, Saria A. Influence of patient-related variables on clozapine plasma levels. Am J Psychiatry. 1990;147:1471–5.

Haring C, Meise U, Humpel C, Saria A, Fleischhacker WW, Hinterhuber H. Dose-related plasma levels of clozapine: influence of smoking, behaviour, sex and age. Psychopharmacology (Berl). 1989;99(Suppl):S38–40.

Harrington CJ, Kreiss J. Successful use of clozapine with immunosuppressive therapy in a renal-transplant patient [letter]. Psychosomatics. 2008;49:546–8.

Hunter R, Gaughan T, Queirazza F, McMillan D, Shankie S. Clozapine-induced interstitial nephritis – a rare but important complication: a case report. J Med Case Reports. 2009;3:8574.

Jann MW, Grimsley SR, Gray EC, Chang W-H. Pharmacokinetics and pharmacodynamics of clozapine. Clin Pharmacokinet. 1993;24:161–76.

Olyaei AJ, Bennett WM. Drug dosing in elderly patients with chronic kidney disease. Clin Geriatr Med. 2009;25:459–527.

Olyaei AJ, Bennett WM. Pharmacologic approach to renal insufficiency. In: Dale DC, Federman DD, Antman K, editors. ACP medicine, WebMD June 2007 update. Hamilton: BC Decker; 2007; NEPHROLOGY IX: Appendix A1–25.

Pettinger WA, Kenton TK, Campbell WB, Harper DC. Evidence for a renal α-adrenergic receptor inhibiting renin release. Circ Res. 1976;38:338–46.

Schaber G, Stevens I, Gaertner HJ, Dietz K, Breyer-Pfaff U. Pharmacokinetics of clozapine and its metabolites in psychiatric patients: plasma protein binding and renal clearance. Br J Clin Pharmacol. 1998;46:453–59.

Sheehan JJ, Sliwa JK, Amatniek JC, Grinspan A, Canuso CM. Atypical antipsychotic metabolism and excretion. Curr Drug Metab. 2010;11:516–25.

Simpson GM, Josiassen RC, Stanilla JK, et al. Double-blind study of clozapine dose response in chronic schizophrenia. Am J Psychiatry. 1999;156:1744–50.

Dosage Adjustment of Medications Eliminated by the Kidneys

Clozapine/Clozaril®, FazaClo® {Atypical antipsychotic; dibenazepine derivative}

Usual initial dose: 12.5 mg orally

Usual maintenance dose: 300–450 mg/day orally in two to three divided doses

Typical maximum dose: 900 mg/day

Proportion eliminated unchanged: 1 % as parent compound, ~13 % as metabolites with limited activity

Adjustment for Kidney Disease

FDA-approved product labeling: *Caution is advisable in using clozapine in patients with renal disease.*

Alternative adjustment:

	GFR >50 mL/min	*300–450 mg/day orally (100 % of usual dose)*
	GFR 10–50 mL/min	*300–450 mg/day orally (100 % of usual dose)*
	GFR <10 mL/min	*300–450 mg/day orally (100 % of usual dose)*
	Hemodialysis	*Data not available. Preferably avoid unless no suitable alternative exists; if indeed necessary, begin with low doses and monitor drug levels.*
	CAPD	*Data not available. Preferably avoid unless no suitable alternative exists; if indeed necessary, begin with low doses and monitor drug levels.*
	CRRT	*Data not available. Preferably avoid unless no suitable alternative exists; if indeed necessary, begin with low doses and monitor drug levels.*

Codeine - Selected References

Aronoff GA, Bennett WM, Berns JS, et al. Drug prescribing in renal failure: dosing guidelines for adults and children. 5th ed. Philadelphia: American College of Physicians; 2007.

Barnes JN, Williams AJ, Tomson MJF, Toseland PA, Goodwin FJ. Dihydrocodeine in renal failure: further evidence for an important role of the kidney in the handling of opioid drugs. Br Med J (Clin Res Ed). 1985;290:740–2.

Chen ZR, Somogyi AA, Reynolds G, Bochner F. Disposition and metabolism of codeine after single and chronic doses in one poor and seven extensive metabolisers. Br J Clin Pharmacol. 1991;31:381–90.

Codeine sulfate tablet [package insert]. Columbus: Roxane Laboratories Inc; 2010.

Davison AN. Pain in hemodialysis patients: prevalence, cause, severity, and management. Am J Kidney Dis. 2003;42: 1239–47.

Dean M. Opioids in renal failure and dialysis patients. J Pain Symptom Manage. 2004;28:497–504.

Findlay JW, Butz RF, Welch RM. Codeine kinetics as determined by radioimmunoassay. Clin Pharmacol Ther. 1977;22:439–46.

Guay DR, Awni WM, Findlay JW, et al. Pharmacokinetics and pharmacodynamics of codeine in end-stage renal disease. Clin Pharmacol Ther. 1988;43:63–71.

Guay DR, Awni WM, Halstenson CE, et al. Pharmacokinetics of codeine after single- and multiple-oral-dose administration to normal volunteers. J Clin Pharmacol. 1987;27:983–7.

McIntyre CW, Owen PJ. Prescribing drugs in kidney disease. In: Brenner BM, editor. Brenner & Rector's the kidney. 8th ed. Philadelphia: Saunders Elsevier; 2008. p. 1930–55.

Mortimer O, Persson K, Ladona MG, et al. Polymorphic formation of morphine from codeine in poor and extensive metabolizers of dextromethorphan: relationship to the presence of immunoidentified cytochrome P-460IID1. Clin Pharmacol Ther. 1990;47:27–35.

Olyaei AJ, Bennett WM. Drug dosing in elderly patients with chronic kidney disease. Clin Geriatr Med. 2009;25:459–527.

Olyaei AJ, Bennett WM. Pharmacologic approach to renal insufficiency. In: Dale DC, Federman DD, Antman K, editors. ACP medicine, WebMD June 2007 update. Hamilton: BC Decker; 2007; NEPHROLOGY IX: Appendix A1–25.

Olyaei AJ, DeMattos AM, Bennett WM. Use of drugs in patients with renal failure. In: Schrier RW, editor. Diseases of the kidney and urinary tract. 8th ed. Philadelphia: Lippincott Williams & Wilkins; 2007. p. 2765–807.

Talbott GA, Lynn AM, Levy FH, Zelikovic I. Respiratory arrest precipitated by codeine in a child with chronic renal failure. Clin Pediatr (Phila). 1997;36:171–3.

Wolfert AI, Sica DA. Narcotic usage in renal failure [editorial]. Int J Artif Organs. 1988;11:411–5.

Yue QY, Hasselström J, Svensson JO, Säwe J. Pharmacokinetics of codeine and its metabolites in Caucasian healthy volunteers: comparisons between extensive and poor hydroxylators of debrisoquine. Br J Clin Pharmacol. 1991;31:635–42.

Dosage Adjustment of Medications Eliminated by the Kidneys

<u>Codeine</u>	{Analgesic; opioid μ-receptor agonist}
Usual initial dose:	15–60 mg orally, subcutaneously, IM, or IV
Usual maintenance dose:	15–60 mg (usually 30 mg) orally, subcutaneously, IM, or IV every 4 h as necessary
Typical maximum dose:	360 mg/24 h
Proportion eliminated unchanged:	Minimal; predominantly excreted in urine as norcodeine and free and conjugated morphine

Adjustment for Kidney Disease

FDA-approved product labeling:	*Use with caution in elderly or debilitated patients and those with severe impairment of renal function.*	
Alternative adjustment:	*GFR >50 mL/min*	*15–60 mg orally, subcutaneously, IM, or IV q4h PRN*
	GFR 10–50 mL/min	*10–45 mg orally, subcutaneously, IM, or IV q4h PRN*
	GFR <10 mL/min	*Preferably avoid unless no suitable alternative exists; if indeed necessary, begin with low doses and monitor carefully.*
	Hemodialysis	*Preferably avoid unless no suitable alternative exists; if indeed necessary, begin with low doses and monitor carefully.*
	CAPD	*Preferably avoid unless no suitable alternative exists; if indeed necessary, begin with low doses and monitor carefully.*
	CRRT	*10–45 mg orally, subcutaneously, IM, or IV q4h PRN*

Dosage Adjustment of Medications Eliminated by the Kidneys

<u>Colchicine</u> - Selected References

Amderspm-Haag T, Patel B. Safety of colchicine in dialysis patients. Semin Dial. 2003;16:412–3.

Aronoff GA, Bennett WM, Berns JS, et al. Drug prescribing in renal failure: dosing guidelines for adults and children. 5th ed. Philadelphia: American College of Physicians; 2007.

Ben-Chetrit E, Backenroth R, Levy M. Colchicine clearance by high-flux polysulfone dialyzers [letter]. Arthritis Rheum. 1998;41:749–50.

Ben-Chetrit E, Scherrmann M-M, Zylber-Katz E, Levy M. Colchicine disposition in patients with familial Mediterranean fever with renal impairment. J Rheumatol. 1994;21:710–3.

Brown D, Sabolic I, Gluck S. Colchicine-induced redistribution of proton pumps in kidney epithelial cells. Kidney Int. 1991;40(Suppl 33):S79–83.

Colcrys® tablet film coated [package insert]. Philadelphia: AR Scientific Inc; 2010.

Cook M, Ramos E, Peterson J, Croker B. Colchicine neuromyopathy in a renal transplant patient with normal muscle enzyme levels [letter]. Clin Nephrol. 1994;42:67–8.

Hanlon JT, Aspinall SL, Semla TP, et al. Consensus guidelines for oral dosing of primarily renally cleared medications in older adults. J Am Geriatr Soc. 2009;57:335–40.

Kaplan MM, Alling DW, Zimmerman HJ, et al. A prospective trial of colchicine for primary biliary cirrhosis. N Engl J Med. 1986;315:1448–54.

Levy M, Spino M, Read SE. Colchicine: a state-of-the-art review. Pharmacotherapy. 1991;11:196–211.

Livneh A, Zemer D, Langevitz P, Laor A, Sohar E, Pras M. Colchicine treatment of AA amyloidosis of familial Mediterranean fever. Arthritis Rheum. 1994;37:1804–11.

Livneh A, Zemer D, Siegal B, Laor A, Sohar E, Pras M. Colchicine prevents kidney transplant amyloidosis in familial Mediterranean fever. Nephron. 1992;60:418–22.

Older SA, Finbloom DS, Pezeshkpour G. Colchicine myoneuropathy and renal dysfunction [letter]. Ann Rheum Dis. 1992;51:1343–4.

Roberts WN. Liang MH, Stern SH. Colchicine in acute gout: reassessment of risks and benefits. JAMA. 1987;257:1920–2.

Sherif AM, Refale AF, Sobh MA-K, Mohamed NA-H, Sheashaa HA, Ghoneim MA. Long-term outcome of live donor kidney transplantation for renal amyloidosis Am J Kidney Dis. 2003;42:370–5.

Simons RJ, Kingma DW. Fatal colchicine toxicity [letter]. Am J Med. 1989;86:356–7.

Skinner M, Anderson JJ, Simms R, et al. Treatment of 100 patients with primary amyloidosis: a randomized trial of melphalan, prednisone, and colchicine versus colchicine only. Am J Med. 1996;100:290–8.

Sobh M, Refaie A. Colchicine could be safely used in renal patients [letter]. Nephrol Dial Transplant. 1997;12:2304.

Tateishi T, Soucek P, Caraco Y, Guengerich FP, Wood AJJ. Colchicine biotransformation by human liver microsomes: identification of CYP3A4 as the major isoform responsible for colchicine demethylation. Biochem Pharmacol. 1997;53:111–6.

Terkeltaub RA. Colchicine update: 2008. Semin Arthritis Rheum. 2009;38:411–9.

Thomas G, Girre C, Scherrmann JM, Francheteau P, Steimer JL. Zero-order absorption and linear disposition of oral colchicine in healthy volunteers. Eur J Clin Pharmacol. 1989;37:79–84.

Ureña P, Nguyen AT, Jehenne G, Descamps-Latscha B, Drüeke T, Basile C. Short-term administration of colchicine to haemodialysis patients: plasma beta-2 microglobulin and phagocyte oxidative response [letter]. Nephron. 1990;55:348–50.

Wallace SL, Omokoku B, Ertel NH. Colchicine plasma levels: implications as to pharmacology and mechanism of action. Am J Med. 1970;48:443–8.

Wallace SL, Singer JX, Duncan GJ, Wigley FM, Kuncl RW. Renal function predicts colchicine toxicity: guidelines for the prophylactic use of colchicine in gout. J Rheumatol. 1991;18:264–9.

Wallace SL, Singer JZ. Review: systemic toxicity associated with the intravenous administration of colchicine – guidelines for use. J Rheumatol. 1985;15:495–9.

Yü T. The efficacy of colchicine prophylaxis in articular gout: a reappraisal after 20 years. Semin Arthritis Rheum. 1982;12:256–64.

Zemer D, Pras M, Sohar E, Modan M, Cabill S, Gafni J. Colchicine in the prevention and treatment of the amyloidosis of familial Mediterranean fever. N Engl J Med. 1986;314:1001–6.

Dosage Adjustment of Medications Eliminated by the Kidneys

Colchicine/Colcrys®   **{Anti-gout agent; antimitotic}**

Usual initial dose:	For acute gout flare: 1.2 mg orally followed by 0.6 mg orally 6 h later
Usual maintenance dose:	0.6 mg orally once or twice daily
Typical maximum dose:	1.2 mg/day orally
Proportion eliminated unchanged:	5–15 %

Adjustment for Kidney Disease

FDA-approved product labeling: *Colchicine dosage adjustment in adults with renal function impairment*

CrCL (mL/min)	Dose
50–80	0.6 mg orally once or twice daily
30–49	0.6 mg orally once or twice daily
<30	0.3 mg orally once daily
Hemodialysis	0.6 mg orally once, followed by 0.3 mg orally once daily

Alternative adjustment:

GFR >50 mL/min	0.6 mg orally once or twice daily
GFR 10–50 mL/min	0.3–0.6 mg orally once or twice daily
GFR <10 mL/min	Due to potential colchicine-related cellular toxicity, preferably avoid unless no suitable alternative exists; if indeed necessary, 0.3 mg orally once daily. Monitor carefully.
Hemodialysis	0.3 mg once daily; monitor carefully.
CAPD	Due to potential colchicine-related cellular toxicity, preferably avoid unless no suitable alternative exists; if indeed necessary, 0.3 mg orally once daily. Monitor carefully.
CRRT	0.3–0.6 mg enterally once or twice daily

Dosage Adjustment of Medications Eliminated by the Kidneys

Colistimethate - Selected References

Adler S, Segel DP. Nonoliguric renal failure secondary to sodium colistimethate: a report of four cases. Am J Med Sci. 1971;262:109–14.

Bulger RJ, Bennett JV, Boen ST. Intraperitoneal administration of broad-spectrum antibiotics in patients with renal failure. JAMA. 1965;194:1198–202.

Colistimethate sodium injection [package insert]. Schaumburg: APP Pharmaceuticals LLC; 2008.

Couet W, Grégoire N, Gobin P, et al. Pharmacokinetics of colistin and colistimethate sodium after a single 80-mg intravenous dose of CMS in young healthy volunteers. Clin Pharmacol Ther. 2011;89:875–9.

Doshi NM, Mount KL, Murphy CV. Nephrotoxicity associated with intravenous colistin in critically ill patients. Pharmacotherapy. 2011;31:1257–64.

Elwood CM, Lucas GD, Muehrcke RC. Acute renal failure associated with sodium colistimethate treatment. Arch Intern Med. 1966;118:326–34.

Evans ME, Feola DJ, Rapp RP. Polymyxin B and colistin: old antibiotics for emerging multiresistant gram-negative bacteria. Ann Pharmacother. 1999;33:960–7.

Goodwin NJ, Friedman EA. The effects of renal impairment, peritoneal dialysis, and hemodialysis on serum sodium colistimethate levels. Ann Intern Med. 1968;68:984–94.

Greenberg PA, Sanford JP. Removal and absorption of antibiotics in patients with renal failure undergoing peritoneal dialysis: tetracycline, chloramphenicol, kanamycin, and colistimethate. Ann Intern Med. 1967;66:465–79.

Hartzell JD, Neff R, Ake J, et al. Nephrotoxicity associated with intravenous colistin (colistimethate sodium) treatment at a tertiary care medical center. Clin Infect Dis. 2009;48:1724–8.

Heintz BH, Matzke GR, Dager WF. Antimicrobial dosing concepts and recommendations for critically ill adult patients receiving continuous renal replacement therapy or intermittent hemodialysis. Pharmacotherapy. 2009;29:562–77.

Kim J, Lee K-H, Yoo S, Pai H. Clinical characteristics and risk factors for colistin-induced nephrotoxicity. Int J Antimicrob Agents. 2009;34:434–8.

Koomanachai P, Tiengrim S, Kiratisin P, Thamlikitkul V. Efficacy and safety of colistin (colistimethate sodium) for therapy of infections caused by multidrug-resistant *Pseudomonas aeruginosa* and *Acinetobacter baumannii* in Siriraj Hospital, Bangkok, Thailand. Int J Infect Dis. 2007;11:402–6.

Li J, Coulthard K, Milne R, et al. Steady-state pharmacokinetics of intravenous colistin methanesulfonate in patients with cystic fibrosis. J Antimicrob Chemother. 2003;52:987–92.

Li J, Nation RL, Owen J, Wong S, Spelman D, Franklin C. Antibiograms of multidrug-resistant clinical *Acinetobacter baumannii*: promising therapeutic options for treatment of infection with colistin-resistant strains. Clin Infect Dis. 2007;45:594–8.

Lim LM, Ly N, Anderson D, et al. Resurgence of colistin: a review of resistance, toxicity, pharmacodynamics, and dosing. Pharmacotherapy. 2010;30:1279–91.

MacKay DN, Kaye D. Sodium colistimethate dosage in renal failure. Ann Intern Med. 1968;69:639–41.

Montero M, Horcajada JP, Sorli L, et al. Effectiveness and safety of colistin for the treatment of multidrug-resistant Pseudomonas aeruginosa infections. Infection. 2009;37:461–5.

Oliveira MS, Prado GVB, Costa SF, Grinbaum RS, Levin AS. Polymyxin B and colistimethate are comparable as to efficacy and renal toxicity. Diagn Microbiol Infect Dis. 2009;65:431–4.

Plachouras D, Karvanen M, Friberg LE, et al. Population pharmacokinetic analysis of colistin methanesulfonate and colistin after intravenous administration in critically ill patients with infections caused by gram-negative bacteria. Antimicrob Agents Chemother. 2009;53:3430–6.

Randall RE, Bridi GS, Setter JG, Brackett NC. Recovery from colistimethate nephrotoxicity. Ann Intern Med. 1970;73:491–2.

Terkoglu M, Dizbay M, Çiftçi A, Aksakal FN, Aygencel G. Colistin therapy in critically ill patients with chronic renal failure and its effect on development of renal dysfunction. Int J Antimicrob Agents. 2011. Epub ahead of print. doi:10.1016/j.ijantimicag.2011.10.006.

Trotman RL, Williamson JC, Shoemaker DM, Salzer WL. Antibiotic dosing in critically ill adult patients receiving continuous renal replacement therapy. Clin Infect Dis. 2005;41:1159–66.

Dosage Adjustment of Medications Eliminated by the Kidneys

Colistimethate (Colistin, Polymyxin E)/Coly-Mycin® M   {Antibacterial; polymyxin derivative}

Usual initial dose:	1.25–2.5 mg/kg IV or IM
Usual maintenance dose:	2.5–5 mg/kg/day IV or IM in two to four divided doses, depending on severity of infection
Typical maximum dose:	5 mg/kg/day IV or IM
Proportion eliminated unchanged:	70 %

Adjustment for Kidney Disease

FDA-approved product labeling:
Colistimethate dosage schedules for adults with impaired renal function

Renal function			Dosage			
Degree of impairment	Serum creatinine (mg/dL)	Urea clearance (% of normal)	Dose (mg)	Frequency (times per day)	Total daily dose (mg)	Approx daily dose (mg/kg)
Normal	0.7–1.2	80–100	100–150	2–4	300	5
Mild	1.3–1.5	40–70	75–115	2	150–230	2.5–3.8
Moderate	1.6–2.5	25–40	66–150	1–2	133–150	2.5
Severe	2.6–4	10–25	100–150	q 36 h	100	1.5

Note: The suggested unit dose is 2.5–5 mg/kg; the time interval between doses should be increased in the presence of impaired renal function

Alternative adjustment:		
	eCrCL >80 mL/min	*2.5–5 mg/kg/day IV in two to three divided doses*
	eCrCL 50–80 mL/min	*2.5–3.8 mg/kg/day IV in two divided doses*
	eCrCL 10–49 mL/min	*2.5 mg/kg/day IV or IM in one or two divided doses*
	CrCL <10 mL/min	*1.5 mg/kg IV or IM every 36 h*
	Hemodialysis	*1.5 mg/kg IV every 24–48 h*
	CVVH	*2.5 mg/kg IV every 48 h*
	CVVHD or CVVHDF	*2.5 mg/kg IV every 48 h*

Dosage Adjustment of Medications Eliminated by the Kidneys

Conivaptan - Selected References

Ali F, Guglin M, Vaitkevicius P, Ghali JK. Therapeutic potential of vasopressin receptor antagonists. Drugs. 2007;67:847–58.

Anderson RJ, Chung HM, Kluge R, Schrier RW. Hyponatremia: a prospective analysis of its epidemiology and the pathogenetic role of vasopressin. Ann Intern Med. 1985;102:164–8.

Burnier M, Fricker AF, Hayoz D, Nussberger J, Brunner HR. Pharmacokinetic and pharmacodynamic effects of YM087, a combined V1/V2 vasopressin receptor antagonists in normal subjects. Eur J Clin Pharmacol. 1999;55:633–7.

DeVita MV, Gardenswartz MH, Konecky A, Zabetakis PM. Incidence and etiology of hyponatremia in an intensive care unit. Clin Nephrol. 1990;34:163–6.

Ellison DH, Berl T. The syndrome of inappropriate antidiuresis. N Engl J Med. 2007;356:2064–72.

Galton C, Deem S, Yanez ND, et al. Open-label randomized trial of the safety and effectiveness of a single dose conivaptan to raise serum sodium in patients with traumatic brain injury. Neurocrit Care. 2011;14:354–60.

Gassanov N, Semmo N, Semmo M, Nia AM, Fuhr U, Er F. Arginine vasopressin (AVP) and treatment with arginine vasopressin receptor antagonists (vaptans) in congestive heart failure, liver cirrhosis and syndrome of inappropriate antidiuretic hormone secretion (SIADH). Eur J Clin Pharmacol. 2011;67:333–46.

Ghali JK, Koren MJ, Taylor JR, et al. Efficacy and safety of oral conivaptan: a V_{1A}/V_2 vasopressin receptor antagonist, assessed in a randomized, placebo-controlled trial in patients with euvolemic or hypervolemic hyponatremia. J Clin Endocrinol Metab. 2006;91:2145–52.

Goldsmith SR, Gilbertson DT, Mackedanz SA, Swan SK. Renal effects of conivaptan, furosemide, and the combination in patients with chronic heart failure. J Card Fail. 2011;17:982–9.

Hawkins RC. Age and gender as risk factors for hyponatremia and hypernatremia. Clin Chem Acta. 2003;337:169–72.

Li-Ng M, Verbalis JG. Conivaptan: evidence supporting its therapeutic use in hyponatremia. Core Evid. 2009;4:83–92.

Mao ZL, Stalker D, Keirns J. Pharmacokinetics of conivaptan hydrochloride, a vasopressin V_{1A}/V_2-receptor antagonist, in patients with euvolemic or hypervolemic hyponatremia and with or without congestive heart failure from a prospective, 4-day open-label study. Clin Ther. 2009;31:1542–50.

Messert B, Orrison WW, Hawkins MJ, Quaglieri CE. Central pontine myelinolysis: considerations on etiology, diagnosis, and treatment. Neurology. 1979;29:147–60.

Oh MS. Management of hyponatremia and clinical use of vasopressin antagonists. Am J Med Sci. 2007;333:101–5.

Potts MB, Deiacomo AF, Deragopian L, Blevins LS Jr. Use of intravenous conivaptan in neurosurgical patients with hyponatremia from syndrome of inappropriate antidiuretic hormone secretion. Neurosurgery. 2011;69:268–73.

Rai A, Whaley-Connell A, McFarlane S, Sowers JR. Hyponatremia, arginine vasopressin dysregulation, and vasopressin receptor antagonism. Am J Nephrol. 2006;26:579–89.

Russell SD, Selaru P, Pyne DA, et al. Rationale for use of an exercise end point and design for the ADVANCE (A Dose evaluation of a Vasopressin ANtagonist in CHF patients undergoing Exercise) trial. Am Heart J. 2003;145:179–86.

Schrier RW. The sea within us: disorders of body water homeostasis. Curr Opin Investig Drugs. 2007;8:304–11.

Sughrue ME, McDermott M, Blevins LS. Extreme correction of hyponatremia in a patient treated with intravenous conivaptan. J Clin Neurosci. 2010;17:1331–4.

Tahara A, Saito M, Sugimoto T, et al. Pharmacological characterization of YM087, a potent, nonpeptide human vasopressin V_{1A} and V_2 receptor antagonist. Naunyn Schmiedebergs Arch Pharmacol. 1998;357:63–9.

Tahara A, Tomura Y, Wada K-I, et al. Pharmacological profile of YM087, a novel potent, nonpeptide vasopressin V_{1A} and V_2 receptor antagonist, in vitro and in vivo. J Pharmacol Exp Ther. 1997;282:301–8.

Udelson JE, Smith WB, Hendrix GH, et al. Acute hemodynamic effects of conivaptan, a dual V_{1A} and V_2 vasopressin receptor antagonist, in patients with advanced heart failure. Circulation. 2001;104:2417–23.

Vaprisol® injection [package insert]. Deerfield: Astellas Pharma US Inc; 2011.

Zeltser D, Rosansky S, van Rensburg H, Verbalis JG, Smith N. Assessment of the efficacy and safety of intravenous conivaptan in euvolemic and hypervolemic hyponatremia. Am J Nephrol. 2007;27:447–57.

Dosage Adjustment of Medications Eliminated by the Kidneys

<u>Conivaptan</u>/Vaprisol®

{Vasopressin receptor antagonist; ℞ for hypovolemic/euvolemic hyponatremia}

Usual initial dose: 20 mg IV over 30 min

Usual maintenance dose: 20 mg/24 h continuous IV infusion for 2–4 days; depending on response, may increase to 40 mg/24 h IV on treatment day 2 and thereafter

Typical maximum dose: 40 mg/day

Proportion eliminated unchanged: 1 % (plus 10 % as minimally active metabolites)

Adjustment for Kidney Disease

FDA-approved product labeling:	*CrCL >60 mL/min*	*20 mg/24 h continuous IV infusion for 2–4 days; monitor fluid status and serum sodium frequently and discontinue if patient develops hypovolemia, hypotension, or an undesirably rapid rate of rise of serum sodium.*
	CrCL 30–60 mg/min	*10 mg IV followed by 10 mg/24 h continuous IV infusion for 2–4 days; if serum sodium is not increasing at a desired rate, may increase to 20 mg/24 h continuous IV infusion.*
	CrCL <30 ml/min, anuria	*Contraindicated (no improvement can be expected.)*
Alternative adjustment:	*Data not available*	

Cycloserine - Selected References

Aronoff GA, Bennett WM, Berns JS, et al. Drug prescribing in renal failure: dosing guidelines for adults and children. 5th ed. Philadelphia: American College of Physicians; 2007.

Bankier RG. Psychosis associated with cycloserine. Can Med Assoc J. 1965;93:35–7.

Conzelman GM. The physiologic disposition of cycloserine in the human subject. Am Rev Tuberc Respir Dis. 1956;74:739–46.

Holdiness MR. Clinical pharmacokinetics of the antituberculosis drugs. Clin Pharmacokinet. 1984;9:511–44.

Jassal M, Rishai WR, Extensively drug-resistant tuberculosis. Lancet Infect Dis. 2009;9:19–30.

Malone RS, Fish DN, Spiegel DM, Childs JM, Peloquin CA. The effect of hemodialysis on cycloserine, ethionamide, para-aminosalicylate, and clofazimine. Chest. 1999;116:984–90.

Peloquin CA. Pharmacology of the antimycobacterial drugs. Med Clin North Am. 1993;77:1253–62.

Seromycin® capsule [package insert]. Indianapolis: Eli Lilly Co; 2005.

Thorsteinsson T, Másson M, Jarvinen T, Nevalainen T, Loftsson T. Cycloserine fatty acid derivatives as prodrugs: synthesis, degradation and in vitro skin permeability. Chem Pharm Bull (Tokyo). 2002;50:554–7.

Zítková L, Toušek J. Pharmacokinetics of cycloserine and terizidone. Chemotherapy. 1974;20:18–28.

Dosage Adjustment of Medications Eliminated by the Kidneys

Cycloserine/Seromycin®   {**Antitubercular; cell wall biosynthesis inhibitor**}

Usual initial dose:	250 mg orally twice daily
Usual maintenance dose:	250–500 mg orally twice daily
Typical maximum dose:	1,000 mg/day orally
Proportion eliminated unchanged:	65 %

Adjustment for Kidney Disease

FDA-approved product labeling:	*Severe renal insufficiency*	*Contraindicated*
Alternative adjustment:	*GFR >50 mL/min*	*250–500 mg orally every 12 h*
	GFR 10–50 mL/min	*250–500 mg orally every 24 h*
	GFR <10 mL/min	*250–500 mg orally every 36–48 h*
	Hemodialysis	*250–500 mg orally three times weekly after hemodialysis*
	CAPD	*Data not available. Preferably avoid unless no suitable alternative exists; if indeed necessary, begin with low doses and monitor carefully.*
	CRRT	*250–500 mg orally every 24 h*

D

L.K. Golightly et al. (eds.), *Renal Pharmacotherapy*,
DOI 10.1007/978-1-4614-5800-5_4, © Springer Science+Business Media New York 2013

Dosage Adjustment of Medications Eliminated by the Kidneys

<u>Dabigatran</u> - Selected References

Alberts MJ, Bernstein RA, Naccarelli GV, Garcia DA. Using dabigatran in patients with stroke: a practical guide for clinicians. Stroke. 2012;43:271–9.

Blech S, Ebner T, Ludwig-Schwellinger E, Stangier J, Roth W. The metabolism of the oral direct thrombin inhibitor, dabigatran, in humans. Drug Metab Dispos. 2008;36:386–99.

Cho Y, Mills K, Sturtevant JM, Pillans PI, Mudge DW. Dabigatran may not be an effective anticoagulant for haemodialysis. Nephrology (Carlton). 2010;15:594–5.

Connolly SJ, Ezekowitz MD, Yusuf S, et al. Dabigatran versus warfarin in patients with atrial fibrillation. N Engl J Med. 2009;361:1139–51.

Cotton BA, McCarthy JJ, Holcomb JB. Acutely injured patients on dabigatran [letter]. N Engl J Med. 2011;365:2039–40.

Ebner T, Wagner K, Wienen W. Dabigatran acylglucuronide, the major human metabolite of dabigatran: in vitro formation, stability, and pharmacological activity. Drug Metab Dispos. 2010;38:1567–75.

Eerenberg ES, Kamphuisen PW, Sijpkens MK, Meijers JC, Buller HR, Levi M. Reversal of rivaroxaban and dabigatran by prothrombin complex concentrate: a randomized, placebo-controlled, crossover study in healthy subjects. Circulation. 2011;124:1573–9.

Ezekowitz MD, Wallentin L, Connolly SJ, et al. Dabigatran and warfarin in vitamin K antagonist-naïve and – experienced cohorts with atrial fibrillation. Circulation. 2010;122:2246–53.

Legrand M, Mateo J, Aribaud A, et al. The use of dabigatran in elderly patients. Arch Intern Med. 2011;171:1285–8.

Lehr T, Haertter S, Liesenfeld K-H, et al. Dabigatran etexilate in atrial fibrillation patients with severe renal impairment: dose identification using pharmacokinetic modeling and simulation. J Clin Pharmacol. 2011. Epub ahead of print. doi:10.1177/0091270011417716.

Liesenfeld K-H, Lehr T, Dansirikul C, et al. Population pharmacokinetic analysis of the oral thrombin inhibitor dabigatran etexilate in patients with non-valvular atrial fibrillation from the RE-LY trial. J Thromb Haemost. 2011;9:2168–75.

Naranjo IC, Portilla-Cuenca JC, Caballero PEJ, Escobar MLC, Sevilla RMR. Fatal intracerebral hemorrhage associated with administration of recombinant tissue plasminogen activator in a stroke patient on treatment with dabigatran. Cerebrovasc Dis. 2011;32:614–5.

Oldgren J, Alings M, Darius H, et al. Risks for stroke, bleeding, and death in patients with atrial fibrillation receiving dabigatran or warfarin in relation to the CHADS$_2$ score: a subgroup analysis of the RE-LY trial. Ann Intern Med. 2011;155:660–7.

Pradaxa® capsule [package insert]. Ridgefield: Boehringer Ingelheim Pharmaceuticals Inc; 2011.

Stangier J. Clinical pharmacokinetics and pharmacodynamics of the oral direct thrombin inhibitor dabigatran etexilate. Clin Pharmacokinet. 2008;47:285–95.

Stangier J, Rathgen K, Stähle H, Gansser D, Roth W. The pharmacokinetics, pharmacodynamics and tolerability of dabigatran etexilate, a new oral direct thrombin inhibitor, in healthy male subjects. Br J Clin Pharmacol. 2007;64:292–303.

Stangier J, Rathgen K, Stähle H, Mazur D. Influence of renal impairment on the pharmacokinetics and pharmacodynamics of oral dabigatran etexilate: an open-label, parallel-group, single center study. Clin Pharmacokinet. 2010;49:259–68.

Stangier J, Stähle H, Rathgen K, Fuhr R. Pharmacokinetics and pharmacodynamics of the direct thrombin inhibitor dabigatran in healthy elderly subjects. Clin Pharmacokinet. 2008;47:47–59.

Trocóniz IF, Tillmann C, Liesenfeld K-H, Schäfer H-G, Stangier J. Population pharmacokinetic analysis of the new oral thrombin inhibitor dabigatran etexilate (BIBR 1048) in patients undergoing primary elective total hip replacement surgery. J Clin Pharmacol. 2007;47:371–82.

van Ryn J, Stangier J, Haertter S, et al. Dabigatran etexilate—a novel, reversible, oral direct thrombin inhibitor: interpretation of coagulation assays and reversal of anticoagulant activity. Thromb Haemost. 2010;103:1116–23.

Wallentin L, Ezekowitz MD, Alings M, et al. Efficacy and safety of dabigatran compared with warfarin at different levels of international normalized ratio control for stroke prevention in atrial fibrillation: an analysis of the RE-LY trial. Lancet. 2010;376:975–83.

Watanabe M, Siddiqui FM, Qureshi AI. Incidence and management of ischemic stroke and intracerebral hemorrhage in patients on dabigatran etexilate treatment. Neurocrit Care. 2011. Epub ahead of print. doi:10.1007/s12028-011-9591-y.

Weitz JI, Eikelboom JW, Samama MM. New antithrombotic drugs: antithrombotic therapy and prevention of thrombosis, 9th ed: American College of Chest Physicians Evidence-Based Clinical Practice Guidelines. Chest 2012;141(2 Suppl):e120–51S. doi:10.1378/chest.11-2294.

Dosage Adjustment of Medications Eliminated by the Kidneys

<u>Dabigatran</u>/Pradaxa®   {Antithrombotic; direct thrombin inhibitor}

Usual initial dose: 150 mg orally

Usual maintenance dose: 150 mg orally twice daily

Typical maximum dose: 300 mg/day orally

Proportion eliminated unchanged: 51–80 %

Adjustment for Kidney Disease

FDA-approved product labeling: *CrCL >30 mL/min*   *150 mg orally twice daily*

                                      CrCL15–30 mL/min   *75 mg orally twice daily*

                                      CrCL <15 mL/min   *Dosing recommendations cannot be provided.*

                                      Hemodialysis   *Dosing recommendations cannot be provided.*

Note: Renal function should be assessed by calculating the CrCL prior to initiation of treatment. While on treatment, renal function should be assessed in clinical situations which may be associated with a decline in renal function. In patients with a CrCL <50 mL/min or >75 years of age, renal function should be assessed at least once a year.

Alternative adjustment: *eCrCL >30 mL/min*   *150 mg orally twice daily*

                                      eCrCL ≤30 mL/min   *Due to the exclusionary lack of clinical trial data and information on patients affected by kidney disease as well as the lack of a clinically effective anticoagulant reversal agent for dabigatran-associated hemorrhage, consider beginning alternative anticoagulation therapy upon hospitalization at a minimum 24 h after patient's last dose of dabigatran:*

                                                             Cardiac failure, hypertension, age, diabetes mellitus, and stroke [doubled] (CHADS) score = 1–2 (low risk) → Suggest prophylactic dose subcutaneous low-molecular-weight heparin (LMWH) or no bridging over bridging with therapeutic dose LMWH or unfractionated heparin (UFH).

                                                             CHADS = 2–3 (moderate risk) → Suggest therapeutic dose subcutaneous or IV UFH or prophylactic dose subcutaneous LMWH over no bridging.

                                                             CHADS = 4–5 (high risk) → Recommend therapeutic dose subcutaneous or IV UFH over no bridging.

                                      Hemodialysis   *Preferably avoid due to hemorrhagic risk*

                                      CRRT   *Data not available*

Dosage Adjustment of Medications Eliminated by the Kidneys

Dalfampridine - Selected References

Ampyra™ tablet film coated extended release [package insert]. Hawthorne: Acorda Therapeutics Inc; 2010.

Dalfampridine (Ampyra) for MS. Med Lett Drugs Ther. 2010;52:73–4.

Dunn J, Blight A. Dalfampridine: a brief review of its mechanism of action and efficacy as a treatment to improve walking in patients with multiple sclerosis. Curr Med Res Opin. 2011;27:1415–23.

Goodman AD, Brown TR, Edwards KR, et al. A phase 3 trial of extended release oral dalfampridine in multiple sclerosis. Ann Neurol. 2010;38:494–502.

Hayes KC. Impact of extended-release dalfampridine on walking ability in patients with multiple sclerosis. Neuropsychiatr Dis Treat. 2011;7:229–39.

Jeffrey DR, Pharr EP. Dalfampridine sustained-release for symptomatic improvement of walking speed in patients with multiple sclerosis. Core Evid. 2010;5:107–12.

Dosage Adjustment of Medications Eliminated by the Kidneys

<u>**Dalfampridine**</u>/Ampyra™   {**Potassium channel blocker; ℞ for improved walking distance in patients with multiple sclerosis (MS)**}

Usual initial dose: 10 mg orally twice daily

Usual maintenance dose: 10 mg orally twice daily

Typical maximum dose: 20 mg/day

Proportion eliminated unchanged: 90 %

Adjustment for Kidney Disease

    FDA-approved product labeling: *CrCL >50 mL/min*   *10 mg orally twice daily (Note: In patients with mild renal impairment [CrCL 51–80 mL/min], this dose was associated serum drug levels equivalent to higher doses in patients with normal renal function that resulted in a fourfold increase in the incidence of drug-induced seizures.)*

                                   CrCL ≤50 mL/min   *Contraindicated*

    Alternative adjustment: *Data not available*

Dosage Adjustment of Medications Eliminated by the Kidneys

Dalteparin - Selected References

Clark NP. Low-molecular-weight heparin use in obese, elderly, and in renal insufficiency. Thromb Res. 2008;123:S58–61.

Cook D, Douketis J, Meade M, et al. Venous thromboembolism and bleeding in critically ill patients with severe renal insufficiency receiving dalteparin thromboprophylaxis: prevalence, incidence and risk factors. Crit Care. 2008;12:R32. doi:10.1186/cc6810.

Douketis J, Cook D, Meade M, et al. Prophylaxis against deep vein thrombosis in critically ill patients with severe renal insufficiency with the low-molecular-weight heparin dalteparin--an assessment of safety and pharmacodynamics: the DIRECT Study. Arch Intern Med. 2008;168:1805–12.

Egger SS, Sawatski MG, Drewe J, Krähenbühl S. Life-threatening hemorrhage after dalteparin therapy in a patient with impaired renal function. Pharmacotherapy. 2005;25:881–5.

Faroq V, Hegarty J, Chandrasekar T, et al. Serious adverse incidents with usage of low molecular weight heparins in patients with chronic kidney disease. Am J Kidney Dis. 2004;43:531–7.

Fragmin® injection [package insert]. New York: Pfizer Inc; 2010.

Frank RD, Brandenburg VM, Lanzmich R, Floege J. Factor Xa-activated whole blood clotting time (Xa-ACT) for bedside monitoring dalteparin anticoagulation during haemodialysis. Nephrol Dial Transplant. 2004;19:1552–8.

Garcia DA, Baglin TP, Weitz JI, Samama MM. Parenteral anticoagulants: antithrombotic therapy and prevention of thrombosis. 9th ed: American College of Chest Physicians Evidence-Based Clinical Practice Guidelines. Chest. 2012;141 (2 Suppl):e24–43S. doi:10.1378/chest.11-2291.

Hofbauer R, Moser D, Frass M, et al. Effect of anticoagulation on blood membrane interactions during hemodialysis. Kidney Int. 1999;56:1578–83.

Jeffrey RF, Khan AA, Douglas JT, Will EJ, Davison AM. Anticoagulation with low molecular weight heparin (Fragmin) during continuous hemodialysis in the intensive care unit. Artif Organs. 1993;17:717–20.

Kani C, Markantonis SL, Nicolaou C, Maggina N. Monitoring of subcutaneous dalteparin in patients with renal insufficiency under intensive care: an observational study. J Crit Care. 2006;21:79–84.

Natescu EA, Spinler SA, Wittkowsky A, Dager WE. Low-molecular-weight heparins in renal impairment and obesity: available evidence and clinical practice recommendations across medical and surgical settings. Ann Pharmacother. 2009;43:1064–83.

Perry SL, O'Shea SI, Byrne S, Szczech LA, Ortel TL. A multi-dose pharmacokinetic study of dalteparin in haemodialysis patients. Thromb Haemost. 2006;96:750–5.

Polkinghorne KR, McMahon LP, Becker GJ. Pharmacokinetic studies of dalteparin (Fragmin), enoxaparin (Clexane), and danaparoid (Orgaran) in stable chronic hemodialysis patients. Am J Kidney Dis. 2002;40:990–5.

Rabbat CG, Cook DJ, Crowther MA, et al. Dalteparin thromboprophylaxis for critically ill medical-surgical patients with renal insufficiency. J Crit Care. 2005;20:357–63.

Reeves JH, Cumming AR, Gallagher L, O'Brien JL, Santamaria JD. A controlled trial of low-molecular-weight heparin (dalteparin) versus unfractionated heparin as anticoagulant during continuous venovenous hemodialysis with filtration. Crit Care Med. 1999;27:2224–8.

Sagedal S, Hartmann A, Sundrtrøm K, Bjørnsen S, Brosstad F. Anticoagulation intensity sufficient for haemodialysis does not prevent activation of coagulation and platelets. Nephrol Dial Transplant. 2001;16:987–93.

Sagedal S, Hartmann A, Sundrtrøm K Bjørnsen S, Fauchald P, Brosstad F. A single dose of dalteparin effectively prevents clotting during haemodialysis. Nephrol Dial Transplant. 1999;14:1493–7.

Schmid P, Brodmann D, Fischer AG, Wuillemin WA. Prospective observational cohort study of bioaccumulation of dalteparin at a prophylactic dose in patients with peritoneal dialysis. J Thromb Haemost. 2010;8:850–2.

Schmid P, Brodmann D, Odermatt Y, Fischer AG, Wuillemin WA. Study of bioaccumulation of dalteparin at a therapeutic dose in patients with renal insufficiency. J Thromb Haemost. 2009;7:1629–32.

Shprecher AR, Cheng-Lai A, Madsen EM, et al. Peak antifactor Xa activity produced by dalteparin treatment in patients with renal impairment compared with controls. Pharmacotherapy. 2005;25:817–22.

Stöbe J, Siegemund A, Achenbach H, Preiss C, Preiss R. Evaluation of the pharmacokinetics of dalteparin in patients with renal insufficiency. Int J Clin Pharmacol Ther. 2006;44:455–64.

Tincani E, Mannucci C, Casolari B, et al. Safety of dalteparin for the prophylaxis of venous thromboembolism in elderly medical patients with renal insufficiency: a pilot study. Haematologica. 2006;91:976–9.

Dosage Adjustment of Medications Eliminated by the Kidneys

<u>Dalteparin</u>/Fragmin®	{Antithrombotic; low-molecular weight heparin}
Usual initial dose:	2,500–5,000 units subcutaneously (prophylaxis)
	200 units/kg subcutaneously (treatment)
Usual maintenance dose:	2,500–5,000 units subcutaneously every 24 h (prophylaxis)
	200 units/kg subcutaneously every 24 h if ≤95 kg or 100 units/kg subcutaneously every 12 h if >95 kg (treatment)
Typical maximum dose:	~30,000 units/day
Proportion eliminated unchanged:	Data not available

Adjustment for Kidney Disease

FDA-approved product labeling:	*CrCL <30 mL/min*	*In patients with symptomatic venous thromboembolism with severely impaired renal function (CrCL <30 mL/min), monitoring for anti-Xa levels is recommended to determine the appropriate dose. Target anti-Xa range is 0.5– 1.5 IU/mL. When monitoring anti-Xa in these patients, sampling should be performed 4–6 h after dosing and only after the patient has received three to four doses.*
Alternative adjustment:	*eGFR <30 mL/min*	*Not recommended, preferably avoid—although substantial data indicate that usual doses of dalteparin provide adequate prophylactic, therapeutic, and intradialytic antithrombotic actions, currently available clinical information suggests that dalteparin effects are highly variable in patients with kidney disease and, accordingly, its use generally should be discouraged in favor of unfractionated heparin, parenteral direct thrombin inhibitors, or warfarin.*

Dosage Adjustment of Medications Eliminated by the Kidneys

Daptomycin - Selected References

Aronoff GA, Bennett WM, Berns JS, et al. Drug prescribing in renal failure: dosing guidelines for adults and children. 5th ed. Philadelphia: American College of Physicians; 2007.

Bahte SK, Bertram A, Burkhardt O, et al. Therapeutic serum concentrations of daptomycin after intraperitoneal administration in a patient with peritoneal dialysis-associated peritonitis [letter]. J Antimicrob Chemother. 2010;65:1312–4.

Benvenuto M, Benziger DP, Yankelev S, Vigliani G. Pharmacokinetics and tolerability of daptomycin at doses up to 12 milligrams per kilogram of body weight once daily in healthy volunteers. Antimicrob Agents Chemother. 2006;50:3245–9.

Benziger DP, Pertel PE, Donovan J, et al. Pharmacokinetics and safety of multiple doses of daptomycin 6 mg/kg in noninfected adults undergoing hemodialysis or continuous ambulatory peritoneal dialysis. Clin Nephrol. 2011;75:63–9.

Bogard KN, Peterson NT, Plumb TJ, Erwin MW, Fuller PD, Olsen KM. Antibiotic dosing during sustained low-efficiency dialysis: special considerations in adult critically ill patients. Crit Care Med. 2011;39:560–70.

Cardone KE, Lodise TP, Patel N, et al. Pharmacokinetics and pharmacodynamics of intravenous daptomycin during continuous ambulatory peritoneal dialysis. Clin J Am Soc Nephrol. 2011. Epub ahead of print. doi:10.2215/CJN.08510910.

Chakraborty A, Roy S, Loeffler J, Chaves RL. Comparison of the pharmacokinetics, safety and tolerability of daptomycin in healthy adult volunteers following intravenous administration by 30 min infusion or 2 min injection. J Antimicrob Chemother. 2009;64:151–8.

Churchwell MD, Mueller BA. Drug dosing during continuous renal replacement therapy. Semin Dial. 2009;22:185–8

Cubicin® injection [package insert]. Lexington: Cubist Pharmaceuticals Inc; 2010.

Dvorchik BH, Brazier D, DeBruin MF, Arbeit RD. Daptomycin pharmacokinetics and safety following administration of escalating doses once daily to healthy subjects. Antimicrob Agents Chemother. 2003;47:1318–23.

Dvorchik BH, Damphousse D. The pharmacokinetics of daptomycin in moderately obese, morbidly obese, and matched nonobese subjects. J Clin Pharmacol. 2005;45:48–56.

Goedecke VA, Clajus C, Burkhardt O, et al. Pharmacokinetics and dialysate levels of daptomycin given intravenously in a peritoneal dialysis patient. Scand J Infect Dis. 2009;41:155–7.

Heintz BH, Matzke GR, Dager WF. Antimicrobial dosing concepts and recommendations for critically ill adult patients receiving continuous renal replacement therapy or intermittent hemodialysis. Pharmacotherapy. 2009;29:562–77.

Huen SC, Hall I, Topal J, Mahnensmith RL, Brewster UC, Abu-Alfa AK. Successful use of daptomycin in the treatment of vancomycin-resistant enterococcus peritonitis. Am J Kidney Dis. 2009;54:538–41.

Kielstein JT, Engbers C, Bode-Boeger SM, et al. Dosing of daptomycin in intensive care unit patients with acute kidney injury undergoing extended dialysis: a pharmacokinetic study. Nephrol Dial Transplant. 2010;25:1537–41.

Kullar R, Davis SL, Levine DP, et al. High-dose daptomycin for treatment of complicated gram-positive infections: a large, multicenter, retrospective study. Pharmacotherapy. 2011;31:527–36.

Liu C, Cosgrove SE, Daum RS, et al. Clinical practice Guidelines by the Infectious Diseases Society of America for the treatment of methicillin-resistant *Staphylococcus aureus* infections in adults and children. Clin Infect Dis. 2011;52:1–38.

Mohr JF III, Ostrosky-Zeichner L, Wainright DJ, Parks DH, Hollenbeck TC, Ericsson Pharmacokinetic evaluation of single-dose intravenous daptomycin in patients with thermal burn injury. Antimicrob Agents Chemother. 2008;52:1891–3.

Oleson FB Jr, Berman CL, Kirkpatrick JB, Regan KS, Lai J-J Tally FP. Once-daily dosing in dogs optimizes daptomycin therapy. Antimicrob Agents Chemother. 2000;44:2948–53.

Patel N, Cardone K, Grabe DW, et al. Use of pharmacokinetic and pharmacodynamic principles to determine optimal administration of daptomycin in patients receiving standardized thrice-weekly hemodialysis. Antimicrob Agents Chemother. 2011;55:1677–83.

Salama NN, Segal JH, Churchwell MD, et al. Intradialytic administration of daptomycin in end stage renal disease patients on hemodialysis. Clin J Am Soc Nephrol. 2009;4:1190–4.

Salama NN, Segal JH, Churchwell MD, et al. Single-dose daptomycin pharmacokinetics in chronic haemodialysis patients. Nephrol Dial Transplant. 2010;25:1279–84.

Vilay AM, Grio M, DePestel DD, et al. Daptomycin pharmacokinetics in critically ill patients receiving continuous veno-venous hemodialysis. Crit Care Med. 2011;39:19–25.

Wenisch JM, Meyer B, Fuhrmann V, et al. Multiple-dose pharmacokinetics of daptomycin during continuous venovenous haemodiafiltration. J Antimicrob Chemother. 2012;67:977–83.

Dosage Adjustment of Medications Eliminated by the Kidneys

Daptomycin/Cubicin®   {Antibacterial, lipopeptide bacterial membrane depolarizer and protein, DNA, and RNA biosynthesis inhibitor}

Usual initial dose:	6 mg/kg IV (actual body weight)
Usual maintenance dose:	6 mg/kg IV every 24 h
Typical maximum dose:	10 mg/kg/day
Proportion eliminated unchanged:	80 %

Adjustment for Kidney Disease

FDA-approved product labeling: *Recommended daptomycin dosage regimen for adult patients*

CrCL (mL/min)	Complicated skin infections	Staphylococcus aureus bloodstream infections
≥30	4 mg/kg once every 24 h	6 mg/kg once every 24 h
<30 (including hemodialysis or CAPD)	4 mg/kg once every 48 h	6 mg/kg once every 48 h

Alternative adjustment:

GFR >50 mL/min	6–10 mg/kg actual body weight IV every 24 h
GFR 10–50 mL/min	4–6 mg/kg IV every 24–48 h
GFR <10 mL/min	4–6 mg/kg IV every 48 h
Hemodialysis	4–6 mg/kg IV every 48 h or 6 mg/kg IV at end of dialysis three times weekly
Sustained low-efficiency dialysis	6 mg/kg IV daily on dialysis days
CAPD	4–6 mg/kg IV every 48 h or addition of 20 mg/L in peritoneal dialysate (limited data)
CVVH	4–6 mg/kg IV every 48 h
CVVHD or CVVHDF	8 mg/kg IV every 48 h

Daunorubicin - Selected References

Bachur NR, Huffman DH. Daunorubicin metabolism: estimation of daunorubicin reductase. Br J Pharmacol. 1971; 43:828–33.

Cerubidine® injection [package insert]. Bedford: Bedford Laboratories; 2007.

Greene W, Huffman D, Wienik PH, Schimpff S, Benjamin R, Bachur N. High-dose daunorubicin for acute nonlymphcytic leukemia: correlation of response and toxicity with pharmacokinetics and intracellular daunorubicin reductase activity. Cancer. 1972;30:1419–27.

Huffman DH, Benjamin RS, Bachur NR. Daunorubicin metabolism in acute nonlymphocytic leukemia. Clin Pharmacol Ther. 1972;13:895–905.

Takanashi S, Bachur NR. Daunorubicin metabolites in human urine. J Pharmacol Exp Ther. 1975;195:41–9.

Dosage Adjustment of Medications Eliminated by the Kidneys

<u>Daunorubicin</u>/Cerubidine®	**{Antineoplastic, anthracycline DNA topoisomerase II, and polymerase blocker}**

Usual initial dose: 25–45 mg/m^2 IV

Usual maintenance dose: 25–45 mg/m^2/day IV for two to three consecutive days of each cycle

Typical maximum dose: 60 mg/m^2 IV

Proportion eliminated unchanged: 20 % (as unchanged drug and active metabolites)

Adjustment for Kidney Disease

    FDA-approved product labeling: *SCr >3.0 mg/dL   Administer 50 % of the usual daily dose.*

    Alternative adjustment: *Data not available*

Dosage Adjustment of Medications Eliminated by the Kidneys

Deferasirox - Selected References

Brosnahan G, Gokden N, Swaminathan S. Acute interstitial nephritis due to deferasirox: a case report. Nephrol Dial Transplant. 2008;23:3356–8.

Even-Or E, Becker-Cohen R, Miskin H. Deferasirox treatment may be associated with reversible renal Fanconi syndrome. Am J Hematol. 2010;85:132–4.

Exjade® tablet for suspension, dispersible oral [package insert]. East Hanover: Novartis Pharmaceuticals Corp; 2011.

Grange S, Bertrand DM, Guerrot D, Eas F, Godin M. Acute renal failure and Fanconi syndrome due to deferasirox. Nephrol Dial Transplant. 2010;25:2376–8.

Kontoghiorghes GJ. Deferasirox: uncertain future following renal failure fatalities, agranulocytosis and other toxicities. Expert Opin Drug Saf. 2007;6:235–9.

Quinn CT, Johnson VL, Kim H-Y, et al. Renal dysfunction in patients with thalassemia. Br J Haematol. 2011;153:111–7.

Rafat C, Fakhouri F, Bibeil J-A, Delarue R, Le Quintrec M. Fanconi syndrome due to deferasirox. Am J Kidney Dis. 2009;54:931–4.

Sánchez-González PD, López-Hernandez FJ, Morales AI, Macía-Nuñez JF, López-Novoa JM. Effects of deferasirox on renal function and renal epithelial cell death. Toxicol Lett. 2011;203:154–61.

Taher A, Cappellini MD, Vichinsky E, et al. Efficacy and safety of deferasirox doses of >30 mg/kg per d in patients with transfusion-dependent anaemia and iron overload. Br J Haematol. 2009;147:752–9.

Vichinsky E, Bernaudin F, Forni GL, et al. Long-term safety and efficacy of deferasirox (Exjade®) for up to 5 years in transfusional iron-overloaded patients with sickle cell disease. Br J Haematol. 2011. Epub ahead of print. doi:10.1111/j.1365-2141.2011.08720.x.

Waldmeier F, Bruin GJ, Glaenzel U, Hazell K, Sechaud R, Warrington S, Porter JB. Pharmacokinetics, metabolism, and disposition of deferasirox in β-thalassemic patients with transfusion-dependent iron overload who are at pharmacokinetic steady state. Drug Metab Dispos. 2010;38:808–16.

Yang LPH, Keam SJ, Keating GM. Deferasirox: a review of its use in the management of transfusional chronic iron overload. Drugs. 2007;67:2211–30.

Yew CT, Talaulikar GS, Falk MC, Clayton P, D'Rozario JD, Brown M. Acute interstitial nephritis secondary to deferasirox causing acute renal injury needing short-term dialysis. Nephrology (Carlton). 2010;15:377.

Dosage Adjustment of Medications Eliminated by the Kidneys

<u>**Deferasirox**</u>/**Exjade**® {**Fe^{3+} chelating agent; ℞ for chronic iron overload caused by blood transfusions (transfusional hemosiderosis)**}

Usual initial dose: 20 mg/kg orally

Usual maintenance dose: 20 mg/kg orally once daily 30 min before food

Typical maximum dose: 40 mg/kg/day

Proportion eliminated unchanged: 8 %

Adjustment for Kidney Disease

FDA-approved product labeling: *Reduce the daily dose by 10 mg/kg if a rise in SCr to >33 % above the average of the pretreatment measurements is seen at two consecutive visits and cannot be attributed to other causes.*

CrCL <40 mL/min or >2 times the age-appropriate upper limit of normal   *Contraindicated*

Alternative adjustment: *Data not available*

Deferoxamine - Selected References

Albalate M, Velasco L, Ortiz A, Monzú B, Casado S, Caramelo C. High risk of retinal damage by desferrioxamine in dialysis patients [letter]. Nephron. 1996;73:726–7.

Allain P, Chaleil D, Mauras Y, et al. Pharmacokinetics of desferrioxamine and of its iron and aluminum chelates in patients on haemodialysis. Clin Chim Acta. 1987;170:331–8.

Allain P, Chaleil D, Mauras Y, et al. Pharmacokinetics of desferrioxamine and of its iron and aluminum chelates in patients on peritoneal dialysis. Clin Chim Acta. 1988;173:316–6.

Allain P, Mauras Y, Chaleil D, et al. Pharmacokinetics and renal elimination of desferrioxamine and ferrioxamine in healthy subjects and patients with haemochromatosis. Br J Clin Pharmacol. 1987;24:207–12.

Aronoff GA, Bennett WM, Berns JS, et al. Drug prescribing in renal failure: dosing guidelines for adults and children. 5th ed. Philadelphia: American College of Physicians; 2007.

Cases A, Kelly Sabater J, et al. Acute visual and auditory neurotoxicity in patients with end-stage renal disease receiving desferrioxamine. Clin Nephrol. 1988;29:176–8.

Clajus C, Becker JU, Stichtenoth DO, Wortmann J, Schwarz A, Kielsterin JT. Acute kidney injury due to deferoxamine in a renal transplant patient. Nephrol Dial Transplant. 2008;23:1061–4.

D'Haese PC, Couttenye M-M, De Broe ME. Diagnosis and treatment of aluminum bone disease. Nephrol Dial Transplant. 1996;11(Suppl 3):74–9.

Desferal® injection [package insert]. East Hanover: Novartis Pharmaceuticals Corp; 2010.

Hakim RM, Stivelman JC, Schulman G, et al. Iron overload and mobilization in long-term hemodialysis patients. Am J Kidney Dis. 1987;10:293–9.

Pengloan J, Dantal J, Rossazza C, Abazza M, Nivet H. Ocular toxicity after a single intravenous dose of desferrioxamine in 2 hemodialyzed patients. Nephron. 1987;46:211–2.

Stivelman J, Schulman G, Fosburg M, Lazarus JM, Hakim RM. Kinetics and efficacy of deferoxamine in iron-overloaded hemodialysis patients. Kidney Int. 1989;36:1125–32.

Weiss LG, Danielson BG, Fellström B, Wikström B. Aluminum removal with hemodialysis, hemofiltration and charcoal hemoperfusion in uremic patients after desferrioxamine infusion: a comparison of efficiency. Nephron. 1989;51:325–9.

<u>**Deferoxamine (Desferrioxamine)**</u>/Desferal®

{**Fe-chelating agent; ℞ for acute iron intoxication and chronic iron overload from multiple transfusions (transfusional hemosiderosis); ℞ for aluminum overload**}

Usual initial dose:	A dose of 1,000 mg IM should be administered initially. This may be followed by 500 mg IM every 4 h for two doses. Depending upon the clinical response, subsequent doses of 500 mg may be administered every 4–12 h. IV administration should be used only for patients in a state of cardiovascular collapse and then only by slow infusion. The rate of infusion should not exceed 15 mg/kg/h for the first 1,000 mg administered. Subsequent IV dosing, if needed, must be at a slower rate, not to exceed 125 mg/h.
Usual maintenance dose:	A daily dose of 1,000–2,000 mg (20–40 mg/kg/day) should be administered subcutaneously over 8–24 h, utilizing a small portable pump capable of providing continuous mini-infusion. The duration of infusion must be individualized. In some patients, as much iron will be excreted after a short infusion of 8–12 h as with the same dose given over 24 h.
Typical maximum dose:	The total amount administered should not exceed 6,000 mg in 24 h.
Proportion eliminated unchanged:	Deferoxamine and the iron chelate are excreted primarily by the kidney.

Adjustment for Kidney Disease

FDA-approved product labeling:	*Severe renal disease or anuria*	*Contraindicated*
Alternative adjustment:	*GFR >50 mL/min*	*1,000 mg IM once, then 500 mg IM every 4–12 h*
	GFR 10–50 mL/min	*500 mg IM once, then 250 mg IM every 4–12 h (50 % decrease)*
	GFR <10 mL/min	*Preferably avoid due to risk for accumulation of deferoxamine and the iron chelate*
	Hemodialysis	*Preferably avoid due to risk for accumulation of deferoxamine and the iron chelate*
	CAPD	*Preferably avoid due to risk for accumulation of deferoxamine and the iron chelate*
	CRRT	*500 mg IM once, then 250 mg IM every 4–12 h (50 % decrease)*

Dosage Adjustment of Medications Eliminated by the Kidneys

Demeclocycline - Selected References

Agwuh KN, MacGowan A. Pharmacokinetics and pharmacodynamics of the tetracyclines including glycylcyclines. J Antimicrob Chemother. 2006;58:256–65.

Demeclocycline hydrochloride tablet [package insert]. Pomona: Barr Laboratories Inc; 2008.

Geheb M, Cox M. Renal effects of demeclocycline [editorial]. JAMA. 1980;243:2519–20.

Miller PD, Línas SL, Schrier RW. Plasma demeclocycline levels and nephrotoxicity: correlation in hyponatremic cirrhotic patients. JAMA. 1980;243:2513–5.

Oster JR, Epstein M. Demeclocycline-induced renal failure [letter]. Lancet. 1977;1:52.

Oster JR, Epstein M, Ulano HB. Deterioration of renal function with demeclocycline administration. Curr Ther Res Clin Exp. 1976;20:794–801.

Padfield PL, Hodsman GP, Morton JJ. Demeclocycline in the treatment of syndrome of inappropriate antidiuretic hormone release: with measurement of plasma ADH. Postgrad Med J. 1978;54:623–7.

Demeclocycline/Declomycin®	**{Antibacterial; tetracycline derivative; ℞ for hyponatremia associated with syndrome of inappropriate antidiuretic hormone (SIADH)}**

Usual initial dose: 150 mg orally

Usual maintenance dose: 150 mg orally four times daily or 300 mg orally twice daily

Typical maximum dose: 1,200 mg/day

Proportion eliminated unchanged: 40 %

Adjustment for Kidney Disease

FDA-approved product labeling: *If renal impairment exists, even usual oral or parenteral doses may lead to excessive systemic accumulation of the drug and possible liver toxicity. Under such conditions, lower than usual total doses are indicated, and if therapy is prolonged, serum level determinations of the drug may be advisable.*

Alternative adjustment: *Data not available*

Desirudin - Selected References

Boyce SW, Bandyk DF, Bartholomew JR, Frame JN, Rice L. A randomized, open-label pilot study comparing desirudin and argatroban in patients with suspected heparin-induced thrombocytopenia with or without thrombosis: PREVENT-HIT study. Am J Ther. 2011;18:14–22.

Desirudin (Iprivask) for DVT prevention. Med Lett Drugs Ther. 2010;52:85–6.

Eriksson BI, Ekman S, Lindbratt S, et al. Prevention of thromboembolism with use of recombinant hirudin. Results of a double-blind, multicenter trial comparing the efficacy of desirudin (Revasc) with that of unfractionated heparin in patients having a total hip replacement. J Bone Joint Surg Am. 1997;79:326–33.

Eriksson BI, Wille-Jørgensen P, Kälebo P, et al. A comparison of recombinant hirudin with a low-molecular-weight heparin to prevent thromboembolic complications after total hip replacement. N Engl J Med. 1997;337:1329–35.

Fisher K-G. The role of recombinant hirudins in the management of thrombotic disorders. BioDrugs. 2004;18:235–68.

Gray E. Watton J, Cesmeli S, Barrowcliffe TW, Thomas DP. Experimental studies on a recombinant hirudin, CGP 39393. Thromb Haemost. 1991;65:355–9.

Iprivask® injection [package insert]. Hunt Valley: Canyon Pharmaceuticals; 2010.

Kaiser B, Simon A, Markwardt F. Antithrombotic effects of recombinant hirudin in experimental angioplasty and intravascular thrombolysis. Thromb Haemost. 1990;63:44–7.

Lefèvre G, Duval M, Gauron S, et al. Effect of renal impairment on the pharmacokinetics and pharmacodynamics of desirudin. Clin Pharmacol Ther. 1997;62:50–9.

Marbet GA, Verstraete M, Kienast J, et al. Clinical pharmacology of intravenously administered recombinant desulfatohirudin (GGP 29393) in healthy volunteers. J Cardiovasc Pharmacol. 1993;22:364–72.

Markwardt F, Nowak G, Bucha E. Hirudin as anticoagulant in experimental hemodialysis. Haemostasis. 1991;21 (Suppl 1):149–55.

Matheson AJ, Goa KL. Desirudin: a review of its use in the management of thrombotic disorders. Drugs. 2000;60: 679–700.

Nafziger AN, Bertino JS Jr. Desirudin dosing and monitoring in moderate renal impairment. J Clin Pharmacol. 2010;50: 614–22.

Rao AK, Sun L, Cheesbro JH, et al. Distinct effects of recombinant desulfatohirudin (Revasc) and heparin on plasma levels of fibrinopeptide A and prothrombin fragment F1.2 in unstable angina: a multicenter trial. Circulation. 1996;94:2389–95.

Topol EJ, Fuster V, Harrington RA, et al. Recombinant hirudin for unstable angina pectoris: a multicenter, randomized angiographic trial. Circulation. 1994;89:1557–66.

Weitz JI, Crowther M. Direct thrombin inhibitors. Thromb Res. 2002;106:V275–83.

Weitz JI, Hudoba M, Massel D, Maraganore J, Hirsch J. Clot-bound thrombin is protected from inhibition by heparin-antithrombin III but is susceptible to inactivation by antithrombin III-independent inhibitors. J Clin Invest. 1990;86:385–91.

Dosage Adjustment of Medications Eliminated by the Kidneys

Desirudin/Iprivask®   {Antithrombotic; direct thrombin inhibitor}

Usual initial dose: 15 mg subcutaneously

Usual maintenance dose: 15 mg subcutaneously every 12 h

Typical maximum dose: 30 mg/day

Proportion eliminated unchanged: 40–50 %

Adjustment for Kidney Disease

FDA-approved product labeling:	*CrCL ≥61 mL/min*	*15 mg subcutaneously every 12 h*
	CrCL ≥30–60 mL/min	*5 mg subcutaneously every 12 h[a]*
	CrCL <31 mL/min	*1.7 mg subcutaneously every 12 h[a]*

[a]Monitor aPTT and SCr at least daily; if aPTT exceeds two times control, interrupt therapy until the value returns to <2 times control. Then resume therapy at a further reduced dose guided by the initial degree of aPTT abnormality

Alternative adjustment:	*GFR <10 mL/min*	*Minimal data available. Preferably avoid due to hemorrhagic risk*
	Hemodialysis	*Data not available*
	CRRT	*Data not available*

Dosage Adjustment of Medications Eliminated by the Kidneys

Desmopressin - Selected References

Agersø H, Larsen LS, Riis A, Lövgren U, Karlsson MO, Senderovitz T. Pharmacokinetics and renal excretion of desmopressin after intravenous administration to healthy subjects and renally impaired patients. Br J Clin Pharmacol. 2004;58:352–8.

Aunsholt NA, Schmidt EB, Stoffersen E. 1-Deamino-8-D-arginine vasopressin lowers protein C activity in uremics. Nephron. 1989;53:6–8.

Byrnes JJ, Larcada A, Moake JL. Thrombosis following desmopressin for uremic bleeding. Am J Hematol. 1988;28:63–5.

DDAVP® nasal spray [package insert]. Bridgewater: Sanofi-Aventis US LLC; 2007.

Desmopressin acetate injection USP [package insert]. Lake Forest: Hospira Inc; 2007.

Escolar G, Cases A, Monteagudo J, et al. Uremic plasma after infusion of desmopressin (DDAVP) improves the interaction of normal platelets with vessel endothelium. J Lab Clin Med. 1989;114:36–42.

Hedges SJ, Dehoney SB, Hooper JS, Amanzadeh J, Busti AJ. Evidence-based treatment recommendations for uremic bleeding. Nat Clin Pract Nephrol. 2007;3:138–53.

Hvistendahl GM, Riis A, Nørgaard JP, Djurhuus JC. The pharmacokinetics of 400 μg of oral desmopressin in elderly patients with nocturia, and the correlation between the absorption of desmopressin and clinical effect. BJU Int. 2005;95:804–9.

Kaufmann JE, Vischer UM. Cellular mechanisms of the hemostatic effects of desmopressin (DDAVP). J Thromb Haemost. 2003;1:682–9.

Köhler M, Harris A. Pharmacokinetics and haematological effects of desmopressin. Br J Clin Pharmacol. 1988;35:281–5.

Lam KSL, Wat MS, Choi KL, Ip TP, Pang WC, Kumana CR. Pharmacokinetics, pharmacodynamics, long-term efficacy and safety of oral 1-deamino-8-D-arginine vasopressin in adult patients with central diabetes insipidus. Br J Clin Pharmacol. 1996;42:379–85.

Lethagen S, Harris AS, Sjörin E, Nilsson IM. Intranasal and intravenous administration of desmopressin: effect on F VIII/vWF, pharmacokinetics and reproducibility. Thromb Haemost. 1987;58:1033–6.

Mannucci PM, Remuzzi G, Pusineri F, et al. Deamino-8-D-arginine shortens bleeding time in uremia. N Engl J Med. 1983;308:8–12.

Mannucci PM, Vicente V, Alberca L, et al. Intravenous and subcutaneous administration of desmopressin (DDAVP) to hemophiliacs: pharmacokinetics and factor VIII responses. Thromb Haemost. 1987;58:1037–9.

Nørgaard JP, Jønler M, Rittig S, Djurhuus JC. A pharmacodynamic study of desmopressin in patients with nocturnal enuresis. J Urol. 1995;153:1984–6.

Pullan PT, Burger HG, Johnston CI. Pharmacokinetics of 1-deamino-8-D-arginine vasopressin (DDAVP) in patients with central diabetes insipidus. Clin Endocrinol (Oxf). 1978;9:273–8.

Ruzicka H, Björkman S, Lethagen S, Sterner G. Pharmacokinetics and antidiuretic effect of high-dose desmopressin in patients with chronic renal failure. Pharmacol Toxicol. 2003;92:137–42.

Sica DA, Gehr TWB. Desmopressin: safety considerations in patients with chronic renal disease. Drug Saf. 2006;29:553–6.

Soslau G, Schwartz AB, Putatunda B, et al. Desmopressin-induced improvement in bleeding times in chronic renal failure patients correlates with platelet serotonin uptake and ATP release. Am J Med Sci. 1990;300:372–9.

Stratton J, Warwicker P, Watkins S, Farrington K. Desmopressin may be hazardous in thrombotic microangiography. Nephrol Dial Transplant. 2001;16:161–2.

Viganò GL, Mannucci PM, Lattuada A, Harris A, Remuzzi G. Subcutaneous desmopressin (DDAVP) shortens the bleeding time in uremia. Am J Hematol. 1989;31:32–5.

Wang C-J, Lin Y-N, Huang S-W, Chang C-H. Low-dose oral desmopressin for nocturnal polyuria in patients with benign prostatic hyperplasia: a double-blind, placebo-controlled, randomized study. J Urol. 2011;185:219–23.

Williams TDM, Dunger DB, Lyon CC, Lewis RJ, Taylor F, Lightman SL. Antidiuretic effect and pharmacokinetics of oral 1-deamino-8-D-arginine vasopressin. 1. Studies in adults and children. J Clin Endocrinol Metab. 1986;63:129–32.

Zeigler AR, Megaludis A, Fraley DS. Desmopressin (d-DAVP) effects on platelet rheology and von Willebrand factor activities in uremia. Am J Hematol. 1992;39:90–5.

Dosage Adjustment of Medications Eliminated by the Kidneys

<u>Desmopressin</u>/DDAVP®, Stimate®   **{Antidiuretic; hemostatic; arginine vasopressin analog; coagulation factor VIII stimulator; ℞ for central diabetes insipidus; ℞ for nocturnal enuresis; ℞ for hemorrhage}**

Usual initial dose: For bleeding, 0.3 mcg/kg IV over 30 min or 300 mcg total dose administered as a single 150 mcg nasal insufflation per nostril; for patients <50 kg body weight, 150 mcg total dose intranasally

Usual maintenance dose: For diabetes insipidus, 0.1–1.2 mg/day orally in two to three divided doses or 10–40 mcg/day intranasally in one to three doses or 2–4 mcg/day IV or subcutaneously in two divided doses

Typical maximum dose: For bleeding, 300 mcg intranasally or 0.4 mcg/kg IV; for diabetes insipidus,1.2 mg/day orally or 40 mcg/day intranasally or 4 mcg/day IV or subcutaneously

Proportion eliminated unchanged: 48 % (subcutaneously), 92 % (intranasal)

Adjustment for Kidney Disease

    FDA-approved product labeling: *CrCL <50 mL/min*   *Contraindicated*

    Alternative adjustment: *CrCL <50 mL/min*   *Although clinical experience and some treatment guidelines suggest that usual parenteral or slightly reduced intranasal single doses of desmopressin are effective for prevention or treatment of uremic bleeding, pharmacological studies and isolated case reports indicate that these patients may be at heightened risk for not only hyponatremia but also stroke, myocardial infarction, and other serious thrombotic complications.*

Desvenlafaxine - Selected References

Dolder C, Nelson M, Stump A. Pharmacological and clinical profile of newer antidepressants: implications for the treatment of elderly patients. Drugs Aging. 2010;27:625–40.

Klamerus KJ, Maloney K, Rudolph RL, Sisenwine SF, Jusko WJ, Chiang ST. Introduction of a composite parameter to the pharmacokinetics of venlafaxine and its active O-desmethyl metabolite. J Clin Pharmacol. 1992;32:716–24.

Nichols AI, Fatato P, Shenouda M, et al. The effects of desvenlafaxine and paroxetine on the pharmacokinetics of the cytochrome P450 2D6 substrate desipramine in healthy adults. J Clin Pharmacol. 2009;49:219–28.

Nichols AI, Richards LS, Behrle JA, Posener JA, McGrory SB, Paul J. The pharmacokinetics and safety of desvenlafaxine in subjects with chronic renal impairment. Int J Clin Pharmacol Ther. 2011;49:3–13.

Perry R, Cassagnol M. Desvenlafaxine: a new serotonin-norepinephrine reuptake inhibitor for the treatment of adults with major depressive disorder. Clin Ther. 2009;31:1374–404.

Preskorn S, Patroneva A, Nichols A, Silman H, Pedersen R, Paul J, Ahmed S. A comparison of the pharmacokinetics of venlafaxine extended release and desvenlafaxine succinate in healthy subjects [abstract]. Eur Neuropsychopharmacol. 2007;17:S339.

Pristiq® tablet extended release [package insert]. Philadelphia: Wyeth Pharmaceuticals Inc; 2011.

Dosage Adjustment of Medications Eliminated by the Kidneys

<u>**Desvenlafaxine**</u>**/Pristiq®**   {**Antidepressant; serotonin and norepinephrine reuptake inhibitor (SRNI)**}

Usual initial dose:	50 mg once daily
Usual maintenance dose:	50–400 mg orally once daily
Typical maximum dose:	400 mg/day
Proportion eliminated unchanged:	49 % plus 4 % as active didesmethylated metabolite

Adjustment for Kidney Disease

    FDA-approved product labeling:

CrCL >50 mL/min	*50–400 mg orally once daily*
CrCL 30–50 mL/min	*50 mg orally once daily*
CrCL <30 mL/min	*50 mg orally every 48 h*
Hemodialysis	*50 mg orally every 48 h (no supplemental dose after dialysis)*

Note: Doses should not be escalated in patients with moderate or severe renal impairment or end-stage renal disease.

    Alternative adjustment: *Data not available*

Dexrazoxane - Selected References

Brier ME, Gaylor SK, McGovern JP, Glue P, Fang A, Aronoff GR. Pharmacokinetics of dexrazoxane in subjects with impaired kidney function. J Clin Pharmacol. 2011;51:731–8.

Chow WA, Synold TW, Tetef ML, et al. Feasibility and pharmacokinetic study of infusional dexrazoxane and dose-intensive doxorubicin administered concurrently over 96 h for the treatment of advanced malignancies. Cancer Chemother Pharmacol. 2004;54:241–8.

Cvetkovi RS, Scott LJ. Dexrazoxane: a review of its use for cardioprotection during anthracycline chemotherapy. Drugs. 2006;65:1005–64.

Dexrazoxane injection [package insert]. Bedford: Bedford Laboratories; 2005.

Earhart RH. Tutsch KD, Koeller JM, et al. Pharmacokinetics of (+)-1,2-di(3,5-dioxopiperazin-i-yl) propane intravenous infusions in adult cancer patients. Cancer Res. 1982;42:5255–61.

Herman EH, El-Hage A, Ferrans VJ. Protective effect of ICRF-187 on doxorubicin-induced cardiac and renal toxicity in spontaneously hypertensive (SHR) and normotensive (WKY) rats. Toxicol Appl Pharmacol. 1988;92:42–53.

Herman EH, Zhang J, Hasinoff BB, Chadwick DP, Clark JR Jr, Ferrans VJ. Comparison of the protective effects against chronic doxorubicin cardiotoxicity and the rates of iron (III) displacement reactions of ICRF-187 and other bisdiketopiperazines. Cancer Chemother Pharmacol. 1997;40:400–8.

Hochster H, Liebes L, Wadler S, et al. Pharmacokinetics of the cardioprotector ADR-529 (ICRF-187) in escalating doses combined with fixed-dose doxorubicin. J Natl Cancer Inst. 1992;84:1725–30.

Johnson SA, Richardson DS. Anthracyclines in haematology: pharmacokinetics and clinical studies. Blood Rev. 1998;12:52–71.

Sargent JM, Williamson CJ, Yardley C, Taylor CG, Hellmann K. Dexrazoxane significantly impairs the induction of doxorubicin resistance in the human leukaemia line, K562. Br J Cancer. 2001;84:959–64.

Tetef ML, Synold TW, Chow W, et al. Phase I trial of 96-hour continuous infusion of dexrazoxane in patients with advanced malignancies. Clin Cancer Res. 2001;7:1569–76.

Vaidyanathan S, Boroujerdi M. Interaction of dexrazoxane with red blood cells and hemoglobin alters pharmacokinetics of doxorubicin. Cancer Chemother Pharmacol. 2000;46:93–100.

Vogel CL, Gorowski E, Davila E, et al. Phase I clinical trial and pharmacokinetics of ICRF-187 (NSC 169780) infusion in patients with solid tumors. Invest New Drugs. 1987;5:187–98.

Dosage Adjustment of Medications Eliminated by the Kidneys

<u>Dexrazoxane</u>/Totect®, Zinecard® {**Cytoprotective agent; ℞ for reducing the incidence of cardiomyopathy associated with anthracyclines; ℞ for extravasation resulting from anthracycline chemotherapy**}

Usual initial dose: Recommended dosage ratio of dexrazoxane:doxorubicin is 10:1 (e.g., 500 mg/m² dexrazoxane IV to 50 mg/m² doxorubicin).

Usual maintenance dose: Ten times the proportional doxorubicin dose (ratio 10:1) IV every 3 weeks

Typical maximum dose: 1,000 mg/m² every 3 weeks

Proportion eliminated unchanged: 11–49 % depending on excretory renal function

Adjustment for Kidney Disease

FDA-approved product labeling: *Moderate to severe renal dysfunction (CrCL <40 mL/min)* *The recommended dosage ratio of dexrazoxane:doxorubicin is 5:1 (e.g., 250 mg/m² dexrazoxane to 50 mg/m² doxorubicin).*

Alternative adjustment: *Data not available*

Diatrizoate - Selected References

Ackrill P, McIntosh CS, Nimmon C, Baker LRI, Cattell WR. A comparison of the clearance of urographic contrast medium (sodium diatrizoate) by peritoneal and haemodialysis. Clin Sci Mol Med. 1976;50:69–74.

Aperia A, Broberger O, Ekengren K. Renal hemodynamics during selective renal angiography. Invest Radiol. 1968;3:389–96.

Bergman LA, Ellison MR, Dunea G. Acute renal failure after drip-infusion pyelography. N Engl J Med. 1968;279:1277.

Carvallo A, Rakowski TA, Argy WP Jr, Schreiner GE. Acute renal failure following drip infusion pyelography. Am J Med. 1978;65:38–45.

Epstein M, Shelp WD, Weinstein AB. Acute renal failure following retrograde pyelography. Invest Urol. 1965;2:355–64.

Feldman HA Goldfarb S, McCurdy DK. Recurrent radiographic dye-induced acute renal failure. JAMA. 1974;229:72.

Gale ME, Robbins AH, Hamburger RJ, Widrich WC. Renal toxicity of contrast agents: iopamidol, iothalamate, and diatrizoate. AJR Am J Roentgenol. 1984;142:333–5.

Goldstein EJ, Feinfeld DA, Fleischner GM, Elkin M. Enzymatic evidence of renal tubular damage following renal angiography. Radiology. 1976;121:617–9.

Hypaque® sodium injection [package insert]. Princeton: Amersham Health Inc; 2006.

Light JA, Hill GS. Acute tubular necrosis in a renal transplant recipient: complication from drip-infusion excretory urography. JAMA. 1975;232:1267–8.

Pillay VKG, Robbins PC, Schwartz FD, Kark RM. Acute renal failure following intravenous urography in patients with long-standing diabetes and azotemia. Radiology. 1970;95:633–6.

Rhea WG Jr, Killen DA, Foster JH. Relative nephrotoxicity of Hypaque and Angio-Conray. Surgery. 1965;57:554–8.

Soejima K, Uozumi J, Kanou T, Fujiyama C, Masaki Z. Nonionic contrast media are less nephrotoxic than ionic contrast media to rat renal cortical slices. Toxicol Lett. 2003;143:17–25.

Talner LB, Davidson AJ. Renal hemodynamic effects of contrast media. Invest Radiol. 1968;3:310–7.

Dosage Adjustment of Medications Eliminated by the Kidneys

Diatrizoate/Hypaque-76™	{Iodinated radiocontrast media}
Usual initial dose:	Excretory urography—20 mL IV
Usual maintenance dose:	N/A
Typical maximum dose:	Excretory urography—40 mL IV
Proportion eliminated unchanged:	94–100 %

Adjustment for Kidney Disease

FDA-approved product labeling:	*Severely impaired renal function*	*Urography should be performed with caution.*
		All other indications—dose adjustment not required
	Azotemia and dehydration	*Urography and large-dose vascular procedures are contraindicated.*
	Anuria	*Urography is contraindicated.*
Alternative adjustment:	*All patients*	*Caution: contrast induced nephropathy*

Dosage Adjustment of Medications Eliminated by the Kidneys

Diclofenac - Selected References

Aronoff GA, Bennett WM, Berns JS, et al. Drug prescribing in renal failure: dosing guidelines for adults and children. 5th ed. Philadelphia: American College of Physicians; 2007.

Bassotti G, Bucaneve G, Betti C, et al. Effects of parenteral diclofenac sodium on upper gastrointestinal motility after food in man. Eur J Clin Pharmacol. 1991;41:497–500.

Bondeson J, Berglund S. Diclofenac-induced thrombocytopenic purpura with renal and hepatic involvement. J Intern Med. 1991;230:543–7.

Davies NM, Anderson KE. Clinical pharmacokinetics of diclofenac: therapeutic insights and pitfalls. Clin Pharmacokinet. 1997;33:184–213.

Degen PH, Dieterle W, Schneider W, Theobald W, Sinterhauf U. Pharmacokinetics of diclofenac and five metabolites after single doses in healthy volunteers and after repeated doses in patients. Xenobiotica. 1988;18:1449–55.

Dilger L. Herrlinger. C. Peters J, Seyberth HW, Schweer H, Klotz U. Effects of celecoxib and diclofenac on blood pressure, renal function, and vasoactive prostanoids in young and elderly subjects. J Clin Pharmacol. 2002;42:985–94.

Fredman B, Zohar E, Golan E, Tillinger M, Bernheim J, Jedeikin R. Diclofenac does not decrease renal blood flow or glomerular filtration in elderly patients undergoing orthopedic surgery. Anesth Analg. 1999;88:149–54.

Kim YK, Hwang MY, Woo JS, Jung JS, Lee SH. Effects of arachidonic acid metabolic inhibitors on hypoxia/reoxygenation-induced renal cell injury. Ren Fail. 2000;22:143–57.

Kim H, Xu M, Lin Y, et al. Renal dysfunction associated with the perioperative use of diclofenac. Anesth Analg. 1999;89:999–1005.

Kinn AC, Elbarouni J, Seideman P, Sollevi A. The effect of diclofenac sodium on renal function. Scand J Urol Nephrol. 1989;23:153–7.

Kulling PEJ, Beckman EA, Skagius ASM. Renal impairment after acute diclofenac, naproxen, and sulindac overdoses. J Toxicol Clin Toxicol. 1995;33:173–7.

Lee A, Cooper MG, Knight JF, Keneally JP. Effects of nonsteroidal anti-inflammatory drugs on postoperative renal function in adults with normal renal function (review). Cochrane Database Syst Rev. 2007;(2):CD002765. doi:10.1002/14651858. CD002765.pub3.

Mohammed EP, Stevens JM. Recurrence of Arthrotec-associated nephritic syndrome with re-challenge. Clin Nephrol. 2000;53:483–5.

Niccoli L, Bellino S, Cantini F. Renal tolerability of three commonly employed non-steroidal anti-inflammatory drugs in elderly patients with osteoarthritis. Clin Exp Rheumatol. 2002;20:201–7.

Power I, Cumming AD, Pugh GC. Effect of diclofenac on renal function and prostacyclin generation after surgery. Br J Anaesth. 1992;69:451–6.

Radford MG, Holley KE, Grande JP, et al. Reversible membranous nephropathy associated with the use of nonsteroidal anti-inflammatory drugs. JAMA. 1996;276:466–9.

Rossi E, Ferraccioli GF, Cavalieri F, Menta R, Dall'Aglio PP, Migone L. Diclofenac-associated renal failure: report of 2 cases. Nephron. 1985;40:491–3.

Sawchuk RJ, Maloney JA, Cartier LL, Rackley RJ, Chan KKH, Lau HSL. Analysis of diclofenac and four of its metabolites. Pharm Res. 1995;12:756–62.

Schwartz J, Altshuler E, Madjar J, Habot B. Acute renal failure associated with diclofenac treatment in an elderly woman [letter]. J Am Geriatr Soc. 1988;36:482.

Schwarz A, Krause PH, Keller F, Offermann G, Mihatsch MJ. Granulomatous interstitial nephritis after nonsteroidal anti-inflammatory drugs. Am J Nephrol. 1988;8:410–6.

Stanziale P, Fuiano G, Balletta MM, et al. A case of relapsing renal micropolyarteritis: a possible association with assumption of non steroidal antiinflammatory drugs (NSAID). Adv Exp Med Biol. 1989;252:303–6.

Todd PA, Sorkin EM. Diclofenac sodium: a reappraisal of its pharmacodynamic and pharmacokinetic properties, and therapeutic efficacy. Drugs. 1988;35:244–85.

Voltaren® tablet delayed release [package insert]. East Hanover: Novartis Pharmaceuticals Corp; 2011.

Dosage Adjustment of Medications Eliminated by the Kidneys

<u>Diclofenac</u>/Voltaren®, Cataflam®   {Anti-inflammatory; nonsteroidal anti-inflammatory drug}

Usual initial dose:	50 mg orally
Usual maintenance dose:	50 mg orally two to three times daily
Typical maximum dose:	200 mg/day
Proportion eliminated unchanged:	65 %

Adjustment for Kidney Disease

  FDA-approved product labeling: *Treatment with diclofenac potassium tablets is not recommended in patients with advanced renal disease; if therapy with diclofenac is undertaken, close monitoring of the patient's renal function is advisable.*

  Alternative adjustment:

GFR >50 mL/min	*50 mg twice daily (50–100 % of usual dose)*
GFR 10–50 mL/min	*25 mg twice daily (50 % of usual dose)*
GFR <10 mL/min	*25 mg once daily (25 % of usual dose)*
Hemodialysis	*Preferably avoid due to potential for gastrointestinal and renal toxicity*
CAPD	*Preferably avoid due to potential for gastrointestinal and renal toxicity*
CRRT	*Not applicable; preferably avoid due to potential for gastrointestinal and renal toxicity*

Dosage Adjustment of Medications Eliminated by the Kidneys

Didanosine - Selected References

Aronoff GA, Bennett WM, Berns JS, et al. Drug prescribing in renal failure: dosing guidelines for adults and children. 5th ed. Philadelphia: American College of Physicians; 2007.

Gupta SK, Eustace JA, Winston JA, et al. Guidelines for the management of chronic kidney disease in HIV-infected patients: recommendations of the HIV Medicine Section of the Infectious Diseases Society of America. Clin Infect Dis. 2005;40:1559–85.

Hoetelmans RWM, van Heeswijk RGP, Profijt M, et al. Comparison of plasma pharmacokinetics and renal clearance of didanosine during once and twice daily dosing in HIV-1 infected individuals. AIDS. 1998;12:F211–6.

Irizarry-Alvarado JM, Dwyer JP, Brumble LM, Alvarez S, Mendez JC. Proximal tubular dysfunction associated with tenofovir and didanosine causing Fanconi syndrome and diabetes insipidus: a report of 3 cases. AIDS Read. 2009;19:114–21.

Jung D, Griffy K Dorr A, et al. Effect of high-dose oral ganciclovir on didanosine disposition in human immunodeficiency virus (HIV)-positive patients. J Clin Pharmacol. 1998;38:1051–6.

Knupp CA, Hak LJ, Coakley DF, et al. Disposition of didanosine in HIV-seropositive patients with normal renal function or chronic renal failure: influence of hemodialysis and continuous ambulatory peritoneal dialysis. Clin Pharmacol Ther. 1996;535–42.

Knupp CA, Milbrath R, Barbhaiya RH. The effect of food administration on the bioavailability of didanosine from a chewable tablet formulation. J Clin Pharmacol. 1993;33:568–73.

Knupp CA, Shyu WC, Dolin R, et al. Pharmacokinetics of didanosine in patients with acquired immunodeficiency syndrome or acquired immunodeficiency syndrome-related complex. Clin Pharmacol Ther. 1991;49:526–35.

McIntyre CW, Owen PJ. Prescribing drugs in kidney disease. In: Brenner BM, editor. Brenner & Rector's the kidney. 8th ed. Philadelphia: Saunders Elsevier; 2008. p. 1930–55.

Murphy MD, O'Hearn M, Chou S. Fatal lactic acidosis and acute renal failure after addition of tenofovir to an antiviral regimen containing didanosine. Clin Infect Dis. 2003;36:1082–5.

Olyaei AJ, Bennett WM. Pharmacologic approach to renal insufficiency. In: Dale DC, Federman DD, Antman K, editors. ACP medicine, WebMD June 2007 update. Hamilton: BC Decker; 2007; NEPHROLOGY IX: Appendix A1–25.

Olyaei AJ, DeMattos AM, Bennett WM. Use of drugs in patients with renal failure. In: Schrier RW, editor. Diseases of the kidney and urinary tract. 8th ed. Philadelphia: Lippincott Williams & Wilkins; 2007. p. 2765–807.

Ostrop NJ, Burgess E, Gill MJ. The use of antiretroviral agents in patients with renal insufficiency. AIDS Patient Care STDS. 1999;13:517–26.

Sahai J, Gallicano K, Garber G, Pakuts A, Cameron W. Pharmacokinetics of simultaneously administered zidovudine and didanosine in HIV-seropositive male patients. J Acquir Immune Defic Syndr Hum Retrovirol. 1995;10:54–60.

Schelling JR, Baum KF, Teitelbaum I. Didanosine administration in a human immunodeficiency virus-positive renal transplant patient. Am J Kidney Dis. 1993;22:60–3.

Seguro AC, de Araujo M, Seguro FS, Rienzo M, Magaldi AJ, Campos SB. Effects of hypokalemia and hypomagnesemia on zidovudine (AZT) and didanosine (ddI) nephrotoxicity in rats. Clin Nephrol. 2003;59:267–72.

Seifert RD, Stewart MB, Sramek JJ, Conrad J, Kaul S, Cutler NR. Pharmacokinetics of co-administered didanosine and stavudine in HIV-seropositive male patients. Br J Clin Pharmacol. 1994;38:405–10.

Shyu WC, Knupp CA, Pittman KA, Dunkle L, Barbhaiya RH. Food-induced reduction in bioavailability of didanosine. Clin Pharmacol Ther. 1991;50:503–7.

Singlas E, Taburet AM, Lebas FB, et al. Didanosine pharmacokinetics in patients with normal and impaired renal function: influence of hemodialysis. Antimicrob Agents Chemother. 1992;36:1519–24.

Videx® EC capsule delayed release [package insert]. Princeton: Bristol-Myers Squibb Co; 2010.

Willig JH, Westfall AO, Allison J, et al. Nucleoside reverse-transcriptase inhibitor dosing errors in an outpatient HIV clinic in the electronic medical record era. Clin Infect Dis. 2007;45:658–61.

Dosage Adjustment of Medications Eliminated by the Kidneys

Didanosine (EC)/ddI, Videx® EC   {Antiretroviral; nucleoside reverse transcriptase inhibitor}

Usual initial dose:	400 mg orally (250 mg if weight <60 kg)
Usual maintenance dose:	400 mg orally every 24 h (250 mg q12h if weight <60 kg)
Typical maximum dose:	400 mg orally
Proportion eliminated unchanged:	60 %

Adjustment for Kidney Disease

FDA-approved product labeling: *Recommended didanosine EC oral dosage in patients with renal impairment by body weight*

	Dosage (mg)	
CrCL (mL/min)	*≥60 kg*	*<60 kg*
≥60	*400 once daily*	*250 once daily*
30–59	*200 once daily*	*125 once daily*
10–29	*125 once daily*	*125 once daily*
<10	*125 once daily*	*Not suitable for use in patients <60 kg with CrCL <10 mL/min* *An alternate formulation of didanosine should be used*

Alternative adjustment:

GFR >50 mL/min	*200 mg orally every 12 h (125 mg q12h if <60 kg)*
GFR 10–50 mL/min	*200 mg orally every 24 h (125 mg q12h if <60 kg)*
GFR <10 mL/min	*125 mg orally every 24 h*
Hemodialysis	*125 mg orally every 24 h*
CAPD	*125 mg orally every 24 h*
CRRT	*200 mg enterally every 24 h (125 mg q12h if <60 kg)*

Note: If taken together with tenofovir, a dose reduction of didanosine EC to 250 mg (adults ≥60 kg with CrCL ≥60 mL/min) or 200 mg (adults <60 kg with CrCL ≥60 mL/min) once daily with a light meal (400 kcal or less, 20 % fat or less) or in the fasted state is recommended.

Dosage Adjustment of Medications Eliminated by the Kidneys

Digoxin - Selected References

Ahmed A, Rich MW, Fleg JL, et al. Effects of digoxin on morbidity and mortality in diastolic heart failure: the Ancillary Digitalis Investigation Group trial. Circulation. 2006;114:397–403.

Aronoff GA, Bennett WM, Berns JS, et al. Drug prescribing in renal failure: dosing guidelines for adults and children. 5th ed. Philadelphia: American College of Physicians; 2007.

Cohen AF, Kroon R, Schoemaker HC, Breimer DD, van Vliet-Verbeek A, Brandenburg HC. The bioavailability of digoxin from three oral formulations measured by specific HPLC assay. Br J Clin Pharmacol. 1993;35:136–42.

Garg R, Gorlin R, Smith T, Yusuf S. The effect of digoxin on mortality and morbidity in patients with heart failure. N Engl J Med. 1997;236:525–33.

Gill J, Malyuk R, Djurdjev O, Levin A. Use of GFR equations to adjust drug doses in an elderly multi-ethnic group: a cautionary tale. Nephrol Dial Transplant. 2007;22:2894–9.

Gjesdal K, Feyzi J, Olsson SB. Digitalis: a dangerous drug in atrial fibrillation? An analysis of the SPORTIF III and V data. Heart. 2008;94:191–6.

Graves SW, Brown B, Valdes R. An endogenous digoxin-like substance in patients with renal impairment. Ann Intern Med. 1983;99:604–8.

Hui J, Wang Y-MC, Chandrasekaran A, et al. Disposition of tablet and capsule formulations of digoxin in the elderly. Pharmacotherapy. 1994;14:607–12.

Lanoxin® injection [package insert]. Research Triangle Park: GlaxoSmithKline; 2009.

Lanoxin® tablets [package insert]. Research Triangle Park: GlaxoSmithKline; 2009.

Lee DC-S, Johnson RAA, Bingham JB, et al. Heart failure in outpatients: a randomized trial of digoxin versus placebo. N Engl J Med. 1982;306:699–705.

Mason DT. Digitalis pharmacology and therapeutics: recent advances. Ann Intern Med. 1974;80:520–30.

McIntyre CW, Owen PJ. Prescribing drugs in kidney disease. In: Brenner BM, editor. Brenner & Rector's the kidney. 8th ed. Philadelphia: Saunders Elsevier; 2008. p. 1930–55.

Meyer P, White M, Mujib M, et al. Digoxin and reduction of heart failure hospitalization in chronic systolic and diastolic heart failure. Am J Cardiol. 2008;102:1681–6.

Mittal MK, Chockalingam P, Chockalingam A. Contemporary indications and therapeutic implications for digoxin use. Am J Ther. 2011;18:280–7.

Olyaei AJ, Bennett WM. Drug dosing in elderly patients with chronic kidney disease. Clin Geriatr Med. 2009;25:459–527.

Olyaei AJ, Bennett WM. Pharmacologic approach to renal insufficiency. In: Dale DC, Federman DD, Antman K, editors. ACP medicine, WebMD June 2007 update. Hamilton: BC Decker; 2007; NEPHROLOGY IX: Appendix A1–25.

Olyaei AJ, DeMattos AM, Bennett WM. Use of drugs in patients with renal failure. In: Schrier RW, editor. Diseases of the kidney and urinary tract. 8th ed. Philadelphia: Lippincott Williams & Wilkins; 2007. p. 2765–807.

Packer M, Gheorghiade M, Young JB, et al. Withdrawal of digoxin from patients with chronic heart failure treated with angiotensin-converting-enzyme inhibitors. N Engl J Med. 1993;329:1–7.

Robert S, Ujhelyi MR, Zarowitz BJ. Reinstitution of digoxin after digoxin fab antibody therapy in a hemodialyzed patient. Crit Care Med. 1993;21:1585–7.

Smith TW. Digitalis glycosides. N Engl J Med. 1973;288:719–22, 942–6.

Smith TW. Digitalis: mechanisms of action and clinical use. N Engl J Med. 1988;318;358–65.

Smith TW, Antman EM. Friedman PL, Blatt CM, Marsh JD. Digitalis glycosides: mechanisms and manifestations of toxicity. Prog Cardiovasc Dis. 1984;26:413–58.

Tzou MC, Reuning RH, Sams RA. Quantitation of interference in digoxin immunoassay in renal, hepatic, and diabetic disease. Clin Pharmacol Ther. 1997;61:429–41.

Uretsky BF, Young JB, Shahidi FE, Yellen LG, Harrison MC, Jolly MK. Randomized study assessing the effect of digoxin withdrawal in patients with mild to moderate chronic congestive heart failure: results of the PROVED Trial. J Am Coll Cardiol. 1993;22:955–62.

Dosage Adjustment of Medications Eliminated by the Kidneys

Digoxin/Lanoxin®, Digitek®   {Inotropic agent; cardiac glycoside}

Usual initial dose:	8–12 μg/kg IV or orally, e.g., 500 μg followed by 125 μg every 6 h ×2 doses
Usual maintenance dose:	125 μg IV or orally once daily
Typical maximum dose:	375 μg IV or orally once daily
Proportion eliminated unchanged:	25 %

Adjustment for Kidney Disease

FDA-approved product labeling: *Usual daily maintenance dose requirements (mcg) of digoxin for estimated peak body stores of 10 mcg/kg*

CrCL (mL/min)	Lean body weight						Number of days before steady state achieved
	50 kg; 110 lb	60 kg; 132 lb	70 kg; 154 lb	80 kg; 176 lb	90 kg; 198 lb	100 kg; 220 lb	
0	62.5	125	125	125	187.5	187.5	22
10	125	125	125	187.5	187.5	187.5	19
20	125	125	187.5	187.5	187.5	250	16
30	125	187.5	187.5	187.5	250	250	14
40	125	187.5	187.5	250	250	250	13
50	187.5	187.5	250	250	250	250	12
60	187.5	187.5	250	250	250	375	11
70	187.5	250	250	250	250	375	10
80	187.5	250	250	250	375	375	9
90	187.5	250	250	250	375	500	8
100	250	250	250	375	375	500	7

Alternative adjustment:	GFR >50 mL/min	125–250 μg IV or orally once daily (100 % of usual dose every 24 h)
	GFR 10–50 mL/min	62.5 μg orally every 24–36 h (25–75 % of usual dose every 24–36 h)
	GFR <10 mL/min	62.5 μg every 48 h (10–25 % of usual dose every 48 h)
	CAPD	62.5 μg every 48 h (10–25 % of usual dose every 48 h)
	Hemodialysis	62.5 μg every 48 h (10–25 % of usual dose every 48 h)
	CRRT	62.5 μg every 48 h (10–25 % of usual dose every 48 h)

Therapeutic drug monitoring

Therapeutic plasma levels: *0.8–2 ng/mL; draw sample 8–24 h after dose.*

Dihydroergotamine - Selected References

Aylward M, Davies DE, Maddock J, Robinson PR, Jones M. On the treatment of migraine: pharmacokinetic-pharmacodynamic relationships for programmed release formulation of dihydroergotamine administered orally in the human. Cephalgia. 1983;3(Suppl 1):146–50.

de Hoon JNJM, Poppe KA, Thjjssen HHW, Struijker-Bouldier HAJ, Van Bortel LMAB. Dihydroergotamine: discrepancy between arterial, arteriolar and pharmacokinetic data. Br J Clin Pharmacol. 2001;52:45–51.

de Marées H, Welzel D, de Marées A, Klotz U, Tiedjeb KU, Jbayo G. Relationship between the venoconstrictor activity of dihydroergotamine and its pharmacokinetics during acute and chronic dosing. Eur J Clin Pharmacol. 1986;30:685–9.

DHE 45® injection [package insert]. Costa Mesa: Valeant Pharmaceuticals North America; 2002.

Kanto J. Bioavailability of dihydroergotamine [letter]. Br Med J. 1980;281:748.

Kanto J, Allonen H, Koulu M, et al. Pharmacokinetics of dihydroergotamine in healthy volunteers and in neurological patients after a single intravenous injection. Int J Clin Pharmacol Ther Toxicol. 1981;19:12730.

Little PJ, Jennings Gl, Skews H, Bobik A. Bioavailability of dihydroergotamine in man. Br J Clin Pharmacol. 1982;13:785–90.

Migranal® nasal spray [package insert]. Aliso Viejo: Valeant Pharmaceuticals North America; 2007.

Olver IN, Jennings GL, Bobik A, Esler M. Low bioavailability as a cause of apparent failure of dihydroergotamine in orthostatic hypotension. Br Med J. 1980;281:275–6.

Saper JR, Silberstein S. Pharmacology of dihydroergotamine and evidence for efficacy and safety in migraine. Headache. 206;46(Suppl 4):S171–81.

Schran HF, Tse FLS. Pharmacokinetics of dihydroergotamine following subcutaneous administration in humans. Int J Clin Pharmacol Ther Toxicol. 1985;23:1–4.

Silberstein SD. The pharmacology of ergotamine and dihydroergotamine. Headache. 1997;37(Suppl 1):S15–25.

Dosage Adjustment of Medications Eliminated by the Kidneys

<u>**Dihydroergotamine**</u>**/DHE 45®, Migranal®**   {Antimigraine; ergotamine derivative}

Usual initial dose: 1 mg (1 mL) intravenously, intramuscularly, or subcutaneously; 1 spray (0.5 mg) in each nostril

Usual maintenance dose: 1 mg (1 mL) intravenously, intramuscularly, or subcutaneously repeated, as needed, at 1-h intervals to a total dose of 3 mg (3 mL) for intramuscular or subcutaneous delivery or 2 mg (2 mL) for intravenous delivery in a 24-h period; 1 spray (0.5 mg) in each nostril repeated if necessary in 15 min for a total of 4 sprays (2 mg)

Typical maximum dose: The total weekly dosage should not exceed 6 mg (6 mL).

Proportion eliminated unchanged: 7 %

Adjustment for Kidney Disease

   FDA-approved product labeling: *Severely impaired renal function*   *Contraindicated*

   Alternative adjustment: *Data not available*

Dosage Adjustment of Medications Eliminated by the Kidneys

Disopyramide - Selected References

Aitio M-L. Plasma concentrations and protein binding of disopyramide and mono-N-dealkyldisopyramide during chronic oral disopyramide therapy. Br J Clin Pharmacol. 1981;11:369–76.

Aitio M-L, Allonen H, Kanto J, Mäntylä R. The pharmacokinetics of disopyramide and mono-N-dealkyldisopyramide in humans. Int J Clin Pharmacol Ther Toxicol. 1982;20:219–26.

Aronoff GA, Bennett WM, Berns JS, et al. Drug prescribing in renal failure: dosing guidelines for adults and children. 5th ed. Philadelphia: American College of Physicians; 2007.

Bonde J, Jensen NM, Pedersen LE, et al. Disposition kinetics and urinary disopyramide in human healthy volunteers described by an open three compartment model. Pharmacol Toxicol. 1989;64:412–6.

Braun J, Sörgel F, Gluth WP, Øie S. Does alpha$_1$-acid glycoprotein reduce the unbound metabolic clearance of disopyramide in patients with renal impairment? Eur J Clin Pharmacol. 1988;35:313–7.

Bryson SM, Cairns CJ, Whiting B. Disopyramide pharmacokinetics during recovery from myocardial infarction. Br J Clin Pharmacol. 1982;13:417–21.

Burk M, Peters U. Disopyramide kinetics in renal impairment: determinants of interindividual variability. Clin Pharmacol Ther. 1983;34:331–40.

Giacomini KM, Nelson WL, Pershe RA, Valdivieso L, Turner-Tamiyasu K, Blaschke TF. In vivo interaction of the enantiomers of disopyramide in human subjects. J Pharmacokinet Biopharm. 1986;14:335–56.

Hasselström J, Enquist M, Hermansson AJ, Dahlqvist R. Enantioselective steady-state kinetics of unbound disopyramide and its dealkylated metabolite in man. Eur J Clin Pharmacol. 1991;41:481–4.

Haughey DB, Kraft CJ, Matzke GR, Keane WF, Halstenson CE. Protein binding of disopyramide and elevated alpha-1-glycoprotein concentrations in serum obtained from dialysis patients and renal transplant recipients. Am J Nephrol. 1985;5:35–9.

Horiuchi T, Johno I, Hasagawa T, Kitazawa S, Goto M, Hata T. Inhibitory effect of free acids on plasma protein binding of disopyramide in haemodialysis patients. Eur J Clin Pharmacol. 1989;36:175–80.

Horiuchi T, Johno I, Kitazawa S, Goto M, Hata T. Plasma free acids and protein binding of disopyramide during haemodialysis. Eur J Clin Pharmacol. 1987;33:327–9.

Inagaki Y, Amano I, Otsu T. Accumulation of a disopyramide metabolite in renal failure. ASAIO J. 1993;39:M609–13.

Jounela AJ, Pentikäinen PJ, Oksanen K. The pharmacokinetics of disopyramide in patients with acute myocardial infarction. Int J Clin Pharmacol Ther Toxicol. 1982;20:276–82.

Kapil RP, Axelson JE, Mansfield IL, et al. Disopyramide pharmacokinetics and metabolism: effect of inducers. Br J Clin Pharmacol. 1987;24:781–91.

Le Corre P, Gibassier D, Sado P, Le Verge R. Stereoselective metabolism and pharmacokinetics of disopyramide enantiomers in humans. Drug Metab Dispos. 1988;16:858–64.

Lima JJ, Boudoulas H, Shields BJ. Stereoselective pharmacokinetics of disopyramide enantiomers in man. Drug Metab Dispos. 1985;13:572–7.

Norpace® capsule [package insert]. New York: GD Searle Div Pfizer Inc; 2006.

Pedersen LE, Bonde J, Graudal NA, Backer NV, Hansen J-ES, Kampmann JP. Quantitative and qualitative binding characteristics of disopyramide in serum from patients with decreased renal and hepatic function. Br J Clin Pharmacol. 1987;23:41–6.

Pentikäinen PJ, Huikuri H, Jounela AJ, Wilen G. Disopyramide pharmacokinetics in patients with acute myocardial infarction. Eur J Clin Pharmacol. 1985;28:45–51.

Siddoway LA, Woosley RL. Clinical pharmacokinetics of disopyramide. Clin Pharmacokinet. 1986;11:214–22.

Stapleton JT, Gillman MW. Hypoglycemic coma due to disopyramide toxicity. South Med J. 1983;76:1453.

Tsuchishita Y, Fukumoto K, Kusumoto M, Ueno K. Effects of serum concentrations of disopyramide and its metabolite mono-n-dealkyldisopyramide on the anticholinergic side effects associated with disopyramide. Biol Pharm Bull. 2008;31:1368–70.

Dosage Adjustment of Medications Eliminated by the Kidneys

Disopyramide/Norpace®   {Antiarrhythmic, class IA}

Usual initial dose:	100 mg orally
Usual maintenance dose:	100 mg orally every 6 h or 200 mg (CR) orally every 12 h (if ≤50 kg)
	150 mg orally every 6 h or 300 mg (CR) orally every 12 h (if >50 kg)
Typical maximum dose:	400 mg orally every 6 h
Proportion eliminated unchanged:	47 % plus 22 % as active oxidative metabolite

Adjustment for Kidney Disease

FDA-approved product labeling: *Disopyramide dosage interval for patients with renal insufficiency*

Following an initial dose of 150 mg orally, administer 100 mg orally at the following intervals

CrCL (mL/min)	*30–40*	*15–30*	*<15*
Approx maintenance–dosing interval	*q 8 h*	*q 12 h*	*q 24 h*

Alternative adjustment:

GFR >50 mL/min	*100–150 mg every 8 h*
GFR 10–50 mL/min	*100 mg orally every 12–24 h; monitor and titrate to clinical effect.*
GFR <10 mL/min	*100 mg orally every 24–48 h; monitor and titrate to clinical effect.*
Hemodialysis	*100 mg orally every 24–48 h; monitor and titrate to clinical effect.*
CAPD	*100 mg orally every 24–48 h; monitor and titrate to clinical effect.*
CRRT	*100 mg enterally every 12–24 h; monitor and titrate to clinical effect.*

Dosage Adjustment of Medications Eliminated by the Kidneys

Dofetilide - Selected References

Coleman CI, Sood N, Chawla D, et al. Intravenous magnesium sulfate enhances the ability of dofetilide to successfully cardiovert atrial fibrillation or flutter: results of the Dofetilide and Intravenous Magnesium Evaluation. Europace. 2009;11:892–5.

Corley SD, Epstein AE, DiMarco JP, et al. Relationships between sinus rhythm, treatment, and survival in the Atrial Fibrillation Follow-up Investigation of Rhythm Management (AFFIRM) Study. Circulation. 2004;109:1509–13.

Gemmill JD, Howie CA, Meredith PA, et al. A dose-ranging study of UK-68,798, a novel class III anti-arrhythmic agent, in normal volunteers. Br J Clin Pharmacol. 1991;32:429–32.

Golightly LK, Matuszewski KA, Kay L. Dofetilide: UHC drug monograph. Oak Brook: University Health-System Consortium; 2000.

Grines CL. Safety and effectiveness of dofetilide for conversion of atrial fibrillation and nesiritide for acute decompensation of heart failure: a report from the Cardiovascular and Renal Advisory Panel of the Food and Drug Administration. Circulation. 2000;101:e200–1.

Jonker DM, Kenna LA, Leishman D, Wallis R, Milligan PA Jonsson EN. A pharmacokinetic-pharmacodynamic model for the quantitative prediction of dofetilide clinical QT prolongation from human ether-a-go-go-related gene current inhibition data. Clin Pharmacol Ther. 2005;77:572–82.

Kim MH, Klingman D, Lin J, Pathak P, Battleman D. Cost of hospitalization for antiarrhythmic drug initiation in atrial fibrillation. Ann Pharmacother. 2009;43:840–8.

Knilans TK, Lathrop DA, Nánási PP, Schwartz A, Varró A. Rate and concentration-dependent effects of UK-68,798, a potent new class III antiarrhythmic, on canine Purkinje fibre action potential duration and V_{max}. Br J Pharmacol. 1991;103:1568–72.

Lande G, Maison-Blanche P, Fayn J, Ghadanfar M, Coumel P, Funck-Brentano C. Dynamic analysis of dofetilide-induced changes in ventricular depolarization. Clin Pharmacol Ther. 1998;64:312–21.

Le Coz F, Funck-Brentano C, Morrill T, Ghadanfar MM, Jaillon P. Pharmacokinetic and pharmacodynamic modeling of the effects of oral and intravenous administrations of dofetilide on ventricular depolarization. Clin Pharmacol Ther. 1995;57:533–42.

McClellan KJ. Markham A. Dofetilide: a review of its use in atrial fibrillation and atrial flutter. Drugs. 1999;58:1043–59.

Møller M, Torp-Pedersen CT, Køber L. Dofetilide in patients with congestive heart failure and left ventricular dysfunction: the Danish Investigators of Arrhythmia and Mortality on Dofetilide (DIAMOND) Study Group. Congest Heart Fail. 2001;7:146–50.

Pedersen HS, Wilming H, Seibæk M, et al. Risk factors and predictors of torsade de pointes ventricular tachycardia in patients receiving dofetilide. Am J Cardiol. 2007;100:876–80.

Sedgwick M, Rasmussen HS, Walker D, Cobbe SM. Pharmacokinetic and pharmacodynamic effects of UK-68,798, a new potential class III antiarrhythmic drug. Br J Clin Pharmacol. 1991;31:515–9.

Tham TCK, MacLennan BA, Burke MT, Harron DWG. Pharmacodynamics and pharmacokinetics of the class III antiarrhythmic agent dofetilide (UK-68,798) in humans. J Cardiovasc Pharmacol. 1993;21:507–12.

Tham TCK, MacLennan BA, Harron DWG, Coates PE, Walker D, Rasmussen HS. Pharmacodynamics and pharmacokinetics of the novel class III antiarrhythmic drug UK-68,798 in man [abstract]. Br J Clin Pharmacol. 1991;31(Suppl):243–4P.

Tikosyn® capsule [package insert]. New York: Pfizer Labs Division of Pfizer Inc; 2006.

Torp-Pedersen C, Møller M, Bloch-Thomsen PE, et al. Dofetilide in patients with congestive heart failure and left ventricular dysfunction. N Engl J Med. 1999;341:857–65.

Tunblad K, Lindbom L, McFadyen L, Jonsson EN, Marshall S, Karlsson MO. The use of clinical irrelevance criteria in covariate modeling with application of dofetilide pharmacokinetic data. J Pharmacokinet Pharmacodyn. 2008;35:503–26.

Walker DK, Alabaster CT, Congrave GS, et al. Significance of metabolism in the disposition and action of the antidysrhythmic drug, dofetilide: in vitro studies and correlation with in vivo data. Drug Metab Dispos. 1996;34:447–55.

Dosage Adjustment of Medications Eliminated by the Kidneys

Dofetilide/Tikosyn®	{**Antiarrhythmic, class III; potassium channel (I_{KR}) blocker**}
Usual initial dose:	500 mcg orally
Usual maintenance dose:	500 mcg orally twice daily
Typical maximum dose:	1,000 mcg/day
Proportion eliminated unchanged:	80 %

Adjustment for Kidney Disease

FDA-approved product labeling:

Dofetilide starting dose determination

Calculated CrCL (mL/min)	Dofetilide dose
>60	500 mcg twice daily
40–60	250 mcg twice daily
20–39	125 mcg twice daily
<20	Contraindicated

Alternative adjustment:

Data not available

Note: Treatment in all patients should be initiated with electrocardiographic monitoring; prolongation of 2-h post-dose corrected QT interval >15 % of baseline or >500 ms indicates need for downward dosage adjustment.

Dosage Adjustment of Medications Eliminated by the Kidneys

Doripenem - Selected References

Abramowicz M, Zuccotti G, Pflomm J-M, et al., editors. Handbook of antimicrobial therapy. 19th ed. New Rochelle: The Medical Letter; 2011.

Cirillo I, Mnnens G, Janssen C, et al. Disposition, metabolism, and excretion of [^{14}C]doripenem after a single 500-mg intravenous infusion in healthy men. Antimicrob Agents Chemother. 2008;52:3478–83.

Cirillo I, Vaccaro N, Balis D, Redman R, Matzke GR. Influence of continuous venovenous hemofiltration and continuous hemodiafiltration on the disposition of doripenem. Antimicrob Agents Chemother. 2011;55:1187–93.

Doribax® injection [package insert]. Raritan: Ortho-McNeil Division of Ortho-McNeil-Jansen Pharmaceuticals; 2010.

Hidaka S, Goto K, Hagiwara S, Wassaka H, Noguchi T. Doripenem pharmacokinetics in critically ill patients receiving continuous hemodiafiltration (CHDF). Yakugaku Zasshi. 2010;130:87–94.

Katsube T, Yano Y, Yamano Y, Munekage T, Kuroda N, Takano M. Pharmacokinetic-pharmacodynamic modeling and simulation for bactericidal effect in an in vitro dynamic model. J Pharm Sci. 2008;97:4108–17.

Keam SJ. Doripenem: a review of its use in the treatment of bacterial infections. Drugs. 2008;68:2021–57.

Nandy P, Samtani M, Lin R. Population pharmacokinetics of doripenem based on data from phase I healthy volunteer studies and phase 2 and 3 studies including critically ill patients. Antimicrob Agents Chemother. 2010;54:2354–9.

Ohchi Y, Kidaka S, Goto K, et al. Effect of hemopurification rate on doripenem pharmacokinetics in critically ill patients receiving high-flow continuous hemodiafiltration. Yakugaku Zasshi. 2011;131:1395–9.

Paterson DL, DePestel DD. Doripenem. Clin Infect Dis. 2009;49:291–8.

Samtani MN, Flamm R, Kaniga K, Nandy P. Pharmacokinetic-pharmacodynamic model guided doripenem dosing in critically ill patients. Antimicrob Agents Chemother. 2010;54:2360–4.

Tanoue K, Nishi K, Kadowaki D, Hirata S. Removal of doripenem during hemodialysis and the optimum dosing regimen or patients undergoing hemodialysis. Ther Apher Dial. 2011;15:327–33.

Van Wart SA, Andes DR, Ambrose PG, Bhavnani SM. Pharmacokinetic-pharmacodynamic modeling to support doripenem dose regimen optimization for critically ill patients. Diagn Microbiol Infect Dis. 2009;63:409–14

Dosage Adjustment of Medications Eliminated by the Kidneys

Doripenem/Doribax®   {**Antibacterial; carbapenem**}

Usual initial dose: 500 mg IV

Usual maintenance dose: 500 mg IV every 8 h

Typical maximum dose: 500 mg IV every 8 h

Proportion eliminated unchanged: 70 %

Adjustment for Kidney Disease

FDA-approved product labeling:

Doripenem dosage in patients with renal function impairment

Estimated CrCL (mL/min)	Recommended dosage
>50	No dosage adjustment necessary
≥30 to ≤50	250 mg IV every 8 h
>10 to <30	250 mg IV every 12 h

Alternative adjustment:

eCrCL >50 mL/min	500 mg IV over 1–4 h every 8 h
eCrCL 30–50 mL/min	250 mg IV over 1–4 h every 8 h
eCrCL 10–29 mL/min	250 mg IV over 1–4 h every 12 h
eCrCL <10 mL/min	250 mg IV every 12 h
Hemodialysis	250 mg IV every 12 h or 500 mg IV every 24 h
CVVHD	250 mg IV every 12 h
High flow CVVHDF	500 mg IV every 12 h

Dosage Adjustment of Medications Eliminated by the Kidneys

Duloxetine - Selected References

Carter NJ, McCormack PL. Duloxetine: a review of its use in generalized anxiety disorder. CNS Drugs. 2009;23:523–41.

Chan C, Yeo KP, Pan AX, Lim M, Knadler MP, Small DS. Duloxetine pharmacokinetics are similar in Japanese and Caucasian patients. Br J Clin Pharmacol. 2007;63:310–4.

Cymbalta® capsule delayed release [package insert]. Indianapolis: Eli Lilly and Company; 2011.

Frampton JE, Plosker GL. Duloxetine: a review of its use in the treatment of major depressive disorder. CNS Drugs. 2007;21:581–609.

Knadler MP, Lobo E, Chappell J, Bergstrom R. Duloxetine: clinical pharmacokinetics and drug interactions. Clin Pharmacokinet. 2011;50:281–94.

Lantz RJ, Gillespie TA, Rash TJ, et al. Metabolism, excretion, and pharmacokinetics of duloxetine in healthy human subjects. Drug Metab Dispos. 2005;31:1142–50.

Lobo ED, Heathman M, Kuan H-Y, et al. Effects of varying degrees of renal impairment on the pharmacokinetics of duloxetine: analysis of a single-dose phase I study and pooled steady-state data from phase II/III trials. Clin Pharmacokinet. 2010;49:311–21.

Lobo ED, Quinlan T, O'Brien L, Knadler MP, Heathman M. Population pharmacokinetics of orally administered duloxetine in patients: implications for dosing recommendations. Clin Pharmacokinet. 2009;48:189–97.

Ormseth MJ, Scholz BA, Boomershine CS. Duloxetine in the management of diabetic peripheral neuropathic pain. Patient Prefer Adherence. 2011;5:343–56.

Sharma A, Goldberg MJ, Cerimele BJ. Pharmacokinetics and safety of duloxetine, a dual-serotonin and norepinephrine reuptake inhibitor. J Clin Pharmacol. 2000;40:161–70.

Skinner MH, Kuan H-Y, Pan A, et al. Duloxetine is both an inhibitor and a substrate of cytochrome P4502D6 in healthy volunteers. Clin Pharmacol Ther. 2003;73:170–7.

Terneou W Jr. Pregabalin and duloxetine for the treatment of neuropathic pain disorders. J Pain Palliat Care Pharmacother. 2007;21:79–84.

Wernicke JF, Gahimer J, Yalcin I, Wulster M, Viktrup L. Safety and adverse event profile of duloxetine. Curr Opin Drug Saf. 2005;4:987–93.

Zhao R-K, Cheng G, Tang J, Song J, Peng W-X. Pharmacokinetics of duloxetine hydrochloride enteric-coated tablets in healthy Chinese volunteers: a randomized, open-label, single- and multiple-dose study. Clin Ther.2009;31:1022–36.

Dosage Adjustment of Medications Eliminated by the Kidneys

<u>Duloxetine</u>/Cymbalta®   {**Antidepressant; anxiolytic; ℞ for neuropathic pain; CNS serotonergic and noradrenergic action potentiator**}

Usual initial dose:	30 mg orally
Usual maintenance dose:	60 mg orally once daily
Typical maximum dose:	120 mg orally once daily
Proportion eliminated unchanged:	Minimal (72 % of an absorbed dose is eliminated in urine as the glucuronide and/or sulfate conjugates of the oxidative duloxetine metabolites)

Adjustment for Kidney Disease

FDA-approved product labeling: *Increased plasma concentration of duloxetine and especially its metabolites occurs in patients with end-stage renal disease (requiring dialysis); duloxetine ordinarily should not be used in patients with end-stage renal disease or severe renal impairment (CrCL <30 mL/min).*

Alternative adjustment:

eCrCL ≥30 mL/min	*30–120 mg orally once daily (no dose adjustment necessary)*
eCrCL <30 mL/min	*Data not available; preferably avoid unless no suitable alternative is available; if indeed necessary, dose conservatively, carefully monitor responses, and cautiously adjust doses.*

Dyphylline - Selected References

Acara M, Carr EA Jr, Terry EN. Probenecid inhibition of the renal excretion of dyphylline in chicken, rat, and man. J Pharm Sci. 1987;39:526–30.

Aronoff GA, Bennett WM, Berns JS, et al. Drug prescribing in renal failure: dosing guidelines for adults and children. 5th ed. Philadelphia: American College of Physicians; 2007.

Gisclon LG, Ayres AW, Ewing GH. Pharmacokinetics of orally administered dyphylline. Am J Hosp Pharm. 1979;36:1179–84.

Lawyer CH, Bardana EJ Jr, Rodgers R, Gerber N. Utilization of intravenous dihydroxypropyl theophylline (dyphylline) in an aminophylline-sensitive patient, and its pharmacokinetic comparison with theophylline. J Allergy Clin Immunol. 1980;65:353–7.

Lee C-SC, Wang LH, Majeske BL, Marbury TC. Pharmacokinetics of dyphylline elimination by uremic patients. J Pharmacol Exp Ther. 1981;217:340–4.

Lufyllin® tablet [package insert]. Somerset: Meda Pharmaceuticals Inc; 2007.

McIntyre CW, Owen PJ. Prescribing drugs in kidney disease. In: Brenner BM, editor. Brenner & Rector's the kidney. 8th ed. Philadelphia: Saunders Elsevier; 2008. p. 1930–55.

Nadai M, Apichartpichean R, Hasegawa T, Nabeshima T. Pharmacokinetics and the effect of probenecid on the renal excretion mechanism of diprophylline. J Pharm Sci. 1992;81:1024–7.

Simons FER, Simons KJ, Bierman CW. The pharmacokinetics of dihydroxypropyltheophylline: a basis for rational therapy. J Allergy Clin Immunol. 1975;56:347–55.

Simons KJ, Simons FER. Urinary excretion of dyphylline in humans. J Pharm Sci. 1979;68:1327–9.

Stablein JJ, Samaan SS, Bukantz SC, Lockey RF. Pharmacokinetics and bioavailability of three dyphylline preparations. Eur J Clin Pharmacol. 1983;25:281–3.

Straughn AB, Wood GC, Raghow G, Meyer MC. Bioavailability of dyphylline and dyphylline-guaifenesin tablets in humans. J Pharm Sci. 1985;74:335–7.

Dosage Adjustment of Medications Eliminated by the Kidneys

<u>Dyphylline</u>/Lufyllin® {Bronchodilator; theophylline derivative; phosphodiesterase and prostaglandin inhibitor}

Usual initial dose:	200 mg orally
Usual maintenance dose:	200–400 mg orally three or four times daily
Typical maximum dose:	15 mg/kg/day
Proportion eliminated unchanged:	83 %

Adjustment for Kidney Disease

FDA-approved product labeling: *Appropriate dosage adjustments should be made in patients with impaired renal function. The renal clearance would be reduced in patients with impaired renal function. In anuric patients, the half-life (approx. 2 h) may be increased three to four times normal.*

Alternative adjustment:

GFR >50 mL/min	*150–300 mg orally three or four times daily (25 % decrease)*
GFR 10–50 mL/min	*100–200 mg orally three or four times daily (50 % decrease)*
GFR <10 mL/min	*50–100 mg orally three or four times daily (75 % decrease)*
Hemodialysis	*50–100 mg orally three or four times daily; administer after hemodialysis on dialysis days.*
CAPD	*Data not available*
CRRT	*100–200 mg orally three or four times daily*

E

L.K. Golightly et al. (eds.), *Renal Pharmacotherapy*,
DOI 10.1007/978-1-4614-5800-5_5, © Springer Science+Business Media New York 2013

Edetate Calcium Disodium - Selected References

Calcium disodium Versenate® injection [package insert]. Northridge: 3M Pharmaceuticals; 2004.

Cory-Slechta DA, Weiss B, Cox C. Mobilization and redistribution of lead over the course of calcium disodium ethylenediamine tetraacetate chelation therapy. J Pharmacol Exp Ther. 1987;243:804–13.

Osterloh J, Becker CE. Pharmacokinetics of CaNa$_2$EDTA and chelation of lead in renal failure. Clin Pharmacol Ther. 1986;40:686–93.

Edetate Calcium Disodium/
Calcium Disodium Versenate®

{**Chelating agent; R for lead poisoning**}

Usual initial dose:	1,000 mg/m² IV or IM
Usual maintenance dose:	If blood lead level is <70 mcg/dL but >20 mcg/dL (World Health Organization recommended upper allowable level), administer 1,000 mg/m²/day IV or IM.
Typical maximum dose:	1,000 mg/m² IV or IM
Proportion eliminated unchanged:	~100 %

Adjustment for Kidney Disease

FDA-approved product labeling:	*Normal renal function*	*500 mg/m² every 24 h for 5 days for patients with SCr levels of 2–3 mg/dL, every 48 h for three doses for patients with SCr levels of 3–4 mg/dL, and once weekly for patients with SCr levels above 4 mg/dL. These regimens may be repeated at 1-month intervals.*
	Active renal disease/ anuria	*Contraindicated*
Alternative adjustment:	*Data not available*	

Note: Edetate calcium disodium may be confused with edetate disodium. Fatal hypocalcemia may result if edetate disodium is used for chelation therapy instead of edetate calcium disodium. Always confirm diagnosis to distinguish between the two drugs prior to dispensing and/or administering either medication.

Efavirenz and Emtricitabine and Tenofovir - Selected References

A once-daily combination tablet (Atripla) for HIV. Med Lett Drugs Ther. 2006;48:78–9.

Atripla® tablet [package insert]. Foster City: Bristol-Myers Squibb & Gilead Sciences LLC; 2011.

Deeks ED, Perry CM. Efavirenz/emtricitabine/tenofovir disoproxil fumarate single-tablet regimen (Atripla®): a review of its use in the management of HIV infection. Drugs. 2010;70:.2315–38.

Feng JY, Ly JK, Myrick F, et al. The triple combination of tenofovir, emtricitabine and efavirenz shows synergistic anti-HIV-1 activity in vitro: a mechanism of action study. Retrovirology. 2009;6:44. doi:10.1186/1742-4690-6-44.

Goicoechea M, Best B. Efavirenz/emtricitabine/tenofovir disoproxil fumarate fixed-dose combination: first-line therapy for all? Expert Opin Pharmacother. 2007;8:371–82.

Gupta SK, Eustace JA, Winston JA, et al. Guidelines for the management of chronic kidney disease in HIV-infected patients: recommendations of the HIV Medicine Section of the Infectious Diseases Society of America. Clin Infect Dis. 2005;40:1559–85.

Jhaveri MA, Browning SR, Bush H, Thornton A, Greenberg RN. Comparison of 3-drug versus 4-drug and PI versus non-PI combinations as initial HAART: experience from 1998 to 2007. J Int Assoc Physicians AIDS Care (Chic). 2009;8:299–307.

Mathias AA, Hinkle J, Menning M, Hui J, Kaul S, Kearney BP. Bioequivalence of efavirenz/emtricitabine/tenofovir disoproxil fumarate single-tablet regimen. J Acquir Immune Defic Syndr. 2007;46:167–73.

Thompson MA, Aberg JA, Cahn P, et al. Antiretroviral treatment of adult HIV infection: 2010 recommendations of the International AIDS Society—USA Panel. JAMA. 2010;304:321–33.

Efavirenz and Emtricitabine and Tenofovir/Atripla®

{Antiretroviral; combination non-nucleoside and nucleoside reverse transcriptase inhibitor}

Usual initial dose:	One tablet
Usual maintenance dose:	One tablet once daily taken orally on an empty stomach; dosing at bedtime may improve the tolerability of nervous system symptoms.
Typical maximum dose:	One tablet daily
Proportion eliminated unchanged:	85 % (emtricitabine)

Adjustment for Kidney Disease

FDA-approved product labeling: *Because efavirenz/emtricitabine/tenofovir is a fixed-dose combination, it should not be prescribed for patients requiring dosage adjustment, such as those with moderate or severe renal impairment (CrCL <50 mL/min).*

Alternative adjustment: *Data not available*

Dosage Adjustment of Medications Eliminated by the Kidneys

Emtricitabine - Selected References

Anderson PL, Kakuda TN, Lichtenstein KA. The cellular pharmacology of nucleoside- and nucleotide-analogue reverse-transcriptase inhibitors and its relationship to clinical toxicities. Clin Infect Dis. 2004;38:743–53.

Aronoff GA, Bennett WM, Berns JS, et al. Drug prescribing in renal failure: dosing guidelines for adults and children. 5th ed. Philadelphia: American College of Physicians; 2007.

Bang LM, Scott LJ. Emtricitabine: an antiretroviral agent for HIV infection. Drugs. 2003;63:2413–24.

Darque A, Valette G, Rousseau F, Wang LH, Sommadossi J-P, Zhou X-J. Quantitation of intracellular triphosphate of emtricitabine in human immunodeficiency virus-infected patients. Antimicrob Agents Chemother. 1999;43:2245–50.

Emtriva® capsule and solution [package insert]. Foster City: Gilead Sciences Inc; 2007.

Gish RG, Leung NWY, Wright TL, et al. Dose range study of pharmacokinetics, safety, and preliminary antiviral activity of emtricitabine in adults with hepatitis B virus infection. Antimicrob Agents Chemother. 2002;46:1734–40.

Gupta SK, Eustace JA, Winston JA, et al. Guidelines for the management of chronic kidney disease in HIV-infected patients: recommendations of the HIV Medicine Section of the Infectious Diseases Society of America. Clin Infect Dis. 2005;40: 1559–85.

Lim SG, Ng TM, Kung N, et al. A double-blind placebo-controlled study of emtricitabine in chronic hepatitis B. Arch Intern Med. 2006;166:49–56.

Parks DA, Jennings HC, Taylor, Acosta EP. Pharmacokinetics of once-daily tenofovir, emtricitabine, ritonavir and fosamprenavir in HIV-infected subjects [letter]. AIDS. 2007;21:1373–5.

Rousseau FS, Kahn JO, Thompson M, et al. Prototype trial design for rapid dose selection of antiretroviral drugs: an example using emtricitabine (Covaricil). J Antimicrob Chemother. 2001;48:507–13.

Saag MS. Emtricitabine, a new antiretroviral agent with activity against HIV and hepatitis B virus. Clin Infect Dis. 2006;42:126–31.

Stevens RC, Blum MR, Rousseau FS, Kearney BP. Intracellular pharmacology of emtricitabine and tenofovir [letter]. Clin Infect Dis. 2004;39:877–8.

Thompson MA, Aberg JA, Cahn P, et al. Antiretroviral treatment of adult HIV infection: 2010 recommendations of the International AIDS Society—USA Panel. JAMA. 2010;304:321–33.

Wang LH, Begley J, St Claire RL III, Harris J, Wakeford C, Rousseau FS. Pharmacokinetic and pharmacodynamic characteristics of emtricitabine support its once daily dosing for the treatment of HIV infection. AIDS Res Hum Retroviruses. 2004;20:1173–82.

Zong J, Chittick GE, Wang LH, Hui J, Begley JA, Blum MR. Pharmacokinetic evaluation of emtricitabine in combination with other nucleoside antivirals in healthy volunteers. J Clin Pharmacol. 2007;47:877–89.

Dosage Adjustment of Medications Eliminated by the Kidneys

Emtricitabine/FTC, Emtriva®   {Antiretroviral; nucleoside reverse transcriptase inhibitor}

Usual initial dose:	200 mg orally
Usual maintenance dose:	200 mg orally once daily
Typical maximum dose:	200 mg orally once daily
Proportion eliminated unchanged:	85 %

Adjustment for Kidney Disease

FDA-approved product labeling: *Emtricitabine dosage adjustment in adult patients with renal impairment*

	CrCL (mL/min)			
Formulation	*≥50*	*30–49*	*15–29*	*<15 or on hemodialysis*
Capsule	*200 mg every 24 h*	*200 mg every 48 h*	*200 mg every 72 h*	*200 mg every 96 h*
Solution	*240 mg every 24 h (24 mL)*	*120 mg every 24 h (12 mL)*	*80 mg every 24 h (8 mL)*	*60 mg every 24 h (6 mL)*

Hemodialysis patients: if dosing on day of dialysis, administer after dialysis

Alternative adjustment:

GFR >50 mL/min	*200 mg every 24 h*
GFR 10–50 mL/min	*200 mg orally every 48–96 h*
GFR <10 mL/min	*200 mg orally every 96 h*
Hemodialysis	*200 mg orally every 96 h; administer after hemodialysis on dialysis days.*
CAPD	*Data not available*
CRRT	*200 mg enterally every 48 h or*
	120 mg (solution) every 24 h

Emtricitabine and Tenofovir - Selected References

Aronoff GA, Bennett WM, Berns JS, et al. Drug prescribing in renal failure: dosing guidelines for adults and children. 5th ed. Philadelphia: American College of Physicians; 2007.

Back DJ, Burger DM, Flexner CW Gerber JG. The pharmacology of antiretroviral nucleoside and nucleotide reverse transcriptase inhibitors: implications for once-daily dosing. J Acquir Immune Defic Syndr. 2005;39(Suppl 1):S1–23.

Blum MR, Chittick GE, Begley JA, Zong J. Steady-state pharmacokinetics of emtricitabine and tenofovir disoproxil fumarate administered alone and in combination in healthy volunteers. J Clin Pharmacol. 2007;47:751–9.

Gallant JE, Dejesus E, Arribas JR, et al. Tenofovir DF, emtricitabine, and efavirenz vs zidovudine, lamivudine, and efavirenz for HIV. N Engl J Med. 2006;354:251–60.

Gupta SK, Eustace JA, Winston JA, et al. Guidelines for the management of chronic kidney disease in HIV-infected patients: recommendations of the HIV Medicine Section of the Infectious Diseases Society of America. Clin Infect Dis. 2005;40:1559–85.

Santos SA, Uriel AJ, Park JS, et al. Effect of switching to tenofovir with emtricitabine in patients with chronic hepatitis B failing to respond to an adefovir-containing regimen. Eur J Gastroenterol Hepatol. 2006;18:1247–53.

Stevens RC, Blum MR, Rousseau FS, Kearney BP. Intracellular pharmacology of emtricitabine and tenofovir [letter]. Clin Infect Dis. 2004;39:877–8.

Thompson MA, Aberg JA, Cahn P, et al. Antiretroviral treatment of adult HIV infection: 2010 recommendations of the International AIDS Society—USA Panel. JAMA. 2010;304:321–33.

Truvada® tablet [package insert]. Foster City: Gilead Sciences Inc; 2009.

Two once-daily fixed dose NRTI combinations for HIV. Med Lett Drugs Ther. 2005;47:19–20.

Dosage Adjustment of Medications Eliminated by the Kidneys

Emtricitabine and Tenofovir/Truvada®	{Antiretroviral; nucleoside/nucleotide analogue reverse transcriptase inhibitor}

Usual initial dose: One tablet

Usual maintenance dose: One tablet (containing 200 mg of emtricitabine and 300 mg of tenofovir disoproxil fumarate) once daily taken orally with or without food

Typical maximum dose: One tablet once daily

Proportion eliminated unchanged: 85 % (emtricitabine)

Adjustment for Kidney Disease

FDA-approved product labeling:

Dosage interval adjustment of Truvada for patients with altered creatinine clearance

CrCL (mL/min)ᵃ	≥50	30–49	<30 (including patients requiring hemodialysis)
Dosing interval	Every 24 h	Every 48 h	Avoid

ᵃCalculated using ideal (lean) body weight

Alternative adjustment:

GFR >50 mL/min	One tablet orally every 24 h
GFR 10–50 mL/min	One tablet orally every 48 h
GFR <10 mL/min	Minimal data available
Hemodialysis	Minimal data available
CAPD	Data not available
CRRT	One tablet enterally every 48 h

Dosage Adjustment of Medications Eliminated by the Kidneys

Enalapril - Selected References

Abraham PA, Opsahl JA, Halstenson CE, Keane WF. Efficacy and renal effects of enalapril therapy for hypertensive patients with chronic renal insufficiency. Arch Intern Med. 1988;148:2358–62.

Ajayi AA, Hockings N, Reid JL. Age and the pharmacodynamics of angiotensin converting enzyme inhibitors enalapril and enalaprilat. Br J Clin Pharmacol. 1986;21:348–57.

Apperloo AJ, de Zeeuw D, de Jong PE. Discordant effects of enalapril and lisinopril on systemic and renal hemodynamics. Clin Pharmacol Ther. 1994;56:647–58.

Aronoff GA, Bennett WM, Berns JS, et al. Drug prescribing in renal failure: dosing guidelines for adults and children. 5th ed. Philadelphia: American College of Physicians; 2007.

Bauer JH, Reams GP, Hewett J, et al. A randomized, double-blind, placebo-controlled trial to evaluate the effect of enalapril in patients with clinical diabetic nephropathy. Am J Kidney Dis. 1992;20:443–57.

Benedict CR, Francis GS, Shelton B, et al. Effect of long-term enalapril therapy on neurohormones in patients with left ventricular failure. Am J Cardiol. 1995;75:1151–7.

Cohn JN, Johnson G, Ziesche S, et al. A comparison of enalapril with hydralazine-isosorbide dinitrate in the treatment of chronic congestive heart failure. N Engl J Med. 1991;325:303–10.

Elung-Jensen T, Heisterberg J, Kamper A-L, Sonne J, Strandgaard S, Larsen NE. High serum enalaprilat in chronic renal failure. J Renin Angiotensin Aldosterone Syst. 2001;2:240–5.

Hockings N, Ajayi AA, Reid JL. Age and the pharmacokinetics of angiotensin converting enzyme inhibitors enalapril and enalaprilat. Br J Clin Pharmacol. 1986;21:341–8.

Karlberg BE, Sjöstrand Å, Öhman P. Different effects of two angiotensin converting enzyme inhibitors in primary hypertension—a comparison of captopril and enalapril. J Hypertens. 1986;4(Suppl 5):S432–4.

Kelly JG, Doyle G, Carmody M, Glover DR, Cooper WD. Pharmacokinetics of lisinopril, enalapril and enalaprilat in renal failure: effects of hemodialysis. Br J Clin Pharmacol. 1988;26:781–6.

Kelly JG, Doyle G, Donohue J, et al. Pharmacokinetics of enalapril in normal subjects and patients with renal impairment. Br J Clin Pharmacol. 1986;21:63–9.

Lees KR, Reid JL. Age and the pharmacokinetics and pharmacodynamics of chronic enalapril treatment. Clin Pharmacol Ther. 1987;41:597–602.

Ljungman S, Kjekshus J, Swedberg K. Renal function in severe congestive heart failure during treatment with enalapril (the Cooperative North Scandinavian Enalapril Survival Study [CONSENSUS] Trial). Am J Cardiol. 1992;70:479–87.

Lowenthal DT, Irvin JD, Merrill D, et al. The effect of renal function on enalapril kinetics. Clin Pharmacol Ther. 1985;38:661–6.

McNabb WR, Noormohamed FH, Brooks BA, Till AE, Lant AF. Effects of repeated doses of enalapril on renal function in man. Br J Clin Pharmacol. 1985;19:353–61.

Prince MJ, Stuart CA, Padia M, Bandi Z, Holland B. Metabolic effects of hydrochlorothiazide and enalapril during treatment of the hypertensive diabetic patient: enalapril for hypertensive diabetics. Arch Intern Med. 1988;148:2363–8.

Scandling JD, Izzo JL Jr, Pabico RC, McKenna BA, Radke KJ, Ornt DB. Potassium homeostasis during angiotensin-converting enzyme inhibition with enalapril. J Clin Pharmacol. 1989;29:916–21.

Shapiro DA, Liss CL, Walker JF, Lewis JL, Lengerich RA, Irvin JD. Enalapril and hydrochlorothiazide as antihypertensive agents in the elderly. J Cardiovasc Pharmacol. 1987;10(Suppl 7):S160–2.

Speirs CJ, Dollery CT, Inman WHW, Rawson NSB, Wilton LV. Postmarketing surveillance of enalapril. II: Investigation of the potential role of enalapril in deaths with renal failure. Br Med J. 1988;297:830–2.

Swedberg K, Kjekshus J. Effects of enalapril on mortality in severe congestive heart failure: results of the Cooperative North Scandinavian Enalapril Survival Study (CONSENSUS). Am J Cardiol. 1988;62:60–6A.

Todd PA, Heel RC. Enalapril: a review of its pharmacodynamic and pharmacokinetic properties and therapeutic use in hypertension and congestive heart failure. Drugs. 1986;31:198–248.

Vasotec® tablet [package insert]. Bridgewater: BTA Pharmaceuticals Subsidiary of Biovail Corp; 2010.

Yusuf S, Probstfield J, Verter J, et al. Effect of enalapril on survival in patients with reduced left ventricular ejection fractions and congestive heart failure: the SOLVD Investigators. N Engl J Med. 1991;293–302.

Dosage Adjustment of Medications Eliminated by the Kidneys

Enalapril/Vasotec® {**Antihypertensive; vasodilator; angiotensin-converting enzyme (ACE)/renin inhibitor**}

Usual initial dose: 2.5 mg

Usual maintenance dose: 5–20 mg orally twice daily

Typical maximum dose: 40 mg/day

Proportion eliminated unchanged: 90 %

Adjustment for Kidney Disease

FDA-approved product labeling: *Dosage adjustments for enalapril in hypertensive patients with renal function impairment*

Renal status	CrCL (mL/min)	Initial dose (mg/day)
Normal renal function	>80	5 mg
Mild impairment	30 to ≤80	5 mg
Moderate to severe impairment	≤30	2.5 mg
Hemodialysis	–	2.5 mg on dialysis day

Alternative adjustment:

GFR >50 mL/min	5–20 mg orally twice daily
GFR 10–50 mL/min	2.5–10 orally twice daily
GFR <10 mL/min	1.25–5 mg orally twice daily
Hemodialysis	1.25–5 mg orally twice daily; dose after hemodialysis on dialysis days
CAPD	1.25–5 mg orally twice daily
CRRT	2.5–10 enterally twice daily; titrate

Dosage Adjustment of Medications Eliminated by the Kidneys

Enalaprilat - Selected References

Ajayi AA, Hockings N, Reid JL. Age and the pharmacodynamics of angiotensin converting enzyme inhibitors enalapril and enalaprilat. Br J Clin Pharmacol. 1986;21:348–57.

Ajayi AA, Hockings N, Reid JL. The relationship between serum enalaprilat concentration and the hypotensive effect in man. Int J Clin Pharmacol Res. 1987;8:1–3.

Aronoff GA, Bennett WM, Berns JS, et al. Drug prescribing in renal failure: dosing guidelines for adults and children. 5th ed. Philadelphia: American College of Physicians; 2007.

De Marco T, Daly PA, Liu M, Kayser S, Parmley WW, Chatterjee K. Enalaprilat: a new parenteral angiotensin-converting enzyme inhibitor: rapid changes in systemic and coronary hemodynamics and humoral profile in chronic heart failure. J Am Coll Cardiol. 1987;9:1131–8.

Elung-Jensen T, Heisterberg J, Kamper A-L, Sonne J, Strandgaard S, Larsen NE. High serum enalaprilat in chronic renal failure. J Renin Angiotensin Aldosterone Syst. 2001;2:240–5.

Elung-Jensen T, Heisterberg J, Sonne J, Strandgaard S, , Kamper A-L. Enalapril dosage in progressive chronic nephropathy: a randomised, controlled trial. Eur J Clin Pharmacol. 2005;61:87–96.

Enalaprilat injection [package insert]. Lake Forest: Hospira Inc; 2010.

Foult J-M, Tavolaro O, Antony I, Nitenberg A. Direct myocardial and coronary effects of enalaprilat in patients with dilated cardiomyopathy: assessment by a bilateral intracoronary infusion technique. Circulation. 1988;77:337–44.

Fruncillo RJ, Rocci ML Jr, Vlasses PH, et al. Disposition of enalapril and enalaprilat in renal insufficiency. Kidney Int. 1987;20(Suppl):S117–22.

Greenbaum R, Zucchelli P, Caspi A, et al. Comparison of pharmacokinetics of fosinoprilat with enalaprilat and lisinopril in patients with congestive heart failure and chronic renal insufficiency. Br J Clin Pharmacol. 2000;49:23–31.

Hirschl MM, Binder M, Bur A, et al. Clinical evaluation of different doses of intravenous enalaprilat in patients with hypertensive crises. Arch Intern Med. 1995;155:2217–23.

Hockings N, Ajayi AA, Reid JL. Age and the pharmacokinetics of angiotensin converting enzyme inhibitors enalapril and enalaprilat. Br J Clin Pharmacol. 1986;21:341–8.

Hornung RS, Hillis WS. The acute haemodynamic effects of intravenous enalaprilic acid (MK422) in patients with left ventricular dysfunction. Br J Clin Pharmacol. 1987;23:29–33.

Kelly JG, Doyle G, Carmody M, Glover DR, Cooper WD. Pharmacokinetics of lisinopril, enalapril and enalaprilat in renal failure: effects of hemodialysis. Br J Clin Pharmacol. 1988;26:781–6.

Kelly JG, Doyle G, Donohue J, et al. Pharmacokinetics of enalapril in normal subjects and patients with renal impairment. Br J Clin Pharmacol. 1986;21:63–9.

Le Jemtel TH, Maskin CS, Chadwick B. Effects of angiotensin converting enzyme inhibition on renal blood flow in patients with stable congestive heart failure. Am J Med Sci. 1986;292:123–7.

Matsukawa S, Suzuki H, Itaya Y, Kumagai H, Saruta T. Antihypertensive action of angiotensin-I converting enzyme inhibitors in the kidney. Clin Exp Hypertens A. 1987;9:391–4.

McNabb WR, Noormohamed FH, Brooks BA, Till AE, Lant AF. Effects of repeated doses of enalapril on renal function in man. Br J Clin Pharmacol. 1985;19:353–61.

Mirenda J, Edwards C. Prolonged hypotension by enalaprilat in a case of renal artery stenosis. Anesth Analg. 1992;75: 1017–20.

Reams GP, Lal SM, Whalen JJ, Bauer JH. Enalaprilat: an intravenous substitute for oral enalapril therapy: humoral and pharmacokinetic effects. J Clin Hypertens. 1986;3:245–53.

Toutain P-L, Lefebvre HP, Laroute V. New insights on effect of kidney insufficiency on disposition of angiotensin-converting enzyme inhibitors: case of enalapril and benazepril in dogs. J Pharmacol Exp Ther. 2000;292:1094–103.

Tunny TJ, Klemm SA, Hamlet SM, Gordon RD. Diagnosis of unilateral renovascular hypertension: comparative effect of intravenous enalaprilat and oral captopril. J Urol. 1988;140:713–5.

van Schaik BAM, Geyskes GG, Mees EJD. The effect of converting enzyme inhibition on the enhanced proximal sodium reabsorption induced by chronic diuretic treatment in patients with essential hypertension. Nephron. 1987;47:167–72.

Dosage Adjustment of Medications Eliminated by the Kidneys

Enalaprilat/Vasotec® IV	{Antihypertensive, vasodilator, angiotensin-converting enzyme (ACE)/renin inhibitor}
Usual initial dose:	0.625 mg IV
Usual maintenance dose:	1.25 mg IV every 6 h over a 5-min period
Typical maximum dose:	2.5 mg IV
Proportion eliminated unchanged:	90 %

Adjustment for Kidney Disease

FDA-approved product labeling: *Dosage adjustments for enalaprilat in hypertensive patients with renal function impairment*

CrCL (mL/min)	Enalaprilat initial dose
≥30 (or SCr <3.0 mg/dL)	1.25 mg IV every 6 h
<30 (or SCr ≥3.0 mg/dL)	0.625 mg IV; if response is inadequate, dose may be repeated in 1 h
	Additional doses of 1.25 mg IV q6h may be given
Hemodialysis	0.625 mg IV

Alternative adjustment:

GFR >50 mL/min	1.25 mg IV every 6 h over a 5-min period
GFR 10–50 mL/min	0.625–1.25 mg IV every 6 h
GFR <10 mL/min	0.312–0.625 mg IV every 6 h
Hemodialysis	0.312–0.625 mg IV every 6 h; dose after hemodialysis on dialysis days
CAPD	0.312–0.625 mg IV every 6 h
CRRT	0.625–1.25 mg IV every 6 h; titrate

Dosage Adjustment of Medications Eliminated by the Kidneys

Enoxaparin - Selected References

Aggarwal A, Whitaker DA, Rimmer JM, et al. Attenuation of platelet reactivity by enoxaparin compared with unfractionated heparin in patients undergoing haemodialysis. Nephrol Dial Transplant. 2004;19:1559–63.

Aronoff GA, Bennett WM, Berns JS, et al. Drug prescribing in renal failure: dosing guidelines for adults and children. 5th ed. Philadelphia: American College of Physicians; 2007.

Bastani B, Gonzalez E. Prolonged anti-factor Xa level in a patient with moderate renal insufficiency receiving enoxaparin [letter]. Am J Nephrol. 2002;22:403–4.

Brophy DF, Sica DA. Use of enoxaparin in patients with chronic kidney disease: safety considerations. Drug Saf. 2007;30:991–4.

Brophy DF, Martin EJ, Gehr TWB, Carr ME Jr. Enhanced anticoagulant activity of enoxaparin in patients with ESRD as measured by thrombin generation time. Am J Kidney Dis. 2004;44:270–7.

Brophy DF, Carr ME Jr, Martin EJ, Venitz J, Gehr TWB. The pharmacokinetics of enoxaparin do not correlate with its pharmacodynamics in patients receiving dialysis therapies. J Clin Pharmacol. 2006;46:887–94.

Busby LT, Weyman A, Rodgers GM. Excessive anticoagulation in patients with mild renal insufficiency receiving long-term therapeutic enoxaparin. Am J Hematol. 2001;67:54–6.

Cadroy Y, Pourrat J, Baladre M-F, et al. Delayed elimination of enoxaparin in patients with chronic renal insufficiency. Thromb Res. 1991;63:385–90

Chow SL, Zammit K, West K, Dannenhoffer MA, Lopez-Candales A. Correlation of antifactor Xa concentration with renal function in patients on enoxaparin. J Clin Pharmacol. 2003;43:586–90.

Garcés EO, Victorino JA, Thomé FS, et al. Enoxaparin versus unfractionated heparin as anticoagulant for continuous venovenous hemodialysis: a randomized open-label trial. Ren Fail. 2010;32:320–7.

Garcia DA, Baglin TP, Weitz JI, Samama MM. Parenteral anticoagulants: antithrombotic therapy and prevention of thrombosis, 9th ed: American college of chest physicians evidence-based clinical practice guidelines. Chest. 2012;141 (2 Suppl):e24–43S. doi:10.1378/chest.11-2291.

Gerlach AT, Pickworth KK, Seth SK, Tanna SB, Barnes JF. Enoxaparin and bleeding complications: a review in patients with and without renal insufficiency. Pharmacotherapy. 2000;20:771–5.

Guillet B, Simon N, Sampol JJ, et al. Pharmacokinetics of the low molecular weight heparin enoxaparin during 48 h after bolus administration as an anticoagulant in haemodialysis. Nephrol Dial Transplant. 2003;18:2348–53.

Hulot J-S, Vantelon C, Urien S, et al. Effect of renal function on the pharmacokinetics of enoxaparin and consequences on dose adjustment. Ther Drug Monit. 2004;26:305–10.

Joannidis M, Kountchev J, Rauchenzauner M, et al. Enoxaparin vs unfractionated heparin for anticoagulation during continuous veno-venous hemofiltration: a randomized controlled crossover study. Intensive Care Med. 2007;33:1571–9.

Lim W, Dentali F, Eikelboom JW, Crowther MA. Meta-analysis: Low-molecular weight heparin and bleeding in patients with severe renal insufficiency. Ann Intern Med. 2006;144:673–84.

Lovenox® injection [package insert]. Bridgewater: Sanofi-Aventis US LLC; 2011.

Naumnik B, Borawski J, Myśliwiec M. Different effects of enoxaparin and unfractionated heparin on extrinsic blood coagulation during haemodialysis: a prospective study. Nephrol Dial Transplant. 2003;18:1376–82.

Polkinghorne KR, McMahon LP, Becker GJ. Pharmacokinetic studies of dalteparin (Fragmin), enoxaparin (Clexane), and danaparoid sodium (Orgaran) in stable chronic hemodialysis patients. Am J Kidney Dis. 2002:40:990–5.

Sanderink G-JCM, Gimart CG, Ozoux M-L, Jariwala N, Shukla UA, Boutouyrie BX. Pharmacokinetics and pharmacodynamics of the prophylactic dose of enoxaparin once daily over 4 days in patients with renal impairment. Thromb Res. 2002;105:225–31.

Sonawane S, Kasbekar N, Berns JS. The safety of heparins in end-stage renal disease. Semin Dial. 2006;19:305–10.

Spinler SA, Inverso SM, Cohen M, Goodman SG, Stringer KA, Antman EM. Safety and efficacy of unfractionated heparin versus enoxaparin in patients who are obese and patients with severe renal impairment: analysis from the ESSENCE and TIMI 11B studies. Am Heart J. 2003;146:33–41.

Thorevska N, Amoateng-Adjepong Y, Sabahi R, et al. Anticoagulation in hospitalized patients with renal insufficiency: a comparison of bleeding rates with unfractionated heparin vs enoxaparin. Chest. 2004;125:856–63.

White HD, Gallo R, Cohen M, et al. The use of intravenous enoxaparin in elective percutaneous coronary intervention in patients with renal impairment: results from the SafeTy and Efficacy of Enoxaparin in PCI patients, an internationaL randomized Evaluation (STEEPLE) trial. Am Heart J. 2009;157:125–31.

Dosage Adjustment of Medications Eliminated by the Kidneys

Enoxaparin/Lovenox®   {Antithrombotic; low-molecular-weight heparin}

Usual initial dose: 30–40 mg subcutaneously (prophylaxis); 1 mg/kg subcutaneously (treatment)

Usual maintenance dose: 30 mg subcutaneously every 12 h or 40 mg subcutaneously every 24 h (prophylaxis); 1 mg/kg subcutaneously every 12 h or 1.5 mg/kg subcutaneously every 24 h (treatment)

Typical maximum dose: 120 mg subcutaneously

Proportion eliminated unchanged: 40 %

Adjustment for Kidney Disease

FDA-approved product labeling:

Enoxaparin dosage regimens for patients with severe renal function impairment (CrCL <30 mL/min)

Indication	Dosage regimen
Acute STEMI[a] in patients <75 years of age	*30-mg single IV bolus plus 1-mg/kg subcutaneous dose followed by 1 mg/kg subcutaneously once daily*
Acute STEMI in patients ≥75 years of age	*1 mg/kg subcutaneously once daily (no initial bolus)*
Prophylaxis of DVT[a], abdominal surgery, hip or knee replacement surgery, medical patients during acute illness	*30 mg subcutaneously once daily*
Treatment of acute DVT with or without PE[a], when administered in conjunction with warfarin	*1 mg/kg subcutaneously once daily*
Unstable angina/non-Q-wave MI, when coadministered with aspirin	*1 mg/kg subcutaneously once daily*

Although no dose adjustment is recommended in patients with moderate (CrCL 30–49 mL/min) and mild (CrCL 50–80 mL/min) renal function impairment, all such patients should be observed carefully for signs and symptoms of bleeding
[a]STEMI ST-elevation myocardial infarction, DVT deep vein thrombosis, PE pulmonary embolism

Alternative adjustment:

GFR >50 mL/min	*30 mg subcutaneously every 12 h or 40 mg subcutaneously every 24 h (prophylaxis) or 1 mg/kg subcutaneously every 12 h or 1.5 mg/kg subcutaneously every 24 h (treatment)*
GFR 10–50 mL/min	*15–20 mg subcutaneously every 12 h (prophylaxis) or 0.5–0.75 mg/kg subcutaneously every 12 h (treatment) (25–50 % decrease); monitor anti-Xa levels.*
GFR <10 mL/min	*15 mg subcutaneously every 12 h (prophylaxis) or 0.5 mg/kg subcutaneously every 12 h (treatment) (50 % decrease); monitor anti-Xa levels.*
Hemodialysis	*0.5 mg/kg subcutaneously every 12 h; monitor anti-Xa levels.*
CAPD	*Data not available*
CVVHD	*0.5–0.7 mg/kg IV every 12 h; monitor anti-Xa levels*

*Note: Patients presenting with STEMI with all levels of kidney function have been successfully managed with IV enoxaparin 0.5 mg/kg ×1 prior to **percutaneous coronary intervention**.*

*Due to **excessive bleeding risk** documented in clinical trials in patients with **eGFR <30 mL/min**, enoxaparin use generally should be discouraged in these individuals in favor of unfractionated heparin or parenteral direct thrombin inhibitors.*

Dosage Adjustment of Medications Eliminated by the Kidneys

Entecavir - Selected References

Baraclude® tablet and oral solution[package insert]. Princeton: Bristol-Myers Squibb Co; 2010.

Bifano M, Yan J-H, Smith RA, Zhang D, Grasela DM, LaCreta F. Absence of a pharmacokinetic interaction between entecavir and adefovir. J Clin Pharmacol. 2007;47:1327–34.

Girndt M. Viral hepatitis in elderly haemodialysis patients: current prevention and management strategies. Drugs Aging. 2008;25:823–40.

Jiménez-Pérez M, Sáez-Gómez AB, Poce LM, Lozano-Rey JM, de la Cruz-Lombardo J, Rodrigo-López JM. Efficacy and safety of entecavir and/or tenofovir for prophylaxis and treatment of hepatitis B recurrence post-liver transplant. Transplant Proc. 2010;42:3167–8.

Kamar N, Milioto O, Alric L, et al. Entecavir therapy for adefovir-resistant hepatitis B virus infection in kidney and liver allograft recipients. Transplantation. 2008;86:611–4.

Liaw Y-F, Sheen I-S, Lee C-M, et al. Tenofovir disoproxil fumarate (TDF), emtricitabine/TDF, and entecavir in patients with decompensated chronic hepatitis B liver disease. Hepatology. 2011;53:62–72.

Robinson DM, Scott LJ, Plosker GL. Entecavir: a review of its use in chronic hepatitis B. Drugs. 2006;66:1605–22.

Tse KC, Yap DYH, Tang CSO, Yung S, Chan TM. Response to adefovir or entecavir in renal allograft recipients with hepatitic flare due to lamivudine-resistant hepatitis B. Clin Transplant. 2010;24:207–12.

Wiegand J, Karlas T, Schiefke I, et al. Resistance management in chronic hepatitis B complicated by renal failure. Clin Nephrol. 2010;74:53–8.

Yan J-H, Bifano M, Olsen S, et al. Entecavir pharmacokinetics, safety, and tolerability after multiple ascending doses in healthy adults. J Clin Pharmacol. 2006;46:1250–8.

Yanxiao C, Ruijuan X, Jin Y, et al. Organic anion and cation transporters are possibly involved in renal excretion of entecavir in rats. Life Sci. 2011. Epub ahead of print. doi:10.1016/j.lfs.2011.03.018.

Yoshitsugu H, Sakurai T, Ishikawa H, et al. Pooled model-based approach to compare the pharmacokinetics of entecavir between Japanese and non-Japanese chronic hepatitis B patients. Diagn Microbiol Infect Dis. 2011;70:91–100.

Zhu M, Bifano M, Xu X, et al. Lack of an effect of human immunodeficiency virus coinfection on pharmacokinetics of entecavir in hepatitis B virus-infected patients. Antimicrob Agents Chemother. 2008;52:2836–41.

Zoutendijk R, Reijnders JGP, Brown A, et al. Entecavir treatment for chronic hepatitis B: adaptation is not needed for the majority of naïve patients with partial virological response. Hepatology. 2011. Epub ahead of print. doi:10.1002/hep.24406.

Dosage Adjustment of Medications Eliminated by the Kidneys

Entecavir/Baraclude®   {Antiviral; ℞ for chronic hepatitis B}

Usual initial dose:	0.5 mg orally
Usual maintenance dose:	0.5–1 mg orally once daily
Typical maximum dose:	1 mg
Proportion eliminated unchanged:	65 %

Adjustment for Kidney Disease

FDA-approved product labeling: *Entecavir oral dosage for adult patients with renal function impairment*

CrCL (mL/min)	Usual dose (nucleoside naïve)	Lamivudine-refractory or decompensated liver disease
≥50	0.5 mg once daily	1 mg once daily
30 to <50	0.25 mg once daily[b] or 0.5 mg every 48 h	0.5 mg once daily or 1 mg every 48 h
10 to <30	0.15 mg once daily[b] or 0.5 mg every 72 h	0.3 mg once daily[b] or 1 mg every 72 h
<10; hemodialysis[a] or CAPD	0.05 mg once daily[b] or 0.5 mg every 7 days	0.1 mg once daily[b] or 1 mg every 7 days

[a]Administer after hemodialysis on dialysis days
[b]Oral solution is recommended for doses <0.5 mg

Alternative adjustment: *Entecavir oral dosage adapted to renal function*

GFR (mL/min)	Naïve patients	Lamivudine-resistant patients
>50	0.5 mg/day	1 mg/day
30–49	0.25 mg/day[b] or 0.5 mg every 48 h	0.5 mg/ day
10–29	0.15 mg/day[b] or 0.5 mg every 72 h	0.3 mg/ day[b] or 0.5 mg every 48 h
Hemodialysis[a]	0.05 mg/day[b] or 0.5 mg every 5–7 days	0.1 mg/ day[b] or 0.5 mg every 72 h

[a]Administer after hemodialysis on dialysis days
[b]Oral solution is recommended for doses <0.5 mg

Dosage Adjustment of Medications Eliminated by the Kidneys

Eplerenone - Selected References

Black HR. Evolving role of aldosterone blockers alone and in combination with angiotensin-converting enzyme inhibitors of angiotensin II receptor blockers n hypertension management: a review of mechanistic and clinical data. Am Heart J. 2004;147:564–72.

Cook CS, Berry LM, Bible RH, Hribar JD, Hajdu E, Liu NW. Pharmacokinetics and metabolism of [^{14}C] eplerenone after oral administration to humans. Drug Metab Dispos. 2003;31:1448–55.

Davis KL, Nappi JM. The cardiovascular effects of eplerenone, a selective aldosterone antagonist. Clin Ther. 2003;25: 2647–68.

Inspra™ tablet [package insert]. New York: GD Searle LLC subsidiary of Pfizer Inc; 2003, 2011.

Levy DG, Rocha R, Funder JW. Distinguishing the antihypertensive and electrolyte effects of eplerenone. J Clin Endocrinol Metab. 2004;89:2736–40.

Pitt B. Aldosterone blockade in patients with systolic left ventricular dysfunction. Circulation. 2003;108:1790–4.

Pitt B, Reichek N, Willenbrock R, et al. Effects of eplerenone, enalapril, and eplerenone/enalapril in patients with essential hypertension and left ventricular hypertrophy: the 4E-left ventricular hypertrophy study. Circulation. 2003;108:1831–8.

Pitt B, Remme W, Zannad F, et al. Eplerenone, a selective aldosterone blocker, in patients with left ventricular dysfunction after myocardial infarction. N Engl J Med. 2003;348:309–21.

White WB, Carr AA, Krause S, et al. Assessment of the novel selective aldosterone blocker eplerenone using ambulatory and clinical blood pressure in patients with systemic hypertension. Am J Cardiol. 2003;92:38–42.

White WB, Duprez D, St Hillaire R, et al. Effects of the selective aldosterone blocker eplerenone versus the calcium antagonist amlodipine in systolic hypertension. Hypertension. 2003;41:1021–6.

Zannad F, McMurray JJV, Krum H, et al (the EMPHASIS-HF Study Group). Eplerenone in patients with systolic heart failure and mild symptoms. N Engl J Med. 2011;364:11–21.

Dosage Adjustment of Medications Eliminated by the Kidneys

Eplerenone/Inspra™   **{Selective aldosterone receptor antagonist; renin inhibitor}**

Usual initial dose:	25 mg orally
Usual maintenance dose:	25–50 mg orally once daily
Typical maximum dose:	100 mg/day
Proportion eliminated unchanged:	7 % (~65 % as metabolites)

Adjustment for Kidney Disease

FDA-approved product labeling:	*CrCL <30 mL/min or SCr >2.0 mg/dL in males or SCr >1.8 mg/dL in females*	*Contraindicated*
Alternative adjustment:	*Data not available*	

Dosage Adjustment of Medications Eliminated by the Kidneys

Eptifibatide - Selected References

Alexander KP, Chen AY, Newby LK, et al. Sex differences in major bleeding with glycoprotein IIb/IIIa inhibitors: results from the CRUSADE (Can Rapid Risk Stratification of Unstable Angina Patients Suppress Adverse Outcomes with Early Implementation of the ACC/AHA Guidelines) initiative. Circulation. 2006;114:1380–7.

Alton KB, Kosoglou T, Baker S, Affrime MB, Cayen MN, Patrick JE. Disposition of ^{14}C-eptifibatide after intravenous administration to healthy men. Clin Ther. 1998;20:307–23.

Anderson JR, Riding D. Glycoprotein IIb/IIIa inhibitors in patients with renal insufficiency undergoing percutaneous coronary intervention. Cardiol Rev. 2008;16:213–8.

Begeiz AG, Dery J-P, Tsiatis AA, et al. Optimal duration of eptifibatide infusion in percutaneous coronary intervention (an ESPRIT substudy). Am J Cardiol. 2004;94:926–9.

Curran MP, Keating GM. Eptifibatide: a review of its use in patients with acute coronary syndromes and/or undergoing percutaneous coronary intervention. Drugs. 2006;65:2009–35.

Donovan JL, Schroeder WS, Tran MT, et al. Assessment of eptifibatide dosing in renal impairment before and after in-service education provided by pharmacists. J Manag Care Pharm. 2007;13:598–605.

Eikelboom JW, Hirsch J, Spencer FA, Baglin TP, Weitz JI. Antiplatelet drugs: antithrombotic therapy and prevention of thrombosis, 9th ed: American College of Chest Physicians Evidence-Based Practice Guidelines. Chest. 2012;141(2 Suppl): e89–119S. doi:10.1378/chest.11.2293.

Gilchrist IC. Platelet glycoprotein IIb/IIIa inhibitors in percutaneous coronary intervention: focus on the pharmacokinetic-pharmacodynamic relationships of eptifibatide. Clin Pharmacokinet. 2003;42:703–20.

Gilchrist IC, O'Shea JC, Kosoglou T, et al. Pharmacodynamics and pharmacokinetics of higher-dose, double-bolus eptifibatide in percutaneous coronary intervention. Circulation. 2001;104:406–11.

Gretler DD. Pharmacokinetic and pharmacodynamic properties of eptifibatide in healthy subjects receiving unfractionated heparin or the low-molecular-weight heparin enoxaparin. Clin Ther. 2003;25:2564–74.

Gretler DD, Guerciolini R, Williams PJ. Pharmacokinetic and pharmacodynamic properties of eptifibatide in subjects with normal and impaired renal function. Clin Ther. 2004;26:390–8.

Harder S, Klinkhardt U, Alvarez JM. Avoidance of bleeding during surgery in patients receiving anticoagulant and/or antiplatelet therapy: pharmacokinetic and pharmacodynamic considerations. Clin Pharmacokinet. 2004;43:963–81.

Hudson JQ, McNeely EB, Green CA, Jennings LK. Assessment of eptifibatide clearance by hemodialysis using an in vitro system. Blood Purif. 2010;30:266–71.

Integrilin® injection [package insert]. Whitehouse Station: Merck & Co, Inc; 2011.

Rasty S, Borzak S, Tisdale JE. Bleeding associated with eptifibatide targeting higher risk patients with acute coronary syndromes: incidence and multivariate risk factors. J Clin Pharmacol. 2002;42:1366–73.

Reddan DN, O'Shea JC, Sarembock IJ, et al. Treatment effects of eptifibatide in planned coronary stent implantation in patients with chronic kidney disease (ESPRIT Trial). Am J Cardiol. 2003;91:17–21.

Sperling RT, Pinto DS, Ho KKL, Carrozza JP Jr. Platelet glycoprotein IIb/IIIa inhibitors with eptifibatide: prolongation of inhibition of aggregation in acute renal failure and reversal with hemodialysis. Catheter Cardiovasc Interv. 2003;59: 459–62.

Tardiff BE, Jennings LK, Harrington RA, et al. Pharmacodynamics and pharmacokinetics of eptifibatide in patients with acute coronary syndromes: prospective analysis from PURSUIT. Circulation. 2001;104:399–405.

Tcheng JE, Talley JD, O'Shea JC, et al. Clinical pharmacology of higher dose eptifibatide in percutaneous coronary intervention (the PRIDE Study). Am J Cardiol. 2001;88:1097–1102.

Tsai TT, Maddox TM, Roe MT, et al. Contraindicated medication use in dialysis patients undergoing percutaneous coronary intervention. JAMA. 2009;302:2458–64.

Dosage Adjustment of Medications Eliminated by the Kidneys

<u>**Eptifibatide**</u>**/Integrilin®** {Platelet aggregation inhibitor; glycoprotein IIb/IIIa antagonist}

Usual initial dose:	180 mcg IV over 1–2 min repeated ×1 10 min after the initial dose
Usual maintenance dose:	2 mcg/kg/min continuous IV infusion
Typical maximum dose:	15 mg/h
Proportion eliminated unchanged:	50 %

Adjustment for Kidney Disease

FDA-approved product labeling: *Acute coronary syndrome*

CrCL ≥50 mL/min — *180 mcg/kg IV followed by continuous infusion of 2 mcg/kg/min until hospital discharge or initiation of coronary bypass surgery, up to 72 h. If the patient undergoes percutaneous coronary intervention while receiving eptifibatide, the infusion should be continued up to hospital discharge (max 96 h) or for up to 18–24 h after the procedure, whichever comes first.*

CrCL <50 mL/min — *180 mcg/kg IV as soon as possible following diagnosis, immediately followed by continuous infusion of 1 mcg/kg/min*

Hemodialysis — *Contraindicated*

Percutaneous coronary intervention

CrCL ≥50 mL/min — *180 mcg/kg IV immediately before initiation of PCI followed by continuous infusion of 2 mcg/kg/min and a second 180 mcg/kg IV bolus 10 min after the first. Infusion should be continued until hospital discharge or for up to 18–24 h, whichever comes first.*

CrCL <50 mL/min — *180 mcg/kg IV administered immediately before initiation of PCI followed by continuous infusion of 1 mcg/kg/min and a second 180 mcg/kg IV bolus 10 min after the first*

Hemodialysis — *Contraindicated*

Alternative adjustment: *Data not available*

Dosage Adjustment of Medications Eliminated by the Kidneys

Eribulin - Selected References

Arnold SM, Moon J, Williamson, et al. Phase II evaluation of eribulin mesylate (E7389, NSC 707389) in patients with metastatic or recurrent squamous cell carcinoma of the head and neck: Southwest Oncology Group trial S0618. Invest New Drugs. 2011;29:352–9.

Cigler T, Vahdat LT. Eribulin mesylate for the treatment of breast cancer. Expert Opin Pharmcother. 2010;11:1587–93.

Cortes J, O'Shaughnessy J, Loesch D, et al. Eribulin monotherapy versus treatment of physician's choice in patients with metastatic breast cancer (EMBRACE): a phase 3 open-label randomised study. Lancet. 2011;377:914–23.

Cortes J, Vahdat L, Blum JL, et al. Phase II study of the halichondrin B analog eribulin mesylate in patients with locally advanced or metastatic breast cancer previously treated with an anthracycline, a taxane, and capecitabine. J Clin Oncol. 2010;3922–8.

Goel S, Mita AC, Mita M, et al. A phase I study of eribulin mesylate (E7389), a mechanistically novel inhibitor of microtubule dynamics, in patients with advanced solid malignancies. Clin Cancer Res. 2009;15:4207–12.

Halaven™ injection [package insert]. Woodcliff Lake: Esai Inc; 2010.

Huyck TK, Gradishar W, Manuguid F, Kirkpatrick P. Eribulin mesylate. Nat Rev Drug Discov. 2011;10:173–4.

Jordan MA, Kamath K, Manna T, et al. The primary antimitotic mechanism of action of the synthetic halichondrin E7389 is suppression of microtubule growth. Mol Cancer Ther. 2005;4:1086–95.

Smith JA, Wilson L, Azarenko O, et al. Eribulin binds at microtubule ends to a single site on tubulin to suppress dynamic instability. Biochemistry. 2010;49:1331–7.

Tan A, Rubin EH, Walton DC, et al. Phase I study of eribulin mesylate administered once every 21 days in patients with advanced solid tumors. Clin Cancer Res. 2009;15:4213–9.

Towle MJ, Salvato KA, Wels BF, et al. Eribulin induces irreversible mitotic blockade: implications of cell-based pharmacodynamics for in vivo efficacy under intermittent dosing conditions. Cancer Res. 2011;71:496–505.

Vahdat LT, Pruitt B, Fabian CJ, et al. Phase II study of eribulin mesylate, a halichondrin B analog, in patients with metastatic breast cancer previously treated with an anthracycline and a taxane. J Clin Oncol. 2009;27:2954–61.

Dosage Adjustment of Medications Eliminated by the Kidneys

Eribulin/Halaven™   {**Antineoplastic; tubulin-based antimitotic; ℞ for refractory metastatic breast cancer**}

Usual initial dose:	1.4 mg/m^2 IV over 2–5 min
Usual maintenance dose:	1.4 mg/m^2 IV over 2–5 min on days 1 and 8 of a 21-day cycle for a minimum of four cycles
Typical maximum dose:	1.4 mg/m^2/dose
Proportion eliminated unchanged:	7 %

Adjustment for Kidney Disease

FDA-approved product labeling:	*Cr CL >50 mL/min*	*1.4 mg/m^2 IV over 2–5 min on days 1 and 8 of a 21-day cycle*
	CrCL 30–50 mL/min	*1.1 mg/m^2 IV over 2–5 min on days 1 and 8 of a 21-day cycle*
	CrCL <30 mL/min	*Not recommended (no data)*
Alternative adjustment:	*Data not available*	

Dosage Adjustment of Medications Eliminated by the Kidneys

Ertapenem - Selected References

Breilh D, Fleureau C, Gordien J-B, et al. Pharmacokinetics of free ertapenem in critically ill septic patients: intermittent versus continuous infusion. Minerva Anestesiol. 2011;77:1–2.

Brink AJ, Richards GA, Schillack V, Kiem S, Schentag J. Pharmacokinetics of once-daily dosing of ertapenem in critically ill patients with severe sepsis. Int J Antimicrob Agents. 2009;33:432–6.

Burkhardt O, Hafer C, Langhoff A, et al. Pharmacokinetics of ertapenem in critically ill patients with acute renal failure undergoing extended daily dialysis. Nephrol Dial Transplant. 2009;24:267–71.

Burkhardt O, Kumar V, Katterwe D, et al. Ertapenem in critically ill patients with early-onset ventilator-associated pneumonia: pharmacokinetics with special consideration of free-drug concentration. J Antimicrob Chemother. 2007;59:277–84.

Burkhardt O, Kumar V, Schmidt S, Kielstein JT, Welte T, Deredorf H. Underdosing of ertapenem in critically ill patients with pneumonia confirmed by Monte Carlo simulations [letter]. Int J Antimicrob Agents. 2010;35:96–7.

Chen M, Nafziger AN, Drusano GL, Ma L, Bertino JS Jr. Comparative pharmacokinetics and pharmacodynamic target attainment of ertapenem in normal-weight, obese, and extremely obese adults. Antimicrob Agents Chemother. 2006;50: 1222–7.

Fica AE, Abusada NJ. Seizures associated with ertapenem use in patients with CNS disorders and renal insufficiency. Scand J Infect Dis. 2008;40:983–5.

Frasc D, Marchand S, Petitpas F, Dahyot-Fizelier C, Couet W, Mimoz O. Pharmacokinetics of ertapenem following intravenous and subcutaneous infusions in patients. Antimicrob Agents Chemother. 2010;54:924–6.

Invanz® injection [package insert]. Whitehouse Station: Merck & Co, Inc; 2010.

Keating GM, Perry CM. Ertapenem: a review of its use in the treatment of bacterial infections. Drugs. 2005;65:2151–78.

Kim A, Kuti JL, Nicolau DP. Probability of pharmacodynamic target attainment with standard and prolonged-infusion antibiotic regimens for empiric therapy in adults with hospital-acquired pneumonia. Clin Ther. 2009;31:2765–78.

Majumdar AK, Musson DG, Birk KL, et al. Pharmacokinetics of ertapenem in healthy young volunteers. Antimicrob Agents Chemother. 2002;46:3506–11.

Mistry GC, Majumdar AK, Swan S, et al. Pharmacokinetics of ertapenem in patients with varying degrees of renal insufficiency and in patients on hemodialysis. J Clin Pharmacol. 2006;46:1128–38,

Musson DG, Majumdar A, Holland S, et al. Pharmacokinetics of total and unbound ertapenem in healthy elderly subjects. Antimicrob Agents Chemother. 2004;48:521–4.

Nix DE, Majumdar AK, DiNubile MJ. Pharmacokinetics and pharmacodynamics of ertapenem: an overview for clinicians. J Antimicrob Chemother. 2004;53(Suppl 2):ii23–8.

Seto AH, Song JC, Guest SS. Ertapenem-associated seizures in a peritoneal dialysis patient. Ann Pharmacother. 2005;39: 352–6.

Stevenson JM, Patel JH, Churchwell MD, et al. Ertapenem clearance during modeled continuous renal replacement therapy. Int J Artif Organs. 2008;31:1027–34.

Wong BK, Xu X, Yu S, et al. Comparative disposition of [^{14}C]ertapenem, a novel carbapenem antibiotic in rat, monkey and man. Xenobiotica. 2004;34:379–89.

Dosage Adjustment of Medications Eliminated by the Kidneys

Ertapenem/Invanz®   {Antibacterial; carbapenem}

Usual initial dose: 1 g IM or IV

Usual maintenance dose: 1 g IM or IV once daily

Typical maximum dose: 1 g/day

Proportion eliminated unchanged: 40 %

Adjustment for Kidney Disease

FDA-approved product labeling:	*CrCL >30 mL/min*	*1 g IV daily*
	CrCL ≤30 mL/min	*500 mg IV daily*
	Hemodialysis	*500 mg IV daily; no supplemental dose is necessary if the daily doses are given within 6 h before dialysis; if given >6 h prior to dialysis, give supplemental dose of 150 mg IV.*
Alternative adjustment:	*GFR >50 mL/min*	*1 g IM or IV every 24 h or 1 g IV followed by continuous IV infusion of 1 g/24 h*
	GFR 10–50 mL/min	*1 g IM or IV every 24 h*
	GFR <10 mL/min	*500 mg IV every 24 h*
	Extended daily dialysis	*1 g IV every 24 h*
	Hemodialysis	*500 mg IV every 24 h; administer supplemental 150 mg IV after hemodialysis on dialysis days.*
	CAPD	*500 mg IM or IV every 24 h*
	CRRT	*1 g IV every 24 h*

Dosage Adjustment of Medications Eliminated by the Kidneys

Ethacrynic Acid - Selected References

Auger RG, Dayton DA, Harrison CE Jr, Tucker RM, Anderson CF. Use of ethacrynic acid in mannitol-resistant oliguric renal failure. JAMA. 1968;206:891–3.

Birtch AG, Zakheim RM, Jones LG, Barger AC. Redistribution of renal blood flow produced by furosemide and ethacrynic acid. Circ Res. 1967;21:869–78.

Bojs G, Lundvall O. Effects of ethacrynic acid on renal function in man. Acta Med Scand. 1966;179:95–100.

Brater DC. Use of diuretics in chronic renal failure and nephrotic syndrome. Semin Nephrol. 1988;8:333–41.

Cannon PJ, Kilcoyne MM. Ethacrynic acid and furosemide: renal pharmacology and clinical use. Prog Cardiovasc Dis. 1969;12:99–118.

Cannon PJ, Heinemann HO, Stason WB, Laragh JH. Ethacrynic acid: effectiveness and mode of diuretic action in man. Circulation. 1965;31:5–18.

Cooperman LB, Rubin IL. Toxicity of ethacrynic acid and furosemide. Am Heart J. 1973;85:831–4.

Earley LE, Friedler RM. Renal tubular effects of ethacrynic acid. J Clin Invest. 1964;43:1495–506.

Edecrin® tablet and Edecrin® sodium injection [package insert]. Whitehouse Station: Merck & Co; 2006.

Edwards KDG, Sinnett PF, Stewart JH. Ethacrynic acid: assessment of saluretic and diuretic potency in patients with severe chronic renal failure. Med J Aust. 1967;1:375–81.

Eide I, Løyning E, Langård Ø, Kiil F. Influence of ethacrynic acid on intrarenal renin release mechanism. Kidney Int. 1975;8:158–65.

Goldberg M, McCurdy DK, Foltz EL, Bluemle LW Jr. Effects of ethacrynic acid (a new saluretic agent) on renal diluting and concentrating mechanisms: evidence for site of action in the Loop of Henle. J Clin Invest. 1964;43:201–16.

Gussin RZ, Cafruny EJ. Renal sites of action of ethacrynic acid. J Pharmacol Exp Ther. 1965;153:148–58.

Hagedorn CW, Kaplan AA, Hulet WH. Prolonged administration of ethacrynic acid in patients with chronic renal disease. N Engl J Med. 1965;272:1152–5.

Hook JB, Blatt AH, Brody MJ, Williamson HE. Effects of several saluretic-diuretic agents on renal hemodynamics. J Pharmacol Exp Ther. 1965;154:667–73.

Hunt JC, Maher FT. Diuretic drugs in patients with impaired renal function. Am J Cardiol. 1966;17:642–7.

Kleeman CR, Okun R, Heller RJ. The renal regulation of sodium and potassium in patients with chronic renal failure (CRF) and the effect of diuretics on the excretion of these ions. Ann N Y Acad Sci. 1966;139:520–39.

Komorn RM, Cafruny EJ. Ethacrynic acid: diuretic property coupled to reaction with sulfhydryl groups in renal cells. Science. 1964;143:133–4.

Lowenthal DT, Dickerman D. The use of diuretics in varying degrees of renal impairment: an overview. Clin Exp Hypertens A. 1983;5:297–307.

Mathog RH, Thomas WG, Hudson WR. Ototoxicity of new and potent diuretics. Arch Otolaryngol Head Neck Surg. 1970;92:7–13.

Matz GJ, Naunton RF. Ototoxic drugs and poor renal function [letter]. JAMA. 1968;206:2119.

Pillay VKG, Schwartz FD, Aimi K, Kark RM. Transient and permanent deafness following treatment with ethacrynic acid in renal failure. Lancet. 1969;1:77–9.

Sloane D, Jick H, Lewis GP, Shapiro S, Miettinen OS. Intravenously given ethacrynic acid gastrointestinal bleeding: a finding resulting from comprehensive drug surveillance. JAMA. 1969;209:1668–71.

Swan SK. Diuretic strategies in patients with renal failure. Drugs. 1994;48:380–5.

Uwai Y, Saito H, Hashimoto Y, Inui K-I. Interaction of thiazide diuretics, loop diuretics, and acetazolamide via rat renal organic anion transporter rOAT1. J Pharmacol Exp Ther. 2000;295:261–5.

Ethacrynic Acid;
Ethacrynate Sodium / Edecrin®   {Diuretic, loop/high ceiling}

Usual initial dose:	25–50 mg orally or 50 mg (0.5–1 mg/kg) IV
Usual maintenance dose:	50 mg once daily after meals to 50–100 mg twice daily after meals orally
	0.5–1 mg/kg IV; dose may be repeated once/24 h if necessary.
Typical maximum dose:	400 mg/day orally or 200 mg/day IV
Proportion eliminated unchanged:	20 %

Adjustment for Kidney Disease

FDA-approved product labeling:	*Anuria or severe progressive renal disease*	*Contraindicated*
Alternative adjustment:	*GFR >50 mL/min*	*50–200 mg/day*
	GFR 10–50 mL/min	*50–200 mg/day*
	GFR <10 mL/min	*Preferably avoid due to risk for gastrointestinal toxicity and ototoxicity*
	Hemodialysis	*Data not available*
	CAPD	*Data not available*
	CRRT	*Data not available*

Dosage Adjustment of Medications Eliminated by the Kidneys

Ethambutol - Selected References

Alffenaar J-W, van der Werf T. Dosing ethambutol in obese patients [letter]. Antimicrob Agents Chemother. 2010;54:4044–5.

Andrew OT, Schoenfeld PY, Hopewell PC, Humphreys MH. Tuberculosis in patients with end-stage renal disease. Am J Med. 1980;68:59–65.

Aronoff GA, Bennett WM, Berns JS, et al. Drug prescribing in renal failure: dosing guidelines for adults and children. 5th ed. Philadelphia: American College of Physicians; 2007.

Chaisson RE, Keiser P, Pierce M, et al. Clarithromycin and ethambutol with or without clofazimine for the treatment of bacteremic *Mycobacterium avium* complex disease in patients with HIV infection. AIDS. 1997;11:311–7.

Christopher TG, Blair AD, Forrey AW, Cutler RE. Hemodialyzer clearances of gentamicin, kanamycin, tobramycin, amikacin, ethambutol, procainamide, and flucytosine, with a technique for planning therapy. J Pharmacokinet Biopharm. 1976;4:427–41.

Deshpande D, Srivastava S, Meek C, Leff R, Gumbo T. Ethambutol optimal clinical dose and susceptibility breakpoint identification by use of a novel pharmacokinetic-pharmacodynamic model of disseminated *Mycobacterium avium*. Antimicrob Agents Chemother. 2010;54:1728–33.

Ethambutol hydrochloride tablet [package insert]. Pomona: Barr Laboratories Inc; 2008.

Gumbo T. New susceptibility breakpoints for first-line antituberculosis drugs based on antimicrobial pharmacokinetic/pharmacodynamic science and population pharmacokinetic variability. Antimicrob Agents Chemother. 2010;54:1481–91.

Gursu M, Tayfur F, Besler M, et al. Tuberculosis in peritoneal dialysis patients in an endemic region. Adv Perit Dial. 2011;27:48–52.

Israili AH, Rogers CM, El-Attar H. Pharmacokinetics of antituberculosis drugs in patients. J Clin Pharmacol. 1987;27:78–83.

Lee CS, Brater DC, Gambertoglio JG, Benet LZ. Disposition kinetics of ethambutol in man. J Pharmacokinet Biopharm. 1980;8:335–46.

Lee CS, Marbury TC, Benet LZ. Clearance calculations in hemodialysis: application to blood, plasma, and dialysate measurements for ethambutol. J Pharmacokinet Biopharm. 1980;8:69–81.

Malone RS, Fish DN, Spiegel DM, Childs JM, Peloquin CA. The effect of hemodialysis on isoniazid, rifampin, pyrazinamide, and ethambutol. Am J Respir Crit Care Med. 1999;159:1580–4.

Peloquin CA, Bulpitt AE, Jaresko GS, Jelliffe RW, Childs JM, Nix DE. Pharmacokinetics of ethambutol under fasting conditions, with food, and with antacids. Antimicrob Agents Chemother. 1999;43:568–72.

Ruslami R, Nijland HMJ, Adhiarta IGN, et al. Pharmacokinetics of antituberculosis drugs in pulmonary tuberculosis patients with type 2 diabetes. Antimicrob Agents Chemother. 2010;54:1068–74.

Sadun AA, Wang MY. Ethambutol optic neuropathy: how we can prevent 100,000 new cases of blindness each year. J Neuroophthalmol. 2008;28:265–8.

Srivastava S, Musuka S, Sherman C Meek C, Leff R, Gumbo T. Efflux-pump derived multiple drug resistance to ethambutol monotherapy in *Mycobacterium tuberculosis* and ethambutol pharmacokinetics-pharmacodynamics. J Infect Dis. 2010;201:1225–31.

Talbert Estlin KA, Sadun AA. Risk factors for ethambutol optic toxicity. Int Ophthalmol. 2010;30:63–72.

Varughese A, Brater DC, Benet LZ, Lee CS. Ethambutol kinetics in patients with impaired renal function. Am Rev Respir Dis. 1986;134:34–8.

Zhu M, Burman WJ, Starke JR, et al. Pharmacokinetics of ethambutol in children and adults with tuberculosis. Int J Tuberc Lung Dis. 2004;8:1360–7.

Dosage Adjustment of Medications Eliminated by the Kidneys

Ethambutol/Myambutol®   {**Antitubercular; metabolite synthesis inhibitor**}

Usual initial dose: 15 mg/kg orally

Usual maintenance dose: 15 mg/kg orally once daily

Typical maximum dose: 25 mg/kg/day

Proportion eliminated unchanged: 50 %

Adjustment for Kidney Disease

> **FDA-approved product labeling:**   *Patients with decreased renal function need the dosage reduced as determined by serum levels of ethambutol, since the main path of excretion of this drug is by the kidneys.*

> **Alternative adjustment:**

GFR >50 mL/min	*15–25 mg/kg orally every 24 h*
GFR 10–50 mL/min	*15 mg/kg orally every 24–36 h or 10 mg/kg orally every 24 h*
GFR <10 mL/min	*15 mg/kg orally every 48 h or 7 mg/kg orally every 24 h*
Hemodialysis	*15–25 mg/kg orally every 48 h; after hemodialysis on dialysis days*
CAPD	*15 mg/kg orally every 48 h*
CRRT	*15–25 mg/kg enterally every 24–36 h*

Dosage Adjustment of Medications Eliminated by the Kidneys

Ethionamide - Selected References

Abramowicz M, Zuccotti G, Pflomm J-M, et al., editors. Handbook of antimicrobial therapy. 19th ed. New Rochelle: The Medical Letter; 2011.

Amsden GW. Tables of antimicrobial agent pharmacology. In: Mandell GL, Bennett JE, Dolin R, editors. Mandell, Douglas, and Bennett's principles and practice of infectious diseases, vol. 1. 6th ed. Philadelphia: Elsevier; 2005. p. 634–700.

Aronoff GA, Bennett WM, Berns JS, et al. Drug prescribing in renal failure: dosing guidelines for adults and children. 5th ed. Philadelphia: American College of Physicians; 2007.

Auclair B, Nix DE, Adam RD, James GT, Peloquin CA. Pharmacokinetics of ethionamide administered under fasting conditions or with orange juice, food, or antacids. Antimicrob Agents Chemother. 2001;45:810–14.

Baulard AR, Betts JC, Engohang-Ndong J, et al. Activation of the pro-drug ethionamide is regulated in mycobacteria. J Biol Chem. 2000;275:28326–31.

Conte JE Jr, Golden JA, McQuitty M, Kipps J, Lin ET, Zurlinden E. Effect of AIDS and gender on steady-state plasma and intrapulmonary ethionamide concentrations. Antimicrob Agents Chemother. 2000;44:1337–41.

Gilbert DN, Moellering RC Jr, Eliopoulos GM, Chambers HF, Saag MS. The sanford guide to antimicrobial therapy. 41st ed. Sperryville: Antimicrobial Therapy Inc; 2011.

Henderson MC, Siddens LK, Morré JT, Krueger SK, Williams DE. Metabolism of the anti-tuberculosis drug ethionamide by mouse and human FMO1, FMO2 and FMO3 and mouse and human lung microsomes. Toxicol Appl Pharmacol. 2008;233:420–7.

Holdiness MR. Clinical pharmacokinetics of the antituberculosis drugs. Clin Pharmacokinet. 1984;9:511–44.

Jenner PJ, Ellard GA, Gruer PJK, Aber VR. A comparison of the blood levels and urinary excretion of ethionamide and prothionamide in man. J Antimicrob Chemother. 1984;13:267–77.

Malone RS, Fish DN, Spiegel DM, Childs JM, Peloquin CA. The effect of hemodialysis on cycloserine, ethionamide, para-aminosalicylate, and clofazimine. Chest. 1999;116:984–90.

McIntyre CW, Owen PJ. Prescribing drugs in kidney disease. In: Brenner BM, editor. Brenner & Rector's the kidney. 8th ed. Philadelphia: Saunders Elsevier; 2008. p. 1930–55.

Trecator® tablet film coated [package insert]. Philadelphia: Wyeth Pharmaceuticals Division of Pfizer Inc; 2007.

Zhu M, Namdar R, Stambaugh JJ, Starke Jr, Bulpitt AE, Berning SE, Peloquin CA. Population pharmacokinetics of ethionamide in patients with tuberculosis. Tuberculosis (Edinb). 2002:82:91–6.

Dosage Adjustment of Medications Eliminated by the Kidneys

<u>**Ethionamide**</u>/Trecator®   {**Antitubercular; peptide synthesis inhibitor**}

Usual initial dose:	250 mg orally
Usual maintenance dose:	500–1,000 mg/day (15–20 mg/kg/day) orally in three to four divided doses
Typical maximum dose:	1,000 mg/day
Proportion eliminated unchanged:	1 %

Adjustment for Kidney Disease

FDA-approved product labeling:	*Data not available*	
Alternative adjustment:	*GFR >50 mL/min*	*500–1,000 mg/day (15–20 mg/kg/day) orally with or without food in two to four divided doses*
	GFR 10–50 mL/min	*500–1,000 mg/day (15–20 mg/kg/day) orally with or without food in two to four divided doses*
	GFR <10 mL/min	*250–500 mg/day (5–10 mg/kg/day) orally with or without food in two to three divided doses*
	Hemodialysis	*250–500 mg orally twice daily with or without food, after hemodialysis on dialysis days*
	CAPD	*250–500 mg/day (5–10 mg/kg/day) orally with or without food in two to three divided doses*
	CRRT	*500–1,000 mg/day (15–20 mg/kg/day) orally with or without food in two to four divided doses*

Etodolac - Selected References

Aronoff GA, Bennett WM, Berns JS, et al. Drug prescribing in renal failure: dosing guidelines for adults and children. 5th ed. Philadelphia: American College of Physicians; 2007.

Benet LZ. Pharmacokinetic profile of etodolac in special populations. Eur J Rheumatol Inflamm. 1994;14(1):15–8.

Brater DC. Evaluation of etodolac in subjects with renal impairment. Eur J Rheumatol Inflamm. 1990;10(1):44–55.

Brater DC, Anderson SA, Brown-Cartwright D, Toto RD, Chen A, Jacob GB. Effect of etodolac in patients with moderate renal impairment compared with normal subjects. Clin Pharmacol Ther. 1985;38:674–9.

Brater DC, Anderson SA, Brown-Cartwright D, Toto RD. Effects of nonsteroidal antiinflammatory drugs on renal function in patients with renal insufficiency and in cirrhotics. Am J Kidney Dis. 1986;8:351–5.

Brater DC, Brown-Cartwright D, Anderson SA, Uaamnuichai M. Effect of high-dose etodolac on renal function. Clin Pharmacol Ther. 1987;42:283–9.

Brocks DR, Jamali F. Etodolac clinical pharmacokinetics. Clin Pharmacokinet. 1994;26:259–74.

Etodolac tablet [package insert]. Hawthorne: Taro Pharmaceuticals USA Inc; 2010.

Kraml M, Hicks DR, McKean M, Panagides J, Furst D. The pharmacokinetics of etodolac in serum and synovial fluid of patients with arthritis. Clin Pharmacol Ther. 1988;43:571–6.

Lee A, Cooper MG, Craig JC, Knight JF, Keneally JP. Effects of nonsteroidal anti-inflammatory drugs on postoperative renal function in adults with normal renal function (review). Cochrane Database Syst Rev. 2007;(2):CD002765. doi: 10.1002/14651858.CD002765.pub3.

McIntyre CW, Owen PJ. Prescribing drugs in kidney disease. In: Brenner BM, editor. Brenner & Rector's the kidney. 8th ed. Philadelphia: Saunders Elsevier; 2008. p. 1930–55.

Neustad DH. Double blind evaluation of the long-term effects of etodolac versus ibuprofen in patients with rheumatoid arthritis. J Rheumatol Suppl. 1997;47:17–22.

Ogiso T, Kitagawa T, Iwaki M, Tanino T. Pharmacokinetic analysis of enterohepatic circulation of etodolac and effect of hepatic and renal injury on the pharmacokinetics. Biol Pharm Bull. 1997;20:405–10.

Shand DG, Epstein C, Kinberg-Calhoun J, Mullane JF, Sanda M. The role of etodolac administration on renal function in patients with arthritis. J Clin Pharmacol. 1986;25:269–74.

Sugimoto T, Aoyama M, Kikuchi K, et al. Membranous nephropathy associated with the relatively selective cyclooxygenase-2 inhibitor, etodolac, in a patient with early rheumatoid arthritis. Intern Med. 2007;46:1055–8.

Svendsen KB, Bech JN, Sørensen, Pedersen EB. A comparison of the effects of etodolac and ibuprofen on renal haemodynamics, tubular function, renin, vasopressin and urinary excretion of albumin and α-glutathione-s-transferase in healthy subjects: a placebo-controlled cross-over study. Eur J Clin Pharmacol. 2000;56:383–8.

Dosage Adjustment of Medications Eliminated by the Kidneys

Etodolac/Lodine® {**Anti-inflammatory; nonsteroidal anti-inflammatory drug**}

Usual initial dose: 200–400 mg orally

Usual maintenance dose: 200–400 mg orally every 6–8 h as needed for pain; 300–500 mg twice daily

Typical maximum dose: 1,200 mg/day

Proportion eliminated unchanged: 1 %

Adjustment for Kidney Disease

FDA-approved product labeling:	*Mild to moderate renal insufficiency (CrCL 37–88 mL/min)*	*No dose adjustment necessary*
	Advanced renal disease	*Use not recommended*
Alternative adjustment:	*GFR >50 mL/min*	*200–400 mg orally every 6–8 h as needed for pain or 300–500 mg orally twice daily*
	GFR 10–50 mL/min	*200–400 mg orally every 6–8 h as needed for pain or 300–500 mg orally twice daily*
	GFR <10 mL/min	*200 mg orally every 6–8 h as needed for pain or 200–300 mg orally twice daily*
	Hemodialysis	*200 mg orally every 6–8 h as needed for pain or 200–300 mg orally twice daily*
	CAPD	*Data not available*
	CRRT	*Not applicable; preferably avoid due to risk for gastrointestinal and/or renal toxicity*

Dosage Adjustment of Medications Eliminated by the Kidneys

Etoposide (VP-16) - Selected References

Aisner J, Van Echo DA, Whitacre M, Wiernik PH. A phase I trial of continuous VP16-213 (etoposide). Cancer Chemother Pharmacol. 1982;7:157–60.

Arbuck SG, Douglass HO, Craom WR, et al. Etoposide pharmacokinetics in patients with normal and abnormal organ function. J Clin Oncol. 1986;4:1690–5.

Aronoff GA, Bennett WM, Berns JS, et al. Drug prescribing in renal failure: dosing guidelines for adults and children. 5th ed. Philadelphia: American College of Physicians; 2007.

Canal P, Chatelut E, Guichard S. Practical treatment guide for dose individualization in cancer chemotherapy. Drugs. 1998;56:1019–38.

D'Incalci M, Rossi C, Zucchetti M, et al. Pharmacokinetics of etoposide in patients with abnormal renal and hepatic function. Cancer Res. 1986;46:2566–71.

English MW, Lowis SP, Peng B, et al. Pharmacokinetically guided dosing of carboplatin and etoposide during peritoneal dialysis and haemodialysis. Br J Cancer. 1996;73:776–80.

Gerritsen-van Schieveen P, Royer B. Level of evidence for therapeutic drug monitoring for etoposide after oral administration. Fundam Clin Pharmacol. 2011;25:277–82.

Hande KR, Wedlund PJ, Noone RM, Wilkinson GR, Greco FA, Wolff SN. Pharmacokinetics of high-dose etoposide (VP-16-213) administered to cancer patients. Cancer Res. 1984;44:379–82.

Holthuis JJM, Van de Vyver FL, van Oort WJ, Verieun H, Bekaert AB, De Broe ME. Pharmacokinetic evaluation of increasing doses of etoposide in a chronic hemodialysis patient. Cancer Treat Rep. 1985;69:2179–82.

Joel SP, Shah R, Slevin ML. Etoposide dosage and pharmacodynamics. Cancer Chemother Pharmacol.1994;34(Suppl): S69–75.

Li YF, Fu S, Hu W, et al. Systemic anticancer therapy in gynecological cancer patients with renal dysfunction. Int J Gynecol Cancer. 2007;17:739–63.

McIntyre CW, Owen PJ. Prescribing drugs in kidney disease. In: Brenner BM, editor. Brenner & Rector's the kidney. 8th ed. Philadelphia: Saunders Elsevier; 2008. p. 1930–55.

Newman EM, Doroshow JH, Forman SJ, Blume KG. Pharmacokinetics of high-dose etoposide. Clin Pharmacol Ther. 1988;43:561–4.

Nguyen L, Chatelut E, Chevreau C, et al. Population pharmacokinetics of total and unbound etoposide. Cancer Chemother Pharmacol. 1998;41:125–32.

Pelsor FR, Allen LM, Creaven PJ. Multicompartment pharmacokinetic model of 4'-demethylepipodophyllotoxin 9-(4,6-O-ethylidene-β-D-glucopyranoside) in humans. J Pharm Sci. 1978;67:1106–8.

Pflüger K-H, Hahn M, Holz J-B, et al. Pharmacokinetics of etoposide: correlation of pharmacokinetic parameters with clinical conditions. Cancer Chemother Pharmacol. 1993;31:350–6.

Ratain MJ, Mick R, Schilsky RL Vogelzang NJ, Berezin F. Pharmacologically based dosing of etoposide: a means of safely increasing dose intensity. J Clin Oncol. 1991;9:1480–6.

Schacter LP, Igwemezie LN, Seyedsadr M, et al. Clinical and pharmacokinetic overview of parenteral etoposide phosphate. Cancer Chemother Pharmacol. 1994;34(Suppl):S58–63.

Slevin M. The clinical pharmacology of etoposide. Cancer. 1991;67:319–29.

Takezawa K, Okamoto I, Fukuoka M, Nakagawa K. Pharmacokinetic analysis of carboplatin and etoposide in a small cell lung cancer patient undergoing hemodialysis. J Thorac Oncol. 2008;3:1073–5.

Toposar™ injection [package insert]. Irvine: Teva Parenteral Medicines Inc; 2010.

Wood JM, Brogden RN. Etoposide: a review of its pharmacodynamic and pharmacokinetic properties, and therapeutic potential in combination chemotherapy of cancer. Drugs. 1990;39:438–90.

You B, Tranchand B, Girard P, et al. Etoposide pharmacokinetics and survival in patients with small cell lung cancer: a multicentre study. Lung Cancer. 2008;62:261–72.

Dosage Adjustment of Medications Eliminated by the Kidneys

Etoposide (VP-16)/Toposar™	{Antineoplastic; podophyllotoxin derivative; antimitotic}

Usual initial dose:	35–100 mg/m² IV
Usual maintenance dose:	50–100 mg/m²/day IV on days 1–5 to 100 mg/m²/day IV on days 1, 3, and 5 (testicular cancer); 35 mg/m²/day for 4 days to 50 mg/m²/day for 5 days (small cell lung cancer). Courses are repeated at 3- to 4-week intervals after adequate recovery from any toxicity.
Typical maximum dose:	100 mg/m²
Proportion eliminated unchanged:	45 %

Adjustment for Kidney Disease

FDA-approved product labeling:	*CrCL >50 mL/min*	*35–100 mg/m² IV according to cancer type or protocol schedule*
	CrCL 15–50 mL/min	*26.25–75 mg/m² IV according to cancer type or protocol (75 % of usual dose)*
	CrCL <15 mL/min	*No data; further dose reduction should be considered.*
Alternative adjustment:	*GFR >50 mL/min*	*35–100 mg/m² IV according to cancer type or protocol schedule*
	GFR 30–50 mL/min	*26.25–75 mg/m² IV according to cancer type or protocol (75 % of usual dose)*
	GFR 10–29 mL/min	*26.25–75 mg/m² IV according to cancer type or protocol (75 % of usual dose)*
	GFR <10 mL/min	*17.5–50 mg/m² IV according to cancer type or protocol (50 % of usual dose)*
	Hemodialysis	*17.5–50 mg/m² IV according to cancer type or protocol (50 % of usual dose)*
	CAPD	*17.5–50 mg/m² IV according to cancer type or protocol (50 % of usual dose)*
	CRRT	*26.25–75 mg/m² IV according to cancer type or protocol (75 % of usual dose)*

Note: Hematological, organ function, and other considerations may suggest further dose adjustments; monitoring drug levels is considered potentially useful, especially in patients with severe renal impairment.

Dosage Adjustment of Medications Eliminated by the Kidneys

Exenatide - Selected References

Byetta® injection [package insert]. San Diego: Amylin Pharmaceuticals Inc; 2010.

Calara F, Taylor K, Han J, et al. A randomized, open-label, crossover study examining the effect of injection site on bioavailability of exenatide (synthetic exendin-4). Clin Ther. 2005;27:210–5.

Copley K, McCowen K, Hiles R, Nielsen LL, Young A, Parkes DG. Investigation of exenatide elimination and its in vivo and in vitro degradation. Curr Drug Metab. 2006;7:367–74.

Cvetković RS, Plosker GL. Exenatide: a review of its use in patients with type 2 diabetes mellitus (as an adjunct to metformin and/or a sulfonylurea). Drugs. 2007;67:935–54.

Drucker DJ, Buse JB, Taylor K, et al. Exenatide once weekly versus twice daily for the treatment of type 2 diabetes: a randomised, open-label, non-inferiority study. Lancet. 2008;372:1240–50.

Ferrer-Garcia JC, Martinez-Chanza N, Tolosa-Torréns M, Sánchez-Juan C. Exenatide and renal failure [letter]. Diabet Med. 2010;27:728–9.

Gedulin BR, Smith PA, Jodka CM, et al. Pharmacokinetics and pharmacodynamics of exenatide following alternate routes of administration. Int J Pharm. 2008;356:231–8.

Iwamoto K, Nasu R, Yamamura A, et al. Safety, tolerability, pharmacokinetics, and pharmacodynamics of exenatide once weekly in Japanese patients with type 2 diabetes. Endocr J. 2009;56:951–62.

Johansen OE, Whitfield R. Exenatide may aggravate moderate diabetic renal impairment: a case report [letter]. Br J Clin Pharmacol. 2008;66:568–9.

Kolterman OG, Buse JB, Fineman MS, et al. Synthetic esendin-4 (exenatide) significantly reduces postprandial and fasting plasma glucose in subjects with type 2 diabetes. J Clin Endocrinol Metab. 2003;88:3082–9.

Kothare PA, Linnebjerg H, Isaka Y, et al. Pharmacokinetics, pharmacodynamics, tolerability, and safety of exenatide in Japanese patients with type 2 diabetes mellitus. J Clin Pharmacol. 2008;48:1389–99.

Linnebjerg H, Kothare PA, Park S, et al. Effect of renal impairment on the pharmacokinetics of exenatide. Br J Clin Pharmacol. 2007;64:317–27.

Linnebjerg H, Kothare PA, Seger M, Wolka AM, Mitchell MI. Exenatide—pharmacokinetics, pharmacodynamics, safety and tolerability in patients ≥75 years of age with type 2 diabetes. Int J Clin Pharmacol Ther. 2011;49:99–108.

López-Ruiz A, del Peso-Gilsanz C, Meoro-Avilés A, et al. Acute renal failure when exenatide is co-administered with diuretics and angiotensin II blockers. Pharm World Sci. 2010;32:559–61.

Neumiller JJ. Clinical pharmacology of incretin therapies for type 2 diabetes mellitus: implications for treatment. Clin Ther. 2011;33:528–76.

Neumiller JJ, Setter SM. Pharmacologic management of the older patient with type 2 diabetes mellitus. Am J Geriatr Pharmacother. 2008;7:324–42.

Ratner R, Han J, Nicewarner D, Yushmanova I, Hoogwerf BJ, Shen L. Cardiovascular safety of exenatide BID: an integrated analysis from controlled clinical trials in participants with type 2 diabetes. Cardiovasc Diabetol. 2011;10:22. doi:10.1186/1475-2840-10-22.

Watson E, Jonker DM, Jacobsen LV, Ingwersen SH. Population pharmacokinetics of liraglutide, a once-daily human glucagon-like peptide-1 analog, in healthy volunteers and subjects with type 2 diabetes, and comparison to twice-daily exenatide. J Clin Pharmacol. 2010;50:886–94.

Weise WJ, Sivanandy MS, Block CA, Comi RJ. Exenatide-associated ischemic renal failure [letter]. Diabetes Care. 2009;32:e22–3.

Dosage Adjustment of Medications Eliminated by the Kidneys

Exenatide/Byetta®, Bydureon®
Extended-Release Suspension   {Antidiabetic; incretin mimetic; glucagon-like peptide (GLP)-1 agonist}

Usual initial dose: 5 mcg subcutaneously or 2 mg extended-release subcutaneously

Usual maintenance Dose: 5 mcg subcutaneously twice daily or 2 mg extended-release subcutaneously once every 7 days

Typical maximum dose: 10 mcg subcutaneously twice daily or 2 mg extended-release subcutaneously once every 7 days

Proportion eliminated unchanged: The kidney appears to be the primary route of elimination and degradation.

Adjustment for Kidney Disease

FDA-approved product labeling:	*CrCL 30–50 mL/min*	*Caution should be applied when initiating treatment or when escalating doses of prompt exenatide from 5 to 10 mcg in patients with moderate renal impairment.*
	CrCL <30 mL/min	*Avoid; prompt or extended-release injection should not be used in patients with severe renal impairment or end-stage renal disease receiving dialysis due to gastrointestinal side effects and intolerance.*
	Renal transplantation	*Use with caution; exenatide may induce nausea and vomiting with transient hypovolemia, and treatment may worsen renal function.*
Alternative adjustment:	*eCrCL <30 mL/min*	*Preferably avoid. As compared with subjects with normal renal function, patients with end-stage renal disease requiring hemodialysis displayed exenatide clearance that was reduced by 84 % and concurrent areas under the plasma concentration-time curve (AUC) that were increased more than 6-fold. Following exenatide administration, most experienced severe nausea and vomiting and some developed headache, tachycardia, and transient increases in systolic and diastolic blood pressure not associated with hypoglycemia. Extended-release exenatide has not been studied in patients with CrCL <30 mL/min, although in patients with moderate renal impairment, exenatide exposure was increased by 62 %.*

F

L.K. Golightly et al. (eds.), *Renal Pharmacotherapy*,
DOI 10.1007/978-1-4614-5800-5_6, © Springer Science+Business Media New York 2013

Famciclovir - Selected References

Famvir® tablet [package insert]. East Hanover: Novartis Pharmaceuticals Corp; 2011.

Filer CW, Allen GD, Brown GD, Brown TA, et al. Metabolic and pharmacokinetic studies following oral administration of ^{14}C-famciclovir to healthy subjects. Xenobiotica. 1994;24:357–68.

Gill KS, Wood MJ. The clinical pharmacokinetics of famciclovir. Clin Pharmacokinet. 1996;31:1–8.

Htwe TH, Bergman S, Koirala J. Famciclovir substitution for patients with acyclovir-associated renal toxicity. J Infect. 2008;57:266–8.

Mubareka S, Leung V, Aoki FY, Vinh DC. Famciclovir: a focus on efficacy and safety. Expert Opin Drug Saf. 2010;9:643–58.

Pue MA, Pratt SK, Fairless AJ, et al. Linear pharmacokinetics of penciclovir following administration of single oral doses of famciclovir 125, 250, 500 and 750 mg to healthy volunteers. J Antimicrob Chemother. 1994;33:119–27.

Simpson D, Lyseng-Williamson KA. Famciclovir: a review of its use in Herpes zoster and genital and orolabial herpes. Drugs. 2006;66:2397–416.

Dosage Adjustment of Medications Eliminated by the Kidneys

Famciclovir/Famvir® {Antiviral; penciclovir prodrug; nucleoside analog; viral DNA polymerase inhibr}

Usual initial dose:	1,500 mg orally
Usual maintenance dose:	500 mg orally every 8–12 h
Typical maximum dose:	1,000 mg orally twice daily
Proportion eliminated unchanged:	60 % (as penciclovir)

Adjustment for Kidney Disease

FDA-approved product labeling:

Famciclovir dosage recommendations for adult patients with renal impairment

Indication and normal dosage regimen	CrCL (mL/min)	Adjusted dosage (mg)	Dosing interval
Single-day dosing regimens			
Recurrent genital herpes 1,000 mg every 12 h for 1 day	≥60	1,000	Every 12 h for 1 day
	40–59	500	Every 12 h for 1 day
	20–39	500	Single dose
	<20	250	Single dose
	Hemodialysis	250	Single dose following dialysis
Recurrent herpes labialis 1,500 mg single dose	≥60	1,500	Single dose
	40–59	750	Single dose
	20–39	500	Single dose
	<20	250	Single dose
	Hemodialysis	250	Single dose following dialysis
Multiple-day dosing regimens			
Herpes zoster 500 mg every 8 h	≥60	500	Every 8 h
	40–59	500	Every 12 h
	20–39	500	Every 24 h
	<20	250	Every 24 h
	Hemodialysis	250	Following each dialysis
Suppression of recurrent genital herpes 250 mg every 12 h	≥40	250	Every 12 h
	20–39	125	Every 12 h
	<20	125	Every 24 h
	Hemodialysis	125	Following each dialysis
Recurrent orolabial or genital herpes in HIV-infected patients 500 mg every 12 h	≥40	500	Every 12 h
	20–39	500	Every 24 h
	<20	250	Every 24 h
	Hemodialysis	250	Following each dialysis

Alternative adjustment:	CRRT	*Not applicable (consider IV ganciclovir)*

Dosage Adjustment of Medications Eliminated by the Kidneys

Famotidine (Oral) - Selected References

Aronoff GA, Bennett WM, Berns JS, et al. Drug prescribing in renal failure: dosing guidelines for adults and children. 5th ed. Philadelphia: American College of Physicians; 2007.

Chremos AN. Clinical pharmacology of famotidine: a summary. J Clin Gastroenterol. 1987;9(Suppl 2):7–12.

Echizen H, Ishizaki T, Clinical pharmacokinetics of famotidine. Clin Pharmacokinet. 1991;21:178–94.

Gitlin N. Famotidine once-a-day in the management of duodenal ulcer: the US placebo-controlled experience. J Clin Gastroenterol. 1987;9(Suppl 2):13.

Hachisu T, Yokoyama T, Oda Y, Ando K, Hattori Y, Yoshida T. Optimal therapeutic regimen of famotidine based on plasma concentrations in patients with chronic renal failure. Clin Ther. 1988;10:656–63.

Heiselman DE, Hulisz DT, Fricker R, Bredle DL, Black LD. Randomized comparison of gastric pH control with intermittent and continuous infusion of famotidine in ICU patients. Am J Gastroenterol. 1995;90:277–9.

Henann NE, Carpenter DU, Janda SM. Famotidine-associated mental confusion in elderly patients. Drug Intell Clin Pharm. 1988;22:976–8.

Inotsume N, Nishimura M, Fujiyama S, et al. Pharmacokinetics of famotidine in elderly patients with and without renal insufficiency and in healthy young volunteers. Eur J Clin Pharmacol. 1989;36:517–20.

Kirch W, Halabi A, Linde M, Santos SR, Ohnhaus EE. Negative effects of famotidine on cardiac performance assessed by noninvasive hemodynamic measurements. Gastroenterology. 1989;96:1388–92.

Kroemer H, Klotz U. Pharmacokinetics of famotidine in man. Int J Clin Pharmacol Ther Toxicol. 1987;25:458–63.

Lin JH, Chremos AN, Kanovsky SM, Schwartz S, Yeh KC, Kann J. Effects of antacids and food on absorption of famotidine. Br J Clin Pharmacol. 1987;24:551–3.

Matsunaga C, Izumi S, Furukubo T, et al. Effect of famotidine and lansoprazole on serum phosphorus levels in hemodialysis patients on calcium carbonate therapy. Clin Nephrol. 2007;68:93–8.

McIntyre CW, Owen PJ. Prescribing drugs in kidney disease. In: Brenner BM, editor. Brenner & Rector's the kidney. 8th ed. Philadelphia: Saunders Elsevier; 2008. p. 930–55.

Odeh M, Oliven A. Central nervous system reactions associated with famotidine: report of five cases. J Clin Gastroenterol. 1998;27:253–4.

Olyaei AJ, Bennett WM. Pharmacologic approach to renal insufficiency. In: Dale DC, Federman DD, Antman K, editors. ACP medicine, WebMD June 2007 update. Hamilton: BC Decker; 2007; NEPHROLOGY IX: Appendix A1–25.

Olyaei AJ, Bennett WM. Drug dosing in elderly patients with chronic kidney disease. Clin Geriatr Med. 2009;25:459–527.

Olyaei AJ, DeMattos AM, Bennett WM. Use of drugs in patients with renal failure. In: Schrier RW, editor. Diseases of the kidney and urinary tract. 8th ed. Philadelphia: Lippincott Williams & Wilkins; 2007. p. 2765–807.

Pepcid® tablet film coated [package insert]. Whitehouse Station; Merck & Co Inc; 2010.

Porro GB, Dicenta C, Cook T, Humphries TJ. Review of an extensive worldwide study of a new H_2-receptor antagonist, famotidine, as compared to ranitidine in the treatment of acute duodenal ulcer. J Clin Gastroenterol. 1987;9(Suppl 2):14–8.

Redmond AM, Pentapaty N, Weibel J, Nolan SF, Hudson JQ, Self T. Use of famotidine in adult patients with end-stage renal disease: assessment of dosing and mental status changes. Am J Med Sci. 2005;330:8–10.

Simon B, Müller P, Dammann H-G. Famotidine once-a-day in the therapy of acute, benign gastric ulcer: a worldwide experience. J Clin Gastroenterol. 1987;9(Suppl 2):19–22.

Dosage Adjustment of Medications Eliminated by the Kidneys

<u>Famotidine (Oral)</u>/Pepcid®	{Antacid; histamine H$_2$ receptor antagonist}

Usual initial dose:	40 mg orally
Usual maintenance dose:	40 mg orally once daily at bedtime or 20 mg twice daily
Typical maximum dose:	Up to 160 mg orally every 6 h
Proportion eliminated unchanged:	40 %

Adjustment for Kidney Disease

FDA-approved product labeling:	*CrCL <50 mL/min*	*20 mg orally daily at bedtime or 40 mg orally every 36–48 h*
Alternative adjustment:	*GFR >50 mL/min*	*20 mg orally at bedtime or 10 mg orally twice daily*
	GFR 10–50 mL/min	*10–20 mg orally at bedtime*
	GFR <10 mL/min	*5–10 mg orally at bedtime*
	Hemodialysis	*10 mg orally at bedtime (after dialysis) or 20 mg orally three times weekly immediately after dialysis*
	CAPD	*5–10 mg orally at bedtime*
	CRRT	*10–20 mg enterally once daily in the evening*

Famotidine (IV) - Selected References

Abraham PA, Opsahl JA, Halstenson CE, Chremos AN, Matzke GR, Keane WF. The effect of famotidine on renal function in patients with renal insufficiency. Br J Clin Pharmacol. 1987;24:385–9.

Aronoff GA, Bennett WM, Berns JS, et al. Drug prescribing in renal failure: dosing guidelines for adults and children. 5th ed. Philadelphia: American College of Physicians; 2007.

Chremos AN. Clinical pharmacology of famotidine: a summary. J Clin Gastroenterol. 1987;9(Suppl 2):7–12.

Echizen H, Ishizaki T. Clinical pharmacokinetics of famotidine. Clin Pharmacokinet. 1991;21:178–94.

Fish DN. Safety and cost of rapid i.v. injection of famotidine in critically ill patients. Am J Health Syst Pharm. 1995;52:1889–94.

Gladziwa U, Klotz U, Krishna DR, Schmitt H, Glöckner WM, Mann H. Pharmacokinetics and dynamics of famotidine in patients with renal failure. Br J Clin Pharmacol. 1988;26:315–21.

Halstenson CE, Abraham PA, Opsahl JA, Chremos AN, Keane WF, Matzke FR. Disposition of famotidine in renal insufficiency. J Clin Pharmacol. 1987;27:782–7.

Kroemer H, Klotz U. Pharmacokinetics of famotidine in man. Int J Clin Pharmacol Ther Toxicol. 1987;25:458–63.

Lin JH, Chremos AN, Yeh KC, Antonello J, Hessey GA II. Effects of age and chronic renal failure on the urinary excretion kinetics of famotidine in man. Eur J Clin Pharmacol. 1988;34:41–6.

Pepcid® injection [package insert]. Whitehouse Station; Merck & Co Inc; 2006.

Saima S, Echizen H, Yoshimoto K, Ishizaki T. Hemofiltrability of H_2-receptor antagonist, famotidine, in renal failure patients. J Clin Pharmacol. 1990;30:159–62.

Takabatake T, Ohta H, Maekawa M, et al. Pharmacokinetics of famotidine, a new H_2-receptor antagonist, in relation to renal function. Eur J Clin Pharmacol. 1985;28:327–31.

Dosage Adjustment of Medications Eliminated by the Kidneys

<u>Famotidine (IV)</u>/Pepcid® IV   {Antacid; histamine H_2 receptor antagonist}

Usual initial dose:	20 mg IV
Usual maintenance dose:	20 mg IV every 12 h
Typical maximum dose:	40 mg/day
Proportion eliminated unchanged:	70 %

Adjustment for Kidney Disease

FDA-approved product labeling:	*CrCL <50 mL/min*	*10 mg IV every 12 h or 20 mg every 36–48 h*
Alternative adjustment:	*GFR >50 mL/min*	*20 mg IV every 12 h or 20 mg IV followed by continuous IV infusion of 1.66 mg/h (40 mg/24 h)*
	GFR 10–50 mL/min	*10 mg IV every 12 h*
	GFR <10 mL/min	*10 mg IV every 24 h*
	Hemodialysis	*10 mg IV every 24 h (after dialysis)*
	CAPD	*10 mg IV every 24 h*
	CRRT	*10 mg IV every 12 h*

Dosage Adjustment of Medications Eliminated by the Kidneys

Felbamate - Selected References

Aronoff GA, Bennett WM, Berns JS, et al. Drug prescribing in renal failure: dosing guidelines for adults and children. 5th ed. Philadelphia: American College of Physicians; 2007.

Banfield CR, Zhu G-RR, Jen JF, et al. The effect of age on the apparent clearance of felbamate: a retrospective analysis using nonlinear mixed-effects modeling. Ther Drug Monit. 1996;18:19–29.

Bourgeois B, Leppik IE, Sackellares JC, et al. Felbamate: a double-blind controlled trial in patients undergoing presurgical evaluation of partial seizures. Neurology. 1993;693–6.

Faught E, Sachdeo RC, Remler MP, et al. Felbamate monotherapy for partial-onset seizures: an active-control trial. Neurology. 1993;43:688–92.

Felbatol® [package insert]. Somerset: MEDA Pharmaceuticals; 2008.

Gareri P, Gravina T, Ferreri G, de Sarro G. Treatment of epilepsy in the elderly. Prog Neurobiol. 1999;58:389–407.

Graves NM. Felbamate. Ann Pharmacother. 1993;27:1073–81.

Graves NM, Ludden TM, Holmes GB, Fuerst RH, Leppik IE. Pharmacokinetics of felbamate, a novel antiepileptic drug: application of mixed-effect modeling to clinical trials. Pharmacotherapy. 1989;9:372–6.

Lacerda G, Krummel T, Sabourdy C, Ryvlin P, Hirsch E. Optimizing therapy of seizures in patients with renal or hepatic dysfunction. Neurology. 2006;67(Suppl 4):S28–33.

Leppik IE, Dreifus FE, Pledger GW, et al. Felbamate for partial seizures: results of a controlled clinical trial. Neurology. 1991;41:1785–9.

Olyaei AJ, Bennett WM. Pharmacologic approach to renal insufficiency. In: Dale DC, Federman DD, Antman K, editors. ACP medicine, WebMD June 2007 update. Hamilton: BC Decker; 2007; NEPHROLOGY IX: Appendix A1–25.

Olyaei AJ, Bennett WM. Drug dosing in elderly patients with chronic kidney disease. Clin Geriatr Med. 2009;25:459–527.

Olyaei AJ, DeMattos AM, Bennett WM. Use of drugs in patients with renal failure. In: Schrier RW, editor. Diseases of the kidney and urinary tract. 8th ed. Philadelphia: Lippincott Williams & Wilkins; 2007. p. 2765–807.

Palmer KJ, McTavish D. Felbamate: a review of its pharmacodynamic and pharmacokinetic properties, and therapeutic efficacy in epilepsy. Drugs. 1993;1041–65.

Perucca E. The clinical pharmacokinetics of the new antiepileptic drugs. Epilepsia. 1999;40(Suppl 9):S7–13.

Rengstorff DS, Milstone AP, Seger DL, Meredith TJ. Felbamate overdose complicated by massive crystalluria and acute renal failure. J Toxicol Clin Toxicol. 2000;38:667–9.

Sachdeo R, Kramer ALD, Rosenberg A, Sachdeo S. Felbamate monotherapy: controlled trial in patients with partial onset seizures. Ann Neurol. 1992;32:386–92.

Theodore WH, Raubertas RF, Porter RJ, et al. Felbamate: a clinical trial for complex partial seizures. Epilepsia. 1991;32:392–7.

Walker MC, Patsalos PN. Clinical pharmacokinetics of new antiepileptic drugs. Pharmacol Ther. 1995;67:351–84.

Wilensky AJ, Friel PN, Ojemann LM, Kupferberg HJ, Levy RH. Pharmacokinetics of W0554 (ADD 03055) in epileptic patients. Epilepsia. 1985;26:602–6.

Dosage Adjustment of Medications Eliminated by the Kidneys

<u>Felbamate</u>/Felbatol®   {**Antiepileptic; N-methyl-D-aspartate (NMDA) antagonist**}

Usual initial dose:	1,200 mg/day orally in three or four divided doses
Usual maintenance dose:	1,200–3,600 mg/day orally in three or four divided doses
Typical maximum dose:	3,600 mg/day
Proportion eliminated unchanged:	25 %

Adjustment for Kidney Disease

FDA-approved product labeling:	*Renal dysfunction*	*Starting and maintenance doses should be reduced by one-half.*
Alternative adjustment:	*GFR >50 mL/min*	*1,200–3,600 mg/day orally in three or four divided doses*
	GFR 10–50 mL/min	*800–2,400 mg/day orally in three or four divided doses (25–50 % dose reduction)*
	GFR <10 mL/min	*600–1,800 mg/day orally in three or four divided doses (50 % dose reduction)*
	Hemodialysis	*600–1,800 mg/day orally in three or four divided doses (50 % dose reduction, dose after dialysis)*
	CAPD	*600–1,800 mg/day orally in three or four divided doses (50 % dose reduction)*
	CRRT	*600–1,800 mg/day enterally in three or four divided doses (50 % dose reduction)*

Fenofibrate - Selected References

Alves de Sousa A, Kronit HS, de Assis Rocha Neves F, Amato AA. Fenofibrate-induced rhabdomyolysis in a patient with chronic kidney disease: an unusual presenting feature of hypothyroidism. Arq Bras Endocrinol Metabol. 2009;53:383–6.

Balfour JA, McTavish D, Heel RC. Fenofibrate: a review of its pharmacodynamic and pharmacokinetic properties and therapeutic use in dyslipidaemia. Drugs. 1990;40:260–90.

Bruno CB, Schaqpiro JM, Saberi P, An increase in serum creatinine after initiation of fenofibrate in an HIV-infected individual: a case report and review of the literature. J Int Assoc Physicians AIDS Care (Chic). 2011. Epub ahead of print. doi:10.1177/1545109711404945.

Chapman MJ. Pharmacology of fenofibrate. Am J Med. 1987;83(Suppl 5B):21–5.

Davidson MH, Armani A, McKenney JM, Jacobson TA. Safety considerations with fibrate therapy. Am J Cardiol. 2007;99(Suppl):3C–18C.

Ireland JH, Eggert CH, Arendt CJ, Williams AW. Rhabdomyolysis with cardiac involvement and acute renal failure in a patient taking rosuvastatin and fenofibrate [letter]. Ann Intern Med. 2005;142:949–50.

Lipscombe J, Lewis GF, Cattran D, Bargman JM. Deterioration in renal function associated with fibrate therapy. Clin Nephrol. 2001;55:39–44.

Miller DB, Spence JD. Clinical pharmacokinetics of fibric acid derivatives (fibrates). Clin Pharmacokinet. 1998;34:155–62.

Tricor® tablet [package insert]. North Chicago: Abbott Laboratories; 2010.

Unal A, Torun E, Sipahioglu MH, et al. Fenofibrate-induced acute renal failure due to massive rhabdomyolysis after coadministration of statin in two patients. Intern Med. 2008;47:1017–9.

Üsküdar Cansu D, Yaşar NS, Korkmaz C. Acute renal failure due to fenofibrate monotherapy. Anadolu Kardiyol Derg. 2011;11:368–7.

Weil A, Caldwell J, Strolin-Benedetti M. The metabolism and disposition of ^{14}C-fenofibrate in human volunteers. Drug Metab Dispos. 1990;18:115–20.

Dosage Adjustment of Medications Eliminated by the Kidneys

<u>Fenofibrate</u>/TriCor®   {**Antihypercholesterolemic; fibric acid derivative; peroxisome proliferator-activated receptor-α activator**}

Usual initial dose: 48–145 mg orally

Usual maintenance dose: 145 mg orally once daily

Typical maximum dose: 145 mg/day

Proportion eliminated unchanged: 60 % (as metabolites fenofibric acid and fenofibrate glucuronide)

Adjustment for Kidney Disease

    FDA-approved product labeling: *Mild to moderate renal impairment (CrCL 30–80 mL/min)*   *48 mg orally once daily; increase only after evaluation of the effects on renal function and lipid levels at this dose.*

        Severe renal dysfunction (CrCL ≤30 mL/min)   *Contraindicated*

    Alternative adjustment: *Data not available*

Dosage Adjustment of Medications Eliminated by the Kidneys

Fenoprofen - Selected References

Aronoff GA, Bennett WM, Berns JS, et al. Drug prescribing in renal failure: dosing guidelines for adults and children. 5th ed. Philadelphia: American College of Physicians; 2007.

Artinano M, Etheridge WB, Stroehlein KB, Barcenas CG. Progression of minimal-change glomerulopathy to focal glomerulosclerosis in a patient with fenoprofen nephropathy. Am J Nephrol. 1986;6:353–7.

Brezin JH, Katz SM, Schwartz AB, Chinitz JL. Reversible renal failure and nephrotic syndrome associated with nonsteroidal anti-inflammatory drugs. N Engl J Med. 1979;301:1271–3.

Carmichael J, Shankel SW. Effects of nonsteroidal anti-inflammatory drugs on prostaglandins and renal function. Am J Med. 1985;78:992–1000.

Caruana RJ, Semble EL. Renal papillary necrosis due to naproxen. J Rheumatol. 1984;11:90–1.

Curt GA, Kaldany A, Whitley LG, et al. Reversible rapidly progressive renal failure with nephrotic syndrome due to fenoprofen calcium [letter]. Ann Intern Med. 1980;62:72–3.

Finkelstein A, Fraley DS, Stachura I, Feldman HA, Gandy DR, Bourke E. Fenoprofen nephropathy: lipoid nephrosis and interstitial nephritis. A possible T-lymphocyte disorder. Am J Med. 1982;72:81–7.

Handy SP. Renal effects of fenoprofen [letter]. Ann Intern Med. 1980;93:508–9.

Handa SP. Drug-induced acute interstitial nephritis: report of 10 cases. CMAJ. 1986;135:1278–81.

Hayball PJ, Meffin PJ. Enantioselective disposition of 2-arylpropionic acid nonsteroidal anti-inflammatory drugs. III. Fenoprofen disposition. J Pharmacol Exp Ther. 1987;240:631–6.

Husserl FE, Lange RK, Kantrow CM Jr. Renal papillary necrosis and pyelonephritis accompanying fenoprofen therapy. JAMA. 1979;242:1896–8.

Lorch J, Lefavour G, Davidson H, Cortell S. Renal effects of fenoprofen [letter]. Ann Intern Med. 1980;93:509.

Nalfon® [package insert]. East Brunswick: Pedinol Pharmacal Inc; 2009.

Nash JF, Bechtol LD, Bunde CA, Bopp RJ, Farid KZ, Spradlin CT. Linear pharmacokinetics of orally administered fenoprofen calcium. J Pharm Sci. 1979;68:1086–90.

Poggi JC, Barissa GR, Donadi EA, et al. Pharmacodynamics, chiral pharmacokinetics, and pharmacokinetic-pharmacodynamic modeling of fenoprofen in patients with diabetes mellitus. J Clin Pharmacol. 2006;46:1328–36.

Radford MG, Holley KE, Grande JP, et al. Reversible membranous nephropathy associated with the use of nonsteroidal anti-inflammatory drugs. JAMA. 1996;276:466–9.

Rubin A, Rodda BE, Warrick P, Ridolfo AS, Gruber CM Jr. Physiological disposition of fenoprofen in man. II: plasma and urine pharmacokinetics after oral and intravenous administration. J Pharm Sci. 1972;61:739–45.

Stachura I, Jayakumar S, Bourke E. T and B lymphocyte subsets in fenoprofen nephropathy. Am J Med. 1983;75:9–16.

Thomsen BS, From A, Jacobsen IA, Starklint H, Pedersen PC. Acute renal failure possibly associated with fenoprofen therapy [letter]. Arthritis Rheum. 1983;26:234–5.

Volland C, Benet LZ. In vitro enantioselective glucuronidation of fenoprofen. Pharmacology. 1991;43:53–60.

Volland C, Sun H, Dammeyer J, Benet LZ. Stereoselective degradation of the fenoprofen acyl glucuronide enantiomers and irreversible binding to plasma proteins. Drug Metab Dispos. 1991;19:1080–6.

Wendland ML, Wagoner RD, Holley KE. Renal failure associated with fenoprofen. Mayo Clin Proc. 1980;55:103–7.

Dosage Adjustment of Medications Eliminated by the Kidneys

<u>**Fenoprofen**</u>/Nalfon®   {**Anti-inflammatory; nonsteroidal anti-inflammatory drug**}

Usual initial dose:	300 mg
Usual maintenance dose:	300–600 mg three to four times daily
Typical maximum dose:	3,200 mg/day
Proportion eliminated unchanged:	30 %

Adjustment for Kidney Disease

FDA-approved product labeling:	*Significantly impaired renal function*	*Contraindicated*
Alternative adjustment:	*GFR >50 mL/min*	*300–600 mg three to four times daily*
	GFR 10–50 mL/min	*300–600 mg three to four times daily*
	GFR <10 mL/min	*Preferably avoid due to risk for gastrointestinal and renal toxicity.*
	Hemodialysis	*Preferably avoid due to risk for gastrointestinal and renal toxicity.*
	CAPD	*Preferably avoid due to risk for gastrointestinal and renal toxicity.*
	CRRT	*Not applicable; preferably avoid.*

Dosage Adjustment of Medications Eliminated by the Kidneys

Fexofenadine - Selected References

Allegra® [package insert]. Bridgewater: Sanofi-Aventis US LLC; 2008.

Aronoff GA, Bennett WM, Berns JS, et al. Drug prescribing in renal failure: dosing guidelines for adults and children. 5th ed. Philadelphia: American College of Physicians; 2007.

Cvetkovic M, Leake B, Fromm MF, Wilkinson GR, Kim RB. OATP and P-glycoprotein transporters mediate the cellular uptake and excretion of fexofenadine. Drug Metab Dispos. 1999;27:866–71.

Devillier P, Roche N, Faisy C. Clinical pharmacokinetics and pharmacodynamics of desloratadine, fexofenadine and levocetirizine: a comparative review. Clin Pharmacokinet. 2008;47:217–30.

Drescher S, Schaeffeler E, Hitzl M, et al. MDR1 gene polymorphisms and disposition of the P-glycoprotein substrate fexofenadine. Br J Clin Pharmacol. 2002;53:526–31.

Golightly LK, Greos LS. Second-generation antihistamines: actions and efficacy in the management of allergic disorders. Drugs. 2005;65:341–84.

Kalliokoski A, Niemi M. Impact of OATP transporters on pharmacokinetics. Br J Pharmacol. 2009;158:693–705.

Lippert C, Ling J, Brown P, et al. Mass balance and pharmacokinetics of MDL 16,455A in healthy male volunteers [abstract 8253]. Pharm Res. 1995;12(Suppl):390.

Liu S, Beringer PM, Hidayat L, et al. Probenecid, but not cystic fibrosis, alters the total and renal clearance of fexofenadine. J Clin Pharmacol. 2008;48:957–65.

Miura M, Uno T. Clinical pharmacokinetics of fexofenadine enantiomers. Expert Opin Drug Metab Toxicol. 2010;6:69–74.

Miura M, Uno T, Tateishi T, Suzuki T. Pharmacokinetics of fexofenadine enantiomers in healthy subjects. Chirality. 2007;19:223–7.

Molimard M, Diquet B, Benedetti MS. Comparison of pharmacokinetics and metabolism of desloratadine, fexofenadine, levocetirizine and mizolastine in humans. Fundam Clin Pharmacol. 2004;18:399–411.

Russell T, Stoltz M, Weir S. Pharmacokinetics, pharmacodynamics, and tolerance of single- and multiple-dose fexofenadine hydrochloride in healthy male volunteers. Clin Pharmacol Ther. 1998;64:612–21.

Shimizu M, Fuse K, Okudaira K, et al. Contribution of OATP (organic anion-transporting polypeptide) family transporters to the hepatic uptake of fexofenadine in humans. Drug Metab Dispos. 2005;33:1477–81.

Tahara H, Kusuhara H, Fuse E, Sugiyama Y. P-glycoprotein plays a major role in the efflux of fexofenadine in the small intestine and blood-brain barrier, but only a limited role in its biliary excretion. Drug Metab Dispos. 2005;33:963–8.

Zhao R, Kalvass JC, Yanni SB, Bridges AS, Pollack GM. Fexofenadine brain exposure and the influence of blood-brain barrier P-glycoprotein after fexofenadine and terfenadine administration. Drug Metab Dispos. 2009;37:529–35.

Dosage Adjustment of Medications Eliminated by the Kidneys

<u>Fexofenadine</u>/Allegra® {**Antihistamine; second-generation histamine H$_1$ blocker**}

Usual initial dose:	60 mg orally
Usual maintenance dose:	60 mg orally twice daily or 180 mg once daily
Typical maximum dose:	180 mg/day
Proportion eliminated unchanged:	11 %

Adjustment for Kidney Disease

FDA-approved product labeling:	*Decreased renal function*	*Starting dose is 60 mg once daily.*
Alternative adjustment:	*GFR >50 mL/min*	*60 mg orally every 12 h*
	GFR 10–50 mL/min	*60 mg orally every 12–24 h*
	GFR <10 mL/min	*60 mg orally every 24 h*
	Hemodialysis	*60 mg orally every 24 h (after dialysis)*
	CAPD	*60 mg orally every 24 h*
	CRRT	*60 mg enterally every 12 h*

Dosage Adjustment of Medications Eliminated by the Kidneys

Flecainide - Selected References

Aronoff GA, Bennett WM, Berns JS, et al. Drug prescribing in renal failure: dosing guidelines for adults and children. 5th ed. Philadelphia: American College of Physicians; 2007.

Baille GR, Waldek S. Pharmacokinetics of flecainide in a patient undergoing continuous ambulatory peritoneal dialysis. J Clin Pharm Ther. 1988;13:121–4.

Borgeat A, Biollaz J Freymond B, Bayer-Berger M, Chiolero R. Hemofiltration clearance of flecainide in a patient with acute renal failure. Intensive Care Med. 1988;14:236–7.

Boriani G, Strocchi E, Capucci A, et al. Flecainide: evidence of non-linear kinetics. Eur J Clin Pharmacol. 1991;41:57–9.

Braun J, Kollert JR, Becker JU. Pharmacokinetics of flecainide in patients with mild and moderate renal failure compared with patients with normal renal function. Eur J Clin Pharmacol. 1987;31:711–4.

Conrad GJ, Ober RE. Metabolism of flecainide. Am J Cardiol. 1984;53(Suppl):B41–B51.

Evers J, Eichelbaum M, Kroemer HK. Unpredictability of flecainide plasma concentrations in patients with renal failure: relationship to side effects and sudden death? Ther Drug Monit. 1994;16:349–51.

Forland SC, Burgess E, Blair AD, et al. Oral flecainide pharmacokinetics in patients with impaired renal function. J Clin Pharmacol. 1988;28:259–67.

Forland SC, Cutler RE, McQuinn RL, et al. Flecainide pharmacokinetics after multiple dosing in patients with impaired renal function. J Clin Pharmacol. 1988;28:727–35.

Gross AS, Mikus G, Fischer C, Eichelbaum M. Polymorphic flecainide disposition under conditions of uncontrolled urine flow and pH. Eur J Clin Pharmacol. 1991;40:155–62.

Hertrampf R, Gundert-Remy U, Beckmann J, Hoppe U, Elsäßer W, Stein H. Elimination of flecainide as a function of urinary flow rate and pH. Eur J Clin Pharmacol. 1991;41:61–3.

Johnston A, Warrington S, Turner P. Flecainide pharmacokinetics in healthy volunteers: the influence of urinary pH. Br J Clin Pharmacol. 1985;20:333–8.

McIntyre CW, Owen PJ. Prescribing drugs in kidney disease. In: Brenner BM, editor. Brenner & Rector's the kidney. 8th ed. Philadelphia: Saunders Elsevier; 2008. p. 1930–55.

Muhiddin KA, Johnston A, Turner P. The influence of urinary pH on flecainide excretion and its serum pharmacokinetics. Br J Clin Pharmacol. 1984;17:447–51.

Roden DM, Woosley RL. Drug therapy: flecainide. N Engl J Med. 1986;315:36–41.

Sangrador G, Sánchez-Alcaraz A, Rodriguez M, Ibánez P. Clinical pharmacokinetics of intravenous flecainide in critically ill patients. J Clin Pharm Ther. 1989;14:309–14.

Tambocor® tablet [package insert]. Northridge: 3M Pharmaceuticals; 2006.

Tjandra-Maga TB, Verbesselt R, Van Hecken A, Mullie A, De Schepper PJ. Flecainide: single and multiple oral dose kinetics, absolute bioavailability and effect of food and antacid in man. Br J Clin Pharmacol. 1986;22:309–16.

Williams AJ, McQuinn RL, Walls J. Pharmacokinetics of flecainide acetate in patients with severe renal impairment. Clin Pharmacol Ther. 1988;43:449–55.

Dosage Adjustment of Medications Eliminated by the Kidneys

Flecainide/Tambocor™	{Antiarrhythmic, class IC}
Usual initial dose:	50 mg orally
Usual maintenance dose:	50–150 mg orally every 12 h
Typical maximum dose:	400 mg/day
Proportion eliminated unchanged:	40 %

Adjustment for Kidney Disease

FDA-approved product labeling:	*Severe renal impairment (CrCL ≤35 mL/min)*	*Initial dosage should be 100 mg orally once daily or 50 mg orally twice daily.*
	Less severe renal disease	*Initial dosage should be 100 mg orally every 12 h.*
Alternative adjustment:	*GFR >50 mL/min*	*50–100 mg orally every 12 h*
	GFR 10–50 mL/min	*50–75 mg orally every 12 h[a]*
	GFR <10 mL/min	*25–50 mg orally every 12 h[a]*
	Hemodialysis	*25–50 mg orally every 12 h[a]*
	CAPD	*25–50 mg orally every 12 h[a]*
	CVVH	*25–50 mg orally every 12 h[a]*

[a]Depending on metabolizer genotype, wide variation in flecainide levels has been documented, particularly in patients with impaired kidney function. Careful electrocardiographic monitoring of PR and QRS intervals and frequent determination of steady-state serum drug levels are recommended.

Dosage Adjustment of Medications Eliminated by the Kidneys

Fluconazole (IV) - Selected References

Abramowicz M, Zuccotti G, Pflomm J-M, et al., editors. Handbook of antimicrobial therapy. 19th ed. New Rochelle: The Medical Letter; 2011.

Aronoff GA, Bennett WM, Berns JS, et al. Drug prescribing in renal failure: dosing guidelines for adults and children. 5th ed. Philadelphia: American College of Physicians; 2007.

Bergner R, Hoffmann M, Riedel K-D, et al. Fluconazole dosing in continuous veno-venous haemofiltration (CVVHF): need for a high daily dose of 800 mg. Nephrol Dial Transplant. 2006;21:1019–23.

Brammer KW, Farrow PR, Faulkner JK. Pharmacokinetics and tissue penetration of fluconazole in humans. Rev Infect Dis. 1990;12(Suppl 3):S318–26.

Bren A. Fungal peritonitis in patients on continuous peritoneal dialysis. Eur J Clin Microbiol Infect Dis. 1998;17:839–43.

Bren A, Kandus A, Lindič J, Varl J. Fluconazole in the treatment of fungal infections in kidney-transplanted patients. Transplant Proc. 1992;24:2765–6.

Cota JM, Burgess DS. Antifungal dose adjustment in renal and hepatic dysfunction: pharmacokinetic and pharmacodynamic considerations. Curr Fungal Infect Rep. 2010;4:120–8. doi:10.1007/s12281-010-0015-9.

Cousin L, Le Berre M, Launay-Vacher V, Izzedine H, Deray G. Dosing guidelines for fluconazole in patients with renal failure. Nephrol Dial Transplant. 2003;18:2227–31.

De Muria D, Forrest A, Rich J, Scavone JM, Cohen LG, Kazanjian PH. Pharmacokinetics and bioavailability of fluconazole in patients with AIDS. Antimicrob Agents Chemother. 1993;37:2187–92.

Debruyne D, Ryckelynck J-P. Clinical pharmacokinetics of fluconazole. Clin Pharmacokinet. 1993;24:10–27.

Diflucan® injection [package insert]. New York: Roerig Division of Pfizer Inc; 2010.

Heintz BH, Matzke GR, Dager WF. Antimicrobial dosing concepts and recommendations for critically ill adult patients receiving continuous renal replacement therapy or intermittent hemodialysis. Pharmacotherapy. 2009;29:562–77.

Humphrey MJ, Jevons S, Tarbit MH. Pharmacokinetic evaluation of UK-49,858, a metabolically stable triazole antifungal drug, in animals and humans. Antimicrob Agents Chemother. 1985;28:648–53.

Kuang D, Verbine A, Ronco C. Pharmacokinetics and antimicrobial dosing adjustment in critically ill patients during continuous renal replacement therapy. Clin Nephrol. 2007;67:267–84.

Menichetti F, Fiorio M, Tosti A, et al. High-dose fluconazole therapy for cryptococcal meningitis in patients with AIDS. Clin Infect Dis. 1996;22:838–40.

Muhl E, Martens T, Iven H, Rob P, Bruch H-P. Influence of continuous veno-venous haemodiafiltration and continuous veno-venous haemofiltration on the pharmacokinetics of fluconazole. Eur J Clin Pharmacol. 2000;56:671–8.

Nicolau DP, Crowe H, Nightingale CH, Quinitilani R. Effect of continuous arteriovenous hemodiafiltration on the pharmacokinetics of fluconazole. Pharmacotherapy. 1994;14:502–5.

Oono S, Tabei K, Tetsuka T, Asano Y. The pharmacokinetics of fluconazole during haemodialysis in uraemic patients. Eur J Clin Pharmacol. 1992;42:667–70.

Rex JH, Bennett JE, Sugar AM, et al. A randomized trial comparing fluconazole with amphotericin B for the treatment of candidemia in patients without neutropenia. N Engl J Med. 1994;331:1325–30.

Schaffner A, Schaffner M. Effect of prophylactic fluconazole on the frequency of fungal infections, amphotericin B use, and health care costs in patients undergoing intensive chemotherapy for hematologic neoplasias. J Infect Dis. 1995;172:1035–41.

Trotman RL, Williamson JC, Shoemaker M, Salzer WL. Antibiotic dosing in critically ill adult patients receiving continuous renal replacement therapy. Clin Infect Dis. 2005;41:1159–66.

Valtonen M, Tiula E, Neuvonen PJ. Effect of continuous venovenous haemofiltration and haemodiafiltration on the elimination of fluconazole in patients with acute renal failure. J Antimicrob Chemother. 1997;40:695–700.

Winston DJ, Hathorn JW, Schuster MG, Schiller GJ, Territo MC. Multicenter, randomized trial of fluconazole versus amphotericin B for empiric antifungal therapy of febrile neutropenic patients with cancer. Am J Med. 2000;108:282–9.

Wolter K, Marggraf G, Dermoumi H, Fritschka E. Elimination of fluconazole during continuous veno-venous haemodialysis (CVVHD) in a single patient [letter]. Eur J Clin Pharmacol. 1994;47:291–2.

Dosage Adjustment of Medications Eliminated by the Kidneys

<u>**Fluconazole (IV)**</u>/**Diflucan® IV**   {Antifungal; triazole ergosterol biosynthesis inhibitor}

Usual initial dose:	400 mg IV
Usual maintenance dose:	400 mg IV every 24 h
Typical maximum dose:	1,200 mg/day
Proportion eliminated unchanged:	80 %

Adjustment for Kidney Disease

FDA-approved product labeling: *Fluconazole dosage in adult patients with impaired renal function*

CrCL (mL/min)	Percent of recommended dose
>50	100 %
≤50 (no dialysis)	50 %
Regular dialysis	100 % after each dialysis

Alternative adjustment:

GFR >50 mL/min	400–800 mg IV every 24 h
GFR 10–50 mL/min	200–400 mg IV every 24 h
GFR <10 mL/min	200 mg every IV 24 h
Hemodialysis	400 mg IV after dialysis
CAPD	200 mg IV every 24 h
CVVH	200–800 mg IV every 24 h
CVVHD	400–800 mg IV every 24 h
CVVHDF	400–800 mg IV every 24 h (consider 800 mg q24h if dialysate flow rate >2 L/h or treating Candida glabrata or other relatively azole-resistant species.)

Fluconazole (Enteral) - Selected References

Abramowicz M, Zuccotti G, Pflomm J-M, et al., editors. Handbook of antimicrobial therapy. 19th ed. New Rochelle: The Medical Letter; 2011.

Back DJ, Tjia JF. Comparative effects of the antimycotic drugs ketoconazole, fluconazole, itraconazole and terbinafine on the metabolism of cyclosporin by human liver microsomes. Br J Clin Pharmacol. 1991;32:624–6.

Berl T, Wilner KD, Gardner M, et al. Pharmacokinetics of fluconazole in renal failure. J Am Soc Nephrol. 1995;6:542–7.

Bozzette SA, Larsen RA, Chiu J, et al. A placebo-controlled trial of maintenance therapy with fluconazole after treatment of cryptococcal meningitis in the acquired immunodeficiency syndrome. N Engl J Med. 1991;324:580–4.

Bren A, Kandus A, Lindič J, Varl J. Fluconazole in the treatment of fungal infections in kidney-transplanted patients. Transplant Proc. 1992;24:2765–6.

Cousin L, Le Berre M, Launay-Vacher V, Izzedine H, Deray G. Dosing guidelines for fluconazole in patients with renal failure. Nephrol Dial Transplant. 2003;18:2227–31.

De Wit S, Weerts D, Goossens H, Clumeck N. Comparison of fluconazole and ketoconazole for oropharyngeal candidiasis in AIDS. Lancet. 1989;1:746–8.

Debruyne D, Ryckelynck J-P. Clinical pharmacokinetics of fluconazole. Clin Pharmacokinet. 1993;24:10–27.

Debruyne D, Ryckelynck J-P, Moulin M, de LIgny BH, Levaltier B, Bigot M-C. Pharmacokinetics of fluconazole in patients undergoing continuous ambulatory peritoneal dialysis. Clin Pharmacokinet. 1990;18:491–8.

Diflucan® tablet and powder for suspension [package insert]. New York: Roerig Division of Pfizer Inc; 2010.

Evans TG, Mayer J, Cohen S, Classen D, Carroll K. Fluconazole failure in the treatment of invasive mycoses. J Infect Dis. 1991;164:1232–5.

Goldie SJ, Kiernan-Troidle L, Torres C, et al. Fungal peritonitis in a large chronic peritoneal dialysis population: a report of 55 episodes. Am J Kidney Dis. 1996;28:86–91.

Koch M, Trapp R, Goepel M. Successful maintenance of continuous ambulatory peritoneal dialysis in a patient after fungal peritonitis and dialysate leakage. Clin Nephrol. 2006;65:294–8.

Laine L, Dretler RH, Conteas CN, et al. Fluconazole compared with ketoconazole for the treatment of candida esophagitis in AIDS: a randomized trial. Ann Intern Med. 1992;117:655–60.

Larsen RA, Leal MA Chan LS. Fluconazole compared with amphotericin B plus flucytosine for cryptococcal meningitis in AIDS: a randomized trial. Ann Intern Med. 1990;113:183–7.

Levine J, Bernard DB, Idelson BA, Farnham H, Saunders C, Sugar AM. Fungal peritonitis complicating continuous ambulatory peritoneal dialysis: successful treatment with fluconazole, a new orally active antifungal agent. Am J Med. 1989;86:825–7.

Michel C, Courdavault L, Al Khayat R, Viron B, Roux P, Mignon F. Fungal peritonitis in patients on peritoneal dialysis. Am J Nephrol. 1994;14:113–20.

Oono S, Tabei K, Tetsuka T, Asano Y. The pharmacokinetics of fluconazole during haemodialysis in uraemic patients. Eur J Clin Pharmacol. 1992;42:667–70.

Toon S, Ross CE, Gokal R, Rowland M. An assessment of the effects of impaired renal function and hemodialysis on the pharmacokinetics of fluconazole. Br J Clin Pharmacol. 1990;29:221–6.

Witt MD, Bayer AS. Comparison of fluconazole and amphotericin B for prevention and treatment of experimental Candida endocarditis. Antimicrob Agents Chemother. 1991;35:2481–5.

Dosage Adjustment of Medications Eliminated by the Kidneys

Fluconazole (Enteral)/Diflucan®   {Antifungal; triazole ergosterol biosynthesis inhibitor}

Usual initial dose:	200 mg
Usual maintenance dose:	50–200 mg enterally every 24 h
Typical maximum dose:	400 mg/day
Proportion eliminated unchanged:	80 %

Adjustment for Kidney Disease

FDA-approved product labeling: *Fluconazole dosage in patients with impaired renal function*

Single-dose treatment of vaginal candidiasis	*No adjustment needed*

Other fungal infections

CrCL (mL/min)	*Percent of recommended dose*
>50	*100 %*
≤50 (no dialysis)	*50 %*
Regular dialysis	*100 % after each dialysis*

Alternative adjustment:

eCrCL >50 mL/min	*50–400 mg enterally every 24 h*
eCrCL 10–50 mL/min	*25–200 mg enterally every 24 h (50 % decrease)*
eCrCL <10 mL/min	*25–100 mg enterally every 24 h (75 % decrease)*
Hemodialysis	*50–400 mg enterally after each dialysis*
CAPD	*100 mg enterally every 24 h or 200 mg intraperitoneally during a 12-h dwell every 48 h*
CRRT	*Not applicable (consider parenteral antifungal)*

Dosage Adjustment of Medications Eliminated by the Kidneys

Flucytosine - Selected References

Ancobon® capsule [package insert]. Costa Mesa: Valeant Pharmaceuticals International; 2007.

Anderson KEH, Olsen H. Candida peritonitis in a patient receiving chronic intermittent peritoneal dialysis. Scand J Infect Dis. 1978;10:91–2.

Aronoff GA, Bennett WM, Berns JS, et al. Drug prescribing in renal failure: dosing guidelines for adults and children. 5th ed. Philadelphia: American College of Physicians; 2007.

Block ER, Bennett JE, Livoti LG, Klein WJ Jr, MacGregor RR, Henderson L. Flucytosine and amphotericin B: hemodialysis effects on the plasma concentration and clearance. Studies in man. Ann Intern Med. 1974;80:613–7.

Christopher TG, Blair AD, Forrey AW, Cutler RE. Hemodialyzer clearances of gentamicin, kanamycin, tobramycin, amikacin, ethambutol, procainamide, and flucytosine, with a technique for planning therapy. J Pharmacokinet Biopharm. 1976;4: 427–41.

Cota JM, Burgess DS. Antifungal dose adjustment in renal and hepatic dysfunction: pharmacokinetic and pharmacodynamic considerations. Curr Fungal Infect Rep. 2010;4:120–8. doi:10.1007/s12281-010-0015-9.

Cutler RE, Blair AD, Kelly MR. Flucytosine kinetics in subjects with normal and impaired renal function. Clin Pharmacol Ther. 1978;24:333–42.

Dawborn JK, Page MD, Schiavone DJ. Use of 5-fluorocytosine in patients with impaired renal function. Br Med J. 1973;4:382–4.

Drouhet E, Babinet P, Chapusot JP, Kleinknecht D. 5-Fluorocytosine in the treatment of candidiasis with acute renal insufficiency: its kinetics during haemodialysis and peritoneal dialysis. Biomedicine. 1973;19:408–14.

Lau AH, Kronfol NO. Elimination of flucytosine by continuous hemofiltration. Am J Nephrol. 1995;15:327–31.

McIntyre CW, Owen PJ. Prescribing drugs in kidney disease. In: Brenner BM, editor. Brenner & Rector's the kidney. 8th ed. Philadelphia: Saunders Elsevier; 2008. p. 1930–55.

Michel C, Courdavault L, Al Khayat R, Viron B, Roux P, Mignon F. Fungal peritonitis in patients on peritoneal dialysis. Am J Nephrol. 1994;14:113–20.

Olyaei AJ, Bennett WM. Pharmacologic approach to renal insufficiency. In: Dale DC, Federman DD, Antman K, editors. ACP medicine, WebMD June 2007 update. Hamilton: BC Decker; 2007; NEPHROLOGY IX: Appendix A1–25.

Olyaei AJ, Bennett WM. Drug dosing in elderly patients with chronic kidney disease. Clin Geriatr Med. 2009;25:459–527.

Olyaei AJ, DeMattos AM, Bennett WM. Use of drugs in patients with renal failure. In: Schrier RW, editor. Diseases of the kidney and urinary tract. 8th ed. Philadelphia: Lippincott Williams & Wilkins; 2007. p. 2765–807.

Phillips I, Eykyn S, MacGregor GA, Jones NF. Candida peritonitis treated with 5-fluorocytosine in a patient receiving hemodialysis. Clin Nephrol. 1973;1:271–2.

Rault RM, Hulme B, Davies RR. 5-Fluorocytosine treatment of candidiasis on a patient receiving regular hemodialysis. Clin Nephrol. 1975;3:225–7.

Schönebeck J, Polak A, Fernex M, Scholer HJ. Pharmacokinetic studies on the oral antimycotic agent 5-fluorocytosine in individuals with normal and impaired kidney function. Chemotherapy. 1973;18:321–36.

Thomson AH, Shankland G, Clareburt C, Binning S. Flucytosine dose requirements in a patient receiving continuous veno-venous haemofiltration [letter]. Intensive Care Med. 2002;28:999.

Vermes A, Guchelaar H-J, Dankert J. Flucytosine: a review of its pharmacology, clinical indications, pharmacokinetics, toxicity and drug interactions. J Antimicrob Chemother. 2000;46:171–9.

Dosage Adjustment of Medications Eliminated by the Kidneys

Flucytosine/Ancobon® {**Antifungal; purine and pyrimidine uptake inhibitor**}

Usual initial dose:	37.5 mg/kg orally (ideal body weight or lean body mass)
Usual maintenance dose:	50–150 mg/kg/day orally in divided doses every 6 h
Typical maximum dose:	150 mg/kg/day
Proportion eliminated unchanged:	90 %

Adjustment for Kidney Disease

FDA-approved product labeling:	*If the BUN or the SCr is elevated or if there are other signs of renal impairment, the initial dose should be at the lower level.*	
Alternative adjustment:	*GFR >50 mL/min*	*37.5 mg/kg orally every 6 h*
	GFR 10–50 mL/min	*25–37.5 mg/kg orally every 12–24 h*
	GFR <10 mL/min	*15–25 mg/kg orally every 24 h*
	Hemodialysis	*15–25 mg/kg orally every 24 h or 25–37.5 mg/kg orally every 48 h (after hemodialysis on dialysis days) or 25–37.5 mg/kg orally three times weekly after dialysis*
	CAPD	*500–1,000 mg orally every 24 h or 50 mg/L of peritoneal dialysis fluid (limited data)*
	CVVH	*25–37.5 mg/kg orally every 24–48 h*

Dosage Adjustment of Medications Eliminated by the Kidneys

off-label: Instagram

Fludarabine - Selected References

Aronoff GA, Bennett WM, Berns JS, et al. Drug prescribing in renal failure: dosing guidelines for adults and children. 5th ed. Philadelphia: American College of Physicians; 2007.

Bonin M, Pursche S, Bergeman T, et al. F-ara-A pharmacokinetics during reduced-intensity conditioning therapy with fludarabine and busulfan. Bone Marrow Transplant. 2007;39:201–6.

Casper ES, Mittelman A, Kelson D, Young CW. Phase I clinical trial of fludarabine phosphate (F-ara-AMP). Cancer Chemother Pharmacol. 1985;15:233–5.

Fludara® injection [package insert]. Cambridge: Genzyme Corp; 2010.

Horwitz ME, Spasojevic I, Morris A, et al. Fludarabine-based nonmyeloablative stem cell transplantation for sickle cell disease with and without renal failure: clinical outcome and pharmacokinetics. Biol Blood Marrow Transplant. 2007;13:1422–6.

Kemena A, Fernandez M, Bauman J, Keating M, Plunkett W. A sensitive fluorescence assay for quantitation of fludarabine and metabolites in biological fluids. Clin Chim Acta. 1991;200:95–106.

Kielstein JT, Stadler M, Czock D, Keller F, Hertenstein B, Radermacher J. Dialysate concentration and pharmacokinetics of 2F-Ara-A in a patient with acute renal failure. Eur J Haematol. 2005;74:533–4.

Lichtman SM, Etcuganas E, Budman DR, et al. The pharmacokinetics and pharmacodynamics of fludarabine phosphate in patients with renal impairment: a prospective dose adjustment study. Cancer Invest. 2002;20:904–13.

Long-Boyle JR, Green KG, Brunstein CG, et al. High fludarabine exposure and relationship with treatment-related mortality after nonmyeloablative hematopoietic cell transplantation. Bone Marrow Transplant. 2011;46:20–6.

Macheta MP, Parapia LA, Gouldesbrough DR. Renal failure in a patient with chronic lymphocytic leukemia treated with fludarabine. J Clin Pathol. 1995;48:181–2.

Malspeis L, Grever MR, Staubus AE, Young D. Pharmacokinetics of 2-F-ara-A (9-β-D-arabinosyl-2-fluoroadenine) in cancer patients during the phase I clinical investigation of fludarabine phosphate. Semin Oncol. 1990;17(Suppl 8):18–32.

Martell RE, Peterson BL, Cohen HJ, et al. Analysis of age, estimated creatinine clearance and pretreatment hematologic parameters as predictors of fludarabine toxicity in patients treated for chronic lymphocytic leukemia: a CALGB (9011) coordinated intergroup study. Cancer Chemother Pharmacol. 2002;50:37–45.

Nunes R, Passos-Coelho JL, Miranda M, Nave M, Leal da Costa F, Abecasis M. Reversible acute renal failure following single administration of fludarabine [letter]. Bone Marrow Transplant. 2004;33:671.

Ogawa Y, Hotta T, Tobinai K, et al. Phase I and pharmacokinetic study of oral fludarabine phosphate in relapsed indolent B-cell non-Hodgkin's lymphoma. Ann Oncol. 2006;17:330–3.

Osborne WL, Lennard AI. Acute renal failure and disseminated intravascular coagulation following an idiosyncratic reaction to alemtuzumab (Campath 1H) or fludarabine. Haematologica. 2005;90:e11–12.

Parikh CR, Sandmaier BM, Storb RF, et al. Acute renal failure after nonmyeloablative hematopoietic cell transplantation. J Am Soc Nephrol. 2004;15:1868–76.

Parikh CR, Schrier RW, Storer B, et al. Comparison of ARF after myeloablative and nonmyeloablative hematopoietic cell transplantation. Am J Kidney Dis. 2005;45:502–9.

Tendas A, Cupelli L, Dentamaro T, et al. Feasibility of a dose-adjusted fludarabine-melphalan conditioning prior to autologous stem cell transplantation in a dialysis-dependent patient with mantle cell lymphoma [letter]. Ann Hematol. 2009;88:285–6.

Timurağaoğlu A, Karadoğan I, Ündar L. Irreversible renal failure in a patient with chronic lymphocytic leukemia treated with fludarabine [letter]. Ann Hematol. 1999;78:109–10.

Weiss AS, Sandmaier BM, Storer B, Storb R, McSweeney PA, Rarikh CR. Chronic kidney disease following non-myeloablative hematopoietic cell transplantation. Am J Transplant. 2006;6:89–94.

Yin W, Karyagina EV, Lundberg AS, Greenblatt DJ, Lister-James J. Pharmacokinetics, bioavailability and effects on electrocardiographic parameters of oral fludarabine phosphate. Biopharm Drug Dispos. 2010;31:72–81.

1:30
Dr. Lavine 292 IP 338 622016-11
3rd.
Medicare Suppl. Plan N.

Dosage Adjustment of Medications Eliminated by the Kidneys

Fludarabine/Fludara®   {Antineoplastic; DNA polymerase-α and ribonucleotide reductase inhibitor}

Usual initial dose: 25 mg/m² IV

Usual maintenance dose: 25 mg/m² IV over 30 min daily for five consecutive days; each 5-day course of treatment should commence every 28 days.

Typical maximum dose: 50 mg/m² IV daily

Proportion eliminated unchanged: 60 %

Adjustment for Kidney Disease

FDA-approved product labeling: *Fludarabine starting dose for renal impairment*

CrCL (mL/min)	Starting dose
≥80	25 mg/m² (full dose)
50–79	20 mg/m²
30–49	15 mg/m²
<30	Do not administer/avoid

Alternative adjustment:

GFR >50 mL/min	30–50 mg/m² IV daily ×3 to 5 prior to hematopoietic stem cell transplantation
GFR 10–50 mL/min	25 mg/m² IV daily ×5 prior to hematopoietic stem cell transplantation
GFR <10 mL/min	12.5 mg/m² IV daily ×5
Hemodialysis	6–12.5 mg/m² IV daily ×5 (after dialysis)
Extended daily dialysis	40 mg/m² IV daily ×3 (limited data)
CAPD	12.5 mg/m² IV daily ×5
CRRT	18.75 mg/m² IV daily ×5

Fomepizole - Selected References

Antizol® injection [package insert]. Dover: Paladin Labs (USA) Inc; 2009.

Aronoff GA, Bennett WM, Berns JS, et al. Drug prescribing in renal failure: dosing guidelines for adults and children. 5th ed. Philadelphia: American College of Physicians; 2007.

Barceloux DG, Bond GR, Krenzelok EP, Cooper H, Vale JA. American Academy of Clinical Toxicology practice guidelines on the treatment of methanol poisoning. J Toxicol Clin Toxicol. 2002;40:415–46.

Baud FJ, Galliot M, Astier A. Treatment of ethylene glycol poisoning with intravenous 4-methylpyrazole. N Engl J Med. 1988;319:97–100.

Bestic M, Blackford M, Reed M. Fomepizole: a critical assessment of current dosing recommendations. J Clin Pharmacol. 2009;49:130–7.

Buchanan JA, Alhelail M, Cetaruk EW, et al. Massive ethylene glycol ingestion treated with fomepizole alone—a viable therapeutic option. J Med Toxicol. 2010;6:131–4.

Corley RA, McMartin KE. Incorporation of therapeutic interventions in physiologically based pharmacokinetic modeling of human clinical case reports of accidental or intentional overdosing with ethylene glycol. Toxicol Sci. 2005;85:495–501.

Faessel H, Houze P, Baud FJ, Scherrmann JM. 4-Methylpyrazole monitoring during haemodialysis of ethylene glycol intoxicated patients. Eur J Clin Pharmacol. 1995;49:211–3.

Hovda KE, Jacobsen D. Expert opinion: fomepizole may ameliorate the need for hemodialysis in methanol poisoning. Hum Exp Toxicol. 2008;27:539–46.

Hovda KE, Andersson KS, Urdal P, Jacobsen D. Methanol and formate kinetics during treatment with fomepizole. Clin Toxicol (Phila). 2005;43:221–7.

Jacobsen D, Barron SK, Sebastian CS, Blomstrand R, McMartin KE. Non-linear kinetics of 4-methylpyrazole in healthy human subjects. Eur J Clin Pharmacol. 1989;37:599–604.

Kerns W II, Tomaszewski C, McMartin K, Ford M, Brent J. Formate kinetics in methanol poisoning. J Toxicol Clin Toxicol. 2002;40:137–43.

Kostic MA, Dart RC. Rethinking the toxic methanol level. J Toxicol Clin Toxicol. 2003;41:793–800.

Kraut JA, Kurtz I. Toxic alcohol ingestions: clinical features, diagnosis, and management. Clin J Am Soc Nephrol. 2008;3: 208–25.

Marraffa J, Forrest A, Grant W, Stork C, McMartin K, Howland MA. Oral administration of fomepizole produces similar blood levels as identical intravenous dose. Clin Toxicol (Phila). 2009;46:181–6

Mégarbane B, Houzé P, Baud FJ. Oral fomepizole administration to treat ethylene glycol and methanol poisonings: advantages and limitations [letter]. Clin Toxicol (Phila). 2008;46:1097.

Sivilotti MLA, Burns MJ, McMartin KE, Brent J. Toxicokinetics of ethylene glycol during fomepizole therapy: implications for management. Ann Emerg Med. 2000;36:114–25.

Wallemacq PE, Vanbinst R, Haufroid V, et al. Plasma and tissue determination of 4-methylpyrazole for pharmacokinetic analysis in acute adult and pediatric methanol/ethylene glycol poisoning. Ther Drug Monit. 2004;26:258–62.

Fomepizole/Antizol®   {**Antidote; ℞ for methanol or ethylene glycol poisoning**}

Usual initial dose: 15 mg/kg IV over 30 min; begin treatment immediately upon suspicion of ethylene glycol or methanol ingestion based on patient history and/or anion gap metabolic acidosis, increased osmolar gap, visual disturbances, or oxalate crystals in the urine or a documented serum ethylene glycol or methanol concentration >20 mg/dL.

Usual maintenance dose: 10 mg/kg IV over 30 min every 12 h for four doses and then 15 mg/kg every 12 h thereafter until ethylene glycol or methanol concentrations are undetectable or have been reduced below 20 mg/dL and the patient is asymptomatic with normal pH

Typical maximum dose: 30 mg/kg/day

Proportion eliminated unchanged: 3 % (metabolites 85 %)

Adjustment for Kidney Disease

FDA-approved product labeling: *Fomepizole dosing in patients requiring hemodialysis*

Dose at the beginning of hemodialysis

If <6 h since last fomepizole dose	*If ≥6 h since last fomepizole dose*
Do not administer dose	*Administer next scheduled dose*

Dosing during hemodialysis

Dose every 4 h

Dosing at the time hemodialysis is completed

Time between last dose and the end of hemodialysis

<1 h	*Do not administer dose at the end of hemodialysis*
1–3 h	*Administer one half of next scheduled dose*
>3 h	*Administer next scheduled dose*

Maintenance dosing off hemodialysis

Give next scheduled dose 12 h from last dose administered

Alternative adjustment: *Data not available*

Dosage Adjustment of Medications Eliminated by the Kidneys

Fondaparinux - Selected References

Arixtra® injection [package insert]. Research Triangle Park: GlaxoSmithKline; 2011.

Bauer KA, Eriksson BI, Lassen MR, et al. Fondaparinux compared with enoxaparin for the prevention of venous thromboembolism after elective major knee surgery. N Engl J Med. 2001;345:1305–10.

Büller HR, Davidson BL, Decousus H, et al. Subcutaneous fondaparinux versus intravenous unfractionated heparin in the initial treatment of pulmonary embolism. N Engl J Med. 2003;349:1695–702.

Büller HR, Davidson BL, Decousus H, et al. Fondaparinux or enoxaparin for the initial treatment of symptomatic deep venous thrombosis: a randomized trial. Ann Intern Med. 2004;140:867–73.

Delavenne X, Zufferey P, Baylot D, et al. Population pharmacokinetics of fondaparinux administered at prophylactic doses after major orthopaedic surgery in everyday practice. Thromb Haemost. 2010;104:252–60.

Dhillon S, Plosker GL. Fondaparinux: use in thromboprophylaxis of acute medical patients. Drugs Aging. 2008;25:81–8.

Donat F, Duret JP, Santoni A, et al. The pharmacokinetics of fondaparinux sodium in healthy volunteers. Clin Pharmacokinet. 2002;41(Suppl 2):1–9.

Eriksson BE, Bauer KA, Lassen R, et al. Fondaparinux compared with enoxaparin for the prevention of venous thromboembolism after hip-fracture surgery. N Engl J Med. 2001;345:1298–304.

Faaij RA, Burggraaf J, Schoemaker RC, van Amsterdam RGM, Cohen AF. Absence of an interaction between the synthetic pentasaccharide fondaparinux and oral warfarin. Br J Clin Pharmacol. 2002;54:304–8.

Fox KAA, Bassand J-P, Mehta SR, et al. Influence of renal function on the efficacy and safety of fondaparinux relative to enoxaparin in non-ST-segment elevation acute coronary syndromes. Ann Intern Med. 2007;147:304–10.

Kearon C, Akl EA, Comerota AJ, et al. Antithrombotic therapy for VTE disease: antithrombotic therapy and prevention of thrombosis, 9th ed: American College of Chest Physicians Evidence-Based Clinical Practice Guidelines. Chest. 2012;141 (2 Suppl):e419–94S. doi:10.1378/chest.11-2301.

Lieu C, Shi J, Donat F, et al. Fondaparinux sodium is not metabolised in mammalian liver fractions and does not inhibit cytochrome P450-mediated metabolism of concomitant drugs. Clin Pharmacokinet. 2002;41(Suppl 2):19–26.

Mehta SR, Steg PG, Granger CB, et al. Randomized, blinded trial comparing fondaparinux with unfractionated heparin in patients undergoing contemporary percutaneous coronary intervention: Arixtra Study in Percutaneous Coronary Intervention: A Randomized Evaluation (ASPIRE) pilot trial. Circulation. 2005;111:1390–7.

Paolucci F, Claviés M-C, Dona F, Necciari J. Fondaparinux sodium mechanism of action: identification of specific binding to purified and human plasma-derived proteins. Clin Pharmacokinet. 2002;41(Suppl 2):11–8.

Sculpher MJ, Lozano-Ortega G, Sambrook J, et al. Fondaparinux versus enoxaparin in non-ST-elevation acute coronary syndromes: short-term cost and long-term cost-effectiveness using data from the Fifth Organization to Assess Strategies in Acute Ischemic Syndromes Investigators (OASIS-5) trial. Am Heart J. 2009;157:845–52.

Steg PG, Jolly SS, Mehta SR, et al. Low-dose vs standard-dose unfractionated heparin for percutaneous coronary intervention in acute coronary syndromes treated with fondaparinux: the FUTURA/OASIS-8 randomized trial. JAMA. 2010;304: 1339–49.

Turpie AGG, Lensing AWA, Fuji T, Boyle DA. Pharmacokinetic and clinical data supporting the use of fondaparinux 1.5 mg once daily in the prevention of venous thromboembolism in renally impaired patients. Blood Coagul Fibrinolysis. 2009;20:114–21.

Vellinga TEvR, Peters RJG, Yusuf S, et al. Efficacy and safety of fondaparinux in patients with ST-segment elevation myocardial infarction across the age spectrum. Results from the Organization to Assess Strategies in Acute Ischemic Syndromes 6 (OASIS-6) trial. Am Heart J. 2010;160:1049–55.

Vogel GMT, Mueleman DG, van Dinther TG, Buijsman R, Princen AWM, Smit MJ. Antithrombotic properties of a direct thrombin inhibitor with a prolonged half-life and AT-mediated factor Xa inhibitory actions. J Thromb Haemost. 2003;1:1945–54.

Yusuf S, Mehta SR, Chrolavicius S, et al. Comparison of fondaparinux and enoxaparin in acute coronary syndromes. N Engl J Med. 2006;354:1464–76.

Dosage Adjustment of Medications Eliminated by the Kidneys

<u>**Fondaparinux**</u>/**Arixtra**®   **{Antithrombotic; selective antithrombin III-mediated coagulation factor Xa inhibitor}**

Usual initial dose: 2.5 mg subcutaneously (prophylaxis), 5–10 mg subcutaneously (treatment)

Usual maintenance dose: 2.5 mg subcutaneously every 24 h after hemostasis has been established but not earlier than 6 h after surgery (prophylaxis)

5 mg (body weight <50 kg), 7.5 mg (body weight 50–100 kg), or 10 mg (body weight >100 kg) subcutaneously every 24 h (treatment)

Typical maximum dose: 10 mg/day

Proportion eliminated unchanged: 77 %

Adjustment for Kidney Disease

FDA-approved product labeling:	*CrCL 30–50 mL/min*	*Use with caution*
	CrCL <30 mL/min	*Contraindicated*
Alternative adjustment:	*GFR >50 mL/min*	*2.5–10 mg subcutaneously once daily*
	GFR 30–50 mL/min	*1.5 mg subcutaneously once daily (prophylaxis)*
	GFR <30 mL/min	*Preferably avoid due to increased hemorrhagic risk.*
	Hemodialysis	*Data not available; preferably avoid due to increased hemorrhagic risk.*
	CAPD	*Data not available; preferably avoid due to increased hemorrhagic risk.*
	CRRT	*Data not available; preferably avoid due to increased hemorrhagic risk.*

Dosage Adjustment of Medications Eliminated by the Kidneys

Foscarnet - Selected References

Alexander ACM, Akers A, Matzke GR, Aweeka FT, Fraley DS. Disposition of foscarnet during peritoneal dialysis. Ann Pharmacother. 1996;30:1106–9.

Amsden GW. Tables of antimicrobial agent pharmacology. In: Mandell GL, Bennett JE, Dolin R, editors. Mandell, Douglas, and Bennett's principles and practice of infectious diseases, vol. 1. 6th ed. Philadelphia: Elsevier; 2005. p. 634–700.

Aweeka F, Gambergoglio J, Mills J, Jacobson MA. Pharmacokinetics of intermittently administered intravenous foscarnet in the treatment of acquired immunodeficiency syndrome patients with serious cytomegalovirus retinitis. Antimicrob Agents Chemother. 1989;33:742–5.

Aweeka FT, Jacobson MA, Martin-Munley S, et al. Effect of renal disease and hemodialysis on foscarnet pharmacokinetics and dosing recommendations. J Acquir Immune Defic Syndr Hum Retrovirol. 1999;20:350–7.

Breganti S, Bertilson S, Tedone E, et al. Foscarnet prophylaxis of cytomegalovirus infections in patients undergoing allogeneic bone marrow transplantation (BMT): a dose-finding study. Bone Marrow Transplant. 2000;26:23–9.

Cacoub P, Deray G, Baumelou A, et al. Acute renal failure induced by foscarnet: 4 cases. Clin Nephrol. 1988;29:315–8.

Castelli F, Tomasoni L, Zeroli C, et al. Comparison of pharmacokinetics and dynamics of two dosage regimens of foscarnet in AIDS patients with Cytomegalovirus retinitis. Eur J Clin Pharmacol. 1997;52:397–401.

Chrisp P, Clissold SP. Foscarnet: a review of its antiviral activity, pharmacokinetic properties and therapeutic use in immunocompromised patients with cytomegalovirus retinitis. Drugs. 1991;41:104–29.

Foscavir® injection [package insert]. Wilmington: AstraZeneca LP; 2006.

Jabs DA, Davis MD, Meinert CL, et al. Mortality in patients with the acquired immunodeficiency syndrome treated with either foscarnet or ganciclovir for cytomegalovirus retinitis. N Engl J Med. 1992;326:213–20.

Jayasekara D, Aweeka FT, Rodriguez R, Kalajian RC, Humphreys MH, Gambertoglio JG. Antiviral therapy for HIV patients with renal insufficiency. J Acquir Immune Defic Syndr. 1999;21:384–95.

Lacy CF, Armstrong LL, Goldman MP, Lance LL, editors. Drug information handbook: a comprehensive source for all clinicians and healthcare professionals. 20th ed. Hudson: Lexi-Comp/American Pharmacists Association; 2011.

MacGregor RR, Graziani AL, Weiss, Grunwald JE, Gambertoglio JG. Successful foscarnet therapy for cytomegalovirus retinitis in an AIDS patient undergoing hemodialysis: rationale for empiric dosing and plasma level monitoring. J Infect Dis. 1991;164:785–7.

Maurice-Estepa L, Daudon M, Katlama C, et al. Identification of crystals in kidneys of AIDS patients treated with foscarnet. Am J Kidney Dis. 1998;32:392–400.

Navarro JF, Quereda C, Quereda C, et al. Nephrogenic diabetes insipidus and renal tubular acidosis secondary to foscarnet therapy. Am J Kidney Dis. 1996;27:431–4.

Noormohamed FH, Youle MS, Giggs CJ, Martin-Munley S, Gazzard BG, Lant AF. Pharmacokinetics and absolute bioavailability of oral foscarnet in human immunodeficiency virus-seropositive patients. Antimicrob Agents Chemother. 1998;42:293–7.

Ringdén O, Lönnqvist B, Paulin T, et al. Pharmacokinetics, safety and preliminary clinical experiences using foscarnet in the treatment of cytomegalovirus infections in bone marrow and renal transplant recipients. J Antimicrob Chemother. 1986; 17:373–87.

Sjövall J, Bergdahl S, Movin G, Ogenstad S, Saarimäki M. Pharmacokinetics of foscarnet and distribution to cerebrospinal fluid after intravenous infusion in patients with human immunodeficiency virus. Antimicrob Agents Chemother. 1989;33:1023–31.

Sjövall J, Karlsson A, Ogenstad S, Sandström E, Saarimäki M. Pharmacokinetics and absorption of foscarnet after intravenous and oral administration to patients with human immunodeficiency virus. Clin Pharmacol Ther. 1988;44:65–73.

Taburet A-M, Katlama C, Blanshard C, et al. Pharmacokinetics of foscarnet after twice-daily administrations for treatment of cytomegalovirus disease in AIDS patients. Antimicrob Agents Chemother. 1992;36:1821–4.

Zanetta G, Maurice-Estepa L, Mousson C, et al. Foscarnet-induced crystalline glomerulonephritis with nephrotic syndrome and acute renal failure after kidney transplantation. Transplantation. 1999;67:1376–8.

Dosage Adjustment of Medications Eliminated by the Kidneys

Foscarnet/Foscavir®	{Antiviral; cytomegalovirus/herpes simplex viral DNA polymerase inhibitor}

Usual initial dose:	60 mg/kg IV
Usual maintenance dose:	40–60 mg/kg IV over a minimum of 1 h every 8–12 h or 90–120 mg/kg IV over 1.5–2 h daily
Typical maximum dose:	180 mg/kg/day
Proportion eliminated unchanged:	88 %

Adjustment for Kidney Disease

FDA-approved product labeling:

Foscarnet dosing guide: Induction

CrCL (mL/min/kg)	Herpes simplex: equivalent to		Cytomegalovirus: equivalent to	
	80 mg/kg/day total (40 mg/kg q12h)	120 mg/kg/day total (40 mg/kg q8h)	180 mg/kg/day total	
			60 mg/kg q8h	90 mg/kg q12h
>1.4	40 mg/kg q12h	40 mg/kg q8h	60 mg/kg q8h	90 mg/kg q12h
>1.0–1.4	30 mg/kg q12h	30 mg/kg q8h	45 mg/kg q8h	70 mg/kg q12h
>0.8–1.0	20 mg/kg q12h	35 mg/kg q12h	50 mg/kg q12h	50 mg/kg q12h
>0.6–0.8	35 mg/kg q24h	25 mg/kg q12h	40 mg/kg q12h	80 mg/kg q24h
>0.5–0.6	25 mg/kg q24h	40 mg/kg q24h	60 mg/kg q24h	60 mg/kg q24h
≥0.4–0.5	20 mg/kg q24h	35 mg/kg q24h	50 mg/kg q24h	50 mg/kg q24h
<0.4	Not recommended	Not recommended	Not recommended	Not recommended

Note that tabulated CrCL units are mL/min/kg; this value may be derived from eCrCL by dividing the value in mL/min by body weight in kg

Foscarnet dosing guide: Maintenance

CrCL (mL/min/kg)	Cytomegalovirus: equivalent to	
	90 mg/kg/day (once daily)	120 mg/kg/day (once daily)
>1.4	90 mg/kg q24h	120 mg/kg q24h
>1.0–1.4	70 mg/kg q24h	90 mg/kg q24h
>0.8–1.0	50 mg/kg q24h	65 mg/kg q24h
>0.6–0.8	80 mg/kg q48h	105 mg/kg q48h
>0.5–0.6	60 mg/kg q48h	80 mg/kg q48h
≥0.4–0.5	50 mg/kg q48h	65 mg/kg q48h
<0.4	Not recommended	Not recommended

Note that tabulated CrCL units are mL/min/kg; this value may be derived from eCrCL by dividing the value in mL/min by body weight in kg

Alternative adjustment:	*GFR >50 mL/min*	*40–60 mg/kg IV every 8–12 h*
	GFR 10–50 mL/min	*45–60 mg/kg IV every 24 h*
	GFR <10 mL/min	*Use not recommended due to lack of experience*
	Hemodialysis	*60–90 mg/kg IV once followed by 45–60 mg/kg IV three times weekly after dialysis*
	CAPD	*45 mg/kg IV every 24 h*
	CRRT	*60 mg/kg IV every 24 h*

Dosage Adjustment of Medications Eliminated by the Kidneys

Fosfomycin - Selected References

Borgia M, Longo A, Lodola E. Relative bioavailability of fosfomycin and of trometamol after administration of single dose by oral route of fosfomycin trometamol in fasting conditions and after a meal. Int J Clin Pharmacol Ther Toxicol. 1989;27:411–7.

Borsa F, Leroy A, Fillastre J-P, Godin M, Moulin B. Comparative pharmacokinetics of tromethamine fosfomycin and calcium fosfomycin in young and elderly adults. Antimicrob Agents Chemother. 1988;32:938–41.

Bouchet JL, Albin H, Quentin C, et al. Pharmacokinetics of intravenous and intraperitoneal fosfomycin in continuous ambulatory peritoneal dialysis. Clin Nephrol. 1988;29:35–40.

Bouchet JL, Quentin C, Albin H, Vinçon G, Guillon J, Martin-Dupont P. Pharmacokinetics of fosfomycin in hemodialyzed patients. Clin Nephrol. 1985;23:218–21.

Brunner M, Reinprecht A, Illievich U, et al. Penetration of fosfomycin into the parenchyma of human brain: a case study of three patients [letter]. Br J Clin Pharmacol. 2002;54:548–50.

Dinh A, Salomon J, Bru JP, Bernard L. Fosfomycin: efficacy against infections caused by multidrug-resistant bacteria. Scand J Infect Dis. 2012;44:182–9.

Fernandez Lastra C, Mariño EL, Barrueco M, Santiago Gervós M, Dominguez-Gil A. Disposition of phosphomycin in patients with pleural effusion. Antimicrob Agents Chemother. 1984;25:458–62.

Fernandez Lastra C, Mariño EL, Dominguez-Gil A, Tabernero JM, Gonzalez Lopez A, Yuste Chavez M. The influence of uremia on the accessibility of phosphomycin into interstitial tissue fluid. Eur J Clin Pharmacol. 1983;25:333–8.

Gattringer R, Meyer B, Heinz G, et al. Single-dose pharmacokinetics of fosfomycin during continuous venovenous haemofiltration. J Antimicrob Chemother. 2006;58:367–71.

Hoyer J, Sack K, Schulz E, Winterhoff R. Improvement of initial graft function after renal transplantation by fosfomycin. Transplant Proc. 1987;19:4043–4.

Joukhadar C, Klein N, Dittrich P, et al. Target site penetration of fosfomycin in critically ill patients. J Antimicrob Chemother. 2003;51:1247–52.

Kühnen E, Pfeifer G, Frenkel C. Penetration of fosfomycin into cerebrospinal fluid across non-inflamed and inflamed meninges. Infection. 1987;15:422–4.

Legat FJ, Maier A, Dittrich P, et al. Penetration of fosfomycin into inflammatory lesions in patients with cellulitis or diabetic foot syndrome. Antimicrob Agents Chemother. 2003;47:371–4.

Mazzei T, Cassetta MI, Falani S, Arrigucci S, Novelli A. Pharmacokinetic and pharmacodynamic aspects of antimicrobial agents for the treatment of uncomplicated urinary tract infections. Int J Antimicrob Agents. 2006;285(Suppl 1):35–41.

Monurol® powder [package insert]. St Louis: Forest Pharmaceuticals Inc; 2011.

Pfausler B, Spiss H, Dittrich P, Zeitlinger MA, Joukhadar C. Concentrations of fosfomycin in the cerebrospinal fluid of neurointensive care patients with ventriculostomy-associated ventriculitis. J Antimicrob Chemother. 2004;53:848–52.

Revert L, López J, Pons J, Olay T. Fosfomycin in patients subjected to periodic hemodialysis. Chemotherapy. 1977;23(Suppl 1):204–9.

Roussos N, Karageorgopoulos DE, Samonis G, Falagas ME. Clinical significance of the pharmacokinetic and pharmacodynamic characteristics of fosfomycin for the treatment of patients with systemic infections. Int J Antimicrob Agents. 2009;34:506–45.

Tobudic S, Matzzneller P, Stoiser B, et al. Pharmacokinetics of intraperitoneal and intravenous fosfomycin in automated peritoneal dialysis patients without peritonitis. Antimicrob Agents Chemother. 2012;56:3992–5.

Tullio V, Cuffini AM, Banche G, et al. Role of fosfomycin tromethamine in modulating non-specific defense mechanisms in chronic uremic patients toward ESBL-producing Escherichia coli. Int J Immunopathol Pharmacol. 2008;21:153–60.

Zeitlinger MA, Marsik C, Georgopoulos A, Müller M, Heinz G Joukhadar C. Target site of bacterial killing of cefpirome and fosfomycin in critically ill patients. Int J Antimicrob Agents. 2003;21:562–7.

Zeitlinger MA, Sauermann R, Traunmüller, Geogopoulous A, Müller M, Joukhadar C. Impact of plasma protein binding on antimicrobial activity using time-killing curves. J Antimicrob Chemother. 2004;54:876–80.

Dosage Adjustment of Medications Eliminated by the Kidneys

Fosfomycin/Monurol®	{Antibacterial; phosphonic acid derivative}
Usual initial dose:	3 g (one sachet) orally dissolved in cool or tepid (not hot) water
Usual maintenance dose:	None (usual ℞ for uncomplicated cystitis is single-dose treatment)
Typical maximum dose:	400 mg/kg/day (for serious systemic infections)
Proportion eliminated unchanged:	38 % (may vary from 11 to 80 % depending on route of administration and GFR)

Adjustment for Kidney Disease

FDA-approved product labeling:	*Renal insufficiency*	*No dosage adjustment is necessary in the elderly (single-dose treatment).*
		In patients with varying degrees of renal impairment (CrCL varying from 55 to 7 mL/min), the half-life of fosfomycin increased from 11 to 50 h. The half-life of fosfomycin during hemodialysis was 40 h.
Alternative adjustment:	*GFR <60 mL/min*	*3 g orally ×1 (no dose adjustment is necessary for single-dose treatment of uncomplicated cystitis with any level of kidney disease)*
	CrCL >80 mL/min	*2–8 g IV every 6–8 h*
	CrCL 40–79 mL/min	*2–4 IV every 12 h*
	CrCL 20–39 mL/min	*2–4 g IV followed by 2–4 g IV every 8 h*
	CrCL 5–19 mL/min	*2–4 g IV followed by 1–2 g IV every 12 h*
	CrCL <5 mL/min	*2–4 g IV followed by 1–2 g IV every 24 h*
	Hemodialysis	*2–4 g IV followed by 1–2 g IV after hemodialysis on dialysis days*
	CAPD	*4 g instilled intraperitoneally with a prolonged dwell ×1 followed by 1 g intraperitoneally every 48 h*
	CVVH	*8 g IV every 12 h*

Note: Parenteral dosage forms of fosfomycin (disodium fosfomycin injection) presently are not commercially available in North America. These are being selectively investigated and used in Europe and elsewhere for serious systemic bacterial infections.

G

L.K. Golightly et al. (eds.), *Renal Pharmacotherapy*,
DOI 10.1007/978-1-4614-5800-5_7, © Springer Science+Business Media New York 2013

Dosage Adjustment of Medications Eliminated by the Kidneys

Gabapentin - Selected References

Aronoff GA, Bennett WM, Berns JS, et al. Drug prescribing in renal failure: dosing guidelines for adults and children. 5th ed. Philadelphia: American College of Physicians; 2007.

Backonja MM, Beydoun A, Edwards KR, et al. Gabapentin for the symptomatic treatment of painful neuropathy in patients with diabetes mellitus: a randomized controlled trial. JAMA. 1998;280:1831–6.

Backonja MM, Canafax SM, Cundy KC. Efficacy of gabapentin enacarbil vs placebo in patients with postherpetic neuralgia and a pharmacokinetic comparison with oral gabapentin. Pain Med. 2011;12(7):1098–108. doi:10.1111/j.1526-4637.2011.01139.x.

Beydoun A, Fischer J, Labar DR, et al. Gabapentin monotherapy: II. A 26-week, double-blind, dose-controlled, multicenter study of conversion from polytherapy in outpatients with refractory complex partial or secondarily generalized seizures. Neurology. 1997;49:746–52.

Blum RA, Comstock TJ, Sica DA, et al. Pharmacokinetics of gabapentin in subjects with various degrees of renal function. Clin Pharmacol Ther. 1994;56:154–9.

Boyd RA, Türck D, Abel RB, Sedman AJ, Bockbrader HN. Effects of age and gender on single-dose pharmacokinetics of gabapentin. Epilepsia. 1999;40:474–9.

Comstock TI, Sica DA, Bockbrader HN, Underwood BA, Sedman AJ. Gabapentin pharmacokinetics in subjects with various degrees of renal function [abstract]. J Clin Pharmacol. 1990;30:862.

Cundy KC, Sastry S, Luo W, et al. Clinical pharmacokinetics of XP13512, a novel transported prodrug of gabapentin. J Clin Pharmacol. 2008;48:1378–88.

Fisher RS, Sachdeo RC, Pellock J, Penovich PE, Magnus L, Bernstein P. Rapid initiation of gabapentin: a randomized, controlled trial. Neurology. 2001;56:743–8.

Goa KL, Sorkin EM. Gabapentin: a review of its pharmacological properties and clinical potential in epilepsy. Drugs. 1993;46:409–27.

Grunze H, Dittert S, Bungert M, Erfurth A. Renal impairment as a possible side effect of gabapentin: a single case report. Neuropsychobiology. 1998;38:198–9.

Hanlon JT, Aspinall SL, Semla TP, et al. Consensus guidelines for oral dosing of primarily renally cleared medications in older adults. J Am Geriatr Soc. 2009;57:335–40.

Horizant® tablet [package insert]. Research Triangle Park: GlaxoSmithKline; 2011.

McLean MJ. Clinical pharmacokinetics of gabapentin. Neurology. 1994;44(Suppl 5):S17–22.

Miller A, Price G. Gabapentin toxicity in renal failure: the importance of dose adjustment. Pain Med. 2009;10:190–2.

Muscas GC, ChiroliS, Luceri F, Del Mastio M, Balestrieri F, Arnetoli G. Conversion from thrice daily to twice daily ad-ministration of gabapentin (GBP) in partial epilepsy: analysis of clinical efficacy and plasma levels. Seizure. 2000;9:47–50.

Neurontin® capsule and suspension [package insert]. New York: Parke-Davis Division of Pfizer Inc; 2011.

Olson WL, Gruenthal M, Mueller ME, Olson WH. Gabapentin for parkinsonism: a double-blind, placebo-controlled, cross-over trial. Am J Med. 1997;102:60–6.

Oommen K, Penry J, Riela A, et al. Gabapentin as add-on therapy in refractory partial epilepsy: a double-blind, placebo-controlled, parallel-group study. Neurology. 1993;43:2292–8.

Pierce DA, Holt SR, Reeves-Daniel A. A probable case of gabapentin-related reversible hearing loss in a patient with acute renal failure. Clin Ther. 2008;30:1681–4.

Rowbotham M, Harden N, Stacey B, Bernstein P, Magnus-Miller L. Gabapentin for the treatment of postherpetic neuralgia: a randomized controlled trial. JAMA. 1998;280:1837–42.

Singh D, Kennedy DH. The use of gabapentin for the treatment of postherpetic neuralgia. Clin Ther. 2003;25:852–89.

Taylor CP. Emerging perspectives on the mechanism of action of gabapentin. Neurology. 1994;44(Suppl 5):S10–6.

Vollmer KO, Türck D, Bockbrader HN, et al. Summary of Neurontin (gabapentin) clinical pharmacokinetics [abstract]. Epilepsia. 1992;33(Suppl 3):77.

Wong MO, Eldon MA, Keane WF, et al. Disposition of gabapentin in anuric subjects on hemodialysis. J Clin Pharmacol. 1995;35:922–6.

Zand L, McKian KP, Qian Q. Gabapentin toxicity in patients with chronic kidney disease: a preventable cause of morbidity. Am J Med. 2010;123:367–73.

Dosage Adjustment of Medications Eliminated by the Kidneys

<u>Gabapentin</u>/Neurontin®   {Antiepileptic; adjunctive analgesic}

Usual initial dose: 100 mg orally

Usual maintenance dose: 300–600 mg orally three times daily

Typical maximum dose: 3,600 mg/day

Proportion eliminated unchanged: 80 %

Adjustment for Kidney Disease

    FDA-approved product labeling: *CrCL ≥60 mL/min*   *600 mg sustained-release orally every evening*

                                                   CrCL 30–59 mL/min   *600 mg sustained-release orally every 48 h*

                                                   CrCL <30 mL/min   *Sustained-release tablets (600 mg) not recommended (℞ for restless legs)*

Gabapentin dosage based on renal function

CrCL (mL/min)	Total daily dose (mg/day)	Dose regimen (mg)				
≥60	900–3,600	300 mg three times daily	400 mg three times daily	600 mg three times daily	800 mg three times daily	1,200 mg three times daily
>30–59	400–1,400	200 mg twice daily	300 mg twice daily	400 mg twice daily	500 mg twice daily	700 mg twice daily
>15–29	200–700	200 mg every day	300 mg every day	400 mg every day	500 mg every day	700 mg every day
<15	100–300	100 mg once daily	125 mg once daily	150 mg once daily	200 mg once daily	300 mg once daily
		Post-hemodialysis supplemental dose (mg)				
Hemodialysis[a]		125	150	200	250	350

[a]For patients on hemodialysis, the maintenance dose should be based upon the estimates of CrCL as indicated in the upper portion of the table under <15 mL/min and a supplemental post-hemodialysis dose administered after each 4 h of hemodialysis as indicated in the lower portion of the table

    Alternative adjustment: *GFR ≥60 mL/min*   *300–1,200 mg enterally every 8 h*

                                              GFR 30–59 mL/min   *600 mg enterally every 12 h*

                                              GFR 10–29 mL/min   *200–600 mg enterally every 24 h*

                                              GFR <10 mL/min   *100 mg enterally every 24 h*

                                              Hemodialysis   *100 mg enterally every 24 h or 200–300 mg enterally after hemodialysis on dialysis days only*

                                              CAPD   *300 mg enterally every 48 h*

                                              CRRT   *300 mg enterally every 12–24 h*

Gadobenate - Selected References

Altun E, Martin DR, Wertman R, Lugo-Somolinos A, Fuller ER III, Semelka RC. Nephrogenic systemic fibrosis: change in incidence following a switch in gadolinium agents and adoption of a gadolinium policy—report from two US universities. Radiology. 2009;253:689–96.

Broome DR. Nephrogenic systemic fibrosis associated with gadolinium based contrast agents: a summary of the medical literature reporting. Eur J Radiol. 2008;66:230–4.

Johnson DBS, Lerner CA, Prince MR, et al. Gadolinium-enhanced magnetic resonance angiography of renal transplants. Magn Reson Imaging. 1997;15:13–20.

MultiHance™ injection [package insert]. Princeton: Bracco Diagnostics Inc; 2008.

Newton BB, Jimenez SA. Mechanism of NSF: new evidence challenging the prevailing theory. J Magn Reson Imaging. 2009;30:1277–83.

Penfield JG, Reilly RF. Nephrogenic systemic fibrosis: is there a difference between gadolinium-based contrast agents? Semin Dial. 2008;21:129–34.

Shellock FG, Parker JR, Venetianer C, Pirovano G, Spinazzi A. Safety of gadobenate dimeglumine (MultiHance): summary of findings from clinical studies and postmarketing surveillance. Invest Radiol. 2006;41:500–9.

Thomsen HS. How to avoid nephrogenic systemic fibrosis: current guidelines in Europe and the United States. Radiol Clin North Am. 2009;47:871–5.

Dosage Adjustment of Medications Eliminated by the Kidneys

Gadobenate/MultiHance™	{**Gadolinium-based contrast agent**}

Usual initial dose:	0.2 mL/kg (0.1 mmol/kg) administered as a rapid bolus IV injection
Usual maintenance dose:	N/A
Typical maximum dose:	0.2 mL/kg (0.1 mmol/kg)
Proportion eliminated unchanged:	78–96 %

Adjustment for Kidney Disease

FDA-approved product labeling:	*GFR ≥30 mL/min/1.73 m²*	*0.2 mL/kg (0.1 mmol/kg) IV*
	GFR <30 mL/min/1.73 m²	*0.2 mL/kg (0.1 mmol/kg) IV; in patients with renal insufficiency, acute renal failure requiring dialysis or worsening renal function has occurred, mostly within 48 h after injection. The risk of these events is higher with increasing doses of contrast. Use the lowest possible dose and evaluate renal function in patients with renal insufficiency.*
Alternative adjustment:	*GFR ≥30 mL/min*	*0.2 mL/kg (0.1 mmol/kg) IV*
	GFR <30 mL/min	*Although it is unclear whether gadobenate has been causally implicated in cases of nephrogenic systemic fibrosis (NSF, a debilitating and potentially life-threatening disease characterized by progressive tissue deposition of collagen and fibroblasts affecting the skin, internal organs, and muscles), its use generally should be **avoided** unless gadolinium-based contrast agent diagnostic information is absolutely essential and not available using non-contrast enhanced magnetic resonance imaging (MRI) or other techniques.*

Dosage Adjustment of Medications Eliminated by the Kidneys

Gadodiamide - Selected References

Agarwal R, Brunelli SM, Williams K, Mitchell MD, Feldman HI, Umscheid CA. Gadolinium-based contrast agents and nephrogenic systemic fibrosis: a systematic review and meta-analysis. Nephrol Dial Transplant. 2009;24:856–63.

Altun E, Martin DR, Wertman R, Lugo-Somolinos A, Fuller ER III, Semelka RC. Nephrogenic systemic fibrosis: change in incidence following a switch in gadolinium agents and adoption of a gadolinium policy—report from two US universities. Radiology. 2009;253:689–96.

Bridges MD, St Amant BS, McNeil RB, Cernigliaro JG, Dwyer JP, Fitzpatrick PM. High-dose gadodiamide for catheter angiography and CT in patients with varying degrees of renal insufficiency: prevalence of subsequent nephrogenic systemic fibrosis and decline in renal function. AJR Am J Roentgenol. 2009;192:1538–43.

Broome DR. Nephrogenic systemic fibrosis associated with gadolinium based contrast agents: a summary of the medical literature reporting. Eur J Radiol. 2008;66:230–4.

Harpur ES, Worah D, Hals P-A, Holtz E, Furuhama K, Nomura H. Preclinical safety assessment and pharmacokinetics of gadodiamide injection, a new magnetic resonance imaging contrast agent. Invest Radiol. 1993;28(Suppl 1):S28–43.

Hoppe H, Spagnuolo S, Froelich JM, et al. Retrospective analysis of patients for development of nephrogenic systemic fibrosis following conventional angiography using gadolinium-based contrast agents. Eur Radiol. 2010;20:595–603.

Johnson DBS, Lerner CA, Prince MR, et al. Gadolinium-enhanced magnetic resonance angiography of renal transplants. Magn Reson Imaging. 1997;15:13–20.

Kallen AJ, Jhung MA, Cheng S, et al. Gadolinium-containing magnetic resonance imaging contrast and nephrogenic systemic fibrosis: a case-control study. Am J Kidney Dis. 2008;51:966–75.

Kane GC, Stanson AW, Kalnicka D, et al. Comparison between gadolinium and iodine contrast for percutaneous intervention in atherosclerotic renal artery stenosis: clinical outcomes. Nephrol Dial Transplant. 2008;23:1233–40.

Kendrick-Jones JC, Voss DM, de Zoysa JR. Nephrogenic systemic fibrosis, in patients with end-state kidney disease on dialysis, in the greater Auckland region, from 2000-2006. Nephrology (Carlton). 2011;16:243–8.

Marckmann P, Nielsen AH, Sloth JJ. Possibly enhanced Gd excretion in dialysate, but no major clinical benefit of 3-5 months of treatment with sodium thiosulfate in late stages of nephrogenic systemic fibrosis. Nephrol Dial Transplant. 2008;23:3280–2.

Newton BB, Jimenez SA. Mechanism of NSF: new evidence challenging the prevailing theory. J Magn Reson Imaging. 2009;30:1277–83.

Omniscan™ injection [package insert]. Princeton: GE Healthcare Inc; 2010.

Penfield JG, Reilly RF. Nephrogenic systemic fibrosis: is there a difference between gadolinium-based contrast agents? Semin Dial. 2008;21:129–34.

Scheitinger BJ, Brammer GM, Wang H, et al. Patterns of late gadolinium enhancement in chronic hemodialysis patients. JACC Cardiovasc Imaging. 2008;1:450–6.

Sieber MA, Lengsfeld P, Walter J, et al. Gadolinium-based contrast agents and their potential role in the pathogenesis of nephrogenic systemic fibrosis: the role of excess ligand. J Magn Reson Imaging. 2008;27:955–62.

Steger-Hartmann T, Raschke M, Riefke B, Pietsch H, Sieber MA, Walter J. The involvement of pro-inflammatory cytokines in nephrogenic systemic fibrosis—a mechanistic hypothesis based on preclinical results from a rat model treated with gadodiamide. Exp Toxicol Pathol. 2009;61:537–52.

Thomsen HS. How to avoid nephrogenic systemic fibrosis: current guidelines in Europe and the United States. Radiol Clin North Am. 2009;47:871–5.

Wertman R, Altun E, Martin DR, et al. Risk of nephrogenic systemic fibrosis: evaluation of gadolinium chelate contrast agents at four American universities. Radiology. 2008;248:799–806.

Dosage Adjustment of Medications Eliminated by the Kidneys

__Gadodiamide__/Omniscan™	__{Gadolinium-based contrast agent}__

__Usual initial dose:__	Kidney—0.1 mL/kg (0.05 mmol/kg) as a bolus IV injection
	CNS, intrathoracic, intra-abdominal, and pelvic cavities—0.2 mL/kg (0.1 mmol/kg) IV
__Usual maintenance dose:__	N/A
__Typical maximum dose:__	0.2 mL/kg (0.1 mmol/kg)
__Proportion eliminated unchanged:__	95 %

Adjustment for Kidney Disease

__FDA-approved product labeling:__	*GFR ≥30 mL/min*	*0.1–0.2 mL/kg IV*
	GFR <30 mL/min	*0.1–0.2 mL/kg IV. In patients with renal insufficiency, acute renal failure requiring dialysis or worsening renal function has occurred, mostly within 48 h after gadopentetate injection. The risk of these events is higher with increasing doses of contrast. Use the lowest possible dose and evaluate renal function in patients with renal insufficiency.*
__Alternative adjustment:__	*GFR ≥30 mL/min*	*0.1–0.2 mL/kg IV*
	GFR <30 mL/min	*Not recommended; preferably avoid. Gadodiamide has been reported in most pharmacodynamic investigations, systematic reviews, cohort studies, and large case series to be associated with a comparatively high incidence of nephrogenic systemic fibrosis (NSF, a debilitating and potentially life-threatening disease characterized by progressive tissue deposition of collagen and fibroblasts affecting the skin, internal organs, and muscles). Its use has been clearly associated with this condition, and it therefore must be avoided unless gadolinium-based contrast agent diagnostic information is absolutely essential and not available using non-contrast enhanced magnetic resonance imaging (MRI) or other techniques.*

Gadopentetate - Selected References

Abujudeh HH, Kaewlai R, KIagan A, et al. Nephrogenic systemic fibrosis after gadopentetate dimeglumine exposure: case series of 36 patients. Radiology. 2009;253:81–9.

Agarwal R, Brunelli SM, Williams K, Mitchell MD, Feldman HI, Umscheid CA. Gadolinium-based contrast agents and nephrogenic systemic fibrosis: a systematic review and meta-analysis. Nephrol Dial Transplant. 2009;24:856–63.

Aime S, Caravan P. Biodistribution of gadolinium-based contrast agents, including gadolinium deposition. J Magn Reson Imaging. 2009;30:1259–67.

Altun E, Martin DR, Wertman R, Lugo-Somolinos A, Fuller ER III, Semelka RC. Nephrogenic systemic fibrosis: change in incidence following a switch in gadolinium agents and adoption of a gadolinium policy—report from two US universities. Radiology. 2009;253:689–96.

Broome DR. Nephrogenic systemic fibrosis associated with gadolinium based contrast agents: a summary of the medical literature reporting. Eur J Radiol. 2008;66:230–4.

Chrysochou C, Power A, Shurrab AE, et al. Low risk for Nephrogenic systemic fibrosis in nondialysis patients who have chronic kidney disease and are investigated with gadolinium-enhanced magnetic resonance imaging. Clin J Am Soc Nephrol. 2010;5:484–9.

Hoffman U, Fischereder M, Reil A, Fischer M, Link J, Krämer BK. Renal effects of gadopentetate dimeglumine in patients with normal and impaired renal function. Eur J Med Res. 2005;10:149–54.

Hoppe H, Spagnuolo S, Froelich JM, et al. Retrospective analysis of patients for development of nephrogenic systemic fibrosis following conventional angiography using gadolinium-based contrast agents. Eur Radiol. 2010;20:595–603.

Janus N, Launay-Vacher V, Karie S, et al. Prevalence of nephrogenic systemic fibrosis in renal insufficiency patients: results of the FINEST study. Eur J Radiol. 2010;73:357–9.

Johnson DBS, Lerner CA, Prince MR, et al. Gadolinium-enhanced magnetic resonance angiography of renal transplants. Magn Reson Imaging. 1997;15:13–20.

Magnevist® injection [package insert]. Wayne: Bayer HealthCare Pharmaceuticals Inc; 2010.

Nakai K, Takeda K, Kimura H, Miura S, Maeda A. Nephrogenic systemic fibrosis in a patient on long-term hemodialysis. Clin Nephrol. 2009;71:217–20.

Newton BB, Jimenez SA. Mechanism of NSF: new evidence challenging the prevailing theory. J Magn Reson Imaging. 2009;30:1277–83.

Penfield JG, Reilly RF. Nephrogenic systemic fibrosis: is there a difference between gadolinium-based contrast agents? Semin Dial. 2008;21:129–34.

Rieger J, Sitter T, Toepfer M, Linsenmaier U, Pfeifer KJ, Schiffl H. Gadolinium as an alternative contrast agent for diagnostic and interventional angiographic procedures in patients with impaired renal function. Nephrol Dial Transplant. 2002;17:824–8.

Rofsky NM, Weinreb JC, Bosniak MA, Libes RB, Birnbaum BA. Renal lesion characterization with gadolinium-enhanced MR imaging: efficacy and safety in patients with renal insufficiency. Radiology. 1991;180:85–9.

Scheitinger BJ, Brammer GM, Wang H, et al. Patterns of late gadolinium enhancement in chronic hemodialysis patients. JACC Cardiovasc Imaging. 2008;1:450–6.

Schuhmann-Giampieri G, Krestin G. Pharmacokinetics of Gd-DPTA in patients with chronic renal failure. Invest Radiol. 1991;26:975–9.

Thomsen HS. How to avoid nephrogenic systemic fibrosis: current guidelines in Europe and the United States. Radiol Clin North Am. 2009;47:871–5.

Wertman R, Altun E, Martin DR, et al. Risk of nephrogenic systemic fibrosis: evaluation of gadolinium chelate contrast agents at four American universities. Radiology. 2008;248:799–806.

Dosage Adjustment of Medications Eliminated by the Kidneys

Gadopentetate/Magnevist®　　　{Gadolinium-based contrast agent}

Usual initial dose:	0.2 mL/kg (0.1 mmol/kg) IV at a rate not to exceed 10 mL/15 s
Usual maintenance dose:	N/A
Typical maximum dose:	0.1 mmol/kg
Proportion eliminated unchanged:	92 %

Adjustment for Kidney Disease

FDA-approved product labeling:	*GFR ≥30 mL/min/1.73 m²*	*0.1 mmol/kg (0.2 mL/kg) IV; in patients with renal insufficiency, acute renal failure requiring dialysis or worsening renal function has occurred, mostly within 48 h after gadopentetate injection. The risk of these events is higher with increasing doses of contrast. Use the lowest possible dose and evaluate renal function in patients with renal insufficiency.*
	GFR <30 mL/min/1.73 m²	*Contraindicated*
Alternative adjustment:	*GFR ≥30 mL/min/1.73 m²*	*0.1 mmol/kg (0.2 mL/kg) IV*
	GFR <30 mL/min/1.73 m² and patients with acute kidney injury of any severity due to hepatorenal syndrome or in the perioperative liver transplant period	*Not recommended; preferably avoid. Although gadopentetate has been reported in systematic reviews, cohort studies, and large case series to be associated with a comparatively modest incidence of nephrogenic systemic fibrosis (NSF, a debilitating and potentially life-threatening disease characterized by progressive tissue deposition of collagen and fibroblasts affecting the skin, internal organs, and muscles), this condition has occurred with administration of this agent, and its use therefore must be avoided unless gadolinium-based contrast agent diagnostic information is absolutely essential and not available using non-contrast enhanced magnetic resonance imaging (MRI) or other techniques.*

Gadoteridol - Selected References

Broome DR. Nephrogenic systemic fibrosis associated with gadolinium based contrast agents: a summary of the medical literature reporting. Eur J Radiol. 2008;66:230–4.

Gemery J, Idelson B, Reid S, et al. Acute renal failure after arteriography with a gadolinium-based contrast agent. AJR Am J Roentgenol. 1998;171:1277–8.

Janus N, Launay-Vacher V, Karie S, et al. Prevalence of nephrogenic systemic fibrosis in renal insufficiency patients: results of the FINEST study. Eur J Radiol. 2010;73:357–9.

Johnson DBS, Lerner CA, Prince MR, et al. Gadolinium-enhanced magnetic resonance angiography of renal transplants. Magn Reson Imaging. 1997;15:13–20.

Kane GC, Stanson AW, Kalnicka D, et al. Comparison between gadolinium and iodine contrast for percutaneous intervention in atherosclerotic renal artery stenosis: clinical outcomes. Nephrol Dial Transplant. 2008;23:1233–40.

Newton BB, Jimenez SA. Mechanism of NSF: new evidence challenging the prevailing theory. J Magn Reson Imaging. 2009;30:1277–83.

Penfield JG, Reilly RF. Nephrogenic systemic fibrosis: is there a difference between gadolinium-based contrast agents? Semin Dial. 2008;21:129–34.

Perazella MA. How should nephrologists approach gadolinium-based contrast imaging in patients with kidney disease? [editorial]. Clin J Am Soc Nephrol. 3:649–51.

ProHance® injection [package insert]. Princeton: Bracco Diagnostics Inc; 2007.

Reilly RF. Risk for nephrogenic systemic fibrosis with gadoteridol (ProHance) in patients who are on long-term hemodialysis. Clin J Am Soc Nephrol. 2008;3:747–51.

Thomsen HS. How to avoid nephrogenic systemic fibrosis: current guidelines in Europe and the United States. Radiol Clin North Am. 2009;47:871–5.

Dosage Adjustment of Medications Eliminated by the Kidneys

Gadoteridol/ProHance® {Gadolinium-based contrast agent}

Usual initial dose: 0.2 mL/kg (0.1 mmol/kg) IV as a rapid bolus (>60 mL/min) or infusion (10–60 mL/min)

Usual maintenance dose: In the presence of negative or equivocal scans and in patients suspected of having poorly enhancing lesions, a second dose of 0.4 mL/kg (0.2 mmol/kg) may be given up to 30 min after the first dose

Typical maximum dose: 0.4 mL/kg (0.2 mmol/kg)

Proportion eliminated unchanged: 98 %

Adjustment for Kidney Disease

FDA-approved product labeling:	*GFR ≥30 mL/min*	*0.2 mL/kg (0.1 mmol/kg) IV as a rapid bolus (>60 mL/min) or infusion (10–60 mL/min)*
	GFR <30 mL/min	*0.2 mL/kg (0.1 mmol/kg) IV as a rapid bolus (>60 mL/min) or infusion (10–60 mL/min)*
Alternative adjustment:	*GFR ≥30 mL/min*	*0.2 mL/kg (0.1 mmol/kg) IV as a rapid bolus (>60 mL/min) or infusion (10–60 mL/min)*
	GFR <30 mL/min/1.73 m² and patients with acute kidney injury of any severity due to hepatorenal syndrome or in the perioperative liver transplant period	*Although gadoteridol has been reported in most pharmacodynamic investigations, systematic reviews, cohort studies, and large case series to be associated with a comparatively modest incidence of nephrogenic systemic fibrosis (NSF, a debilitating and potentially life-threatening disease characterized by progressive tissue deposition of collagen and fibroblasts affecting the skin, internal organs, and muscles), its use has been associated with this condition, and it therefore must be avoided unless gadolinium-based contrast agent diagnostic information is absolutely essential and not available using non-contrast enhanced magnetic resonance imaging (MRI) or other techniques.*

Gadoversetamide - Selected References

Broome DR. Nephrogenic systemic fibrosis associated with gadolinium based contrast agents: a summary of the medical literature reporting. Eur J Radiol. 2008;66:230–4.

Johnson DBS, Lerner CA, Prince MR, et al. Gadolinium-enhanced magnetic resonance angiography of renal transplants. Magn Reson Imaging. 1997;15:13–20.

Kadiyala D, Roer DA, Perazella MA. Nephrogenic systemic fibrosis associated with gadoversetamide exposure: treatment with sodium thiosulfate. Am J Kidney Dis. 2009;53:133–7.

Kallen AJ, Jhung MA, Cheng S, et al. Gadolinium-containing magnetic resonance imaging contrast and nephrogenic systemic fibrosis: a case-control study. Am J Kidney Dis. 2008;51:966–75.

Newton BB, Jimenez SA. Mechanism of NSF: new evidence challenging the prevailing theory. J Magn Reson Imaging. 2009;30:1277–83.

OptiMARK™ injection [package insert]. St Louis: Mallinckrodt Inc; 2010.

Penfield JG, Reilly RF. Nephrogenic systemic fibrosis: is there a difference between gadolinium-based contrast agents? Semin Dial. 2008;21:129–34.

Sieber MA, Lengsfeld P, Walter J, et al. Gadolinium-based contrast agents and their potential role in the pathogenesis of nephrogenic systemic fibrosis: the role of excess ligand. J Magn Reson Imaging. 2008;27:955–62.

Thomsen HS. How to avoid nephrogenic systemic fibrosis: current guidelines in Europe and the United States. Radiol Clin North Am. 2009;47:871–5.

Dosage Adjustment of Medications Eliminated by the Kidneys

<u>Gadoversetamide</u>/OptiMARK™   {Gadolinium-based contrast agent}

Usual initial dose: 0.2 mL/kg (0.1 mmol/kg) IV at a rate of 1–2 mL/s

Usual maintenance dose: N/A

Typical maximum dose: 0.2 mL/kg (0.1 mmol/kg)

Proportion eliminated unchanged: 96 %

Adjustment for Kidney Disease

FDA-approved product labeling:	*GFR ≥30 mL/min/1.73 m²*	*0.2 mL/kg (0.1 mmol/kg) IV; in patients with renal insufficiency, acute renal failure requiring dialysis or worsening renal function has occurred, mostly within 48 h after gadoversetamide injection. The risk of these events is higher with increasing doses of contrast. Use the lowest possible dose and evaluate renal function in patients with renal insufficiency.*
	GFR <30 mL/min/1.73 m²	*Contraindicated*
Alternative adjustment:	*GFR ≥30 mL/min*	*0.2 mL/kg (0.1 mmol/kg) IV*
	GFR <30 mL/min	*Not recommended; preferably avoid. Although gadoversetamide has been reported in most pharmacodynamic investigations, systematic reviews, cohort studies, and large case series to be associated with a comparatively modest incidence of nephrogenic systemic fibrosis (NSF, a debilitating and potentially life-threatening disease characterized by progressive tissue deposition of collagen and fibroblasts affecting the skin, internal organs, and muscles), its use has been associated with this condition, and it therefore must be avoided unless gadolinium-based contrast agent diagnostic information is absolutely essential and not available using non-contrast enhanced magnetic resonance imaging (MRI) or other techniques.*

Gadoxetate - Selected References

Bluemke DA, Sahani D, Amendola M, et al. Efficacy and safety of MR imaging with liver-specific contrast agent; US multicenter phase III study. Radiology. 2005;237:89–98.

Bollow M, Taupitz M, Hamm B, Staks T, Wolf KJ, Weinmann HJ. Gadolinium-ethoxybenzyl-DTPA as a hepatobiliary contrast agent for use in MR cholangiography: results of an in vivo phase-I clinical investigation. Eur Radiol. 1997;7:126–32.

Broome DR. Nephrogenic systemic fibrosis associated with gadolinium based contrast agents: a summary of the medical literature reporting. Eur J Radiol. 2008;66:230–4.

Cheng KT. Gadoxetate. Molecular Imaging and Contrast Agent Database (MICAD). Bethesda: National Center for Biotechnology Information (US); 2008.

Cruite I, Schreder M, Merkle EM, Sirlin CB. Gadoxetate sodium-enhanced MRI of the liver: part 2, protocol optimization and lesion appearance in the cirrhotic liver. AJR Am J Roentgenol. 2010;195:29–41.

Eovist® injection [package insert]. Wayne: Bayer HealthCare Pharmaceuticals Inc; 2010.

Johnson DBS, Lerner CA, Prince MR, et al. Gadolinium-enhanced magnetic resonance angiography of renal transplants. Magn Reson Imaging. 1997;15:13–20.

Marin D, Bova V, Agnello F, Youngblood R, Midiri M, Brancatelli G. Gadoxetate disodium-enhanced magnetic resonance cholangiography for the noninvasive detection of an active bile leak after laparoscopic cholecystectomy. J Comput Assist Tomogr. 2010;34:213–6.

Newton BB, Jimenez SA. Mechanism of NSF: new evidence challenging the prevailing theory. J Magn Reson Imaging. 2009;30:1277–83.

Penfield JG, Reilly RF. Nephrogenic systemic fibrosis: is there a difference between gadolinium-based contrast agents? Semin Dial. 2008;21:129–34.

Ringe KI, Husrik DB, Sirlin CB, Merkle EM. Gadoxetate sodium-enhanced MRI of the liver: part 1, protocol optimization and lesion appearance in the noncirrhotic liver. AJR Am J Roentgenol. 2010;195:13–28.

Schuhmann-Giampieri G, Frenzel T, Schmitt-Willich H. Pharmacokinetics in rats, dogs and monkeys of a gadolinium chelate used as a liver-specific agent for magnetic resonance imaging. Arzneimittelforschung. 1993;43:927–31.

Schuhmann-Giampieri G, Mahler M, Röll G, Maibauer R, Schmitz S. Pharmacokinetics of the liver-specific contrast agent Gd-EOB-DTPA in relation to contrast-enhanced liver imaging in humans. J Clin Pharmacol. 1997;37:587–96.

Thomsen HS. How to avoid nephrogenic systemic fibrosis: current guidelines in Europe and the United States. Radiol Clin North Am. 2009;47:871–5.

Van Montfoort JE, Stieger B, Meijer DKF, Weinmann H-J, Meier PJ, Fattinger KE. Hepatic uptake of the magnetic resonance contrast agent gadoxetate by the organic anion transporting polypeptide OATP1. J Pharmacol Exp Ther. 1999;290:153–7.

Dosage Adjustment of Medications Eliminated by the Kidneys

<u>Gadoxetate</u>/Eovist®	{Gadolinium-based contrast agent}
Usual initial dose:	0.1 mL/kg (0.025 mmol/kg) IV at a flow rate of 2 mL/s
Usual maintenance dose:	N/A
Typical maximum dose:	0.1 mL/kg
Proportion eliminated unchanged:	44–59 %

Adjustment for Kidney Disease

FDA-approved product labeling: *GFR ≥30 mL/min/1.73 m²* *0.1 mL/kg IV*

GFR <30 mL/min/1.73 m² *0.1 mL/kg IV. Warning: Gadolinium-based contrast agents (GBCAs) increase the risk for nephrogenic systemic fibrosis (NSF) among patients with impaired elimination of the drugs. The risk for NSF appears to be highest among patients with chronic severe kidney disease (GFR <30 mL/min/1.73 m²) or acute kidney injury. For patients at risk for chronically reduced renal function (e.g., age >60 years, hypertension, or diabetes), estimate the glomerular filtration rate (GFR) through laboratory testing. For patients at highest risk for NSF, do not exceed the recommended dose and allow a sufficient period of time for elimination of the drug from the body prior to re-administration.*

Alternative adjustment: *GFR ≥30 mL/min* *0.1 mL/kg IV*

GFR <30 mL/min and/or acute kidney injury of any severity due to hepatorenal syndrome or in the perioperative liver transplant period *Although it is unclear whether gadoxetate has been causally implicated with nephrogenic systemic fibrosis (NSF, a debilitating and potentially life-threatening disease characterized by progressive tissue deposition of collagen and fibroblasts affecting the skin, internal organs, and muscles), its use should be avoided unless gadolinium-based contrast agent diagnostic information is absolutely essential and not available using non-contrast enhanced magnetic resonance imaging (MRI) or other techniques.*

Galantamine - Selected References

Bickel U, Thomsen T, Weber W, et al. Pharmacokinetics of galanthamine in humans and corresponding cholinesterase inhibition. Clin Pharmacol Ther. 1991;50:420–8.

Di Stefano A, Iannitelli A, Laserra S, Sozio P. Drug delivery strategies for Alzheimer's disease treatment. Expert Opin Drug Deliv. 2011;8:581–603.

Farlow MR. Clinical pharmacokinetics of galantamine. Clin Pharmacokinet. 2003;42:1383–92.

Grossberg GT, Edwards KR, Zhao Q. Rationale for combination therapy with galantamine and memantine in Alzheimer's disease. J Clin Pharmacol. 2006;46(7 Suppl 1):17S–26S.

Huang F, Fu Y. A review of clinical pharmacokinetics and pharmacodynamics of galantamine, a reversible acetylcholinesterase inhibitor for the treatment of Alzheimer's disease, in healthy subjects and patients. Curr Clin Pharmacol. 2010;5:115–24.

Huang F, Lasseter KC, Janssens L, Verhaeghe T, Lau H, Zhao Q. Pharmacokinetic and safety assessments of galantamine and risperidone after the two drugs are administered alone and together. J Clin Pharmacol. 2002;42:1341–51.

Maelicke A. Pharmacokinetic rationale for switching from donepezil to galantamine. Clin Ther. 2001;23(Suppl A):A8–12.

Mihailova D, Yamboliev I, Zhivkova A, Tehcheva J, Jonovich V. Pharmacokinetics of galanthamine hydrobromide after single subcutaneous and oral dosage in humans. Pharmacology. 1989;39:50–8.

Piotrovsky V, Van Peer A, Van Osselaer N, Armstrong M, Aerssens J. Galantamine population pharmacokinetics in patients with Alzheimer's disease: modeling and simulations. J Clin Pharmacol. 2003;43:514–23.

Razadyne® capsule extended release, solution, and tablet film coated [package insert]. Titusville: Ortho-McNeil Neurologics Inc Division of Ortho-McNeil-Janssen Pharmaceuticals Inc; 2010.

Scott LJ, Goa KL. Galantamine: a review of its use in Alzheimer's disease. Drugs. 2000;60:1095–122.

Wilcock G, Howe I, Coles H, et al. A long-term comparison of galantamine and donepezil in the treatment of Alzheimer's disease. Drugs Aging. 2003;20:777–89.

Zhang LJ, Fang XL, Li XN, et al. Pharmacokinetics and bioequivalence studies of galantamine hydrobromide dispersible tablet in healthy male Chinese volunteers. Drug Dev Ind Pharm. 2007;33:335–40.

Zhao Q, Brett M, Van Osselaer N, et al. Galantamine pharmacokinetics, safety, and tolerability profiles are similar in healthy Caucasian and Japanese subjects. J Clin Pharmacol. 2002;42:1002–10.

Zhao Q, Janssens L, Verhaeghe T, Brashear HR, Truyen L. Pharmacokinetics of extended-release and immediate-release formulations of galantamine at steady state in healthy volunteers. Curr Med Res Opin. 2005;21:1547–54.

Dosage Adjustment of Medications Eliminated by the Kidneys

<u>Galantamine</u>/Razadyne®	{Reversible competitive acetylcholinesterase inhibitor; ℞ for Alzheimer's disease}
Usual initial dose:	4 mg orally twice daily (8 mg/day)
Usual maintenance dose:	8–12 mg orally twice daily (16–24 mg/day) or 16–24 mg orally extended-release capsules once daily
Typical maximum dose:	32 mg/day
Proportion eliminated unchanged:	32 %

Adjustment for Kidney Disease

FDA-approved product labeling:	*Moderately impaired renal function*	*Titration should proceed cautiously; dose not to exceed 16 mg/day*
	Severe renal impairment (CrCL <9 mL/min)	*Use not recommended; avoid*
Alternative adjustment:	*Data not available*	

Gallium Nitrate - Selected References

Bockman R. The effects of gallium nitrate on bone resorption. Semin Oncol. 2003;30(Suppl 5):5–12.

Bockman RS. Studies on the mechanism of action of gallium nitrate. Semin Oncol. 1991;18(Suppl 5):21–5.

Bockman RS, Bepo MA, Warrell RP Jr, et al. Distribution of trace levels of therapeutic gallium in bone as mapped by synchrotron x-ray microscopy. Proc Natl Acad Sci. 1990;87:4149–53.

Ganite™ injection [package insert]. Berkeley Heights: Genta Inc; 2003.

Hall SW, Yeung K, Benjamin RS, et al. Kinetics of gallium nitrate, a new anticancer agent. Clin Pharmacol Ther. 1979;25:82–7.

Keller J, Bartolucci A, Carpenter JT Jr, Feagler J. Phase II evaluation of bolus gallium nitrate in lymphoproliferative disorders: a Southeastern Cancer Study Group trial. Cancer Treat Rep. 1986;70:1221–3.

Kelsen DP, Alcock N, Yeh S, Brown J, Young C. Pharmacokinetics of gallium nitrate in man. Cancer. 1980;46:2009–13.

Krakoff IH, Newman RA, Goldberg RS. Clinical toxicologic and pharmacologic studies of gallium nitrate. Cancer. 1979;44:1722–7.

Leyland-Jones B. Treatment of cancer-related hypercalcemia: the role of gallium nitrate. Semin Oncol. 2003;30(Suppl 5): 13–19.

Leyland-Jones B. Pharmacokinetics and therapeutic index of gallium nitrate. Semin Oncol. 1991;18(Suppl 5):16–20.

Leyland-Jones B, Bhalla RB, Farag F, Williams L, Coonley CJ, Warrell RP Jr. Administration of gallium nitrate by continuous infusion: lack of chronic nephrotoxicity confirmed by studies of enzymuria and β2 microglobulin. Cancer Treat Rep. 1983;67:941–2.

Schwartz S, Yagoda A. Phase I-II trial of gallium nitrate for advanced hypernephroma. Anticancer Res. 1984;4:317–8.

Senderowicz AM, Reid R, Headlee D, et al. A phase II trial of gallium nitrate in patients with androgen-metastatic prostate cancer. Urol Int. 1999;63:120–5.

Warrell RP Jr. Clinical trials of gallium nitrate in patients with cancer-related hypercalcemia. Semin Oncol. 1991;18 (Suppl 5):26–31.

Warrell RP Jr, Issacs M, Alcock NW, Bockman RS. Gallium nitrate for treatment of refractory hypercalcemia from parathyroid carcinoma. Ann Intern Med. 1987;107:683–6.

Webster LK, Olver IN, Stokes KH, Sephton RG, Hillcoat BL, Bishop JF. A pharmacokinetic and phase II study of gallium nitrate in patients with non-small cell cancer. Cancer Chemother Pharmacol. 2000;45:55–8.

Zojer N, Keck AV, Pecherstorfer M. Comparative tolerability of drug therapies for hypercalcemia of malignancy. Drug Saf. 1999;21:389–406.

Dosage Adjustment of Medications Eliminated by the Kidneys

<u>Gallium Nitrate</u>/Ganite™   {Hypocalcemic agent; bone resorption inhibitor}

Usual initial dose:	200 mg/m² IV daily
Usual maintenance dose:	200 mg/m² continuous IV infusion over 24 h daily for 5 consecutive days or until normalization of serum calcium levels
Typical maximum dose:	200 mg/m² IV daily
Proportion eliminated unchanged:	50 %

Adjustment for Kidney Disease

FDA-approved product labeling:	*Moderate renal impairment (SCr 2.0–2.5 mg/dL)*	*Frequently monitor the patient's renal status.*
	Severe renal impairment (SCr >2.5 mg/dL)	*Contraindicated*
Alternative adjustment:	*Data not available*	

Dosage Adjustment of Medications Eliminated by the Kidneys

<u>Ganciclovir (IV)</u> - Selected References

Aronoff GA, Bennett WM, Berns JS, et al. Drug prescribing in renal failure: dosing guidelines for adults and children. 5th ed. Philadelphia: American College of Physicians; 2007.

Bastien O, Boulieu R, Bleyzac N, Estanove S. Clinical use of ganciclovir during renal failure and continuous hemodialysis. Intensive Care Med. 1994;20:47–8.

Boulieu R, Bastien O, Bleyzac N. Pharmacokinetics of ganciclovir in heart transplant patients undergoing continuous venovenous hemodialysis. Ther Drug Monit. 1993;15:105–7.

Brennan DC, Garlock KA, Lipmann BA, et al. Control of cytomegalovirus-associated morbidity in renal transplant patients using intensive monitoring and either preemptive or deferred therapy. J Am Soc Nephrol. 1997;8:118–25.

Caldés A, Colom H, Armendariz Y, et al. Population pharmacokinetics of ganciclovir after intravenous ganciclovir and oral valganciclovir administration in solid organ transplant patients infected with cytomegalovirus. Antimicrob Agents Chemother. 2009;53:4816–24.

Combarnous F, Fouque D, Bernard N, et al. Pharmacokinetics of ganciclovir in a patient undergoing chronic haemodialysis. Eur J Clin Pharmacol. 1994;46:379–81.

Crumpacker CS. Drug therapy: ganciclovir. N Engl J Med. 1996;335:721–9.

Cytovene® IV injection [package insert]. South San Francisco: Genentech USA Inc; 2010.

Czock D, Rasche FM. New AUC-based method to estimate drug fraction removed by hemodialysis. Kidney Blood Press Res. 2004;27:172–6.

De Keyser K, Van Laecke S, Peeters P, Vanholder R. Human cytomegalovirus and kidney transplantation: a clinician's update. Am J Kidney Dis. 2011;58:118–26.

Erice A, Jordan C, Chac BA, Fletcher C, Chinnock BJ, Balfour JJ Jr. Ganciclovir treatment of cytomegalovirus disease in transplant recipients and other immunocompromised hosts. JAMA. 1987;257:3082–7.

Fletcher C, Sawchuck R, Chinnock B, de Miranda P, Balfour HH Jr. Human pharmacokinetics of the antiviral drug DHPG. Clin Pharmacol Ther. 1986;40:281–6.

Gando S, Kameue T, Nanzaki S, Hayakawa T, Kakanishi Y. Pharmacokinetics and clearance of ganciclovir during continuous hemodiafiltration. Crit Care Med. 1998;26:184–7.

Gilbert DN, Moellering RC Jr, Eliopoulos GM, Chambers HF, Saag MS. The Sanford Guide to Antimicrobial Therapy. 41st ed. Sperryville: Antimicrobial Therapy Inc; 2011.

Heintz BH, Matzke GR, Dager WF. Antimicrobial dosing concepts and recommendations for critically ill adult patients receiving continuous renal replacement therapy or intermittent hemodialysis. Pharmacotherapy. 2009;29:562–77.

Hrebinko R, Jordan ML, Dummer JS, et al. Ganciclovir for invasive cytomegalovirus infection in renal allograft recipients. Transplant Proc. 1991;23:1346–7.

Jabs DA, Cavis MD, Mowery R, et al. Mortality in patients with the acquired immunodeficiency syndrome treated with either foscarnet or ganciclovir for cytomegalovirus retinitis. N Engl J Med. 1992;326:213–20.

Jassal SV, Roscoe JM, Zaltzman JS, et al. Clinical practice guidelines: prevention of cytomegalovirus disease after renal transplantation. J Am Soc Nephrol. 1998;9:1697–708.

Jordan ML, Hrebinko RL Jr, Dummer JS, Therapeutic use of ganciclovir for invasive cytomegalovirus infection in cadaveric renal allograft recipients. J Urol. 1992;148:1388–92.

Lake KD, Fletcher CV, Love KR, Brown DC, Joyce LD, Pritzker MR. Ganciclovir pharmacokinetics during renal impairment. Antimicrob Agents Chemother. 1988;32:1899–900.

Maiwald J, Sperschneider H, Stein G. The problem of cytomegalovirus (CMV) prophylaxis in high-risk renal transplant recipients [letter]. Nephrol Dial Transplant. 1996;11:1897.

Noble S, Faulds D. Ganciclovir: an update of its use in the prevention of cytomegalovirus infection and disease in transplant recipients. Drugs. 1998;56:115–46.

Peddi VR, Hariharan S, Schroeder TJ, First MR. Impact of ganciclovir prophylaxis on cytomegalovirus infection in recipients of cadaveric renal allografts. Nephron. 1997;76:49–55.

Sommadossi J-P, Bevan R, Ling T, et al. Clinical pharmacokinetics of ganciclovir in patients with normal and impaired renal function. Rev Infect Dis. 1988;10(Suppl 3):S507–14.

Tornatore KM, Garey KW, Saigal N, et al. Ganciclovir pharmacokinetics and cytokine dynamics in renal transplant recipients with cytomegalovirus infection. Clin Transplant. 2001;15:297–308.

Dosage Adjustment of Medications Eliminated by the Kidneys

Ganciclovir (IV)/Cytovene® IV	{Antiviral; nucleoside analog; ℞ cytomegalovirus}
Usual initial dose:	5 mg/kg IV
Usual maintenance dose:	5 mg/kg IV every 12 h for 7–14 days (induction), 5 mg/kg IV daily (maintenance)
Typical maximum dose:	10 mg/kg/day
Proportion eliminated unchanged:	95 %

Adjustment for Kidney Disease

FDA-approved product labeling:

Ganciclovir IV dosing in renal function impairment

	Induction		Maintenance	
CrCL (mL/min)	IV induction dose (mg/kg)	Dosing interval (h)	IV maintenance dose (mg/kg)	Dosing interval (h)
≥70	5	12	5	24
50–69	2.5	12	2.5	24
25–49	2.5	24	1.25	24
10–24	1.25	24	0.625	24
<10	1.25	Three times per week, after hemodialysis	0.625	Three times per week, after hemodialysis

Alternative adjustment:

GFR >70 mL/min	*5 mg/kg IV over 1 h every 12 h for 14–21 days (induction) followed by 5 mg/kg IV every 24 h (maintenance)*
GFR 50–69 mL/min	*2.5 mg/kg IV every 12 h for 14–21 days (induction) followed by 2.5 mg/kg IV every 24 h (maintenance)*
GFR 25–49 mL/min	*2.5 mg/kg IV every 24 h for 14–21 days (induction) followed by 1.25 mg/kg IV every 24 h (maintenance)*
GFR 10–24 mL/min	*1.25 mg/kg IV every 24 h for 14–21 days (induction) followed by 0.625 mg/kg IV every 24 h (maintenance)*
GFR <10 mL/min	*1.25 mg/kg IV every 48 h*
Hemodialysis	*1.25 mg/kg IV every 48–72 h or 3 times weekly, after hemodialysis on dialysis days*
CAPD	*1.25 mg/kg IV every 48 h*
CVVH	*2.5 mg/kg IV every 24 h*
CVVHD or CVVHDF	*2.5 mg/kg IV every 12 h*

Dosage Adjustment of Medications Eliminated by the Kidneys

<u>Ganciclovir</u> (Oral) - Selected References

Aronoff GA, Bennett WM, Berns JS, et al. Drug prescribing in renal failure: dosing guidelines for adults and children. 5th ed. Philadelphia: American College of Physicians; 2007.

Buturović-Ponikvar J, Kandus A, Malovrh KM, Ponikvar R, Kveder R. Ganciclovir treatment of cytomegalovirus infections in renal transplant recipients. Transplant Proc. 1992;24:1921–3.

Crumpacker CS. Drug therapy: ganciclovir. N Engl J Med. 1996;335:721–9.

De Keyser K, Van Laecke S, Peeters P, Vanholder R. Human cytomegalovirus and kidney transplantation: a clinician's update. Am J Kidney Dis. 2011;58:118–26.

Ganciclovir capsule [package insert]. Hightstown: Ranbaxy Laboratories Ltd; 2008.

Gilbert DN, Moellering RC Jr, Eliopoulos GM, Chambers HF, Saag MS. The Sanford Guide to Antimicrobial Therapy. 41st ed. Sperryville: Antimicrobial Therapy Inc; 2011.

Griffy KG. Pharmacokinetics of oral ganciclovir capsules in HIV-infected persons. AIDS. 1996;10(Suppl 4):53–6.

Jassal SV, Roscoe JM, Zaltzman JS, et al. Clinical practice guidelines: prevention of cytomegalovirus disease after renal transplantation. J Am Soc Nephrol. 1998;9:1697–708.

McIntyre CW, Owen PJ. Prescribing drugs in kidney disease. In: Brenner BM. Brenner & Rector's the kidney. 8th ed. Philadelphia: Saunders/Elsevier; 2008. p. 1930–55.

Morse GD, Shelton MJ, O'Donnell AM. Comparative pharmacokinetics of antiviral nucleoside analogues. Clin Pharmacokinet. 1993;24:100–23.

Noble S, Faulds D. Ganciclovir: an update of its use in the prevention of cytomegalovirus infection and disease in transplant recipients. Drugs. 1998;56:115–46.

Olyaei AJ, Bennett WM. Drug dosing in elderly patients with chronic kidney disease. Clin Geriatr Med. 2009;25:459–527.

Olyaei AJ, Bennett WM. Pharmacologic approach to renal insufficiency. In: Dale DC, Federman DD, Antman K, editors. ACP medicine, WebMD June 2007 update. Hamilton: BC Decker; 2007. Nephrology IX: Appendix A1–25.

Olyaei AJ, DeMattos AM, Bennett WM. Use of drugs in patients with renal failure. In: Schrier RW, editor. Diseases of the kidney and urinary tract. 8th ed. Philadelphia: Lippincott Williams & Wilkins; 2007. p. 2765–807.

Pescovitz MD, Pruett TL, Gonwa T, et al. Oral ganciclovir dosing in transplant recipients and dialysis patients based on renal function. Transplantation. 1998;66:1104–7.

Tornatore KM, Garey KW, Saigal N, et al. Ganciclovir pharmacokinetics and cytokine dynamics in renal transplant recipients with cytomegalovirus infection. Clin Transplant. 2001;15:297–308.

Wiltshire H, Hirankarn S, Farrell C, et al. Pharmacokinetic profile of ganciclovir after its oral administration and from its prodrug, valganciclovir, in solid organ transplant recipients. Clin Pharmacokinet. 2005;44:495–507.

Dosage Adjustment of Medications Eliminated by the Kidneys

<u>Ganciclovir (Oral)</u>/Cytovene®   **{Antiviral; nucleoside analog; ℞ cytomegalovirus}**

Usual initial dose:	1,000 mg orally
Usual maintenance dose:	1,000 mg orally three times daily with food
Typical maximum dose:	3 g/day
Proportion eliminated unchanged:	95 % of absorbed dose (oral bioavailability 6–9 %)

Adjustment for Kidney Disease

FDA-approved product labeling:

Ganciclovir oral dosing in renal function impairment

CrCL (mL/min)	Ganciclovir capsule doses
≥ 70	1,000 mg 3 times daily or 500 mg every 3 hours, 6 times daily
50 to 69	1,500 mg once daily or 500 mg 3 times daily
25 to 49	1,000 mg once daily or 500 mg twice daily
10 to 24	500 mg once daily
< 10	500 mg 3 times per week following hemodialysis

Alternative adjustment:

GFR >50 mL/min	1,000 mg orally three times daily
GFR 10–50 mL/min	1,000 mg orally twice daily
GFR <10 mL/min	500 mg orally every 48 h
Hemodialysis	500 mg orally three times/week after dialysis
CAPD	500 mg orally every 48 h
CRRT	Not applicable (consider IV ganciclovir)

Note: Oral ganciclovir should be used only for prophylaxis (not treatment) of cytomegalovirus disease.

Dosage Adjustment of Medications Eliminated by the Kidneys

Gemfibrozil - Selected References

Akoglu H, Yilmaz R, Kirkpantur A, Arici M, Altun B, Turgan C. Combined organ failure with combination antihyperlipidemic treatment: a case of hepatic injury and acute renal failure. Ann Pharmacother. 2007;41:143–7.

Broeders N, Knoop C, Antoine M, Tielemans C, Abramowicz D. Fibrate-induced increase in blood urea and creatinine: is gemfibrozil the only innocuous agent. Nephrol Dial Transplant. 2000;15:1993–9.

Davidson MH, Armani A, McKenney JM, Jacobson TA. Safety considerations with fibrate therapy. Am J Cardiol. 2007;99(Suppl 6A):3C–18C.

de Miguel D, García-Suáez J, Martín Y, Gil-Fernández JJ, Burgaleta C. Severe acute renal failure following high-dose methotrexate therapy in adults with haematological malignancies: a significant number result from unrecognized co-administration of several drugs. Nephrol Dial Transplant. 2008;23:3762–6.

Evans JR, Forland SC, Cutler RE. The effect of renal function on the pharmacokinetics of gemfibrozil. J Clin Pharmacol. 1987;27:994–1000.

Górriz JL, Sancho A, Lopez-Martín JM, Alcoy E, Catalán C, Pallardó LM. Rhabdomyolysis and acute renal failure associated with gemfibrozil therapy. Nephron. 1996;74:437–8.

Irish AB, Thompson CH. The effect of gemfibrozil upon the hypercoagulable state in dyslipidaemic patients with chronic renal failure. Nephrol Dial Transplant. 1996;11:2223–8.

Kasiske BL, Heim-Duthoy KL, Singer GG, Watschinger B, Germain MJ, Bastani B. The effects of lipid-lowering agents on acute renal allograft rejection. Transplantation. 2001;72:223–7.

Knauf H, Kölle EU, Mutschler E. Gemfibrozil absorption and elimination in kidney and liver disease. Klin Wochenschr. 1990;68:692–8.

Layne RD, Sehbai AS, Stark LJ. Rhabdomyolysis and renal failure associated with gemfibrozil monotherapy. Ann Pharmacother. 2004;38:232–4.

Lipscombe J, Lewis GF, Cattran D, Bargman JM. Deterioration in renal function associated with fibrate therapy. Clin Nephrol. 2001;55:39–44.

Lopid® tablet [package insert]. New York: Pfizer Inc; 2010.

Mänttäri M, Tiula E, Alikoski T, Manninen V. Effects of hypertension and dyslipidemia on the decline in renal function. Hypertension. 1995;26:670–5.

Miller DB, Spence JD. Clinical pharmacokinetics of fibric acid derivatives (fibrates). Clin Pharmacokinet. 1998;34:155–62.

Ok E, Kuraat S, Alev M, et al. Further evidence of favorable effects of gemfibrozil on the lipid profile in renal allograft recipients. Nephron. 1996;73:491–2.

Oldemeyer JB, Lund RJ, Koch M, Meares AJ, Dunlay R. Rhabdomyolysis and acute renal failure after changing statin-fibrate combinations. Cardiology. 2000;94:127–8.

Rubins HB, Robins SJ, Collins D, et al. Gemfibrozil for the secondary prevention of coronary heart disease in men with low levels of high-density lipoprotein cholesterol. N Engl J Med. 1999;341:410–8.

Samuelson O, Attman P-O, Knight-Gibson C, et al. Effect of gemfibrozil on lipoprotein abnormalities in chronic renal insufficiency: a controlled study in human chronic renal disease. Nephron. 1997;75:286–94.

Schech S, Graham D, Staffa J, et al. Risk factors for statin-associated rhabdomyolysis. Pharmacoepidemiol Drug Saf. 2007;16:352–8.

Spencer CM, Barradell LB. Gemfibrozil: a reappraisal of its pharmacological properties and place in the management of dyslipidaemia. Drugs. 1996;51:982–1016.

Toneli M, Collins D, Robins S, et al. Effect of gemfibrozil on change in renal function in men with moderate chronic renal insufficiency and coronary disease. Am J Kidney Dis. 2004;44:832–9.

Toneli M, Collins D, Robins S, et al. Gemfibrozil for secondary prevention of cardiovascular events in mild to moderate chronic renal insufficiency. Kidney Int. 2004;68:1123–30.

Yen T-H, Chang C-T, Wu M-S, Huang C-C. Acute rhabdomyolysis after gemfibrozil therapy in a pregnant patient complicated with acute pancreatitis and hypertriglyceridemia while receiving continuous veno-venous hemofiltration therapy. Ren Fail. 2003;25:139–43.

Dosage Adjustment of Medications Eliminated by the Kidneys

<u>Gemfibrozil</u>/Lopid®   {Antihypercholesterolemic; fibric acid derivative}

Usual initial dose:	600 mg orally
Usual maintenance dose:	600 mg orally twice daily before meals
Typical maximum dose:	1,200 mg/day
Proportion eliminated unchanged:	1 % (7–14 % as conjugates)

Adjustment for Kidney Disease

FDA-approved product labeling:	*Mild to moderate renal impairment*	*Use with caution.*
	Severe renal impairment	*Contraindicated.*
Alternative adjustment:	*GFR >50 mL/min*	*600 mg orally twice daily.*
	GFR 10–50 mL/min	*300 mg orally twice daily for 6 weeks with careful monitoring; if no symptomatic, biochemical, or metabolic adverse effects arise, increase to 600 mg orally twice daily.*
	GFR <10 mL/min	*Preferably avoid or 300 mg orally once daily for 6 weeks with careful monitoring; if no symptomatic, biochemical, or metabolic adverse effects arise, increase to 300 mg orally twice daily.*
	Hemodialysis	*Preferably avoid or 300 mg orally once daily for 6 weeks with careful monitoring; if no symptomatic, biochemical, or metabolic adverse effects arise, increase to 300 mg orally twice daily.*
	CAPD	*Preferably avoid or 300 mg orally once daily for 6 weeks with careful monitoring; if no symptomatic, biochemical, or metabolic adverse effects arise, increase to 300 mg orally twice daily.*
	CRRT	*Not applicable; preferably avoid.*

Dosage Adjustment of Medications Eliminated by the Kidneys

Gemifloxacin - Selected References

Allen A, Bygate E, Clark D, Lewis A, Pay V. The effect of food on the bioavailability of oral gemifloxacin in healthy volunteers. Int J Antimicrob Agents. 2000;16:45–50.

Allen A, Bygate E, Oliver S, et al. Pharmacokinetics and tolerability of gemifloxacin (SB-265805) after administration of single doses to healthy volunteers. Antimicrob Agents Chemother. 2000;44:1604–8.

Allen A, Bygate E, Vousden M, et al. Multiple-dose pharmacokinetics and tolerability of gemifloxacin administered orally to healthy volunteers. Antimicrob Agents Chemother. 2001;45:540–5.

Ball P, Mandell L, Patou G, Dankner W, Tillotson G. A new respiratory fluoroquinolone, oral gemifloxacin: a safety profile in context. Int J Antimicrob Agents. 2004;23:421–9.

Bhavani SM, Andes DR. Gemifloxacin for the treatment of respiratory tract infections: in vitro susceptibility, pharmacokinetics and pharmacodynamics, clinical efficacy, and safety. Pharmacotherapy. 2005;25:717–40.

Brenwald NP, Appelbaum P, Davies T, Gill MJ. Evidence for efflux pumps, other than PmrA, associated with fluoroquinolone resistance in *Streptococcus pneumoniae*. Clin Microbiol Infect. 2003;9:140–3.

Factive® tablet [package insert]. Waltham: Oscient Pharmaceuticals; 2008.

Firsov AA, Lubenko IY, Portnoy YA, Zinner SH, Vostrov SN. Relationships of the area under the curve/MIC ratio to different integral endpoints of the antimicrobial effect: gemifloxacin pharmacodynamics in an in vitro dynamic mode. Antimicrob Agents Chemother. 2001;45:927–31.

Firsov AA, Zinner SH, Lubenko IY, Vostrov SN. Gemifloxacin and ciprofloxacin pharmacodynamics in an in-vitro dynamic model: prediction of the equivalent AUC/MIC breakpoints and doses. Int J Antimicrob Agents. 2000;16:407–14.

García-Calvo G, Parra A, Aguilar L, et al. Antibacterial properties of gemifloxacin and trovafloxacin in urine ex vivo: phase I study. Antimicrob Agents Chemother. 2001;45:1876–8.

Gee T, Andrews JM, Ashby JP, Marshall G, Wise R. Pharmacokinetics and tissue penetration of gemifloxacin following a single oral dose. J Antimicrob Chemother. 2001;47:431–4.

Gilbert DN. Urinary tract infections in patients with chronic renal insufficiency. Clin J Am Soc Nephrol. 2006;1:327–31.

Gilbert DN, Moellering RC Jr, Eliopoulos GM, Chambers HF, Saag MS. The Sanford Guide to Antimicrobial Therapy. 41st ed. Sperryville: Antimicrobial Therapy Inc; 2011.

Hansen GT, Metzler K, Drilica K, Blondeau JM. Mutant prevention concentration of gemifloxacin for clinical isolates of *Streptococcus pneumoniae* [letter]. Antimicrob Agents Chemother. 2003;47:440–1.

Islinger F, Bouw R, Stahl M, et al. Concentrations of gemifloxacin at the target site in healthy volunteers after a single dose. Antimicrob Agents Chemother. 2004;48:4246–9.

Landersdorfer CB, Kirkpatrick CMJ, Kinzig M, et al. Competitive inhibition of renal tubular secretion of gemifloxacin by probenecid. Antimicrob Agents Chemother. 2009;53:3902–7.

MacGowan AP, Bowker KE. Mechanism of fluoroquinolone resistance is an important factor in determining the antimicrobial effect of gemifloxacin against *Streptococcus pneumoniae* in an in vitro pharmacokinetic model. Antimicrob Agents Chemother. 2003;47:1096–100.

Norreddin AM, Reese AA, Ostroski M, Hoban DJ, Zhanel GG. Comparative pharmacokinetics of garenoxacin, gemifloxacin, and moxifloxacin in community-acquired pneumonia caused by *Streptococcus pneumoniae*: a Monte-Carlo simulation analysis. Clin Ther. 2007;29:2685–9.

Owens RC Jr, Bhavnani SM, Ambrose PG. Assessment of pharmacokinetic-pharmacodynamic target attainment of gemifloxacin against *Streptococcus pneumoniae*. Diagn Microbiol Infect Dis. 2005;51:45–9.

Prieto J, Aguilar L, Fuentes F, et al. Influence of diminished susceptibility of *Streptococcus pneumoniae* to ciprofloxacin on the serum bactericidal activity of gemifloxacin and trovafloxacin after a single dose in healthy volunteers. Int J Antimicrob Agents. 2001;18:231–8.

Smith HJ, Noreddin AM, Siemens CG, et al. Designing fluoroquinolone breakpoints for Streptococcus pneumoniae by using genetics instead of pharmacokinetics-pharmacodynamics. Antimicrob Agents Chemother. 2004;48:3630–5.

Stahlmann R, Lode H. Safety considerations of fluoroquinolones in the elderly: an update. Drugs Aging. 2010;27:193–209.

Dosage Adjustment of Medications Eliminated by the Kidneys

Gemifloxacin/Factive®   {**Antibacterial; fluoroquinolone**}

Usual initial dose: 320 mg orally

Usual maintenance dose: 320 mg orally once daily

Typical maximum dose: 320 mg/day

Proportion eliminated unchanged: 25–40 %

Adjustment for Kidney Disease

FDA-approved product labeling:	*CrCL >40 mL/min*	*320 mg orally once daily*
	CrCL ≤40 mL/min	*160 mg orally every 24 h*
	Hemodialysis	*160 mg orally every 24 h*
	Peritoneal dialysis (CAPD)	*160 mg orally every 24 h*
Alternative adjustment:	*GFR >50 mL/min*	*320 mg orally every 24 h*
	GFR 10–50 mL/min	*160–320 mg orally every 24 h*
	GFR <10 mL/min	*160 mg every 24 h*
	Hemodialysis	*160 mg every 24 h; administer after hemodialysis on dialysis days*
	CAPD	*160 mg every 24 h*
	CRRT	*160–320 mg every 24 h*

Dosage Adjustment of Medications Eliminated by the Kidneys

Gentamicin - Selected References

Aronoff GA, Bennett WM, Berns JS, et al. Drug prescribing in renal failure: dosing guidelines for adults and children. 5th ed. Philadelphia: American College of Physicians; 2007.

Bartal C, Danon A, Schlaeffer F, et al. Pharmacokinetic dosing of aminoglycosides: a controlled trial. Am J Med. 2003;114:194–8.

Barza M, Brown RB, Shen D, Gibaldi M, Weinstein L. Predictability of blood levels of gentamicin in man. J Infect Dis. 1975;132:165–74.

Bennett WM, Hartnett MN, Craven R, Gilbert DN, Porter GA. Gentamicin concentrations in blood, urine, and renal tissue of patients with end-stage renal disease. J Lab Clin Med. 1977;90:389–93.

Christopher TG, Korn D, Blair AD, Forrey QW, O'Neill MA, Cutler RE. Gentamicin pharmacokinetics during hemodialysis. Kidney Int. 1974;6:38–44.

Dahlgren JG, Anderson ET, Hewitt WL. Gentamicin blood levels: a guide to nephrotoxicity. Antimicrob Agents Chemother. 1975;8:58–62.

Danish M, Schultz R, Jusko WJ. Pharmacokinetics of gentamicin and kanamycin during hemodialysis. Antimicrob Agents Chemother. 1974;6:841–7.

Gentamicin Sulfate Injection Solution Concentrate [package insert]. Lake Forest: Hospira; 2004.

Gingell JC, Chisholm GD, Calnan JS, Waterworth PM. The dose, distribution, and excretion of gentamicin with special reference to renal failure. J Infect Dis. 1969;119:396–401.

Gyselynck AM, Forrey A, Cutler R. Pharmacokinetics of gentamicin: distribution and plasma and renal clearance. J Infect Dis. 1971;124(Suppl):S70–6.

Heintz BH, Matzke GR, Dager WF. Antimicrobial dosing concepts and recommendations for critically ill adult patients receiving continuous renal replacement therapy or intermittent hemodialysis. Pharmacotherapy. 2009;29:562–77.

Helps A, Deighan C, Gourlay Y, Seaton RA. Gentamicin and acute kidney injury requiring renal replacement therapy in the context of a restrictive antibiotic policy [letter]. J Antimicrob Chemother. 2011;e-pub ahead of print. doi:10.1093/jac/dkr177.

Hilmer SN, Tran K, Rubie P, et al. Gentamicin pharmacokinetics in old age and frailty. Br J Clin Pharmacol. 2011;71:224–31.

Hitala R, Dinh T, Cook DJ. Once-daily aminoglycoside dosing in immunocompetent adults: a meta-analysis. Ann Intern Med. 1996;124:717–25.

Kaye D, Levison ME, Labovitz ED. The unpredictability of serum concentrations of gentamicin: pharmacokinetics of gentamicin in patients with normal and abnormal renal function. J Infect Dis. 1974;130:150–4.

Kuang D, Verbine A, Ronco C. Pharmacokinetics and antimicrobial dosing adjustment in critically ill patients during continuous renal replacement therapy. Clin Nephrol. 2007;67:267–84.

Lockwood WR, Bower JD. Tobramycin an gentamicin concentrations in the serum of normal and anephric patients. Antimicrob Agents Chemother. 1973;3:125–9.

McHenry MC, Gavan TL, Gifford RW Jr, et al. Gentamicin dosages for renal insufficiency: adjustments based on endogenous creatinine clearance and serum creatinine concentration. Ann Intern Med. 1971;74:192–7.

Moore RC, Leitman PS, Smith CR. Clinical response to aminoglycoside therapy: importance of the ratio of peak concentration to minimal inhibitory concentration. J Infect Dis. 1987;155:93–9.

Moore RC, Smith CR, Leitman PS. Association of aminoglycoside plasma levels with therapeutic outcome in gram-negative pneumonia. Am J Med. 1984;77:657–62.

Nicolau DP, Freeman CD, Belliveau PP, Nightingale CH, Ross JW, Qunitillani R. Experience with a once-daily aminoglycoside program administered to 2,184 adult patients. Antimicrob Agents Chemother. 1995;39:650–5.

Pai MP, Nafziger AN, Bertino JS Jr. Simplified estimation of aminoglycoside pharmacokinetics in underweight and obese adult patients. Antimicrob Agents Chemother. 2011;55:4006–11.

Sarrubbi FA Jr, Hull JH. Amikacin serum concentrations: prediction of levels and dosage guidelines. Ann Intern Med. 1978;89:612–8.

Schentag JJ, Jusko WJ. Renal clearance and tissue accumulation of gentamicin. Clin Pharmacol Ther. 1977;22:364–70.

Sowinski KM, Magner SJ, Lucksiri A, Scott MK, Hamburger RJ, Mueller BA. Influence of hemodialysis on gentamicin pharmacokinetics, removal during hemodialysis, and recommended dosing. Clin J Am Soc Nephrol. 2008;3:355–61.

Dosage Adjustment of Medications Eliminated by the Kidneys

<u>Gentamicin</u>/Garamycin®	{Antibacterial; aminoglycoside}
Usual initial dose:	2–7 mg/kg IV (actual body weight [ABW] or ideal [IBW] + 0.4(ABW − IBW) if ABW > IBW)
Usual maintenance dose:	3–5 mg/kg/day in two to three divided doses or 4–7 mg/kg IV every 24 h
Typical maximum dose:	10 mg/kg/day
Proportion eliminated unchanged:	95 %

Adjustment for Kidney Disease

FDA-approved product labeling: *Dosage adjustment guide for patients with renal impairment[a] (dosage at 8-h intervals after the usual initial dose)*

Serum creatinine (mg/dL)	CrCL (mL/min)	Percent of usual dose
≤1.0	>100	100
1.1–1.3	70–100	80
1.4–1.6	55–70	65
1.7–1.9	45–55	55
2.0–2.2	40–45	50
2.3–2.5	35–40	40
2.6–3.0	30–35	35
3.1–3.5	25–30	30
3.6–4.0	20–25	25
4.1–5.1	15–20	20
5.2–6.6	10–15	15
6.7–8.0	< 10	10

Hemodialysis: 1–1.7 mg/kg at the end of each dialysis

Alternative adjustment:

GFR >50 mL/min	*2–2.5 mg/kg IV once followed by 1.7 mg/kg every 8–12 h or 4–7 mg/kg (9 mg/kg lean body mass in obese patients) IV every 24 h[a]*
GFR 10–50 mL/min	*2–2.5 mg/kg IV once followed by 1.7 mg/kg IV every 24–48 h[a] (if pre-dose plasma level is within desired range, usually ≤1 mg/L)[a]*
GFR <10 mL/min	*1.7 mg/kg IV every 72 h (if pre-dose plasma level is within desired range, usually ≤1 mg/L)[a]*
Hemodialysis	*1–1.7 mg/kg IV at the end of each dialysis (if pre-dose plasma level is within desired range, usually ≤1 mg/L)[a]*
CAPD	*Add to dialysate qs 4–8 mg/L[a]*
CVVHD or CVVHDF	*1.5–2.5 mg/kg IV every 24–48 h (if pre-dose plasma level is within desired range, usually ≤1 mg/L)[a]*

[a]Therapeutic Drug Monitoring

Therapeutic plasma levels: *Peak: 6–10 mg/L (conventional dosing).*

Trough: <2 mg/L; patients on extended-interval dosing generally should be re-dosed when levels fall below 1 mg/L.

Dosage Adjustment of Medications Eliminated by the Kidneys

Glipizide - Selected References

Abe M, Okada K, Soma M. Antidiabetic agents in patients with chronic kidney disease and end-stage renal disease on dialysis: metabolism and clinical practice. Curr Drug Metab. 2011;12:57–69

Asplund K, Wiholm BE, Lundman B. Severe hypoglycaemia during treatment with glipizide. Diabet Med. 1991;8:726–31.

Balant L, Zahnd G, Gorgía A, Schwartz R, Fabre J. Pharmacokinetics of glipizide in man: influence of renal insufficiency. Diabetologia. 1973;9(Suppl):331–8.

Bitzén P-O, Melander A, Scherstén B, Wåhlin-Boll E. The influence of glipizide on early insulin release and glucose disposal before and after dietary regulation in diabetic patients with different degrees of hyperglycaemia. Eur J Clin Pharmacol. 1988;35:31–7.

Chan JCN, Scott R, Ferreira JCA, et al. Safety and efficacy of sitagliptin in patients with type 2 diabetes and chronic renal insufficiency. Diabetes Obes Metab. 2008;10:545–55.

Courtois P, Sener A, Herband C, Turc A, Malaisse WJ. Pharmacokinetics of gliquidone, glibenclamide, gliclazide and glipizide in middle-aged and aged subjects. Res Commun Mol Pathol Pharmacol. 1999;103:211–22.

Davis SN, Mann S, Briscoe VJ, Ertl AC, Tate DB. Effects of intensive therapy and antecedent hypoglycemia on counterregulatory responses to hypoglycemia in type 2 diabetes. Diabetes. 2009;58:701–9.

Glucotrol® tablet [package insert]. New York: Roerig Division of Pfizer Inc; 2011.

Groop L, Groop P-H, Stenman S, et al. Comparison of pharmacokinetics, metabolic effects and mechanisms of action of glyburide and glipizide during long-term treatment. Diabetes Care. 1987;10:671–8.

Groop L, Wåhlin-Boll E, Groop P-H, Tötterman K-J, Melander A, Tolppanen E-M, Fyhrqvist F. Pharmacokinetics and metabolic effects of glibenclamide and glipizide in type 2 diabetics. Eur J Clin Pharmacol. 1985;28:697–704.

Jaber LA, Ducharme MP, Edwards DJ, Slaughter RL, Grunberger G. The influence of multiple dosing and age on the pharmacokinetics and pharmacodynamics of glipizide in patients with type II diabetes mellitus. Pharmacotherapy. 1996;16:760–8.

Kobayashi KA, Bauer LA, Horn JR, Opheim K, Wood F Jr, Kradjan WA. Glipizide pharmacokinetics in young and elderly volunteers. Clin Pharm. 1988;7:224–8.

Kradjan WA, Kobayashi KA, Bauer LA, Horn JR, Opheim KE, Wood FJ Jr. Glipizide pharmacokinetics: effects of age, diabetes, and multiple dosing. J Clin Pharmacol. 1989;29:1121–7.

Kradjan WA, Takeuchi KY, Opheim K, Wood F Jr. Pharmacokinetics and pharmacodynamics of glipizide after once-daily and divided doses. Pharmacotherapy. 1995;15:465–71.

Lebovitz HE. Glipizide: a second-generation sulfonylurea hypoglycemic agent: pharmacology, pharmacokinetics and clinical use. Pharmacotherapy. 1985;5:63–77.

McIntyre CW, Owen PJ. Prescribing drugs in kidney disease. In: Brenner BM. Brenner & Rector's the kidney. 8th ed. Philadelphia: Saunders/Elsevier; 2008. p. 1930–55.

Melander A, Wåhlin-Boll E. Clinical pharmacology of glipizide. Am J Med. 1985;75(Suppl 5B):41–5.

Pentikäinen PJ, Neuvonen PJ, Penttilä A. Pharmacokinetics and pharmacodynamics of glipizide in healthy volunteers. Int J Clin Pharmacol Ther Toxicol. 1983;21:98–107.

Peterson CM, Sims RV, Jones RL, Rieders F. Bioavailability of glipizide and its effects on blood glucose and insulin levels in patients with non-insulin-dependent diabetes. Diabetes Care. 1982;5:497–500.

Schmidt HAE, Schoog M, Schweer KH, Winkler E. Pharmacokinetics and pharmacodynamics as well as metabolism following orally and intravenously administered C^{14}-glipizide, a new antidiabetic. Diabetologia. 1973;9(Suppl):320–30.

Simonson DC, Fischette CT, Kourides IA, et al. Efficacy, safety, and dose-response characteristics of glipizide gastrointestinal therapeutic system on glycemic control and insulin secretion in NIDDM. Diabetes Care. 1997;20:597–606.

Tan B, Zhang Y-F, Chen X-Y, Zhao X-H, Li G-X, Zhong D-F. The effects of *CYP2C9* and *CYP2C19* genetic polymorphisms on the pharmacokinetics and pharmacodynamics of glipizide in Chinese subjects. Eur J Clin Pharmacol. 2010;66:145–51.

Wåhlin-Boll E, Almér L-O, Melander A. Bioavailability, pharmacokinetics and effects of glipizide in type 2 diabetics. Clin Pharmacokinet. 1982;7:363–72.

Dosage Adjustment of Medications Eliminated by the Kidneys

Glipizide/Glucotrol®   {**Antidiabetic; sulfonylurea**}

Usual initial dose: 5 mg orally once daily before breakfast

Usual maintenance dose: 2.5–15 mg orally once or twice daily according to blood glucose levels

Typical maximum dose: 40 mg/day

Proportion eliminated unchanged: 10 %

Adjustment for Kidney Disease

FDA-approved product labeling: *With impaired renal function, initial and maintenance dosing should be conservative to avoid hypoglycemic reactions.*

Alternative adjustment:

GFR >50 mL/min	*2.5–15 mg once or twice daily according to blood glucose levels.*
GFR 10–50 mL/min	*2.5–7.5 mg once or twice daily according to blood glucose levels.*
GFR <10 mL/min	*Preferably avoid due to risk of severe hypoglycemia.*
Hemodialysis	*Preferably avoid due to risk of severe hypoglycemia.*
CAPD	*Preferably avoid due to risk of severe hypoglycemia.*
CRRT	*Not applicable; preferably avoid due to risk of severe hypoglycemia.*

Dosage Adjustment of Medications Eliminated by the Kidneys

Glyburide - Selected References

Abe M, Okada K, Soma M. Antidiabetic agents in patients with chronic kidney disease and end-stage renal disease on dialysis: metabolism and clinical practice. Curr Drug Metab. 2011;12:57–69

Aspinall SL, Zhao X, Good CB, et al. Intervention to decrease glyburide use in elderly patients with renal insufficiency. Am J Geriatr Pharmacother. 2011;9:58–68.

Balant L, Zahnd GR, Weber F, Fabre J. Behaviour of glibenclamide on repeated administration to diabetic patients. Eur J Clin Pharmacol. 1977;11:19–25.

Ben-Ami H, Nagachandran P, Mendelson A, Edoute Y. Drug-induced hypoglycemic coma in 102 diabetic patients. Arch Intern Med. 1999;159:281–4.

Brier ME, Bays H, Sloan R, Stalker DJ, Welshman I, Aronoff GR. Pharmacokinetics of oral glyburide in subjects with non-insulin-dependent diabetes mellitus and renal failure. Am J Kidney Dis. 1997;29:907–11.

Diaβeta® tablet [package insert]. Bridgewater: Sanofi-Aventis US LLC; 2009.

Groop L, Melander A, Ratheiser K, Simonson DC, DeFronzo RA. Different effects of glyburide and glipizide on insulin secretion and hepatic glucose production in normal and NIDDM subjects. Diabetes. 1987;36:1320–8.

Groop L, Wåhlin-Boll E, Groop P-H, Tötterman K-J, Melander A, Tolppanen E-M, Fyhrqvist F. Pharmacokinetics and metabolic effects of glibenclamide and glipizide in type 2 diabetics. Eur J Clin Pharmacol. 1985;28:697–704.

Hanlon JT, Aspinall SL, Semla TP, et al. Consensus guidelines for oral dosing of primarily renally cleared medications in older adults. J Am Geriatr Soc. 2009;57:335–40.

Hartmann B, Czock D, Keller F. Drug therapy in patients with chronic renal failure. Dtsch Ärztebl Int. 2010;107:647–55.

Holsterin A, Egberts E-H. Risk of hypoglycaemia with oral antidiabetic agents in patients with type 2 diabetes. Exp Clin Endocrinol Diabetes. 2003;111;405–14.

Holstein A, Hammer C, Hahn M, Kulamadayil NSA, Kovacs P. Severe sulfonylurea-induce hypoglycemia: a problem of uncritical prescription and deficiencies of diabetes care in geriatric patients. Expert Opin Drug Saf. 2010;9:675–81.

Jaber LA, Wenzloff NJ, Komanicky P, Antal EJ. An evaluation of the therapeutic effects and dosage equivalence glyburide and glipizide. J Clin Pharmacol. 1990;181:181–8.

Johnson A, Rydberg T, Ekberg G, Hallengren B, Melander A. slow elimination of glyburide in NIDDM subjects. Diabetes Care. 1994; 17:142–5.

Lachin JM, Viberti G, Zinman B, et al. Renal function in type 2 diabetes with rosiglitazone, metformin, and glyburide monotherapy. Clin J Am Soc Nephrol. 2011;6:1032–40.

Lardinois CK, Liu GC, Reaven GM. Glyburide in non-insulin dependent diabetes: its therapeutic effect in patients with disease poorly controlled by insulin alone. Arch Intern Med. 1985;145:1028–32.

McIntyre CW, Owen PJ. Prescribing drugs in kidney disease. In: Brenner BM. Brenner & Rector's the kidney. 8th ed. Philadelphia: Saunders/Elsevier; 2008. p. 1930–55.

Pearson JG. Pharmacokinetics of glyburide. Am J Med. 1985;79(Suppl 3B):67–71.

Pearson JG, Antal EJ, Raehl CL, et al. Pharmacokinetic disposition of ^{14}C-glyburide in patients with varying renal function. Clin Pharmacol Ther. 1986;39:318–24.

Rogers HJ, Spector RG, Morrison PJ, Bradbrook ID. Pharmacokinetics of intravenous glibenclamide investigated by a high performance liquid chromatographic assay. Diabetologia. 1982;23:37–40.

Rydberg R, Jönsson A, Melander A. Comparison of the kinetics of glyburide and its active metabolites in humans. J Clin Pharm Ther. 1995;20:283–95.

Scheen AJ, Jaminet C, Luyckx AS, Lefebvre PJ. Pharmacokinetics and pharmacological properties of two galenical preparations of glibenclamide, HB419 and HB420, in non-insulin-dependent (type 2) diabetes. Int J Clin Pharmacol Ther Toxicol. 1987;25:70–6.

Schwinghammer TL, Antal EJ, Kubacka RT, Hackimer ME, Johnston JM. Pharmacokinetics and pharmacodynamics of glyburide in young and elderly nondiabetic adults. Clin Pharm. 1991;10:532–8.

Seltzer HS. Drug-induced hypoglycemia: a review of 1418 cases. Endocrinol Metab Clin North Am. 1989;18:163–83.

Weir MA, Gomes T, Mamdani M, et al. Impaired renal function modifies the risk of severe hypoglycemia among users of insulin but not glyburide: a population-based nested case-control study. Nephrol Dial Transplant. 2011;26:1888–94.

Dosage Adjustment of Medications Eliminated by the Kidneys

<u>Glyburide</u>/Micronase®, Diaβeta®   {Antidiabetic; sulfonylurea}

Usual initial dose: 2.5–5 mg orally once daily before breakfast

Usual maintenance dose: 1.25–20 mg/day orally in single or divided doses

Typical maximum dose: 20 mg/day

Proportion eliminated unchanged: 50 % (as metabolites)

Adjustment for Kidney Disease

FDA-approved product labeling: *The risk of toxic reactions may be greater in patients with impaired renal function; the initial and maintenance dosing should be conservative to avoid hypoglycemic reactions.*

Alternative adjustment:

GFR >50 mL/min	*1.25–10 mg once or twice daily according to blood glucose levels*
GFR 30–50 mL/min	*1.25–5 mg once or twice daily according to blood glucose levels*
GFR <30 mL/min	*Preferably avoid due to risk of severe hypoglycemia.*
Hemodialysis	*Preferably avoid due to risk of severe hypoglycemia.*
CAPD	*Preferably avoid due to risk of severe hypoglycemia.*
CRRT	*Not applicable; preferably avoid due to risk of severe hypoglycemia.*

H

L.K. Golightly et al. (eds.), *Renal Pharmacotherapy*,
DOI 10.1007/978-1-4614-5800-5_8, © Springer Science+Business Media New York 2013

Dosage Adjustment of Medications Eliminated by the Kidneys

Hetastarch - Selected References

Baldassarre S, Vincent J-L. Coagulopathy induced by hydroxyethyl starch. Anesth Analg. 1997;84:449–50.

Blaicher AM, Reiter WJ, Blaicher W, et al. The effect of hydroxyethyl starch on platelet aggregation in vitro. Anesth Analg. 1998;86:1318–21.

Boldt J, Haisch G, Suttner S, Kumle B, Schellhaass A. Effects of a new modified, balanced hydroxyethyl starch preparation (Hextend®) on measures of coagulation. Br J Anaesth. 2002;89:722–8 (Note—Prof Boldt has been associated in other media with questionable authenticity of certain clinical data).

Cittanova ML, Leblanc I, Legendre C, Mouquet C, Riou B, Coriat P. Effect of hydroxyethylstarch in brain-dead kidney donors on renal function in kidney-transplant recipients. Lancet. 1996;348:1620–22.

Conroy JM, Fishman RL, Pinosky ML, Lazarchick J. The effects of desmopressin and 6% hydroxyethyl starch on factor VIII:C. Anesth Analg. 1996;83:804–7.

Cope JT, Banks D, Mauney MC, et al. Intraoperative hetastarch infusion impairs hemostasis after cardiac operations. Ann Thorac Surg. 1997;63:78–83.

Dart AB, Mutter TC, Ruth CA, Taback SP. Hydroxyethyl starch (HES) versus other fluid therapies: effects on kidney function. Cochrane Database Syst Rev. 2010;(1):CD007594. doi:10.1002/14651858.CD007594.pub2.

Deman A, Peeters P, Sennesael J. Hydroxyethyl starch does not impair immediate renal function in kidney transplant recipients: a retrospective, multicentre analysis. Nephrol Dial Transplant. 1999;14:1517–20.

Dickenmann M, Oettl T, Mihatsch MJ. Osmotic nephrosis: Acute kidney injury with accumulation of proximal tubular lysosomes due to accumulation of exogenous solutes. Am J Kidney Dis. 2008;51:491–503.

Dienes HP, Gerharz C-D, Wagner R, Weber M, John H-D. Accumulation of hydroxyethyl starch (HES) in the liver of patients with renal failure and portal hypertension. J Hepatol. 1986;3:223–7.

Egli GA, Zollinger A, Seifert B, Popovic D, Pasch T, Spahn DR. Effect of progressive haemodilution with hydroxyethyl starch, gelatin, and albumin on blood coagulation. Br J Anaesth. 1997;78:684–9.

Gan TJ, Bennett-Guerrero E, Phillips-Bute B, et al. Hextend®, a physiologically balanced plasma expander for large volume use in major surgery: a randomized phase III clinical trial. Anesth Analg. 1999;88:992–8.

6% Hetastarch in 0.9% Sodium Chloride injection [package insert]. Irvine: Teva Parenteral Medicines Inc; 2008.

Hextend® 6% Hetastarch in Lactated Electrolyte Injection [package insert]. Lake Forest: Hospira Inc; 2008.

Innerhofer P, Fries D, Martreiter J, et al. The effects of perioperatively administered colloids and crystalloids on primary platelet-mediated hemostasis and clot formation. Anesth Analg. 2002;95:858–65.

Niemi TT, Kuttunen AH. Hydroxyethyl starch impairs in vitro coagulation. Acta Anaesthesiol Scand. 1998;42:1104–9.

Perel P, Roberts I. Colloids versus crystalloids for fluid resuscitation in critically ill patients. Cochrane Database Syst Rev. 2011;(3):CD000567. doi:10.1002/14651858.CD000567.pub4.

Petroianu GA, Maleck WH, Mattnger C, Bergler WF. The effect of in vitro hemodilution with gelatin, dextran, hydroxyethyl starch, or Ringer's solution on Thromboelastograph®. Anesth Analg. 2000;90:795–800.

Roche AM, James MFM, Grocott MPW, Mythen MG, Coagulation effects of in vitro serial haemodilution with a balanced electrolyte hetastarch solution compared with a saline-based hetastarch solution and lactated Ringer's solution. Anaesthesia. 2002;57:950–5.

Siegmund M. 10% Hydroxyethylstarch impairs renal function and induces interstitial proliferation, macrophage infiltration and tubular damage [letter]. Crit Care. 2009;13:413.

Wiedermann CJ. Systematic review of randomized clinical trials on the use of hydroxyethyl starch for fluid management in sepsis. BMC Emerg Med. 2008;8:1. doi:10.1186/1471-227X-8-1.

Wiedermann CJ, Dunzendorfer S, Gaioni LU, Zaraca F, Joannidis M. Hyperoncotic colloids and acute kidney injury: a meta-analysis of randomized trials. Crit Care. 2010;14LR191. doi:10.1186/cc9308.

Zhao HJ, Chen HP, Meng ZY, Wang Q. A case of acute renal failure due to hydroxyethyl starch. Clin Nephrol. 2009;71:329–32.

Dosage Adjustment of Medications Eliminated by the Kidneys

6% Hetastarch in 0.9% Sodium Chloride/
Hespan® 6% Hetastarch in Lactated
Electrolyte Injection/Hextend®   {Plasma volume expander; colloid}

Usual initial dose: 500 mL IV

Usual maintenance dose: 500–1,000 mL/day IV

Typical maximum dose: 20 mL/kg ($\approx$1,500 mL) per day

Proportion eliminated unchanged: 33 %

Adjustment for Kidney Disease

    FDA-approved product labeling: *Renal disease with oliguria or anuria   Contraindicated*
                                           not related to hypovolemia

    Alternative adjustment: *Data not available*

                                   Note: Use of hetastarch may be of particular concern for worsening kidney function in patients with serious illness and preexisting chronic or acute kidney disease; those undergoing kidney, kidney-pancreas, or liver transplantation; and those with hypoalbuminemia and/or sepsis.

Hydrochlorothiazide - Selected References

Ackerman GL, Flanigan WJ. Reversible insufficiency in chronic renal disease. JAMA. 1966;197:749–53.

Barbhaiya RH, Craig WA, Corrick-West HP, Welling PG. Pharmacokinetics of hydrochlorothiazide in fasted and nonfasted subjects: a comparison of plasma level and urinary excretion methods. J Pharm Sci. 1982;71:245–8.

Beermann B, Groschinsky-Grind M. Pharmacokinetics of hydrochlorothiazide in man. Eur J Clin Pharmacol. 1977;12:297–303.

Beermann B, Groschinsky-Grind M. Pharmacokinetics of hydrochlorothiazide in patients with congestive heart failure. Br J Clin Pharmacol. 1979;7:579–83.

Bello CT, Sevy RW, Harakal C. Renal and hemodynamic effects of combination therapy in hypertension. J Clin Pharmacol. 1974;14:630–7.

Cassin S, Vogh B. Effect of hydrochlorothiazide on renal blood flow and clearance of para-aminohippurate and creatinine. Proc Soc Exp Biol Med. 1966;122:970–3.

Gifford RW Jr. A guide to the practical use of diuretics. JAMA. 1976;235:1890–3.

Hook JB, Blatt AH, Brody MJ, Williamson HE. Effects of several saluretic-diuretic agents on renal hemodynamics. J Pharmacol Exp Ther. 1966;154:667–73.

Hydrochlorothiazide capsule [package insert]. Sellersville: Teva Pharmaceuticals USA Inc; 2011.

Januszewicz W, Heinemann HO, Demartini FE, Laragh JH. A clinical study of the effects of hydrochlorothiazide on the renal excretion of electrolytes and free water. N Engl J Med. 1959;261:264–9.

Kluza RB, Ronfeld RA, Yakatan GJ. Bioavailability monograph: hydrochlorothiazide. J Am Pharm Assoc. 1976;16(1):47–50.

Morgan T, Adam W, Hodgson M. Adverse reactions to long-term diuretic therapy for hypertension. J Cardiovasc Pharmacol. 1984;6(Suppl 1):S269–73.

Niemeyer C, Hasenfuß G, Wais U, Knauf H, Schäfer-Korting M, Mutschler E. Pharmacokinetics of hydrochlorothiazide in relation to renal function. Eur J Clin Pharmacol. 1983;24:661–5.

Patel RB, Patel UR, Hogge MC, et al. Bioavailability of hydrochlorothiazide from tablets and suspensions. J Pharm Sci. 1984;73:359–61.

Sackner MA, Wallack AA, Bellet S. The diuretic effects of hydrochlorothiazide in congestive heart failure, cirrhosis, chronic renal disease and hypertension: preliminary report based on a study of 28 cases. Am J Med Sci. 1959;237:575–84.

Dosage Adjustment of Medications Eliminated by the Kidneys

<u>Hydrochlorothiazide</u>/Microzide®, Hydrodiuril®   {Diuretic, thiazide}

Usual initial dose:	12.5–25 mg orally
Usual maintenance dose:	12.5–50 mg orally once or twice daily
Typical maximum dose:	100 mg/day
Proportion eliminated unchanged:	65–72 %

Adjustment for Kidney Disease

FDA-approved product labeling:	*Severe renal disease*	*Use with caution*
	Anuria	*Contraindicated*
Alternative adjustment:	*GFR >50 mL/min*	*12.5–50 mg orally once or twice daily*
	GFR 10–50 mL/min	*12.5–25 mg orally once daily*
	GFR <10 mL/min	*Usually ineffective, preferably avoid*
	Hemodialysis	*Usually ineffective, preferably avoid*
	CAPD	*Usually ineffective, preferably avoid*
	CRRT	*Not applicable; preferably avoid*

Hydroxyethyl Starch 130/0.4 in 0.9 % Sodium Chloride - Selected References

Boldt J, Brosch C, Ducke M, Papsdorf M, Lehmann A. Influence of volume therapy with a modern hydroxyethylstarch preparation on kidney function in cardiac surgery patients with compromised renal function: a comparison with human albumin. Crit Care Med. 2007;35:2740–6 (Note—Prof Boldt has been associated in other media with questionable authenticity of certain clinical data).

Boussekey N, Darmon R, Langlois J, et al. Resuscitation with low volume hydroxyethylstarch 130 kDa/0.4 is not associated with acute kidney injury. Crit Care. 2010;14:R40. doi:10.1186/cc8920.

Bunn F, Trivedi D, Ahraf S. Colloid solutions for fluid resuscitation. Cochrane Database Syst Rev. 2011;(3):CD001319. doi:10.1002/14651858.CD001319.pub3.

Godet G, Lehot JJ, Janvier G, Steib A, De Castro V, Coriat P. Safety of HES 130/0.1 (Voluven®) in patients with preoperative renal dysfunction undergoing abdominal aortic surgery: a prospective, randomized, controlled, parallel-group multicentre trial. Eur J Anaesth. 2008;25:986–94.

Hüter L, Simon T-P, Weinmann L, et al. Hydroxyethylstarch impairs renal function and induces interstitial proliferation, macrophage infiltration and tubular damage in an isolated renal perfusion model. Crit Care. 2009;13:R23. doi:10.1186/cc7726.

Jungheinrich C, Neff TA. Pharmacokinetics of hydroxyethyl starch. Clin Pharmacokinet. 2005;44:681–99.

Jungheinrich C, Scharpf R, Wargenau M, Bepperling F, Baron J-F. The pharmacokinetics and tolerability of an intravenous infusion of the hydroxyethyl starch 130/0.4 (6 %, 500 mL) in mild-to-severe renal impairment. Anesth Analg. 2002;95:544–51.

Kozek-Langenecker SA, Jungheinrich C, Sauermann W, Van der Linden P. The effects of hydroxyethyl starch 130/0.4 (6 %) on blood loss and use of blood products in major surgery: a pooled analysis of randomized trials. Anesth Analg. 2008;107:382–90.

Mukhtar A, Aboulfetouh F, Obayah G, et al. The safety of modern hydroxyethyl starch in living donor liver transplantation: a comparison with human albumin. Anesth Analg. 2009;109:924–30.

Perel P, Roberts I. Colloids versus crystalloids for fluid resuscitation in critically ill patients. Cochrane Database Syst Rev. 2011;(3):CD000567. doi:10.1002/14651858.CD000567.pub4.

Schabinski F, Oishi J, Tuche F, et al. Effects of a predominantly hydroxyethyl starch (HES)-based and a predominantly non HES-based fluid therapy on renal function in surgical ICU patients. Intensive Care Med. 2009;35:1539–47.

Schick MA, Isbary TJ, Schlegel N, et al. The impact of crystalloid and colloid infusion on the kidney in rodent sepsis. Intensive Care Med. 2010;36:541–8.

Schramko AA, Suojaranta-Ylinen R, Kuitunen AH, Kukkonen SI, Niema TT. Rapidly degradable hydroxyethyl starch solutions impair blood coagulation after cardiac surgery: a prospective randomized trial. Anesth Analg. 2009;108:30–6.

Voluven® injection [package insert]. Lake Forest: Hospira Inc; 2010.

Wiedermann CJ. Iatrogenic hypoalbuminemia due to hydroxyethyl starch 130/0.4: a risk factor for acute kidney injury? [letter]. Anesth Analg. 2010;110:1242.

Wiedermann CJ. Hydroxyethyl starch 130/0.4: does modern mean safe? [letter]. Anesth Analg. 2009;109:1346–7.

Wittlinger M, Schläpfer M, De Conno E, et al. The effect of hydroxyethyl starches (HES 130/0.42 and HES 200/0.5) on activated renal tubular epithelial cells. Anesth Analg. 2010;110:531–40.

6 % Hydroxyethyl Starch 130/0.4 in
0.9 % Sodium Chloride /Voluven®   {Plasma volume expander; colloid}

Usual initial dose: 10–20 mL IV infused slowly with observation for possible anaphylactoid reactions followed by IV infusion of the remainder of a 500-mL container at a relatively rapid rate (e.g., over 30 min) dependent on the patient's blood loss, hemodynamics, and hemodilution effects

Usual maintenance dose: ≤50 mL/kg (3 g/kg) per day (equivalent to 3,500 mL in a 70-kg patient)

Typical maximum dose: 50 mL/kg/day (~3,500 mL/day)

Proportion eliminated unchanged: 59–70 %

Adjustment for Kidney Disease

FDA-approved product labeling:	*Renal dysfunction*	*Adjust dosage, avoid fluid overload*
	Renal failure with oliguria or anuria not associated with hypovolemia	*Contraindicated*
Alternative adjustment:	*eCrCL 30–50 mL/min*	*≤500 mL/24 h IV*
	eCrCL 15–30 mL/min	*≤500 mL/24 h IV*
	Hemodialysis	*Data not available; preferably avoid due to risk for accumulation and possible nephrotoxicity*
	CAPD	*Data not available; preferably avoid due to risk for accumulation and possible nephrotoxicity*
	CRRT	*Data not available; preferably avoid due to risk for accumulation and possible nephrotoxicity*

Dosage Adjustment of Medications Eliminated by the Kidneys

Hydroxyurea - Selected References

Allen A, Scoble J, Snowden S, Hambley H, Bellingham A. Hydroxyurea, sickle cell disease and renal transplantation [letter]. Nephron. 1997;75:106–7.

Belt RJ, Haas CD, Kennedy J, Taylor S. Studies of hydroxyurea administered by continuous infusion: toxicity, pharmacokinetics, and cell synchronization. Cancer. 1980;46:455–62.

Charache S, Terrin ML, Moore RD, et al. Effect of hydroxyurea on the frequency of painful crises in sickle cell anemia. N Engl J Med. 1995;332:1317–22.

de Montalembert M, Bachir D, Hulin A, et al. Pharmacokinetics of hydroxyurea 1,000 mg coated breakable tablets and 500 mg capsules in pediatric and adult patients with sickle cell disease. Haematologica. 2006;91:1685–8.

Droxia® [package insert]. Princeton: Bristol-Myers Squibb Co; 2010.

Gandhi V, Plunkett W, Kantarjian H, Talpaz M, Robertson LE, O'Brien S. Cellular pharmacodynamics and plasma pharmacokinetics of parenterally infused hydroxyurea during a phase I clinical trial in chronic myelogenous leukemia. J Clin Oncol. 1998;16:2321–31.

Gwilt PR, Maouilov KK, McNabb JC, Swindells SS. Pharmacokinetics of hydroxyurea in plasma and cerebrospinal fluid of HIV-1-infected patients. J Clin Pharmacol. 2003;43:1003–7.

Gwilt PR, Tracewell WG. Pharmacokinetics and pharmacodynamics of hydroxyurea. Clin Pharmacokinet. 1998;34:347–58.

Hydrea® capsule [package insert]. Princeton: Bristol-Myers Squibb Co; 2010.

Lanzkron S, Strouse JJ, Wilson R, et al. Systematic review: hydroxyurea for the treatment of adults with sickle cell disease. Ann Intern Med. 2008;148:939–55.

Lisziewicz J, Foli A, Wainberg M, Lori F. Hydroxyurea in the treatment of HIV infection: clinical efficacy and safety concerns. Drug Saf. 2003;26:605–24.

Luzzati R, Di Perri G, Fendt D, Ramarli D, Broccali G, Concia E. Pharmacokinetics, safety and anti-human immunodeficiency virus (HIV) activity of hydroxyurea in combination with didanosine [letter]. J Antimicrob Chemother. 1998;42:565–6.

McIntyre CW, Owen PJ. Prescribing drugs in kidney disease. In: Brenner BM, editor. Brenner & Rector's the kidney. 8th ed. Philadelphia: Saunders/Elsevier; 2008. p. 1930–55.

Newman EM, Carroll M, Akman SA, et al. Pharmacokinetics and toxicity of 120-hour continuous-infusion hydroxyurea in patients with advanced solid tumors. Cancer Chemother Pharmacol. 1997;39:254–8.

Paule I, Sassi H, Habibi A, et al. Population pharmacokinetics and pharmacodynamics of hydroxyurea in sickle cell anemia patients, a basis for optimizing the dosing regimen. Orphanet J Rare Dis. 2011;6:30. doi:10.1186/1750-1172-6-30

Reardon DA, Dresemann G, Taillibert S, et al. Multicentre phase II studies evaluating Imatinib plus hydroxyurea in patients with progressive glioblastoma. Br J Cancer. 2009;101:1993–2004.

Rodriguez GI, Kuhm JG, Weiss GR, et al. A bioavailability and pharmacokinetic study of oral and intravenous hydroxyurea. Blood. 1998;91:1533–41.

Skirvin JA, Lichtman SM. Pharmacokinetic considerations of oral chemotherapy in elderly patients with cancer. Drugs Aging. 2002;19:25–42.

Tracewell WG, Trump DL, Vaughan WP, Smith DC, Gwilt PR. Population pharmacokinetics of hydroxyurea in cancer patients. Cancer Chemother Pharmacol. 1995;35:417–22.

Tracewell WG, Vaughan WP, Gwilt PR. Nonlinear disposition of hydroxyurea [letter]. J Pharm Sci. 1994;83:1060–1.

Villani P, Maserati R, Regazzi MB, Giacchino R, Lori F. Pharmacokinetics of hydroxyurea in patients with human immunodeficiency virus type I. J Clin Pharmacol. 1996;36:117–21.

Yan J-H, Ataga AK, Kaul S, et al. The influence of renal function on hydroxyurea pharmacokinetics in adults with sickle cell disease. J Clin Pharmacol. 2005;45:434–45.

Hydroxyurea (Hydroxycarbamide)/
Hydrea®, Droxia®   {Antineoplastic; ribonucleotide reductase inhibitor}

Usual initial dose:	Malignancy, 20–30 mg/kg orally; sickle cell disease, 15 mg/kg orally
Usual maintenance dose:	Malignancy, 20–30 mg/kg orally once daily or 80 mg/kg orally as a single dose every third day; sickle cell disease, 15 mg/kg orally once daily
Typical maximum dose:	35 mg/kg/day
Proportion eliminated unchanged:	36 %

Adjustment for Kidney Disease

FDA-approved product labeling:	*Malignancy*	Use with caution in patients with marked renal dysfunction. As renal excretion is a pathway of elimination, consideration should be given to decreasing dosage in patients with renal impairment. Close monitoring of hematologic parameters is advised in these patients.
	Sickle cell disease	
	CrCL ≥60 mL/min	15 mg/kg orally once daily
	CrCL <60 or end-stage renal disease	7.5 mg/kg orally once daily, after dialysis on hemodialysis days
Alternative adjustment:	*Malignancy*	
	GFR >50 mL/min	20–30 mg/kg orally every 24 h
	GFR 10–50 mL/min	10–15 mg/kg orally every 24 h (50 % decrease)
	GFR <10 mL/min	4–6 mg/kg orally every 24 h (80 % decrease)
	Hemodialysis	4–6 mg/kg orally every 24 h; administer after hemodialysis on dialysis days.
	CAPD	4–6 mg/kg orally every 24 h
	CRRT	10–15 mg/kg orally every 24 h

Note: Hematological and other considerations may suggest further dosage adjustments.

I

L.K. Golightly et al. (eds.), *Renal Pharmacotherapy*,
DOI 10.1007/978-1-4614-5800-5_9, © Springer Science+Business Media New York 2013

Dosage Adjustment of Medications Eliminated by the Kidneys

Ibandronate - Selected References

Barrett J, Worth E, Bauss F, Epstein S. Ibandronate: a clinical pharmacological and pharmacokinetic update. J Clin Pharmacol. 2004;44:951–65.

Bergner R, Dill K, Boerner D, Uppenkamp M. Elimination of intravenously administered ibandronate in patients on haemodialysis: a monocentre open study. Nephrol Dial Transplant. 2002;17:1281–5.

Bergner R, Henrich DM, Hoffmann M, et al. Renal safety and pharmacokinetics of ibandronate in multiple myeloma patients with or without impaired renal function. J Clin Pharmacol. 2007;47:942–50.

Body JJ, Diel IJ, Lichinitzer M, et al. Oral ibandronate reduced the risk of skeletal complications in breast cancer patients with metastatic bone disease: results from two randomised, placebo-controlled phase III studies. Br J Cancer. 2004; 90:1133–7.

Body JJ, Diel IJ, Tripathy D, Bergstrom B. Intravenous ibandronate does not affect time to renal function deterioration in patients with skeletal metastases from breast cancer: phase III trial results. Eur J Cancer Care (Engl). 2006;15:299–302.

Boniva® injection [package insert]. South San Francisco: Genentech USA Inc; 2011.

Boniva® tablet [package insert]. South San Francisco: Genentech USA Inc; 2010.

Diel IJ, Weide R, Köppler H, et al. Risk of renal impairment after treatment with ibandronate versus zoledronic acid: a retrospective medical records review. Support Care Cancer. 2009;17:719–25.

Grotz W, Nagel C, Poeschel D, et al. Effect of ibandronate on bone loss and renal function after kidney transplantation. J Am Soc Nephrol. 2001;12:1530–7.

Miller PD. The kidney and bisphosphonates. Bone. 2011;49:77–81.

Musso CG, Guelman R, Varela F, et al. Ibandronate improves hyperphosphatemia in dialysis patients with hyperparathyroidism. Int J Urol Nephrol. 2004;36:625–7.

Pecherstorfer M, Diel IJ. Rapid administration of ibandronate does not affect renal functioning: evidence from clinical studies in metastatic bone disease and hypercalcaemia of pregnancy. Support Care Cancer. 2004;12:877–81.

Perazella MA, Markowitz GS. Bisphosphonate nephrotoxicity. Kidney Int. 2008;74:1385–93.

Pivot X, Lortholary A, Avadie-Lacourtoisie S, et al. Renal safety of ibandronate 6 mg infused over 15 min versus 60 min in breast cancer patients with bone metastases: a randomized open-label equivalence trial. Breast. 2011;20(6):510–4. doi:10.1016/j.breast.2011.05.006.

von Moos R, Caspar CB, Thürlimann B, et al. Renal safety profiles of ibandronate 6 mg infused over 15 and 60 min: a randomized, open-label study. Ann Oncol. 2008;19:1266–70.

Weide R, Köppler H, Antràs L, et al. Renal toxicity in patients with multiple myeloma receiving zoledronic acid vs ibandronate: a retrospective medical records review. J Cancer Res Ther. 2010.6:31–5.

Dosage Adjustment of Medications Eliminated by the Kidneys

Ibandronate/Boniva®	{Anti-osteoporotic; bisphosphonate}
Usual initial dose:	2.5 mg or 150 mg orally or 3 mg IV
Usual maintenance dose:	2.5 mg orally once daily or 150 mg orally once monthly or 3 mg IV over 15–30 s every 3 months
Typical maximum dose:	150 mg/month orally or 6 mg IV over 15–60 min every 3 months
Proportion eliminated unchanged:	50–60 % of an IV dose within 24 h

Adjustment for Kidney Disease

FDA-approved product labeling:	*Mild or moderate renal impairment*	*No dose adjustment needed*
	Severe renal impairment (SCr >2.3 mg/dL or CrCL <30 mL/min)	*Use not recommended*
Alternative adjustment:	*GFR ≥30 mL/min*	*150 mg orally once monthly or 3–6 mg IV every 3 months*
	GFR <30 mL/min	*Preferably avoid due to (1) risk (presently theoretical and/or undocumented) for renal adverse effects, (2) minimal safety evidence, and (3) only limited experience available with reduced dose regimens (1 mg IV once monthly) in patients on chronic hemodialysis*

Dosage Adjustment of Medications Eliminated by the Kidneys

Idarubicin - Selected References

Aronoff GA, Bennett WM, Berns JS, et al. Drug prescribing in renal failure: dosing guidelines for adults and children. 5th ed. Philadelphia: American College of Physicians; 2007.

Bárdi Bobok I, Oláh AV, Kappelmayer J, Kiss C. Anthracycline antibiotics induce acute renal tubular toxicity in children with cancer. Pathol Oncol Res. 2007;13:249–53.

Camaggi CM, Strocchi E, Carisi P, et al. Idarubicin metabolism and pharmacokinetics after intravenous and oral administration in cancer patients: a crossover study. Cancer Chemother Pharmacol. 1992;30:307–16.

Eksborg S, Söderberg M, Nilsson B, Antila K. Plasma pharmacokinetics of idarubicin and its 13-hyroxymetabolite after intravenous and oral administration under fasting and non-fasting conditions. Acta Oncol. 1990;29:921–5.

Elbæk K, Effehøj E, Jakobsen A, et al. Pharmacokinetics of oral idarubicin in breast cancer patients with reference to anti-tumour activity and side effects. Clin Pharmacol Ther. 1989;45:627–34.

Gillies HC, Herriott D, Liang R, Ohashi K, Rogers HJ, Harper PG. Pharmacokinetics of idarubicin (4-demethoxydaunorubicin; IMI-30; NSC 256439) following intravenous and oral administration in patients with advanced cancer. Br J Clin Pharmacol. 1987;23:303–10.

Hollingshead LM, Faulds D. Idarubicin: a review of its pharmacodynamic and pharmacokinetic properties, and therapeutic potential in the chemotherapy of cancer. Drugs. 1991;42:690–719.

Idamycin PFS® injection [package insert]. New York: Pharmacia & Upjohn Co Division of Pfizer Inc; 2006.

Leoni F, Ciolli S, Giuliani G, et al. Attenuated-dose idarubicin in acute myeloid leukaemia of the elderly: pharmacokinetic study and clinical results. Br J Haematol. 1995;90:169–74.

Lu K, Savaraj N, Kavanagh J, et al. Clinical pharmacology of 4-demethoxydaunorubicin (DMDR). Cancer Chemother Pharmacol. 1986;17:143–8.

Pannuti F, Camaggi CM, Strocchi E, Comparsi R, Angelelli B, Pacciarini MA. Low dose oral administration of 4-demethoxy-daunorubicin (idarubicin) in advanced cancer patients. Cancer Chemother Pharmacol. 1986;16:295–9.

Robert J. Clinical pharmacokinetics of idarubicin. Clin Pharmacokinet. 1993;24:275–88.

Robert J, Rigal-Huguet F, Harousseau JL, et al. Pharmacokinetics of idarubicin after daily intravenous administration in leukemic patients. Leuk Res. 1987;11:961–4.

Robert J, Rigal-Huguet F, Hurteloup P. Comparative pharmacokinetic study of idarubicin and daunorubicin in leukemia patients. Hematol Oncol. 1992;10:111–6.

Smith DB, Margison JM, Lucas SB, Wilkinson PM, Howell A. Clinical pharmacology of oral and intravenous 4-demethoxy-daunorubicin. Cancer Chemother Pharmacol. 1987;19:138–42.

Speth PAJ, van de Loo FAJ, Linssen PCM, Wessels HMC, Haanen C. Plasma and human leukemic cell pharmacokinetics of oral and intravenous 4-demethoxydaunorubicin. Clin Pharmacol Ther. 1986;40:643–9.

Tamassia V, Pacciarini MA, Moro E, Piazza E, Vago G, Libretti A. Pharmacokinetic study of intravenous and oral idarubicin in cancer patients. Int J Clin Pharmacol Res. 1987;7:419–26.

Tidefelt U, Sundman-Engberg B, Paul C. Comparison of the intracellular pharmacokinetics of daunorubicin and idarubicin in patients with acute leukemia. Leuk Res. 1994;18:293–7.

Zanette L, Zucchetti M, Freshi A, Erranti D, Tirelli U, D'Incalci M. Pharmacokinetics of 4-demethoxydaunorubicin in cancer patients. Cancer Chemother Pharmacol. 1990;25:445–8.

Dosage Adjustment of Medications Eliminated by the Kidneys

<u>Idarubicin</u>/Idamycin®　　　　　　　　{Antineoplastic; anthracycline}

Usual initial dose: 12 mg/m² IV

Usual maintenance dose: 12 mg/m² IV daily for 3 days

Typical maximum dose: 12 mg/m²/day

Proportion eliminated unchanged: 3–5 % in 24 h, 16 % in 4 days (8 % of active hydroxylated metabolite, idarubicinol)

Adjustment for Kidney Disease

FDA-approved product labeling:	*Renal impairment*	*Dose reduction should be considered.*
Alternative adjustment:	*GFR >50 mL/min*	*12 mg/kg IV daily for 3 days*
	GFR 10–50 mL/min	*8 mg/kg IV daily for 3 days (~25 % decrease)*
	GFR <10 mL/min	*6 mg/kg IV daily for 3 days (50 % decrease)*
	Hemodialysis	*Data not available*
	CAPD	*Data not available*
	CRRT	*Data not available*

Note: Hematological and other considerations may suggest further dosage adjustments.

Dosage Adjustment of Medications Eliminated by the Kidneys

Ifosfamide - Selected References

Aleksa K, Ito S, Koren G. Enantioselective metabolism of ifosfamide by the kidney. Chirality. 2006;18:398–405.

Aleksa K, Ito S, Koren G. Renal-tubule metabolism of ifosfamide to the nephrotoxic chloroacetaldehyde: pharmacokinetic modeling for estimation of intracellular levels. J Lab Clin Med. 2004;143:159–62.

Allen LM, Creaven PJ. Pharmacokinetics of ifosfamide. Clin Pharmacol Ther. 1975;17:492–8.

Antman KH, Elias A, Ryan L. Ifosfamide and mesna: response and toxicity at standard- and high-dose schedules. Semin Oncol. 1990;17(Suppl 4):68–73.

Brade WP, Herdrich K, Kachel-Fischer U, Araujo CE. Dosing and side-effects of ifosfamide plus mesna. J Cancer Res Clin Oncol. 1991;117(Suppl 4):S164–86.

Chen N, Aleksa K, Woodland C, Rieder M, Koren G. Prevention of ifosfamide nephrotoxicity by N-acetylcysteine: clinical pharmacokinetic considerations. Can J Clin Pharmacol. 2007;14: 246–50.

Ciarimboli G, Holle SK, Vollenbröcker B, et al. New clues for nephrotoxicity induced by ifosfamide: preferential renal uptake via the human organic cation transporter 2. Mol Pharm. 2011;8:270–9.

Elias A, Eder JP, Shea T, Begg CB, Frei E III, Antman KH. High-dose ifosfamide with mesna uroprotection: a phase I study. J Clin Oncol. 1990;8:170–8.

Granvil CP, Ducharme J, Leyland-Jones B, Trudeau M, Wainer IW. Stereoselective pharmacokinetics of ifosfamide and its 2- and 3-N-dechlorethylated metabolites in female cancer patients. Cancer Chemother Pharmacol. 1996;37:451–6.

Hanley L, Chen N, Rieder M, Koren G. Ifosfamide nephrotoxicity in children: a mechanistic base for pharmacological prevention. Expert Opin Drug Saf. 2009;8:155–68.

Ifex® [package insert]; Deerfield: Baxter Healthcare Corp; 2009.

Ingemi AI, Bota VM, Pegurero A, Charpentier M. Fanconi's syndrome and nephrogenic diabetes insipidus in an adult treated with ifosfamide. Pharmacotherapy. 2012;32:e12–16. doi:10.1002/PHAR.1013.

Kurowski V, Wagner T. Urinary excretion of ifosfamide, 4-hydroxyifosfamide, 3- and 2-dechloroethylifosfamide, mesna, and dimesna in patients on fractionated intravenous ifosfamide and concomitant mesna therapy. Cancer Chemother Pharmacol. 1997;39:431–9.

Latcha S, Maki RG, Schwartz GK, Flombaum CD. Ifosfamide may be safely used in patients with end stage renal disease on hemodialysis. Sarcoma. 2009;2009:575629. doi:10.1155/2009/575629.

Lewis LD. A study of 5 day fractionated ifosfamide pharmacokinetics in consecutive treatment cycles. Br J Clin Pharmacol. 1996;42:179–86.

McIntyre CW, Owen PJ. Prescribing drugs in kidney disease. In: Brenner BM, editor. Brenner & Rector's the kidney. 8th ed. Philadelphia: Saunders/Elsevier; 2008. p. 1930–55.

Nelson RL, Allen LM, Creaven PJ. Pharmacokinetics of divided-dose ifosfamide. Clin Pharmacol Ther. 1976;19:365–70.

Nissim I, Horyn O, Daikhin Y, et al. Ifosfamide-induced nephrotoxicity: mechanism and prevention. Cancer Res. 2006;66:7824–31.

Patterson WP, Khojasteh A. Ifosfamide-induced renal tubular defects. Cancer. 1989;63:649–51.

Rodriguez V, Bodey G, Freireich EJ, McCredie KB, McKelvey EM, Tashima CK. Reduction of ifosfamide toxicity using dose fractionation. Cancer Res. 1976;36:2945–8.

Skinner R, Parry A, Price L, Cole M, Craft AW, Pearson ADJ. Glomerular toxicity persists 10 years after ifosfamide treatment in childhood and is not predictable by age or dose. Pediatr Blood Cancer. 2010;54:983–9.

Springate JE. Ifosfamide metabolite chloroacetaldehyde causes renal dysfunction in vivo. J Appl Toxicol. 1996;17:75–9.

Springate JE, Zamlauski-Tucker MJ, Lu H, Chan KK. Renal clearance of ifosfamide. Drug Metab Dispos. 1997;25:1081–2.

Willemse PHB, de Jong PE, Elema JD, Mulder NH. Severe renal failure following high-dose ifosfamide and mesna. Cancer Chemother Pharmacol. 1989;23:239–30.

Woodland C, Ito S, Granvil C, Wainer IW, Klein J, Koren G. Evidence of renal metabolism of ifosfamide to nephrotoxic metabolites. Life Sci. 2000;68:109–17.

Wright JE, Elias A, Tretyakov O, et al. High-dose ifosfamide, carboplatin, and etoposide pharmacokinetics: correlation of plasma drug levels with renal toxicity. Cancer Chemother Pharmacol. 1995;36:345–51.

Zhang J, Hongjuan L. Ifosfamide induces acute renal failure via inhibition of the thioredoxin reductase activity. Free Radic Biol Med. 2007;43:1574–83.

Dosage Adjustment of Medications Eliminated by the Kidneys

Ifosfamide/Ifex®   {Antineoplastic; alkylating agent}

Usual initial dose: 1.2 g/m²

Usual maintenance dose: 1.2 g/m² IV over 1–2 h daily for 5 consecutive days every 3 weeks or after hematological recovery (with mesna)

Typical maximum dose: May be limited by hematological toxicity

Proportion eliminated unchanged: 14 % (Stereoselective renal metabolism may contribute to production of nephrotoxic metabolites such as chloroacetaldehyde.)

Adjustment for Kidney Disease

FDA-approved product labeling:	*Compromised renal function*	*Studies to establish optimal dose schedules in such patients have not been conducted.*
Alternative adjustment:	*GFR >50 mL/min*	*1.2 g/m² IV daily for 5 days every 3 weeks or after hematological recovery*
	GFR 10–50 mL/min	*0.9 g/m² IV daily for 5 days every 3 weeks or after hematological recovery (25 % decrease)*
	GFR <10 mL/min	*0.6 g/m² IV daily for 5 days every 3 weeks or after hematological recovery (50 % decrease)*
	Hemodialysis	*0.0.4–0.6 g/m² IV daily for 5 days every 3 weeks or after hematological recovery (~50 % decrease)*
	CAPD	*0.6 g/m² IV daily for 5 days every 3 weeks or after hematological recovery (50 % decrease)*
	CRRT	*0.9 g/m² IV daily for 5 days*

Note: Urological, hematological, and/or other considerations may suggest further dosage adjustments.

Dosage Adjustment of Medications Eliminated by the Kidneys

Imatinib - Selected References

Ali Y, Lin Y, Gharibo MM, et al. Phase I and pharmacokinetic study of imatinib mesylate (Gleevec) and gemcitabine in patients with refractory solid tumors. Clin Cancer Res. 2007;13:5876–82.

Chandran S, Petersen J. Jacobs C, Fiorentino D, Doeden K, Lafayette RA. Imatinib in the treatment of nephrogenic systemic fibrosis. Am J Kidney Dis. 2009;53:129–32.

Foringer JR, Verani RR, Tjia VM, Finkel KW, Samuels JA, Guntupalli JS. Acute renal failure secondary to imatinib mesylate treatment in prostate cancer. Ann Pharmacother. 2005;69:2136–8.

Gafter-Gvili A, Ram R, Gafter U, Shpilberg O, Raanani P. Renal failure associated with tyrosine kinase inhibitors: case report and review of the literature. Leuk Res. 2010;34:123–7.

Gibbons J, Egorin MJ, Ramanathan RK, et al. Phase I and pharmacokinetic study of imatinib mesylate in patients with advanced malignancies and varying degrees of renal dysfunction: a study of the National Cancer Institute Organ Dysfunction working group. J Clin Oncol. 2008;26:570–6.

Gleevec® tablet [package insert]. East Hanover: Novartis Pharmaceuticals Inc; 2011.

Kay J. Nephrogenic systemic fibrosis: a gadolinium-associated fibrosing disorder in patient with renal dysfunction. Ann Rheum Dis. 2008;67(Suppl 3):iii66–9.

Kitiyakara C, Atichartakarn V. Renal failure associated with a specific inhibitor of BCR-ABL tyrosine kinase, STI 571 [letter]. Nephrol Dial Transplant. 2002;17:685–7.

Marcolino MS, Boersma E, Clementino NCD, et al. Imatinib treatment duration is related to decreased estimated glomerular filtration rate in chronic myeloid leukemia patients. Ann Oncol. 2011;22(9):2073–9. doi:10.1093/annonc/mdq715.

Ozdemir E, Koc Y, Kansu E. Successful treatment of chronic myeloid leukemia with imatinib mesylate in a patient with chronic renal failure on hemodialysis [letter]. Am J Hematol. 2008;81:474.

Pappas P, Karavasilis V, Briasoulis E, Pavlidis N, Marselos M. Pharmacokinetics of imatinib mesylate in end stage renal disease: a case study. Cancer Chemother Pharmacol. 2005;56:358–60.

Peng B, Lloyd P, Schran H. Clinical pharmacokinetics of imatinib. Clin Pharmacokinet. 2005;44:879–94.

Pou M, Saval N, Vera M, et al. Acute renal failure secondary to imatinib mesylate treatment in chronic myeloid leukemia. Leuk Lymphoma. 2003;44:1239–41.

Ramanathan RK, Egorin MJ, Takimoto CHM, et al. Phase I and pharmacokinetic study of imatinib mesylate in patients with advanced malignancies and varying degrees of liver dysfunction: a study of the National Cancer Institute Organ Dysfunction working group. J Clin Oncol. 2008;26:563–9.

Reardon DA, Desjardins A, Vredenburgh JJ, et al. Safety and pharmacokinetics of dose-intensive imatinib mesylate plus temozolomide: phase I trial in adults with malignant glioma. Neuro Oncol. 2008;10:330–40.

Ryan CW, Vuky J, Chang JS, Chen Z, Beer TM, Nauman D. A phase II study of everolimus in combination with imatinib for previously treated advanced renal carcinoma. Investig New Drugs. 2011;29:374–9.

Thierry A, Dreyfus B, Bridoux F, et al. Long-term molecular efficacy and safety of imatinib in a patient with chronic myeloid leukaemia after renal transplantation [letter]. Nephrol Dial Transplant. 2007;22:1791–2.

Tong W-G, Kantarjian H, O'Brien S, et al. Imatinib front-line therapy is safe and effective in patients with chronic myelogenous leukemia with pre-existing liver and/or renal dysfunction. Cancer. 2010;116:3152–9.

van Erp NP, Gelderblom H, Guchelaar H-J. Clinical pharmacokinetics of tyrosine kinase inhibitors. Cancer Treat Rev. 2009;35:692–75.

Vuky J, Isacson C, Fotoohi M, et al. Phase II trial of imatinib (Gleevec®) in patients with metastatic renal cell carcinoma. Investig New Drugs. 2006;24:85–8.

Yuzawa Y, Sato W, Masuda T, et al. Acute kidney injury presenting a feature of leukemic infiltration during therapy for chronic myelogenous leukemia. Intern Med. 2010;49:1139–42.

Dosage Adjustment of Medications Eliminated by the Kidneys

<u>**Imatinib**</u>/Gleevec®   {**Antineoplastic; protein-tyrosine kinase inhibitor**}

Usual initial dose:	400–600 mg orally with a meal
Usual maintenance dose:	400–600 mg orally once daily or 400 mg orally twice daily with meals
Typical maximum dose:	1,200 mg/day
Proportion eliminated unchanged:	5 %

Adjustment for Kidney Disease

FDA-approved product labeling: *CrCL ≥60 mL/min*   *400–600 mg orally once daily with a meal or 400 mg orally twice daily with meals*

     CrCL 40–59 mL/min   *400–600 mg orally once daily with a meal*

     CrCL 20–39 mL/min   *200–300 mg orally once daily with a meal (50 % starting dose reduction; future doses may be increased as tolerated, not to exceed 400 mg/day)*

     CrCL <20 mL/min   *100 mg orally once daily with a meal*

Alternative adjustment: *eCrCL ≥60 mL/min*   *400–600 mg orally once daily with a meal or 400 mg orally twice daily with meals was generally well tolerated in a phase I study, although edema was prevalent (64 % of patients); the incidence of all other serious adverse effects was unrelated to kidney function.*

     eCrCL 40–59 mL/min   *400–600 mg orally once daily with a meal or 400 mg orally twice daily with meals was generally well tolerated in most patients, although edema was commonly reported (27 % of patients); investigators advised that dose adjustment was unnecessary with mild renal dysfunction.*

     eCrCL 20–39 mL/min   *400–600 mg orally once daily with a meal was well generally tolerated in most patients although edema was commonly reported (27 % of patients); investigators advised that dose adjustment was unnecessary with moderate renal dysfunction.*

     eCrCL <20 mL/min   *100 mg orally once daily was generally well tolerated in two patients.*

     Hemodialysis   *400 mg orally once daily with a meal was effective and well tolerated in at least two patients.*

Dosage Adjustment of Medications Eliminated by the Kidneys

Imipenem/Cilastatin - Selected References

Alarabi AA, Cars O, Danielson BG, Salmonson T, Wikström B. Pharmacokinetics of intravenous imipenem/cilastatin during intermittent haemofiltration. J Antimicrob Chemother. 1990;26:91–8.

Anwar N, Merchant M, Were T, Tooth A, Uttley L, Gokal R. A prospective, randomized study of the comparative safety and efficacy of intraperitoneal imipenem versus vancomycin and netilmicin in the treatment of peritonitis on CAPD. Perit Dial Int. 1995;15:167–71.

Aronoff GA, Bennett WM, Berns JS, et al. Drug prescribing in renal failure: dosing guidelines for adults and children. 5th ed. Philadelphia: American College of Physicians; 2007.

Berman SJ, Sugihara JG, Nakamura JM, et al. Multiple-dose study of imipenem/cilastatin in patients with end-stage renal disease undergoing long-term hemodialysis. Am J Med. 1985;78(Suppl 6A):113–6.

Finch RG, Craddock C, Kelly J, Deaney NB. Pharmacokinetic studies of imipenem/cilastatin in elderly patients. J Antimicrob Chemother. 1986;18(Suppl E):103–7.

Fish DN, Teitelbaum I, Abraham E. Pharmacokinetics and pharmacodynamics of imipenem during continuous renal replacement therapy in critically ill patients. Antimicrob Agents Chemother. 2005;49:2421–8.

Gibson TP, Demetriades JL, Bland JA. Imipenem/cilastatin: pharmacokinetic profile in renal insufficiency. Am J Med. 1985;78(Suppl 6A):54–61.

Hashimoto S, Honda M, Yamaguchi M, Sekimoto M, Tanaka Y. Pharmacokinetics of imipenem and cilastatin during continuous venovenous hemodialysis in patients who are critically ill. ASAIO J. 1997;43:84–8.

Heintz BH, Matzke GR, Dager WF. Antimicrobial dosing concepts and recommendations for critically ill adult patients receiving continuous renal replacement therapy or intermittent hemodialysis. Pharmacotherapy. 2009;29:562–77.

Joos B, Schmidli M, Keusch G. Pharmacokinetics of antimicrobial agents in anuric patients during continuous venovenous haemofiltration. Nephrol Dial Transplant. 1996;11:1582–5.

Keller E, Fecht H, Böhler J, Schollmeyer P. Single-dose kinetics of imipenem/cilastatin during continuous arteriovenous haemofiltration in intensive care patients. Nephrol Dial Transplant. 1989;4:640–5.

Kihara M, Ikeda Y, Shibata K, et al. Pharmacokinetic profiles of intravenous imipenem/cilastatin during slow hemodialysis in critically ill patients. Clin Nephrol. 1994;42:193–7.

Kihara M, Ikeda Y, Shiratori K, et al. A serial application study on twice daily dose of imipenem/cilastatin in patients undergoing slow hemodialysis [letter]. Nephron. 1994;68:406–7.

Mueller BA, Scarim SK, Macias WL. Comparison of imipenem pharmacokinetics in patients with acute or chronic renal failure treated with continuous hemofiltration. Am J Kidney Dis. 1993;21:172–9.

Norrby SR, Alestig K, Björnegård B, et al. Urinary recovery of N-formimidoyl thienamycin (MK0787) as affected by co-administration of N-formimidoyl thienamycin dehydropeptidase inhibitors. Antimicrob Agents Chemother. 1983;23:300–7.

Norrby SR, Alestig K, Ferber F, et al. Pharmacokinetics and tolerance of N-formimidoyl thienamycin (MK0787) in humans. Antimicrob Agents Chemother. 1983;23:293–9.

Pietroski NA, Gaziani AL, Lawson LA, Bland JA, Rogers JD, MacGregor RR. Steady-state pharmacokinetics of intramuscular imipenem-cilastatin in elderly patients with various degrees of renal function. Antimicrob Agents Chemother. 1991;35:972–5.

Primaxin® IV injection [package insert]. Whitehouse Station: Merck & Co Inc; 2010.

Somani P, Freimer EH, Gross EL, Higgins JT Jr. Pharmacokinetics of imipenem-cilastatin in patients with renal insufficiency undergoing continuous ambulatory peritoneal dialysis. Antimicrob Agents Chemother. 1988;32:530–4.

Tegeder I, Bremer F, Oelders R, et al. Pharmacokinetics of imipenem-cilastatin in critically ill patients undergoing continuous venovenous hemofiltration. Antimicrob Agents Chemother. 1997;41:2640–5.

Tegeder I, Schmidtko A, Bräutigam L, Kirchbaum A, Geisslinger G, Lötsch J. Tissue distribution of imipenem in critically ill patients. Clin Pharmacol Ther. 2002;71:325–3.

Verbist L, Verpooten GA, Giuliano RA, et al. Pharmacokinetics and tolerance after repeated doses of imipenem/cilastatin in patients with severe renal failure. J Antimicrob Chemother. 1986;18(Suppl E):115–20.

Verpooten GA, Verbist L, Buntinx AP, Entwistle LA, Jones KH, De Broe ME. The pharmacokinetics of imipenem (thienamycin-formamidine) and the renal dehydropeptidase inhibitor cilastatin sodium in normal subjects and patients with renal failure. Br J Clin Pharmacol. 1984;18:183–93.

Dosage Adjustment of Medications Eliminated by the Kidneys

Imipenem/Cilastatin/Primaxin®   {Antibacterial; carbapenem}

Usual initial dose:	500 mg IV
Usual maintenance dose:	500 mg IV every 6 h
Typical maximum dose:	4,000 mg/day
Proportion eliminated unchanged:	70 %

Adjustment for Kidney Disease

FDA-approved product labeling:

Imipenen-cilastatin reduced IV dosage in adult patients with impaired renal function

CrCL (mL/min)	Body weight (kg)				
	≥70	60	50	40	30
	If total daily dose for normal renal function is 1 g/day, use:				
≥71	250 mg q 6 h	250 mg q 8 h	125 mg q 6 h	125 mg q 6 h	125 mg q 8 h
41–70	250 mg q 8 h	125 mg q 6 h	125 mg q 6 h	125 mg q 8 h	125 mg q 8 h
21–40	250 mg q 12 h	250 mg q 12 h	125 mg q 8 h	125 mg q 12 h	125 mg q 12 h
6–20	250 mg q 12 h	125 mg q 12 h	125 mg q 12 h	125 mg q 12 h	125 mg q 12 h
	If total daily dose for normal renal function is 1.5 g/day, use:				
≥71	500 mg q 8 h	250 mg q 6 h	250 mg q 6 h	250 mg q 8 h	125 mg q 6 h
41–70	250 mg q 6 h	250 mg q 8 h	250 mg q 8 h	125 mg q 6 h	125 mg q 8 h
21–40	250 mg q 8 h	250 mg q 8 h	250 mg q 12 h	125 mg q 8 h	125 mg q 8 h
6–20	250 mg q 12 h	250 mg q 12 h	250 mg q 12 h	125 mg q 12 h	125 mg q 12 h
	If total daily dose for normal renal function is 2 g/day, use:				
≥71	500 mg q 6 h	500 mg q 8 h	250 mg q 6 h	250 mg q 6 h	250 mg q 8 h
41–70	500 mg q 8 h	250 mg q 6 h	250 mg q 6 h	250 mg q 8 h	125 mg q 6 h
21–40	250 mg q 6 h	250 mg q 8 h	250 mg q 8 h	250 mg q 12 h	125 mg q 8 h
6–20	250 mg q 12 h	250 mg q 12 h	250 mg q 12 h	250 mg q 12 h	125 mg q 12 h
	If total daily dose for normal renal function is 3 g/day, use:				
≥71	1,000 mg q 8 h	750 mg q 8 h	500 mg q 6 h	500 mg q 8 h	250 mg q 6 h
41–70	500 mg q 6 h	500 mg q 8 h	500 mg q 8 h	250 mg q 6 h	250 mg q 8 h
21–40	500 mg q 8 h	500 mg q 8 h	250 mg q 6 h	250 mg q 8 h	250 mg q 8 h
6–20	500 mg q 12 h	500 mg q 12 h	250 mg q 12 h	250 mg q 12 h	250 mg q 12 h
	If total daily dose for normal renal function is 4 g/day, use:				
≥71	1,000 mg q 6 h	1,000 mg q 8 h	750 mg q 8 h	500 mg q 6 h	500 mg q 8 h
41–70	750 mg q 8 h	750 mg q 8 h	500 mg q 6 h	500 mg q 8 h	250 mg q 6 h
21–40	500 mg q 6 h	500 mg q 8 h	500 mg q 8 h	250 mg q 6 h	250 mg q 8 h
6–20	500 mg q 12 h	500 mg q 12 h	500 mg q 12 h	250 mg q 12 h	250 mg q 12 h

Use dosage for CrCL 6–20 mL/m in hemodialysis; give after hemodialysis on dialysis days. Patients with CrCL ≤5 mL/min should not receive imipenem unless hemodialysis is initiated within 48 h

Alternative adjustment:	*GFR >50 mL/min*	*500 mg IV every 8 h*
	GFR 10–50 mL/min	*250–500 mg IV every 8–12 h (~50 % decrease)*
	GFR <10 mL/min	*250 mg IV every 12 h (~75 % decrease)*
	Hemodialysis	*250–500 mg IV every 12 h, after hemodialysis on dialysis days*
	CAPD	*250 mg IV every 12 h or 1 g intraperitoneally every other exchange*
	CVVH	*250 mg IV every 6 h or 500 mg IV every 6–8 h*
	CVVHD or CVVHDF	*500 mg IV every 6–8 h*
	Caution—Increased seizure potential in patients with renal impairment	

Dosage Adjustment of Medications Eliminated by the Kidneys

Indapamide - Selected References

Acchiardo SR, Skoutakis VA. Clinical efficacy, safety, and pharmacokinetics of indapamide in renal impairment. Am Heart J. 1983;106:237–44.

Beerman B, Grind M. Clinical pharmacokinetics of some newer diuretics. Clin Pharmacokinet. 1987;13:254–66.

Brennan L, Wu MJ, Laquer UJ. A multicenter study of indapamide in hypertensive patients with impaired renal function. Clin Ther. 1982;5:1218.

Burke TI, Nobles EM, Wolf PS, Erickson AI. Effect of indapamide on volume-dependent hypertension, renal haemodynamics, solute excretion and proximal Nephron fractional reabsorption in the dog. Curr Med Res Opin. 1983;8(Suppl 3):25–37.

Campbell DB, Moore RA. The pharmacology and clinical pharmacology of indapamide. Postgrad Med J. 1981;57(Suppl 2): 7–17.

Caruso FS, Szabadi RR, Vukovich RA. Pharmacokinetics and clinical pharmacology of indapamide. Am Heart J. 1983;106: 212–20.

Danielsen H, Pedersen EB, Spencer ES. Effect of indapamide on the renin-aldosterone system, and urinary excretion of potassium and calcium in essential hypertension. Br J Clin Pharmacol. 1984;18:229–31.

Klunk LJ, Ringel S, Neiss ES. The disposition of ^{14}C-indapamide in man. J Clin Pharmacol. 1983;23:37–84.

Leenen FHH, Smith DL, Farkas RM, Boer AH, Reeves RA, Marquez-Julio A. Cardiovascular effects of indapamide in hypertensive patients with or without renal failure: a dose–response curve. Am J Med. 1988;84(Suppl 1B):76–85.

Lozol® tablet [package insert]. Bridgewater: Aventis Pharmaceuticals Inc; 2005.

Madkour H, Ali K, Nosrati S, Massry SG. Efficacious response with low-dose indapamide therapy in the treatment of type II diabetic patients with normal renal function or moderate renal insufficiency and moderate hypertension. Am J Nephrol. 2002;22:2–5.

Madkour H, Gadallah M, Riveline B, Plante GE, Massry SG. Comparison of the effects of indapamide and hydrochlorothiazide on creatinine clearance in patients with impaired real function and hypertension. Am J Nephrol. 1995;15:251–5.

Madkour H, Gadallah M, Riveline B, Plante GE, Massry SG. Indapamide is superior to thiazide in the preservation of renal function in patients with renal insufficiency and systemic hypertension. Am J Cardiol. 1996;77(Suppl 6B):23B–25B.

McIntyre CW, Owen PJ. Prescribing drugs in kidney disease. In: Brenner BM, editor. Brenner & Rector's the kidney. 8th ed. Philadelphia: Saunders/Elsevier; 2008. p. 1930–55.

Morledge JH. Clinical efficacy and safety of indapamide in essential hypertension. Am Heart J. 1983;106:229–32.

Pedersen EB, Danielsen H, Spencer ES. Effect of indapamide on the renal plasma flow, glomerular filtration rate and arginine vasopressin in plasma in essential hypertension. Eur J Clin Pharmacol. 1984;26:543–7.

Robinson DM, Wellington K. Indapamide sustained release: a review of its use in the treatment of hypertension. Drugs. 2006;66:257–71.

Schaeffer P, Vigne P, Frelin C, Lazdunski M. Identification and pharmacological properties of binding sites for the atypical thiazide diuretic, indapamide. Eur J Pharmacol. 1990;182:503–8.

Villarreal H, Nuñez-Poissot E, Anguas MC, Degandarías L, Meza U. Effects of the acute and chronic administration of indapamide on systemic and renal haemodynamics in essential hypertension. Curr Med Res Opin. 1983;8(Suppl 3):135–9.

Dosage Adjustment of Medications Eliminated by the Kidneys

Indapamide/Lozol®   {Diuretic; thiazide-like}

Usual initial dose: 2.5 mg orally

Usual maintenance dose: 1.25–5 mg orally once daily

Typical maximum dose: 5 mg/day

Proportion eliminated unchanged: 7 %

Adjustment for Kidney Disease

    FDA-approved product labeling:

	Severe renal disease	*Use with caution.*
	Anuria	*Contraindicated*

    Alternative adjustment:

	GFR >50 mL/min	*2.5 mg orally once daily*
	GFR 10–50 mL/min	*1.25–2.5 mg orally once daily*
	GFR <10 mL/min	*1.25–2.5 mg orally once daily (limited data available)*
	Hemodialysis	*1.25–2.5 mg orally once daily (limited data available)*
	CAPD	*Data not available; preferably avoid due to potentially limited effectiveness*
	CRRT	*Not applicable; preferably avoid*

Dosage Adjustment of Medications Eliminated by the Kidneys

Indomethacin - Selected References

Basivireddy J, Jacob M, Pulimood AB, Balasubramanian KA. Indomethacin-induced renal damage: role of oxygen free radicals. Biochem Pharmacol. 2004;67:587–99.

Bernheim JL, Korzets Z. Indomethacin-induced renal failure [letter]. Ann Intern Med. 1979;792.

Brater DC, Anderson SA, Brown-Cartwright D, Toto RD. Effects of nonsteroidal antiinflammatory drugs on renal function in patients with renal insufficiency and in cirrhotics. Am J Kidney Dis. 1986;8:351–5.

Davis HA, Horton EW. Output of prostaglandins from the rabbit kidney, its increase on renal nerve stimulation and its inhibition by indomethacin. Br J Pharmacol. 1972;46:658–75.

Douma CE, de Waart DR, Zemel D, Struijk DG, Krediet RT. Prostaglandin inhibition by intraperitoneal indomethacin has no effect on peritoneal permeability during stable CAPD. Nephrol Dial Transplant. 2001;16:803–8.

Favre L, Glasson P, Vallotton MB. Reversible acute renal failure from combined triamterene and indomethacin. Ann Intern Med. 1982;96:317–20.

Fawaz-Estrup F, Ho G Jr. Reversible acute renal failure induced by indomethacin. Arch Intern Med. 1981;141:1870–1.

Fox DA, Jick H. Nonsteroidal anti-inflammatory drugs and renal disease. JAMA. 1984;251:1299–300.

Frölich JC, Hollifield JW, Cormois JC, et al. Suppression of plasma renin activity by indomethacin in man. Circ Res. 1976;39:447–52.

Galler M, Folkert VW, Schlondorff D. Reversible acute renal insufficiency and hyperkalemia following indomethacin therapy. JAMA. 1981;246:154–5.

Gary NE, Dodelson R, Eisinger RP. Indomethacin-associated renal failure. Am J Med. 1988;69:135–6.

Handa SP. Drug-induced acute interstitial nephritis: report of 10 cases. Can Med Assoc J. 1986;135:1278–81.

Helleberg L. Clinical pharmacokinetics of indomethacin. Clin Pharmacokinet. 1981;6:245–81.

Indomethacin capsule [package insert]. Sellersville: Teva Pharmaceuticals USA; 2010.

Kharasch MS, Johnson KM, Strange GR. Cardiac arrest secondary to indomethacin-induced renal failure: a case report. J Emerg Med. 1990;8:51–4.

Kleinknecht C, Broyer M, Gubler M-C, Palcoux J-B. Irreversible renal failure after indomethacin in steroid-resistant nephrosis [letter]. N Engl J Med. 1980;302:691.

Minuth ANW, Nottebohm GA, Eknoyan G, Suki WN. Indomethacin treatment of pericarditis in chronic hemodialysis patients. Arch Intern Med. 1975;135:807–10.

Miyamori I, Ikeda M, Matsubara T, et al. The renal, cardiovascular and hormonal actions of human atrial natriuretic peptide in man: effects of indomethacin. Br J Clin Pharmacol. 1987;23:425–31.

Mujovic VM, Fisher JW. The effects of indomethacin on erythropoietin production in dogs following renal artery constriction. I. The possible role of prostaglandins in the generation of erythropoietin by the kidney. J Pharmacol Exp Ther. 1974;191:575–80.

Neeleman P, Douglas JR Jr, Jakschik B, Stoecklein PB, Johnson EM Jr. Release of renal prostaglandin by catecholamines: relationship to renal endocrine function. J Pharmacol Exp Ther. 1974;188:453–60.

O'Meara ME, Eknoyan G. Acute renal failure associated with indomethacin administration. South Med J. 1983;73:587–9.

Schlondorff D. Renal complications of nonsteroidal anti-inflammatory drugs. Kidney Int. 1993;44:643–53.

Schneider R, Jeusel M, Renker S, et al. Low-dose indomethacin after ischemic acute kidney injury prevents downregulation of Oat1/3 and improves renal outcome. Am J Physiol Renal Physiol. 2009;297:F1614–21.

Skoutakis V, Acchiardo SR, Carter CA, Wojciechowski NJ, Straughn AB, Meyer MC. Dialyzability and pharmacokinetics of indomethacin in adult patients with end-stage renal disease. Drug Intell Clin Pharm. 1986;20:956–60.

Toto RD, Anderson SA, Brown-Cartwright D, Kokko JP, Brater DC. Effects of acute and chronic dosing of NSAIDs in patients with renal insufficiency. Kidney Int. 1986;30:760–8.

Walshe JJ, Venuto RC. Acute oliguric renal failure induced by indomethacin: possible mechanism. Ann Intern Med. 1979;91:47–9.

Weinberg MS, Quigg RJ, Salant DJ, Bernard DB. Anuric renal failure precipitated by indomethacin and triamterene. Nephron. 1985;40:216–8.

Dosage Adjustment of Medications Eliminated by the Kidneys

<u>**Indomethacin**</u>/**Indocin**®   {**Anti-inflammatory; nonsteroidal anti-inflammatory drug**}

Usual initial dose:	25 mg
Usual maintenance dose:	25–50 mg twice or three times daily
Typical maximum dose:	200 mg/day
Proportion eliminated unchanged:	15 %

Adjustment for Kidney Disease

FDA-approved product labeling:	*Advanced renal disease*	*Not recommended, avoid*
Alternative adjustment:	*Hemodialysis*	*25 mg orally three times daily*

Dosage Adjustment of Medications Eliminated by the Kidneys

Insulins - Selected References

Abe M, Okada K, Ikeda K, Matsumoto S, Soma M, Matsumoto K. Characterization of insulin adsorption behavior of dialyzer membranes used in hemodialysis. Artif Organs. 2011;35:398–403.

American Diabetes Association. Standards of medical care in diabetes—2012. Diabetes Care. 2012;35(Suppl 1):S11–63.

Aronoff GA, Bennett WM, Berns JS, et al. Drug prescribing in renal failure: dosing guidelines for adults and children. 5th ed. Philadelphia: American College of Physicians; 2007.

Asche C, LaFleur J, Conner C. A review of diabetes treatment adherence and the association of clinical and economic outcomes. Clin Ther. 2011;33:74–109.

Bhattacharyya A, Christodoulides C, Kaushal K, New JP, Young RJ. In-patient management of diabetes and patient satisfaction. Diabet Med. 2002;19:412–6.

Dagogo-Jack S, Santiago JV. Pathophysiology of type 2 diabetes and modes of action of therapeutic interventions. Arch Intern Med. 1997;157:1802–17.

DeWitt DE, Dugdale DC. Using new insulin strategies in the outpatient treatment of diabetes: clinical applications. JAMA. 2003;289:2265–9.

Golightly LK, Jones MA, Hamamura D, Stolpman NM, McDermott MT. Management of diabetes mellitus in hospitalized patients: efficiency and efficacy of sliding-scale insulin therapy. Pharmacotherapy. 2006;26:1421–32.

Grunberger G, Bailey TS, Cohen AJ, et al. Statement of the American Association of Clinical Endocrinologists on insulin pump management. Endocr Pract. 2010;16:746–62.

Hirsch IB, Bergenstal RM, Parkin CG, Wright E Jr, Buse JB. A real-world approach to insulin therapy in primary care practice. Clin Diabetes. 2005;23(2):78–86.

Kansagara D, Fu R, Freeman M, Wolf F, Helfand M. Intensive insulin therapy in hospitalized patients: a systematic review Ann Intern Med. 2011;154:268–82.

Kitabchi AE, Murphy MB, Umpierrez GE, Kreisberg RA. Hyperglycemic crises in adult patients with diabetes: a consensus statement from the American Diabetes Association. Diabetes Care. 2006;29:2739–48.

Lassmann-Vague V, Clavel S, Guerci B, et al. When to treat a diabetic patient using an external insulin pump. Expert consensus: Société Francophone du Diabète (ex ALFEDIAM) 2009. Diabetes Metab. 2010;36:79–85.

Maynard G, Lee J, Phillips G, Fink E, Renvall M. Improved inpatient use of basal insulin, reduced hypoglycemia, and improved glycemic control: effect of structured subcutaneous insulin orders and an insulin management algorithm. J Hosp Med. 2009;4:3–15.

Moghissi ES, Hirsch IB, Korytkowski MT, et al. American Association of Clinical Endocrinologists and American Diabetes Association consensus statement on inpatient glycemic control. Diabetes Care. 2009;32:1119–31.

Mooradian AD, Bernbaum M, Alber SG. A rational approach to starting insulin therapy. Ann Intern Med. 2006;145:125–34.

Nathan DM, Holman RR, Buse JB, et al. Management of hyperglycemia in type 2 diabetes: a consensus algorithm for the initiation and adjustment of therapy: a consensus statement from the American Diabetes Association and the European Association for the Study of Diabetes. Diabetes Care. 2006;29:1963–72.

Nyenwe EA, Jerkins TW, Umpierrez GE, Kitabchi AE. Management of type 2 diabetes: evolving strategies for the treatment of patients with type 2 diabetes. Metabolism. 2011;60:1–23.

Savage MW, Dhatariya KK, Kilvert A, et al. Joint British Diabetes Societies guideline for the management of diabetic ketoacidosis. Diabet Med. 2011;28:508–15.

Smiley D, Rhee M, Peng L, et al. Safety and efficacy of continuous insulin infusion in noncritical care settings. J Hosp Med. 2010;5:212–7.

Smiley D, Umpierrez GE. Management of hyperglycemia in hospitalized patients. Ann N Y Acad Sci. 2010;1212:1–11.

Trence DL, Kelly JL, Hirsch IB. The rationale and management of hyperglycemia for in-patients with cardiovascular disease: time for change. J Clin Endocrinol Metab. 2003;88:2430–7.

Umpierrez GE, Mulligan P, Smiley D, et al. Randomized study of basal-bolus insulin therapy in the inpatient management of patients with type 2 diabetes undergoing general surgery (RABBIT 2 Surgery). Diabetes Care. 2011;34:256–61.

Umpierrez GE, Palacio A, Smiley D, et al. Randomized study of basal-bolus insulin therapy in the management of patients with type 2 diabetes (RABBIT 2 Trial). Diabetes Care. 2007;30:2181–6.

Dosage Adjustment of Medications Eliminated by the Kidneys

<u>Insulins</u>/Apidra® (Glulisine), Humalog® (Lispro), Humulin N® (Isophane/NPH), Humulin R® (Regular), Lantus® (Glargine), Levemir® (Detemir), Novolin N® (Isophane /NPH), Novolin R® (Regular), NovoLog® (Aspart)

{Antidiabetic; hormone}

Usual initial dose:

0.2–0.4 units/kg/day subcutaneously in divided amounts; 0.1–14 units/h IV

Usual maintenance dose:

0.5–2 units/kg/day subcutaneously in divided amounts, often 40–60 % as basal insulin with the remainder as prandial rapid-acting insulin

Typical maximum dose:

Widely variable

Proportion eliminated unchanged:

None

Adjustment for Kidney Disease

FDA-approved product labeling:

The requirements for insulin may be reduced in patients with renal impairment.

Alternative adjustment:

GFR >50 mL/min	*100 % of usual dose; monitor and titrate.*	
GFR 10–50 mL/min	*75 % of usual dose; monitor and titrate.*	
GFR <10 mL/min	*50 % of usual dose; monitor and titrate.*	
Hemodialysis	*50 % of usual dose; no supplemental dose after dialysis; monitor and titrate.*	
CAPD	*50 % of usual dose; monitor and titrate.*	
CRRT	*75 % of usual dose; monitor and titrate.*	

Interferon Alfa-2b and Ribavirin - Selected References

Berenguer M. Treatment of chronic hepatitis C in hemodialysis patients. Hepatology. 2008;48:1690–9.

Ghany MG, Strader DB, Thomas DL, Seeff LB. American Association for the Study of Liver Diseases Practice Guidelines. Diagnosis, management, and treatment of hepatitis C: an update. Hepatology. 2009;49:1335–74.

Jen JF, Glue P, Ezzet F, et al. Population pharmacokinetic analysis of pegylated interferon alfa-2b and interferon alfa-2b in patients with chronic hepatitis B. Clin Pharmacol Ther. 2001;69:407–21.

Jen JF, Glue P, Gupta S, Zambas D, Hajian G. Population pharmacokinetic and pharmacodynamic analysis of ribavirin in patients with chronic hepatitis C. Ther Drug Monit. 2000;22:555–65.

Jen J, Laughlin M, Chung C, et al. Ribavirin dosing in chronic hepatitis C: application of population pharmacokinetic-pharmacodynamic models. Clin Pharmacol Ther. 2002;72:349–61.

Khakoo S, Glue P, Grellier L, et al. Ribavirin and interferon alfa-2b in chronic hepatitis C: assessment of possible pharmacokinetic and pharmacodynamic interactions. Br J Clin Pharmacol. 1998;46:563–70.

Kramer TH, Gaar GG, Ray CG, Minnich L, Copeland JG, Connor JD. Hemodialysis clearance of intravenously administered ribavirin. Antimicrob Agents Chemother. 1990;34:489–90.

Lertora JJL, Rege AB, Lacour JT, et al. Pharmacokinetics and long-term tolerance to ribavirin in asymptomatic patients infected with human immunodeficiency virus. Clin Pharmacol Ther. 1991;50:442–9.

Mutimer D, Naoumov N, Honkoop P, et al. Combination alpha-interferon and lamivudine therapy for alpha-interferon-resistant chronic hepatitis B infection: results of a pilot study. J Hepatol. 1998;28:923–9.

Paroni R, Del Puppo M, Borghi C, Sirtori CR, Kienle MG. Pharmacokinetics of ribavirin and urinary excretion of the major metabolite 1,2,4-triazole-3-carboxamide in normal volunteers. Int J Clin Pharmacol Ther Toxicol. 1989;27:302–7.

Preston SL, Drusano GL, Glue P, Nash J, Gupta SK, McNamara P. Pharmacokinetics and absolute bioavailability of ribavirin in healthy volunteers as determined by stable-isotope methodology. Antimicrob Agents Chemother. 1999;43:2451–6.

Rabih SA, Agudo RG. Management of HCV infection in chronic kidney disease. Nefrologia. 2011;31:260–7.

Rebetron™ [package insert]. Kenilworth: Schering Corp; 2001.

Rostaing L, Chatelut E, Payen J-L, et al. Pharmacokinetics of αIFN-2b in chronic hepatitis C virus patients undergoing chronic hemodialysis or with normal renal function: clinical implications. J Am Soc Nephrol. 1998;9:2344–8.

Sawyer LA, Metcalf JA, Zoon KC, et al. Effects of interferon-α in patients with AIDS-associated Kaposi's sarcoma are related to blood interferon levels and dose. Cytokine. 1990;2:247–52.

Schüller J, Czejka MJ, Schernthaner G, et al. Pharmacokinetic aspects of interferon alfa-2b after intrahepatic or intraperitoneal administration. Semin Oncol. 1992;19(Suppl 3):98–104.

Scott LJ, Perry CM. Interferon-α-2b plus ribavirin: a review of its use in the management of chronic hepatitis C. Drugs. 2002;62:507–56.

Tsubota A, Akuta N, Suzuki F, et al. Viral dynamics and pharmacokinetics in combined interferon alfa-2b and ribavirin therapy for patients infected with hepatitis C virus of genotype 1b and high pretreatment viral load. Intervirology. 2002.45:33–42.

Tsubota A, Hirose Y, Izumi N, Kumada H. Pharmacokinetics of ribavirin in combined interferon-alpha 2b and ribavirin therapy of chronic hepatitis C infection. Br J Clin Pharmacol. 2003;55:360–7.

van Vlerken LG, van Oijen MGH, van Erpecum KJ. Ribavirin concentration is a more important predictor of sustained viral response than anemia in hepatitis C patients [letter]. Gastroenterology. 2011;140:1693–4.

Wade JR, Snoeck E, Duff F, Lamb M, Jorga K. Pharmacokinetics of ribavirin in patients with hepatitis C virus. Br J Clin Pharmacol. 2006;62:710–4.

Interferon Alfa-2b and Ribavirin/Rebetron™   {Antiviral; ℞ for hepatitis C}

Usual initial dose:	Interferon alfa-2b three million units intramuscularly or subcutaneously three times weekly plus ribavirin 1,000–1,200 mg/day in two divided doses
Usual maintenance dose:	Interferon alfa-2b three million units intramuscularly or subcutaneously three times weekly plus ribavirin 1,000–1,200 mg/day in two divided doses
Typical maximum dose:	Interferon alfa-2b three million units intramuscularly or subcutaneously three times weekly plus ribavirin 1,200 mg/day in two divided doses
Proportion eliminated unchanged:	Interferon alfa-2b = nil; ribavirin 5–15 %

Adjustment for Kidney Disease

FDA-approved product labeling:	*CrCL <50 mL/min*	*Contraindicated (ribavirin)*
Alternative adjustment:	*Hemodialysis*	*Three million units subcutaneously three times weekly with ribavirin 200 mg orally once daily*

Isocarboxazid - Selected References

Blackwell B, Taylor D. An operational evaluation of monoamine oxidase inhibitors. Proc R Soc Med. 1967;60:830–4.

Colvin LB. Metabolic fate of hydrazines and hydrazides. J Pharm Sci. 1969;58:1433–43.

Kurland AA, Destounis N, Shaffer JW, Pinto A. A critical study of isocarboxazid (Marplan) in the treatment of depressed patients. J Nerv Ment Dis. 1967;145:292–305.

Marplan® tablet [package insert]. Parsippany: Validus Pharmaceuticals LLC; 2012.

Preskorn SH. Recent pharmacologic advances in antidepressant therapy for the elderly. Am J Med. 1993;94(Suppl 5A):2–12S.

Satoh T, Moroi K. Enzymatic hydrolysis of isocarboxazid in rat tissues. Biochem Pharmacol. 1971;20:504–7.

Satoh T, Moroi K. Species and age differences in the activity of isocarboxazid hydrolyzing enzyme. Arch Int Pharmacodyn Ther. 1971;192:128–34.

Dosage Adjustment of Medications Eliminated by the Kidneys

<u>Isocarboxazid</u>/Marplan®   {Antidepressant; monoamine oxidase inhibitor}

Usual initial dose:	10 mg orally twice daily
Usual maintenance dose:	20 mg orally twice daily
Typical maximum dose:	60 mg/day
Proportion Eliminated Unchanged:	Unknown (hydrolytic cleavage and further oxidation to benzoate are believed to be the foremost means of elimination)

Adjustment for Kidney Disease

FDA-approved product labeling:	*Impaired renal function*	*Use cautiously to prevent accumulation.*
	Severe impairment of renal function	*Contraindicated*
Alternative adjustment:	*Data not available*	

Dosage Adjustment of Medications Eliminated by the Kidneys

Itraconazole - Selected References

Aronoff GA, Bennett WM, Berns JS, et al. Drug prescribing in renal failure: dosing guidelines for adults and children. 5th ed. Philadelphia: American College of Physicians; 2007.

Billaud EM, Guillemain R, Berge M, et al. Pharmacological considerations for azole antifungal drug management in cystic fibrosis lung transplant patients. Med Mycol. 2010;48(Suppl 1):S52–9.

Boelaert J, Schurgers M, Matthys E, et al. Itraconazole pharmacokinetics in patients with renal dysfunction. Antimicrob Agents Chemother. 1988;32:1595–7.

Brüggemann RJM, Alffenaar J-WC, Blijlevens NMA, et al. Clinical relevance of the pharmacokinetic interactions of azole antifungal drugs with other coadministered agents. Clin Infect Dis. 2009;48:1441–58.

Buchanan CM, Buchanan NL, Edgar KJ, et al. Pharmacokinetics of itraconazole after intravenous and oral dosing of itraconazole-cyclodextrin formulations. J Pharm Sci. 2007;96:3100–16.

Buchkowsky SS, Partovi N, Ensom MHH. Clinical pharmacokinetic monitoring of itraconazole is warranted in only a subset of patients. Ther Drug Monit. 2005;27:322–33.

Conway SP, Etherington C, Peckham DG, Brownlee K, Whitehead A, Cunliffe H. Pharmacokinetics and safety of itraconazole in patients with cystic fibrosis. J Antimicrob Chemother. 2004;53:841–7.

Coronel B, Levron J-C, Dorez D, Van Devenne A, Archimbaud E, Mercatello A. Itraconazole lung concentrations in haematological patients. Mycoses. 2000;43:125–7.

Googaerts MA, Maertens J, van der Geest R, et al. Pharmacokinetics and safety of a 7-day administration of intravenous itraconazole followed by 14-day administration of itraconazole oral solution in patients with hematologic malignancy. Antimicrob Agents Chemother. 2001;45:981–5.

Hagihara M, Kasai H, Umemura T, Kato T, Haseawa T, Mikamo H. Pharmacokinetic-pharmacodynamic study of itraconazole in patients with fungal infections in intensive care units. J Infect Chemother. 2011;17:224–30.

Hardin TC, Graybill JR, Fetchick R, Woestenborghs R, Rinaldi MG, Kuhn JG. Pharmacokinetics of itraconazole following oral administration to normal volunteers. Antimicrob Agents Chemother. 1988;32:1310–3.

Hassan HA, Al-Marzouqi AH, Jobe B, Hamza AA, Ramadan GA. Enhancement of dissolution amount and in vivo bioavailability of itraconazole by complexation with β-cyclodextrin using supercritical carbon dioxide. J Pharm Biomed Anal. 2007;45:243–50.

Heintz BH, Matzke GR, Dager WF. Antimicrobial dosing concepts and recommendations for critically ill adult patients receiving continuous renal replacement therapy or intermittent hemodialysis. Pharmacotherapy. 2009;29:562–77.

Hope WW, Billaud EM, Lestner J, Denning DW. Therapeutic monitoring for triazoles. Curr Opin Infect Dis. 2008;21:580–6.

Lestner JM, Roberts SA, Moore CB, Howard SJ, Denning DW, Hope WW. Toxicodynamics of itraconazole: implications for therapeutic drug monitoring. Clin Infect Dis. 2009;49:928–30.

Mohr JF, Finkel KW, Rex JH, Rodriguez JR, Leitz GJ, Ostrosky-Zeichner L. Pharmacokinetics of intravenous itraconazole in stable hemodialysis patients. Antimicrob Agents Chemother. 2004;48:3151–3.

Prentice AG, Warnock DW, Johnson SAN, Phillips MJ, Oliver DA. Multiple dose pharmacokinetics of an oral solution of itraconazole in autologous bone marrow transplant recipients. J Antimicrob Chemother. 1994;34:247–52.

Reynes J, Bazin C, Ajana F, et al. Pharmacokinetics of itraconazole (oral solution) in two groups of human immunodeficiency virus-infected adults with oral candidiasis. Antimicrob Agents Chemother. 1997;41:2554–8.

Sporanox® capsules [package insert]. Raritan: PriCara Division of Ortho-McNeil-Janssen Pharmaceuticals Inc; 2011.

Sporanox® solution [package insert]. Raritan: Centocor Ortho Biotech Products LP; 2011.

Van de Velde VJS, Van Peer AP, Heykants JJP, et al. Effect of food on the pharmacokinetics of a new hydroxypropyl-β-cyclodextrin formulation of itraconazole. Pharmacotherapy. 1996;16:424–8.

Vandewoude AK, Vogelaers D, Decruyenaere J, et al. Concentrations in plasma and safety of 7 days of intravenous itraconazole solution in patients in intensive care units. Antimicrob Agents Chemother. 1997;41:2714–8.

Willems L, van der Geest R, de Beule K. Itraconazole oral solution and intravenous formulations: a review of pharmacokinetics and pharmacodynamics. J Clin Pharm Ther. 2001;26:159–69.

Zhao Q, Zhou H, Pesco-Koplowitz L. Pharmacokinetics of intravenous itraconazole followed by itraconazole oral solution in patients with human immunodeficiency virus infection. J Clin Pharmacol. 2001;41:1319–28.

Dosage Adjustment of Medications Eliminated by the Kidneys

<u>Itraconazole/Sporanox®</u>	{Antifungal; triazole ergosterol biosynthesis inhibitor}
Usual initial dose:	Capsules, 200 mg orally three times daily with food for the first 3 days of treatment; oral solution, 100–200 mg orally once daily without food
Usual maintenance dose:	Capsules, 200 mg orally once or twice daily with food; oral solution, 100 mg orally twice daily without food
Typical maximum dose:	600 mg/day
Proportion eliminated unchanged:	<1 % (35 % as inactive metabolites)

Adjustment for Kidney Disease

FDA-approved product labeling:	*Renal impairment*	*Caution should be exercised when this drug is administered in this patient population.*
Alternative adjustment:	*GFR >50 mL/min*	*Capsules, 200 mg orally three times daily with food for the first 3 days of treatment followed by 100–200 mg orally once or twice daily with food; oral solution, 100–200 mg (2.5 mg/kg in cystic fibrosis patients) enterally every 12 h given without food*
	GFR 10–50 mL/min	*Oral solution: 100 mg enterally every 12 h given without food*
	GFR <10 mL/min	*Oral solution: 50–100 mg enterally every 12 h given without food (50 % decrease)*
	Hemodialysis	*Oral solution: 100 mg enterally every 12 h given without food*
	CAPD	*Oral solution: 50–100 mg enterally every 12 h given as an oral solution without food*
	CVVH	*Oral solution: 100 mg enterally every 12 h given without food*
	CVVHD or CVVHDF	*Oral solution: 100–200 mg enterally every 12 h given without food*

K

L.K. Golightly et al. (eds.), *Renal Pharmacotherapy*,
DOI 10.1007/978-1-4614-5800-5_10, © Springer Science+Business Media New York 2013

Dosage Adjustment of Medications Eliminated by the Kidneys

Kanamycin - Selected References

Aronoff GA, Bennett WM, Berns JS, et al. Drug prescribing in renal failure: dosing guidelines for adults and children. 5th ed. Philadelphia: American College of Physicians; 2007.

Buck AC, Cohen SL. Absorption of antibiotics during peritoneal dialysis in patients with renal failure. J Clin Pathol. 1968;21:88–92.

Cabana BE, Taggart JG, Comparative pharmacokinetics of BB-K8 and kanamycin in dogs and humans. Antimicrob Agents Chemother. 1973;3:478–83.

Christopher TG, Blair AD, Forrey AW, Cutler RE. Hemodialyzer clearances of gentamicin, kanamycin, tobramycin, amikacin, ethambutol, procainamide, and flucytosine, with a technique for planning therapy. J Pharmacokinet Biopharm. 1976;4:427–41.

Clarke JT, Libke RD, Regamey C, Kirby WMM. Comparative pharmacokinetics of amikacin and kanamycin. Clin Pharmacol Ther. 1974;15:610–6.

Cutler RE, Orme BM. Correlation of serum creatinine concentration and kanamycin half-life. JAMA. 1969;209:539–42.

Danish M, Schultz R, Jusko WJ. Pharmacokinetics of gentamicin and kanamycin during hemodialysis. Antimicrob Agents Chemother. 1974;6:841–7.

Ericsson CD, Duke JH Jr, Pickering LK. Clinical pharmacology of intravenous and intraperitoneal aminoglycoside antibiotics in the prevention of wound infections. Ann Surg. 1978;188:66–70.

Greenberg PA, Sanford JP. Removal and absorption of antibiotics in patients with renal failure undergoing peritoneal dialysis: tetracycline, chloramphenicol, kanamycin, and colistimethate. Ann Intern Med. 1967;66:465–79.

Healy JK, Drum PJ, Elliott AJ. Kanamycin dosage in renal failure. Aust NZ J Med. 1973;3:474–9.

Hollenberg NK, Adams DF, Oken DE, Abrams HL, Merrill JP. Acute renal failure due to nephrotoxins: renal hemodynamic and angiographic studies in man. N Engl J Med. 1970;282:1329–34.

Kanamycin injection USP [package insert]. Schaumburg: APP Pharmaceuticals LLC; 2008.

Kirby WM, Clarke JT, Libke RD, Regamey C. Clinical pharmacology of amikacin and kanamycin. J Infect Dis. 1976;134(Suppl):S312–5.

Kunin CM. Nephrotoxicity of antibiotics. JAMA. 1967;202:204–8.

Kunin CM, Finland M. Persistence of antibiotics in blood of patients with acute renal failure. III. Penicillin, streptomycin, erythromycin and kanamycin. J Clin Invest. 1959;38:1509–19.

Mawer GE, Knowles BR, Lucas SB, Stirland RM, Tooth JA. Computer-assisted prescribing of kanamycin for patients with renal insufficiency. Lancet. 1972;1:12–5.

Mingeot-Leclercq M-P, Glupczynski Y, Tulkens PM. Aminoglycosides: activity and resistance. Antimicrob Agents Chemother. 1999;43:727–37.

Neu HC. Clinical use of aminoglycosides. In: Whelton A, Neu HC, editors. The aminoglycosides: microbiology, clinical use, and toxicology. New York: Marcel Dekker; 1982:611–28.

Nielsen B, Sørensen AWS, Szabo L, Aagaard Pedersen E, Scharff A. Kanamycin serum half-life and renal function: age and sex. Dan Med Bull. 1973;20:144–9.

Orme RM, Cutler RE. The relationship between kanamycin pharmacokinetics: distribution and renal function. Clin Pharmacol Ther. 1969;10:543–50.

Ory EM, Williams TW Jr, Camp FA, Regester RF, Morgen RO. Kanamycin in the treatment of patients with diminished kidney function. Ann NY Acad Sci. 1966;132:933–40.

Perrier D, Gibaldi M. Estimation of drug elimination in renal failure. J Clin Pharmacol. 1973;13:458–62.

Sarubbi FA, Hull JH, Amikacin serum concentrations: prediction of levels and dosage guidelines. Ann Intern Med. 1978;89:612–8.

Sørensen AWS, Szabo L, Pedersen A, Scharff A. Correlation between renal function and serum half-life of kanamycin and its application to dosage adjustment. Postgrad Med J. 1967;73(Suppl):37–43.

Toyoda Y, Tachibana M. Tissue levels of kanamycin in correlation with oto- and nephrotoxicity. Acta Otolaryngol. 1978;86:9–14.

Dosage Adjustment of Medications Eliminated by the Kidneys

Kanamycin/Kantrex®	{Antibacterial; aminoglycoside}
Usual initial dose:	7.5 mg/kg IV
Usual maintenance dose:	7.5 mg/kg IV every 12 h
Typical maximum dose:	1,500 mg/day
Proportion eliminated unchanged:	95 %

Adjustment for Kidney Disease

FDA-approved product labeling:	*7.5 mg/kg IV every (9 × SCr [mg/dL]) h[a]*	
Alternative adjustment:	*GFR >50 mL/min*	*7.5 mg/kg IM or IV every 12–24 h[a]*
	GFR 10–50 mL/min	*7.5 mg/kg IM or IV every 24–72 h[a]*
	GFR <10 mL/min	*7.5 mg/kg IM or IV every 48–72 h[a]*
	Hemodialysis	*3.75 mg/kg IM or IV after hemodialysis on dialysis days only[a]*
	CAPD	*Add to dialysate qs 15–20 mg/L[a]*
	CRRT	*7.5 mg/kg IM or IV every 24–72 h[a]*

[a]Therapeutic Drug Monitoring

Therapeutic plasma levels:	*Peak: 25–35 mg/L*
	Trough: 4–8 mg/L

Dosage Adjustment of Medications Eliminated by the Kidneys

Ketoprofen - Selected References

Abas A, Meffin PJ. Enantioselective disposition of 2-arylpropionic acid nonsteroidal anti-inflammatory drugs. IV. Ketoprofen disposition. J Pharmacol Exp Ther. 1987;240:637–41.

Aronoff GA, Bennett WM, Berns JS, et al. Drug prescribing in renal failure: dosing guidelines for adults and children. 5th ed. Philadelphia: American College of Physicians; 2007.

Brater DC, Anderson SA, Brown-Cartwright D, Toto RD Effects of nonsteroidal antiinflammatory drugs on renal function in patients with renal insufficiency and in cirrhotics. Am J Kidney Dis. 1986;8:351–5.

de Souza Silva M, Castiglia YMM, Vianna PTG, Viero RM, Braz JRC, Xassetari ML. Rat model of depending prostaglandin renal state: effect of ketoprofen. Ren Fail. 2006;28:77–84.

Debruyne D, de Ligny BH, Ryckelynck J-P, Albessard F, Moulin M. Clinical pharmacokinetics of ketoprofen after single intravenous administration as a bolus or infusion. Clin Pharmacokinet. 1987;12:214–21.

Dennis MJ, French PC, Crome P, Babiker M, Shillingford J, Hopkins R. Pharmacokinetic profile of controlled release ketoprofen in elderly patients. Br J Clin Pharmacol. 1985;20:567–73.

Grubb NG, Rudy DW, Brater DC, Hall SD. Stereoselective pharmacokinetics of ketoprofen and ketoprofen glucuronide in end-stage renal disease: evidence for a 'futile cycle' of elimination. Br J Clin Pharmacol. 1999;48:494–500.

Grubb NG, Rudy DW, Hall SD. Stereoselective high-performance liquid chromatographic analysis of Ketoprofen and its acyl glucuronides in chronic renal insufficiency. J Chromatogr B Biomed Appl. 1996;678:237–44.

Hayball PJ, Nation RL, Bochner F, Sansom LN, Ahern MJ, Smith MD. The influence of renal function on the enantioselective pharmacokinetics and pharmacodynamics of ketoprofen in patients with rheumatoid arthritis. Br J Clin Pharmacol. 1993;36:185–93.

Ishizaki T, Sasaki T, Suganuma T, Pharmacokinetics of ketoprofen following single oral, intramuscular and rectal doses and after repeated oral administration. Eur J Clin Pharmacol. 1980;18:407–14.

Jamali F, Brocks DR. Clinical pharmacokinetics of ketoprofen and its enantiomers. Clin Pharmacokinet. 1990;19:193–217.

Ketoprofen capsule [package insert], Morgantown: Mylan Pharmaceuticals Inc; 2009.

Krummel T, Dimitrov Y, Moulin B, Hannedouche T. Acute renal failure induced by topical ketoprofen. BMJ. 2000;320:93.

Lee A, Cooper MG, Knight JF, Keneally JP. Effects of nonsteroidal anti-inflammatory drugs on postoperative renal function in adults with normal renal function (review). Cochrane Database Syst Rev. 2007;(2):CD002765. doi:10.1002/14651858.CD002765.pub3.

Pazmiño PA, Pazmiño PB. Ketoprofen-induced irreversible renal failure [letter]. Nephron. 1988;50:70–1.

Sakai T, Maruyama T, Imamura H, Shimada H, Otagiri M. Mechanism of Stereoselective serum binding of ketoprofen after hemodialysis. J Pharmacol Exp Ther. 1996;278:786–92.

Skeith KJ, Dasgupta M, Lange R, Jamali F. The influence of renal function on the pharmacokinetics of unchanged and acyl-glucuroconjugated ketoprofen enantiomers after 50 and 100 mg racemic ketoprofen. Br J Clin Pharmacol. 1996;42:163–9.

Skeith KJ, Russell AS, Jamali F. Ketoprofen pharmacokinetics in the elderly: influence of rheumatic disease, renal function, and dose. J Clin Pharmacol. 1993;33:1052–9.

Stafanger G, Larsen HW, Hansen H, Sørensen K. Pharmacokinetics of ketoprofen in patients with chronic renal failure. Scand J Rheumatol. 1981;10:189–92.

Toto RD, Anderson SA, Brown-Cartwright D, Kokko JP, Brater DC. Effects of acute and chronic dosing of NSAIDs in patients with renal insufficiency. Kidney Int. 1986;30:760–8.

Dosage Adjustment of Medications Eliminated by the Kidneys

<u>**Ketoprofen**</u>**/Orudis®**   {**Anti-inflammatory; analgesic; nonsteroidal anti-inflammatory drug**}

Usual initial dose:	50 mg orally
Usual maintenance dose:	25–50 mg orally every 6–8 h
Typical maximum dose:	300 mg/day
Proportion eliminated unchanged:	<1 % (63–75 % of dose as metabolites in urine)

Adjustment for Kidney Disease

FDA-approved product labeling:	*Mildly impaired renal function*	*Max 150 mg/day*
	Severe/end-stage renal impairment (GFR <25 mL/min/1.73 m²)	*Max 100 mg/day*
Alternative adjustment:	*GFR >50 mL/min*	*25–75 mg orally three times daily*
	GFR 10–50 mL/min	*25–50 mg orally three times daily (~25 % decrease)*
	GFR <10 mL/min	*12.5–25 mg orally two to three times daily (~50 % decrease)*
	Hemodialysis	*12.5–25 mg orally two to three times daily (~50 % decrease)*
	CAPD	*12.5–25 mg orally two to three times daily (~50 % decrease)*
	CRRT	*Not applicable; preferably avoid*

Dosage Adjustment of Medications Eliminated by the Kidneys

Ketorolac - Selected References

Adverse Drug Reactions Advisory Committee. Ketorolac and renal failure. Med J Aust. 1993;159:488.

Aitken HA, Burns JW, McArdle CS, Kenny GC. Effects of ketorolac trometamol on renal function. Br J Anaesth. 1992;62:481–5.

Aronoff GA, Bennett WM, Berns JS, et al. Drug prescribing in renal failure: dosing guidelines for adults and children. 5th ed. Philadelphia: American College of Physicians; 2007.

Boras-Uber LA, Brackett NC Jr. Ketorolac-induced acute renal failure [letter]. Am J Med. 1992;92:450–2.

Brocks DR, Jamali F. Clinical pharmacokinetics of ketorolac tromethamine. Clin Pharmacokinet. 1992;23:415–27.

Brown J, Diagnostic and treatment patterns for renal colic in US emergency departments. Int Urol Nephrol. 2006;38:87–92.

Buller GK, Perazella MA. Acute renal failure and ketorolac [letter]. Ann Intern Med. 1997;127:493–4.

Corelli RL, Gericke KR. Renal insufficiency associated with intramuscular administration of ketorolac tromethamine. Ann Pharmacother. 1993;27:1055–7.

Feldman HI, Kinman JL, Berlin JA, et al. Parenteral ketorolac: the risk for acute renal failure. Ann Intern Med. 1997;126:193–9.

Forse A, El-Beheiry H, Butler PD, Pace RF. Indomethacin and Ketorolac given preoperatively are equally effective in reducing early postoperative pain after laparoscopic cholecystectomy. Can J Surg. 1996;39:26–30.

Freedland SJ, Blanco-Yarosh M, Sun JC, et al. Effect of ketorolac on renal function after donor nephrectomy. Urology. 2002;59:826–30.

Freedland SJ, Blanco-Yarosh M, Sun JC, et al. Ketorolac-based analgesia improves outcomes for living kidney donors. Transplantation. 2002;73:741–5.

Haragsim L, Dalai R, Bagga H, Bastani B. Ketorolac-induced acute renal failure and hyperkalemia: report of three cases. Am J Kidney Dis. 1994;24:578–80.

Jones SF, Ulyatt D, Ketorolac and renal failure [letter]. Anaesth Intensive Care. 1994;22:113–4.

Kelley M, Bastaini B. Ketorolac-induced acute renal failure and hyperkalemia [letter]. Clin Nephrol. 1995;44:276–7.

Ketorolac tromethamine injection [package insert]. Lake Forest: Hospira Inc; 2008.

Laisalmi M, Teppo A-M, Koivusalo A-M, Honkanen E, Valta P, Lindgren L. The effect of ketorolac and sevoflurane anesthesia on renal and glomerular function. Anesth Analg. 2001;93:1210–3.

Lee A, Cooper MG, Craig JC, Knight JF, Keneally JP. The effects of nonsteroidal anti-inflammatory drugs (NSAIDs) on postoperative renal function: a meta-analysis. Anaesth Intensive Care. 1999;27:574–80.

Oosterlink W, Philp NH, Charig C, Gillies G, Hetherington JW, Lloyd J. A double-blind single dose comparison of intramuscular ketorolac tromethamine and pethidine in the treatment of renal colic. J Clin Pharmacol. 1990;30:336–41.

Pearce CJ, Gonzalez FM, Wallin JD. Renal failure and hyperkalemia associated with ketorolac tromethamine. Arch Intern Med. 1993;153:1000–2.

Perazella MA, Buler K. NSAID nephrotoxicity revisited: acute renal failure due to parenteral ketorolac. South Med J. 1993;86:1421–4.

Quan DJ, Kayser SR. Ketorolac induced acute renal failure following a single dose. J Toxicol Clin Toxicol. 1994;32:305–9.

Reinhart DJ. Minimising the adverse effects of ketorolac. Drug Saf. 2000;22:487–97.

Riddle MC, McDaniel PA. Acute reduction of renal 11β-hydroxysteroid dehydrogenase activity by several antinatriuretic stimuli. Metabolism. 1993;42:1370–4.

Safdar B, Degutis LC, Landry K, Vedere SR, Moscovitz HC, D'Onofrio G. Intravenous morphine plus ketorolac is superior to either drug alone for treatment of acute renal colic. Ann Emerg Med. 2006;48:173–81.

Smith K, Halliwell RMAT, Lawrence S, Klineberg PL, O'Connell P. Acute renal failure associated with intramuscular ketorolac. Anaesth Intensive Care. 1993;21:700–3.

Steinberg PL, Nangia AK, Curtis K. A standardized pain management protocol improves timeliness of analgesia among emergency department patients with renal colic. Qual Manag Health Care. 2011;20:30–6.

Toradol® tablet film coated [package insert]. Nutley: Roche Laboratories Inc; 2009.

Dosage Adjustment of Medications Eliminated by the Kidneys

<u>Ketorolac</u>/Toradol®	{Anti-inflammatory; analgesic; nonsteroidal anti-inflammatory drug}	

Usual initial dose: 30–60 mg IM or IV or 20 mg orally

Usual maintenance dose: 15–30 mg IM or IV every 6 h as needed for pain or 10 mg orally every 4–6 h as needed for pain

Typical maximum dose: 120 mg/day IV or IM or 40 mg/day orally, not to exceed 5 days duration

Proportion eliminated unchanged: 60 %

Adjustment for Kidney Disease

FDA-approved product labeling:	*Renally impaired patients*	*15 mg IM or IV every 6 h as needed for pain (max 60 mg/day) or 10 mg orally once, then 10 mg orally every 4–6 h prn not >40 mg/day*
	Advanced renal impairment or patients at risk for renal failure due to volume depletion	*Contraindicated*
Alternative adjustment:	*GFR >50 mL/min*	*15–30 mg IM or IV every 6 h, not to exceed 5 days duration*
	GFR 10–50 mL/min	*Preferably avoid or 7.5–15 mg IM or IV every 6 h, not to exceed 5 days duration (50 % decrease)*
	GFR <10 mL/min	*Preferably avoid due to risk for gastrointestinal and renal toxicity*
	Hemodialysis	*Preferably avoid due to risk for gastrointestinal and renal toxicity*
	CAPD	*Preferably avoid due to risk for gastrointestinal and renal toxicity*
	CRRT	*7.5–15 mg IM or IV every 6 h, not to exceed 5 days duration*

L

L.K. Golightly et al. (eds.), *Renal Pharmacotherapy*,
DOI 10.1007/978-1-4614-5800-5_11, © Springer Science+Business Media New York 2013

Dosage Adjustment of Medications Eliminated by the Kidneys

Lacosamide - Selected References

Andurkar SV, Stables JP, Kohn H. The anticonvulsant activities of N-benzyl 3-methoxypropionamides. Bioorg Med Chem. 1999;7:2381–9.

Ben-Menachem E, Biton V, Jatuzis D, Abou-Khalil B, Doty P, Rudd GD. Efficacy and safety of oral lacosamide as adjunctive therapy in adults with partial-onset seizures. Epilepsia. 2007;48:1308–17.

Beyreuther BK, Callizot N, Brot MD, Feldman R, Bain SC, Stöhr T. Antinociceptive efficacy of lacosamide in rat models for tumor- and chemotherapy-induced cancer pain. Eur J Pharmacol. 2007;565:98–104.

Beyreuther BK, Freitag J, Heers C, Krebsfänger N, Scharfenecker U, Stöhr T. Lacosamide: a review of preclinical properties. CNS Drug Rev. 2007;13:21–42.

Biton V, Rosenfeld WE, Whitesides J, Fountain NB, Vaiciene N, Rudd GD. Intravenous lacosamide as replacement for oral lacosamide in patients with partial-onset seizures. Epilepsia. 2008;49:418–24.

Chung S, Sperling MR, Biton V, et al. Lacosamide as adjunctive therapy for partial-onset seizures: a randomized controlled trial. Epilepsia. 2010;51:958–67.

Costa J, Fareleira F, Ascenção R, Borges M, Sampaío C, Vaz-Carneiro A. Clinical comparability of the new antiepileptic drugs in refractory partial epilepsy: a systematic review and meta-analysis. Epilepsia. 2011;52:1280–91.

Duncan GE, Kohn H. The novel antiepileptic drug lacosamide blocks behavioral and brain metabolic manifestations of seizure activity in the 6 Hz psychomotor seizure model. Epilepsy Res. 2005;67:81–7.

Greenaway C, Ratnaraj N, Sander JW, Patsalos PN. Saliva and serum lacosamide concentrations in patients with epilepsy. Epilepsia. 2011;52:258–63.

Halász P, Kälviäinen R, Mazurkiewicz-Beldzi ska M, et al. Adjunctive lacosamide for partial-onset seizures: efficacy and safety results from a randomized controlled trial. Epilepsia. 2009;50:443–53.

Kelemen A, Halász P. Lacosamide for the prevention of partial onset seizures in epileptic adults. Neuropsychiatr Dis Treat. 2010.6:465–71.

Koubeissi MZ, Mayor CL, Estephan B, Rashid S, Azar NJ. Efficacy and safety of intravenous lacosamide in refractory nonconvulsive status epilepticus. Acta Neurol Scand. 2011;123:142–6.

Krause LU, Brodowski KO, Kellinghaus C. Atrioventricular block following lacosamide intoxication. Epilepsy Behav. 2011;20:725–7.

Łuszcki JJ. Third-generation antiepileptic drugs : mechanisms of action, pharmacokinetics and interactions. Pharmacol Rep. 2009;61:197–216.

Maschio M, Dinapoli L, Mingoia M, et al. Lacosamide as add-on in brain tumor-related epilepsy : preliminary report on efficacy and tolerability. J Neurol. 2011;258(11):2100–4. doi:10.1007/s00415-011-6132-8.

Nizam A, Mylavarapu K, Thomas T, et al. Lacosamide-induced second-degree atrioventricular block in a patient with partial epilepsy. Epilepsia. 2011;52(10):e153–5. doi:10.1111/j.1528-1167.2011.03212.x.

Parkerson KA, Reinsberger C, Chou SH, Dworetzky BA, Lee JW. Lacosamide in the treatment of acute recurrent seizures and periodic epileptiform patterns in critically ill patients. Epilepsy Behav. 2011;20:48–51.

Tilz C, Resch R, Hofer T, Eggers C. Successful treatment for refractory convulsive status epilepticus by non-parenteral lacosamide. Epilepsia. 2010;51:316–7.

Vimpat® tablet film coated, injection for intravenous use, solution [package insert]. Smyrna: UCB Inc; 2010.

Wehner T, Bauer S, Hamer HM, et al. Six months of postmarketing experience with adjunctive lacosamide in patients with pharmacoresistant focal epilepsy at a tertiary care epilepsy center in Germany. Epilepsy Behav. 2009;16:423–5.

Wymer JP, Simpson J, Sen D, Bongardt S. Efficacy and safety of lacosamide in diabetic neuropathic pain: an 18-week double-blind placebo-controlled trial of fixed-dose regimens. Clin J Pain. 2009;25:376–85.

Ziegler D, Sen D, Hidvégi T, et al. Efficacy and safety of lacosamide in painful diabetic neuropathy. Diabetes Care. 2010;33:839–41.

Dosage Adjustment of Medications Eliminated by the Kidneys

<u>Lacosamide</u>/Vimpat®	{Antiepileptic; neuronal voltage-gated sodium channel blocker; collapsing response mediator protein-2 (CRIMP-2) inhibitor}
Usual initial dose:	50 mg orally or IV twice daily
Usual maintenance dose:	100–200 mg orally or IV twice daily
Typical maximum dose:	400 mg/day
Proportion eliminated unchanged:	40 %

Adjustment for Kidney Disease

FDA-approved product labeling:	*Mild to moderate renal impairment (CrCL >30 mL/min)*	*100–200 mg enterally or IV twice daily (no dose adjustment necessary)*
	Severe renal impairment (CrCL ≤30 mL/min)	*100–150 mg enterally or IV twice daily (max 300 mg/day)*
	Hemodialysis	*Give supplemental dose (50 % of single maintenance dose amount) after each dialysis.*
Alternative adjustment:	*GFR ≤30 mL/min*	*100–150 mg enterally or IV twice daily (max 300 mg/day; cardiac monitoring is recommended during dose titration and intercurrent acute illness)*

Dosage Adjustment of Medications Eliminated by the Kidneys

Lamivudine - Selected References

Aronoff GA, Bennett WM, Berns JS, et al. Drug prescribing in renal failure: dosing guidelines for adults and children. 5th ed. Philadelphia: American College of Physicians; 2007.

Asari A, Iles-Smith H, Chen Y-C, et al. Pharmacokinetics of lamivudine in subjects receiving peritoneal dialysis in end-stage renal failure. Br J Clin Pharmacol. 2007;64:738–44.

Bohjanen PR, Johnson MD, Szezech LA, et al. Steady-state pharmacokinetics of lamivudine in human immunodeficiency virus-infected patients with end-stage renal disease receiving chronic dialysis. Antimicrob Agents Chemother. 2002;46:2387–92.

Bruno R, Regazzi MB, Ciappina V, et al. Comparison of plasma pharmacokinetics of lamivudine during twice and once daily administration in patients with HIV. Clin Pharmacokinet. 2001;40:695–700.

de Muys J-M, Gourdeau H, Nguyen-Ba N, et al. Anti-human immunodeficiency virus type 1 activity, intracellular metabolism, and pharmacokinetic evaluation of 2'-deoxy-3'-oxa-4'-thiocytidine. Antimicrob Agents Chemother. 1999;43:1835–44.

de Silva HJ, Herath CA, Sheriff MHR. Lamivudine therapy for hepatitis B infection in post-renal transplant patients: results after 36 months follow-up [letter]. Liver Int. 2005;25:1074–5.

Epivir-HBV® tablet and solution [package insert]. Research Triangle Park: GlaxoSmithKline; 2011.

Epivir® tablet film coated and solution [package insert]. Research Triangle Park: GlaxoSmithKline; 2009.

Filik L, Karakayali H, Moray G, et al. Lamivudine therapy in kidney allograft recipients who are seropositive for hepatitis B surface antigen. Transplant Proc. 2006;38:496–8.

Gupta SK, Eustace JA, Winston JA, et al. Guidelines for the management of chronic kidney disease in HIV-infected patients: recommendations of the HIV Medicine Section of the Infectious Diseases Society of America. Clin Infect Dis. 2005;40:1559–85.

Heald AE, Hsyu PH, Yuen GJ, Robinson P, Mydlow P, Bartlett JA. Pharmacokinetics of lamivudine in human immunodeficiency virus-infected patients with renal dysfunction. Antimicrob Agents Chemother. 1996;40:1514–9.

Izzedine H, Launay-Vacher V, Deray G. Dosage of lamivudine in a haemodialysis patient [letter]. Nephron. 2000;86:553.

Johnson MA, Moore KHP, Yuen GJ, Bye A, Pakes GE. Clinical pharmacokinetics of lamivudine. Clin Pharmacokinet. 1999;36:41–66.

Johnson MA, Verpooten GA, Daniel MJ, et al. Single dose pharmacokinetics of lamivudine in subjects with impaired renal function and the effects of haemodialysis. Br J Clin Pharmacol. 1998;46:21–7.

Moore KHP, Barrett JE, Shaw S, et al. The pharmacokinetics of lamivudine phosphorylation in peripheral mononuclear cells from patients with HIV-1. AIDS. 1999;13:2239–50.

Motta JS, Mello FC, Lago BV, Perez RM, Gomes SA, Figueiredo FF. Occult hepatitis B virus infection and lamivudine-resistant mutations in isolates from renal patients undergoing hemodialysis. J Gastroenterol Hepatol. 2010;25:101–6.

Okuse C, Yotsuyanagi H, Yamada N, et al. Successful treatment of hepatitis B virus-associated membranous nephropathy with lamivudine. Clin Nephrol. 2008;65:53–6.

Perry GM, Faulds D. Lamivudine: a review of its antiretroviral activity, pharmacokinetic properties and therapeutic efficacy in the management of HIV infection. Drugs. 1997;53:657–80.

Pluda JM, Cooley TP, Montaner JSG, et al. A phase I/II study of 2'-deoxy-3'-thiacytidine (lamivudine) in patients with advanced human immunodeficiency virus infection. J Infect Dis. 1995;171:1438–7.

Tang S, Lai FM-M, Lui YH, et al. Lamivudine in hepatitis B-associated membranous nephropathy. Kidney Int. 2005;68:1750–8.

Thompson MA, Aberg JA, Cahn P, et al. Antiretroviral treatment of adult HIV infection: 2010 recommendations of the International AIDS Society—USA Panel. JAMA. 2010;304:321–33.

van Leeuwen R, Lange JMA, Hussey EK, et al. The safety and pharmacokinetics of a reverse transcriptase inhibitor, 3TC, in patients with HIV infection: a phase I study. AIDS. 1992;6:1471–5.

Yuen GJ, Lou Y, Bumgarner NF, et al. Equivalent steady-state pharmacokinetics of lamivudine in plasma and lamivudine triphosphate within cells following administration of lamivudine 300 milligrams once daily and 150 milligrams twice daily. Antimicrob Agents Chemother. 2004;48:176–82.

Yuen GJ, Morris DM, Mydlow PK, Haidar S, Hall ST, Hussey EK. Pharmacokinetics, absolute bioavailability, and absorption characteristics of lamivudine. J Clin Pharmacol. 1995;35:1174–80.

Dosage Adjustment of Medications Eliminated by the Kidneys

Lamivudine (3TC)/Epivir®   {Antiretroviral; nucleoside analog; ℞ for hepatitis B}

Usual initial dose:	150 mg orally
Usual maintenance dose:	150 mg orally twice daily or 300 mg once daily
Typical maximum dose:	300 mg/day
Proportion eliminated unchanged:	70 %

Adjustment for Kidney Disease

FDA-approved product labeling: *Adjustment of dosage of lamivudine in adults and adolescents (≥30 kg)*

CrCL (mL/min)	Recommended dosage of lamivudine
Human immunodeficiency virus (HIV-1) infection	
≥50	150 mg twice daily or 300 mg once daily
30–49	150 mg once daily
15–29	150 mg first dose, then 100 mg once daily
5–14	150 mg first dose, then 50 mg once daily
<5	50 mg first dose, then 25 mg once daily
Hepatitis B virus HBV infection	
≥50	100 mg once daily
30–49	100 mg first dose, then 50 mg once daily
15–29	100 mg first dose, then 25 mg once daily
5–14	35 mg first dose, then 15 mg once daily
<5	35 mg first dose, then 10 mg once daily

Alternative adjustment:

GFR >50 mL/min	150 mg orally every 12 h or 300 mg orally once daily
GFR 10–50 mL/min	150 mg orally every 24 h
GFR <10 mL/min	20 mg orally every 24 h
Hemodialysis	25 mg orally once daily or 75 mg orally every other day; administer after hemodialysis on dialysis days.
CAPD	10 mg orally once daily
CRRT	150 mg orally every 24 h

Lanreotide - Selected References

Antonjian RM, Barbanoj MJ, Cordero JA, et al. Pharmacokinetics of a new Autogel formulation of the somatostatin analogue lanreotide after a single subcutaneous dose in healthy volunteers. J Pharm Pharmacol. 2004;56:471–6.

Astruc B, Marbac P, Bouterfa H, et al. Long-acting octreotide and prolonged-release lanreotide formulations have different pharmacokinetic profiles. J Clin Pharmacol. 2005;45:836–44.

Barbanoj M, Antonijoan R, Morte A, et al. Pharmacokinetics of the somatostatin analog lanreotide in patients with severe renal insufficiency. Clin Pharmacol Ther. 1999;66:485–91.

Bornschein J, Drozdov I, Malferetheiner P. Octreotide LAR: safety and tolerability issues. Expert Opin Drug Saf. 2009;8:755–68.

Bronstein M, Musolino N, Jallad R, et al. Pharmacokinetic profile of lanreotide Autogel® in patients with acromegaly after four deep subcutaneous injections of 60, 90 or 120 mg every 28 days. Clin Endocrinol (Oxf). 2005;63:514–9.

Cendros JM, Peraire C, Fernández-Trocóniz I, Obach R. Pharmacokinetics and population pharmacodynamic analysis of lanreotide Autogel. Metabolism. 2005;54:1276–81.

Croxtall JD, Scott LJ. Lanreotide Autogel®: a review of its use in the management of acromegaly. Drugs. 2008;68:711–23.

Heron I, Thomas F, Dero M, et al. Pharmacokinetics and efficacy of a long-acting formulation of the new somatostatin analog BIM 23014 in patients with acromegaly. J Clin Endocrinol Metab. 1993;76:721–7.

Jacobs ML, Derkx FH, Stijnen T, Lamberts SW, Weber RF. Effects of long-acting somatostatin analog (Somatulin) on renal hyperfiltration in patients with IDDM. Diabetes Care. 1997;20:632–6.

Kuhn JM, Legrand A, Ruiz JM, Obach R, De Ronzan J, Thomas F. Pharmacokinetic and pharmacodynamic properties of a long-acting formulation of the new somatostatin analogue, lanreotide, in normal healthy volunteers. Br J Clin Pharmacol. 1994;38:213–9.

Motet C, Sieber CC, Nauer A, et al. Hemodynamic effects of somatostatin analog lanreotide in humans : placebo-controlled, cross-over dose-ranging echo-Doppler study. Hepatology. 1998;27:920–5.

Somatuline® depot injection [package insert]. Brisbane: Tercica Inc subsidiary of the Ibsen Group; 2011.

Tomlinson B, Thomas NG, Lan IW, et al. Pharmacokinetic profile of the somatostatin analogue lanreotide in individuals with chronic hepatic insufficiency. Clin Pharmacokinet. 2006;45:1003–11.

Trocóniz IF, Cendrós JM, Peraire C, et al. Population pharmacokinetic analysis of lanreotide Autogel® in healthy subjects: evidence for injection interval of up to 2 months. Clin Pharmacokinet. 2009;48:51–62.

Dosage Adjustment of Medications Eliminated by the Kidneys

<u>Lanreotide</u>/Somatuline® Depot	{Somatostatin analog; ℞ for acromegaly}

Usual initial dose: 90 mg every 4 weeks for 3 months administered as a deep subcutaneous injection in the superior external quadrant of the buttock

Usual maintenance dose: 60–120 mg subcutaneously every 4 weeks, with dose adjusted based on growth hormone (GH) and insulin-like growth factor (IGF-1) levels

Typical maximum dose: 120 mg every 4 weeks

Proportion eliminated unchanged: Unknown

Adjustment for Kidney Disease

FDA-approved product labeling: *Lanreotide starting dose in patients with moderate and severe renal impairment should be 60 mg every 4 weeks for 3 months administered as a deep subcutaneous injection in the superior external quadrant of the buttock, with subsequent dosage adjusted based on growth hormone (GH) and insulin-like growth factor (IGF-1) levels as tabulated below*

Patient response	Dose
GH >1 to ≤2.5 ng/mL; normalized IGF-1; and/or controlled clinical symptoms	*90 mg every 28 days*
GH >2.5 ng/ml; IGF-1 elevated; and/or clinical symptoms uncontrolled	*120 mg every 28 days*
GH ≤1 ng/mL; IGF-1 normal clinical symptoms controlled	*60 mg every 28 days*

Alternative adjustment: *Data not available*

Dosage Adjustment of Medications Eliminated by the Kidneys

<u>Lenalidomide</u> - Selected References

Andrisitos LA, Johnson AJ, Lozanski G, et al. Higher doses of lenalidomide are associated with unacceptable toxicity including life-threatening tumor flare in patients with chronic lymphocytic leukemia. J Clin Oncol. 2008;26:2519–25.

Batts ED, Sanchorawala V, Hegerfeldt Y, Lazarus HM. Azotemia associated with use of lenalidomide in plasma cell dyscrasias. Leuk Lymphoma. 2008;49:1108–15.

Borrello I. Lenalidomide in renal insufficiency: balancing the risks and benefits [letter]. Br J Haematol. 2008;144:446–7.

Chen N, Lau H, Kong L, et al. Pharmacokinetics of lenalidomide in subjects with various degrees of renal impairment and in subjects on hemodialysis. J Clin Pharmacol. 2007;47:1466–75.

Dahut WL, Aragon-Ching JB, Woo S, et al. A phase I study of oral lenalidomide in patients with refractory metastatic cancer. J Clin Pharmacol. 2009;49:650–60.

de la Rubia J, Roig M, Ibáñez Á, et al. Activity and safety of lenalidomide and dexamethasone in patients with multiple myeloma requiring dialysis: a Spanish multicenter retrospective study [letter]. Eur J Haematol. 2010;85:363–5.

Dimopoulos M, Alegre A, Stadtmauer EA, et al. The efficacy and safety of lenalidomide plus dexamethasone in relapsed and/or refractory multiple myeloma patients with impaired renal function. Cancer. 2010;116:3807–14.

Dimopoulos MA, Christoulas C, Roussou M, et al. Lenalidomide and dexamethasone for the treatment of refractory/relapsed multiple myeloma: dosing of lenalidomide according to renal function and effect on renal impairment. Eur J Haematol. 2010;85:1–5.

Dimopoulos MA, Kastritis E, Rosinol L, Bladé J, Ludwig H. Pathogenesis and treatment of renal failure in multiple myeloma. Leukemia. 2008;22:1485–93.

Dimopoulos MA, Palumbo A, Attal M, et al. Optimizing the use of lenalidomide in relapsed or refractory multiple myeloma: consensus statement. Leukemia. 2011;25:749–60.

Dimopoulos MA, Terpos E. Renal insufficiency an failure. Hematology Am Soc Hematol Educ Program. 2010;2010:431–6.

Dimopoulos MA, Terpos E, Chanan-Khan A, et al. Renal impairment in patients with multiple myeloma: a consensus statement on behalf of the International Myeloma Working Group. J Clin Oncol. 2010;28:4976–84.

Gay F, Palmbo A. Management of disease- and treatment-related complication in patients with multiple myeloma. Med Oncol. 2010;27(Suppl 1):S43–52.

González Rodríguez AP. Management of the adverse effects of lenalidomide in multiple myeloma. Adv Ther. 2011;28 (Suppl 1):1–10.

Knop S, Einsele H, Bargou R, Cosgrove D, List A. Adjusted dose lenalidomide is safe and effective in patients with deletion (5q) myelodysplastic syndrome and severe renal impairment [letter]. Leuk Lymphoma. 2008;49:346–9.

Meletios-Athanasios D, Terpos E. Lenalidomide: an update on evidence from clinical trials. Blood Rev. 2010;24(Suppl 1): S21–6.

Niesvizky R, Badros AZ. Complications of multiple myeloma therapy, part 2: risk reduction and management of venous thromboembolism, osteonecrosis of the jaw, renal complications, and anemia. J Natl Compr Cancer Netw. 2010;8(Suppl 1): S13–20.

Niesvizky R, Naib T, Christos PJ, et al. Lenalidomide-induced myelosuppression is associated with renal dysfunction: adverse events evaluation of treatment-naïve patients undergoing front-line lenalidomide and dexamethasone therapy. Br J Haematol. 2007;138:640–3.

Offidani M, Corvatta L, Polloni C, et al. Thalidomide, dexamethasone, Doxil and Velcade (ThaDD-V) followed by consolidation/maintenance therapy in patients with relapsed-refractory multiple myeloma. Ann Hematol. 2011;90:429–39.

Revlimid® capsule [package insert]. Summit: Celgene Corp; 2010.

Roussou M, Kastritis E, Christoulas D, et al. Reversibility of renal failure in newly diagnosed patients with multiple myeloma and the role of novel agents. Leuk Res. 2010;34:1395–7.

Specter R, Sanchorawala V, Seldin DC, et al. Kidney dysfunction during lenalidomide treatment for amyloidosis. Nephrol Dial Transplant. 2011;26:881–6.

Zeldis JB, Knight RD, Jacques C, Tozer A, Bizzari J-P. Lenalidomide in multiple myeloma: current role and future directions. Expert Opin Pharmacother. 2010;11:829–42.

Dosage Adjustment of Medications Eliminated by the Kidneys

<u>Lenalidomide</u>/Revlimid®   {Immunomodulator; ℞ for myelodysplastic syndromes, multiple myeloma, Behçet syndrome}

Usual initial dose:	10–25 mg orally
Usual maintenance dose:	Myelodysplastic syndromes, 10 mg orally once daily; multiple myeloma, 25 mg orally once daily for 21 days of repeated 28-day cycles
Typical maximum dose:	25 mg/day
Proportion eliminated unchanged:	65 %

Adjustment for Kidney Disease

FDA-approved product labeling:

Lenalidomide renal function impairment starting dose

Category	Renal function	Multiple myeloma	Myelodysplastic syndrome
Moderate renal impairment	*CrCL 30–59 mL/min*	*10 mg every 24 h*	*5 mg every 24 h*
Severe renal impairment	*CrCL <30 mL/min (not requiring dialysis)*	*15 mg every 48 h*	*5 mg every 48 h*
End-stage renal disease	*CrCL <30 mL/min (requiring dialysis)*	*5 mg once daily; on dialysis days, administer following dialysis*	*5 mg three times per week following each dialysis*

Alternative adjustment:

Myelodysplastic syndromes

eCrCL ≥50 mL/min	*10 mg orally every 24 h*
eCrCL 30–49 mL/min	*5 mg orally every 24 h*
eCrCL <30 mL/min	*5 mg orally every 48 h*
Hemodialysis	*5 mg orally three times weekly; administer after hemodialysis on dialysis days.*
CRRT	*Data not available*

Multiple myeloma

eCrCL ≥50 mL/min	*25 mg orally every 24 h*
eCrCL 30–49 mL/min	*10 mg orally every 24 h*
eCrCL <30 mL/min	*15 mg orally every 48 h*
Hemodialysis	*15 mg orally three times weekly; administer after hemodialysis on dialysis days.*
CRRT	*Data not available*

Dosage Adjustment of Medications Eliminated by the Kidneys

<u>Lepirudin</u> - Selected References

Benz K, Nauck MA, Böhler J, Fischer K-G. Hemofiltration of recombinant hirudin by different hemodialyzer membranes: implications for clinical use. Clin J Am Soc Nephrol. 2007;2:470–6.

Chuang P, Parikh C, Reilly RF. A case review: anticoagulation in hemodialysis patients with heparin-induced thrombocytopenia. Am J Nephrol. 2001;21:226–31.

Desconclois C, Ract C, Boutekedjiret T, et al. Heparin-induced thrombocytopenia: Successful biological and clinical management with lepirudin despite severe renal impairment [letter]. Thromb Haemost. 2011;105:568–9.

Fischer K-G. Hirudin in renal insufficiency. Semin Thromb Hemost. 2002;28:467–82.

Fischer K-G, van de Loo A, Böhler J. Recombinant hirudin (lepirudin) as anticoagulant in intensive care patients treated with continuous hemodialysis. Kidney Int. 1999;56(Suppl 72):S46–50.

Frank RD, Farber H, Stefanidis I, Lanzmich R, Kierdorf HP. Hirudin elimination by hemofiltration: a comparative study of different membranes. Kidney Int. 1999;56(Suppl 72):S41–5.

Gajra A, Vajpayee N, Smith A, Poiesz BJ, Narsipur S. Lepirudin for anticoagulation in patients with heparin-induced thrombocytopenia treated with continuous renal replacement therapy. Am J Hematol. 2007;82:391–3.

Garcia DA, Baglin TP, Weitz JI, Samama MM. Parenteral anticoagulants: antithrombotic therapy and prevention of thrombosis, 9th ed: American College of Chest Physicians Evidence-Based Clinical Practice Guidelines. Chest. 2012;141(2 Suppl):e24–43S. doi:10.1378/chest.11-2291.

Gay BE, Räz H-R, Schmid H-R, Beer JH. Long-term application of lepirudin on chronic haemodialysis over 34 months after heparin-induced thrombocytopenia [letter]. Nephrol Dial Transplant. 2007;22:1790–1.

Hartman V, Malbrain M Daelemans R, Meersman P, Zachée P. Pseudo-pulmonary embolism as a sign of acute heparin-induced thrombocytopenia in hemodialysis patients: safety of resuming heparin after disappearance of HIT antibodies. Nephron Clin Pract. 2006;104:C143–8. doi:10.1159/000094959.

Hein OV, von Heymann C, Diehl T, et al. Intermittent hirudin versus continuous heparin for anticoagulation in continuous renal replacement therapy. Ren Fail. 2004;26:297–303.

Hein OV, von Heymann C, Morgra S, Konertz W, Ziemer S, Spies C. Protracted bleeding after hirudin anticoagulation for cardiac surgery in a patient with HIT II and chronic renal failure. Artif Organs. 2005;29:507–10.

Kim Y-G. Anticoagulation during haemodialysis in patients at high-risk of bleeding. Nephrology (Carlton). 2003;8(Suppl): S23–7.

Lubenow N, Eichler P, Lietz T, Farner B, Breinacher A. Lepirudin for prophylaxis of thrombosis in patients with acute isolated heparin-induced thrombocytopenia: an analysis of 3 prospective studies. Blood. 2004;104:3072–7.

Mon C, Moreno G, Ortiz M, et al. Treatment of hirudin overdosage in a dialysis patient with heparin-induced thrombocytopenia with mixed hemodialysis and hemofiltration treatment. Clin Nephrol. 2006;66:302–5.

Patel VB, Snyder J, Shopnick RI. Successful use of low-dose r-hirudin (Refludan®) for recurrent dialysis catheter thrombosis in a patient with heparin induced thrombocytopenia [letter]. Thromb Haemost. 1999;82:1205–6.

Refludan® injection [package insert]. Wayne: Bayer HealthCare Pharmaceuticals Inc; 2006.

Schneider T, Heuer B, Deller A, Boesken WH. Continuous haemofiltration with r-hirudin (lepirudin) as anticoagulant in a patient with heparin induced thrombocytopenia (HIT II). Wien Klin Wochenschr. 2000;112:552–5.

Tardy B, Lecompte T, Boelhen F, et al. Predictive factors for thrombosis and major bleeding in an observational study in 181 patients with heparin-induced thrombocytopenia treated with lepirudin. Blood. 2006;108:1492–6.

Tardy-Poncet B, Charier D, Diconne E, et al. Extremely low doses of lepirudin in a patient with heparin-induced thrombocytopenia, high bleeding risk and renal insufficiency [letter]. Br J Haematol. 2009;146:456–64.

Tscyudi M, Lämmie B, Alberio L. Dosing lepirudin in patients with heparin-induced thrombocytopenia and normal or impaired renal function: a single-center experience with 68 patients. Blood. 2009;113:2402–9.

Vanholder Camez A, Veys NM, et al. Recombinant hirudin: a specific thrombin inhibiting anticoagulant for hemodialysis. Kidney Int. 1994;45:1754–9.

Vanholder Camez A, Veys N, Van Loo A, Dhondt AM, Ringoir S. Pharmacokinetics of recombinant hirudin in hemodialyzed end-stage renal failure patients. Thromb Haemost. 1997;77:650–5.

Willey ML, de Denus S, Spinler SA. Removal of lepirudin, a recombinant hirudin, by hemodialysis, hemofiltration, or plasmapheresis. Pharmacotherapy. 2002;22:492–9.

Wittkowsky AK, Kondo M. Lepirudin dosing in dialysis-dependent renal failure. Pharmacotherapy. 2000;20:1123–8.

Dosage Adjustment of Medications Eliminated by the Kidneys

<u>Lepirudin</u>/Refludan®	{Antithrombotic; direct thrombin inhibitor}
Usual initial dose:	0.4 mg/kg IV bolus (max 44 mg)
Usual maintenance dose:	0.15 mg/kg/h IV (max 16.5 mg/h)
Typical maximum dose:	0.21 mg/kg/h
Proportion eliminated unchanged:	40 %

Adjustment for Kidney Disease

FDA-approved product labeling: *Lepirudin reduction of infusion rate in patients with renal impairment*

		Adjusted infusion rate	
CrCL [mL/min]	*SCr [mg/dL]*	*% of standard initial rate*	*mg/kg/h*
45–60	*1.6–2.0*	*50*	*0.075*
30–44	*2.1–3.0*	*30*	*0.045*
15–29	*3.1–6.0*	*15*	*0.0225*
<15	*>6.00*	*Avoid or STOP infusion*	*-0-*

The target range (therapeutic window) for the aPTT ratio should be 1.5–2.0 times the mean of the normal laboratory range (corresponding to lepirudin plasma levels of 600–700 μg/L); monitoring should be performed at 4-h intervals until it is apparent that steady state within the target range is achieved

In all patients with renal insufficiency, the bolus dose is to be reduced to 0.2 mg/kg IV

In hemodialysis patients or in acute renal failure (CrCL <15 mL/min or SCr >6.0 mg/dL), infusion of lepirudin is to be avoided or stopped

Alternative adjustment: *The target range (therapeutic window) for the aPTT ratio usually should be 1.5–2.0 times the mean of the normal laboratory range (corresponding to lepirudin plasma levels of 600–700 μg/L); monitoring should be performed at 4-h intervals until it is apparent that steady-state values within the target range are attained.*

eCrCL >60 mL/h or SCr <1.0 mg/dL	*0.08–0.10 mg/kg/h IV (no initial bolus)*
eCrCL 30–60 mL/h or SCr 1.0–1.67 mg/dL	*0.04–0.05 mg/kg/h IV (no initial bolus)*
eCrCL 15–30 mL/h or SCr 1.68–4.80 mg/dL	*0.01 mg/kg/h IV (no initial bolus)*
eCrCL <15 mL/h or SCr >4.80 mg/dL	*0.005 mg/kg/h IV (no initial bolus)*
Hemodialysis	*0.025–0.1 mg/kg IV bolus; repeat doses may be administered when aPTT values fall below 1.5 times the patient's baseline (intervals between doses may be as long as 6–12 days).*
CVVHD	*0.004–0.025 mg/kg/h continuous IV infusion (removal of lepirudin from plasma is dependent on membrane material and wide variations in rate are reported; removal is negligible with some low-flux membranes)*

Dosage Adjustment of Medications Eliminated by the Kidneys

Levetiracetam - Selected References

Aronoff GA, Bennett WM, Berns JS, et al. Drug prescribing in renal failure: dosing guidelines for adults and children. 5th ed. Philadelphia: American College of Physicians; 2007.

Brockmöller J, Thomsen T, Wittstock M, Coupez R, Lochs H, Roots I. Pharmacokinetics of levetiracetam n patients with moderate to severe liver cirrhosis (Child-Pugh classes A, B, and C): characterization by dynamic liver function tests. Clin Pharmacol Ther. 2005;77:529–41.

Chaluvadi S, Chiang S, Tran L, Goldsmith CE, Friedman DE. Clinical experience with generic levetiracetam in people with epilepsy. Epilepsia. 2011;52:810–5.

French J. Use of levetiracetam in special populations. Epilepsia. 42(Suppl 4):40–3.

French JA, Kanner AM, Bautista J, et al. Efficacy and tolerability of the new antiepileptic drugs. I: treatment of new onset epilepsy. Report of the Therapeutics and Technology Assessment Subcommittee and Quality Standards Subcommittee of the American Academy of Neurology and the American Epilepsy Society. Neurology. 2004;62:1252–60.

Hirsch LJ, Arif H, Buchsbaum R, et al. Effect of age and comedication on levetiracetam pharmacokinetics and tolerability. Epilepsia. 2007;48:1351–9.

Hurwitz KA, Ingulli EG, Krous HF. Levetiracetam induced interstitial nephritis and renal failure. Pediatr Neurol. 2009;41:57–8.

Ishherranin N, Roeder M, Sobck S, Yagen B, Schurig V, Bialer M. Enantioselective analysis of levetiracetam and its enantiomer R-α-ethyl-2-oxo-pyrrolidine acetamide using gas chromatography and ion trap mass spectrometric detection. J Chromatogr B Biomed Sci Appl. 2000;745:325–32.

Keppra® injection [package insert]. Smyrna: UCB Inc; 2008.

Keppra® tablet film coated and solution [package insert]. Smyrna: UCB Inc; 2009.

Lacerda G, Krummel T, Sabourdy C, Ryvlin P, Hirsch E. Optimizing therapy of seizures in patients with renal or hepatic dysfunction. Neurology. 2006;67(Suppl 4):S28–33.

Leppik IE, Goel V, Rarick J, Nixdorf DR, Cloyd JC. Intramuscular and intravenous levetiracetam in humans: safety and pharmacokinetics. Epilepsy Res. 2010;91:289–92.

Lo BWY, Kyu HH, Jichici D, Upton AM, Akl EA, Meade MO. Meta-analysis of randomized trials on first line and adjunctive levetiracetam. Can J Neurol Sci. 2011;38:475–86.

Löscher W, Hönack D. Development of tolerance during chronic treatment of kindled rats with the novel antiepileptic drug levetiracetam. Epilepsia. 2000;41:1499–506.

Löscher W, Hönack D, Bloms-Funke P. The novel antiepileptic drug levetiracetam (UCB L059) induces alterations in GABA metabolism and turnover in discrete areas of rat brain and reduces neuronal activity in substantia nigra pars reticulata. Brain Res. 1996;735:208–16.

Löscher W, Hönack D, Rundfeldt C. Antiepileptogenic effects of the novel anticonvulsant levetiracetam (UCB L059) in the kindling model of temporal lobe epilepsy. J Pharmacol Exp Ther. 1998;284:474–9.

Lyseng-Williamson KA. Levetiracetam: a review of its use in epilepsy. Drugs. 2011;71:489–514.

Nau KM Divertie GD, Valentino AK, Freeman WD. Safety and efficacy of levetiracetam for critically ill patients with seizures. Neurocrit Care. 2009;11:34–7.

Patsalos PN. Clinical pharmacokinetics of levetiracetam. Clin Pharmacokinet. 2004;43:707–24.

Patsalos PN. Pharmacokinetic profile of levetiracetam: toward ideal characteristics. Pharmacol Ther. 2000;85:77–85.

Perucca E, Gidal BE, Baltès E. Effects of antiepileptic comedication on levetiracetam pharmacokinetics: a pooled analysis of data from randomized adjunctive therapy trials. Epilepsy Res. 2003;53:47–56.

Radtke RA. Pharmacokinetics of levetiracetam. Epilepsia. 2001;42(Suppl 4):24–7.

Spencer DD, Jacobi J, Juenke JM, Fleck JD, Kays MB. Steady-state pharmacokinetics of intravenous levetiracetam in neurocritical care patients. Pharmacotherapy. 2011;31:934–41.

Strolin Benedetti M, Whomsley R, Nicolas J-M, Young C, Baltes E. Pharmacokinetics and metabolism of ^{14}C-levetiracetam, a new antiepileptic agent, in healthy volunteers. Eur J Clin Pharmacol. 2003;59:621–30.

Vulliemoz S, Iwanowski P, Landis T, Jallon P. Levetiracetam accumulation in renal failure causing myoclonic encephalopathy with triphasic waves. Seizure. 2009;18:376–8.

Dosage Adjustment of Medications Eliminated by the Kidneys

Levetiracetam/Keppra®   {Antiepileptic; synaptic vesicle protein SV2A modulator; N-type calcium current blocker}

Usual initial dose: 500 mg orally or IV twice daily

Usual maintenance dose: 1,500 mg orally twice daily or 1,000 mg IV every 12 h

Typical maximum dose: 4,000 mg/day orally or 3,000 mg/day IV

Proportion eliminated unchanged: 66 %

Adjustment for Kidney Disease

FDA-approved product labeling: *Levetiracetam dosage adjustment for adults with renal function impairment*

Renal function status	CrCL (mL/min)	Oral or IV dose (mg)	Frequency
Healthy	>80	500–1,500	Every 12 h
Mild	50–80	500–1,000	Every 12 h
Moderate	30–50	250–750	Every 12 h
Severe	<30	250–500	Every 12 h
ESRD patients on dialysis	–	500–1,000	Every 24 h

Alternative adjustment:

GFR >50 mL/min	*500–1,000 mg orally or IV every 12 h*
GFR 10–50 mL/min	*250–750 mg orally or IV every 12 h*
GFR <10 mL/min	*500–1,000 mg orally or IV every 24 h*
Hemodialysis	*500–1,000 mg orally or IV every 24 h plus 250–500 mg after hemodialysis on dialysis days*
CAPD	*500–1,000 mg orally or IV every 24 h*
CRRT	*250–750 mg orally or IV every 12 h*

Dosage Adjustment of Medications Eliminated by the Kidneys

Levocetirizine - Selected References

Bachert C, Bousquet J, Canonica GW, et al. Levocetirizine improves quality of life and reduces costs in long-term management of persistent allergic rhinitis. J Allergy Clin Immunol. 2004;114:838–44.

Baltes E, Coupez R, Giezek H, Voss G, Meyerhoff C, Strolin Benedetti M. Absorption and disposition of levocetirizine, the eutomer of cetirizine, administered alone or as cetirizine to healthy volunteers. Fundam Clin Pharmacol. 2001;15:269–77.

Bree F, Thiault L, Gautiers G, et al. Blood distribution of levocetirizine, a new non-sedating histamine H_1-receptor antagonist, in humans. Fundam Clin Pharmacol. 2002;16:471–8.

Denham KJ, Boutsiouki P, Clough GF, Church MK. Comparison of the effects of desloratadine and levocetirizine on histamine-induced wheal, flare and itch in human skin. Inflamm Res. 2003;52:424–7.

Devillier P, Roche N, Faisy C. Clinical pharmacokinetics and pharmacodynamics of desloratadine, fexofenadine and levocetirizine: a comparative review. Clin Pharmacokinet. 2008;47:217–30.

Ferrer M. Pharmacokinetic evaluation of levocetirizine. Expert Opin Drug Metab Toxicol. 2011;7:1035–47.

Gandon JM, Allain H. Lack of effect of single and repeated doses of levocetirizine, a new antihistamine drug, on cognitive and psychomotor functions in healthy volunteers. Br J Clin Pharmacol. 2002;54:51–8.

Gupta A, Gillard M, Christophe B, Chatelain P, Massingham R, Hammarlund-Udenaes M. Peripheral and central H_1 histamine receptor occupancy by levocetirizine, a non-sedating antihistamine; a time course study in the guinea pig. Br J Pharmacol. 2007;151:1129–36.

Hair PI, Scott LJ. Levocetirizine: a review of its use in the management of allergic rhinitis and skin allergies. Drugs. 2006;66:973–96.

Hulhoven R, Rosillon D, Letiexhe M, Meeus M-A, Daoust A, Stockis A. Levocetirizine does not prolong the AT/QTc interval in healthy subjects results from a thorough QT study. Eur J Clin Pharmacol. 2007;63:1011–7.

Lee DKC, Gardiner M, Haggaart K, Fujihara S, Lipworth BJ. Comparative effects of desloratadine, fexofenadine, and levocetirizine on nasal adenosine monophosphate challenge in patients with perennial allergic rhinitis. Clin Exp Allergy. 2004;34:650–3.

Lee DKC, Gray RD, Wilson AM, Robb FM, Soutar PC, Lipworth BJ. Single and short-term dosing effects of levocetirizine on adenosine monophosphate bronchoprovocation in atopic asthma. Br J Clin Pharmacol. 2004;58:34–9.

Srinivas NR. Steroselective renal tubular secretion of cetirizine enantiomers: initial plasma and urine data analysis may hold the key [letter]. Fundam Clin Pharmacol. 2009;23:537–8.

Strolin Benedetti M, Plisnier M, Kaise J, et al. Absorption, distribution, metabolism and excretion of [^{14}C]levocetirizine, the R enantiomer of cetirizine, in healthy volunteers. Eur J Clin Pharmacol. 2001;57:571–82.

Strolin Benedetti M, Whomsley R, Mathy F-X, Jaques P, Espie P, Canning M. Stereoselective renal tubular secretion of levocetirizine and dextrocetirizine, the two enantiomers of the H_1-antihistamine cetirizine. Fundam Clin Pharmacol. 2008;22:19–23.

Tillement J-P, Testa B, Brée F. Compared pharmacological characteristics in humans of racemic cetirizine and levocetirizine, two histamine H_1-receptor antagonists. Biochem Pharmacol. 2003;66:1123–6.

Verster JC, de Weert AM, Bijtjes SIR, et al. Driving ability after acute and sub-chronic administration of levocetirizine and diphenhydramine: a randomized, double-blind, placebo-controlled trial. Psychopharmacology (Berl). 2003;169:84–90.

Walsh GM. A review of the role of levocetirizine as an effective therapy for allergic disease. Expert Opin Pharmacother. 2008;9:859–67.

Zyzal® tablet film coated and solution [package insert]. Smyrna: UCB Inc; 2010.

Dosage Adjustment of Medications Eliminated by the Kidneys

<u>Levocetirizine</u>/Xyzal®	{Antihistamine; second-generation histamine H₁ blocker}

Usual initial dose:	5 mg orally
Usual maintenance dose:	2.5–5 mg orally once daily
Typical maximum dose:	10 mg
Proportion eliminated unchanged:	77 %

Adjustment for Kidney Disease

FDA-approved product labeling:	*Mild renal impairment (CrCL 50–80 mL/min)*	*2.5 mg orally once daily in the evening*
	Moderate renal impairment (CrCL 30–50 mL/min)	*2.5 mg orally every other day in the evening*
	Severe renal impairment (CrCL 10–30 mL/min)	*2.5 mg orally twice weekly in the evening*
	End-stage renal disease (CrCL <10 mL/min)	*Contraindicated*
	Hemodialysis	*Contraindicated*
Alternative adjustment:	*CRRT*	*Not applicable*

Dosage Adjustment of Medications Eliminated by the Kidneys

Levofloxacin - Selected References

Aronoff GA, Bennett WM, Berns JS, et al. Drug prescribing in renal failure: dosing guidelines for adults and children. 5th ed. Philadelphia: American College of Physicians; 2007.

Bellmann R, Egger P, Gritsch W, et al. Elimination of levofloxacin in critically ill patients with renal failure: influence of continuous veno-venous hemofiltration. Int J Clin Pharmacol Ther. 2002;40:142–9.

Czock D, Hüsig-Linde C, Langhoff A, et al. Pharmacokinetics of moxifloxacin and levofloxacin in intensive care unit patients who have acute renal failure and undergo extended daily dialysis. Clin J Am Soc Nephrol. 2006;1:1263–8.

Davis R, Bryson HM. Levofloxacin: a review of its antibacterial activity, pharmacokinetics and therapeutic efficacy. Drugs. 1994;47:677–700.

Fish DN, Chow AT. The clinical pharmacokinetics of levofloxacin. Clin Pharmacokinet. 1997;32:101–19.

Gabardi S, Waikar SS, Martin S, et al. Evaluation of fluoroquinolones for the prevention of BK viremia after renal transplantation. Clin J Am Soc Nephrol. 2010.5:1298–304.

Gilbert DN. Urinary tract infections in patients with chronic renal insufficiency. Clin J Am Soc Nephrol. 2006;1:327–31.

Goodwin SD, Gallis HA, Chow AT, Wong FA, Flor SC, Bartlett JA. Pharmacokinetics and safety of levofloxacin in patients with human immunodeficiency infection. Antimicrob Agents Chemother. 1994;38:799–804.

Guenter SG, Iven H, Boos C, Bruch H-P, Muhl E. Pharmacokinetics of levofloxacin during continuous venovenous hemodiafiltration and continuous venovenous hemofiltration in critically ill patients. Pharmacotherapy. 2002;22:175–83.

Hansen E, Bucher M, Jakob W, Lemberger P, Kees F. Pharmacokinetics of levofloxacin during continuous veno-venous hemofiltration. Intensive Care Med. 2001;27:371–5.

Heintz BH, Matzke GR, Dager WF. Antimicrobial dosing concepts and recommendations for critically ill adult patients receiving continuous renal replacement therapy or intermittent hemodialysis. Pharmacotherapy. 2009;29:562–77.

Korzets A, Gafter U, Dicker D, Herman M, Ori Y. Levofloxacin and rhabdomyolysis in a renal transplant patient. Nephrol Dial Transplant. 2006;21:3304–5.

Lee CKK, Boyle MP, Diener-West M, Brass-Ernst L, Noschese M, Zeitlin PL. Levofloxacin pharmacokinetics in adult cystic fibrosis. Chest. 2007;131:796–802.

Levaquin® tablet film coated, solution, injection [package insert]. Raritan: PriCara Div Ortho-Janssen-McNeil Pharmaceuticals Inc; 2009.

Malone RS, Fish DN, Abraham E, Teitelbaum I. Pharmacokinetics of levofloxacin and ciprofloxacin during continuous renal replacement therapy in critically ill patients. Antimicrob Agents Chemother. 2001;45:2949–54.

Pea F, Viale P, Pavan F, Furlanut M. Pharmacokinetic considerations for antimicrobial therapy in patients receiving renal replacement therapy. Clin Pharmacokinet. 2007;46:997–1038.

Preston SL, Drusano GL, Berman AL, et al. Levofloxacin population pharmacokinetics and creation of a demographic model for prediction of individual drug clearance in patients with serious community-acquired infection. Antimicrob Agents Chemother. 1998;42:1098–104.

Preston SL, Drusano GL, Berman AL, et al. Pharmacodynamics of levofloxacin: a new paradigm for early clinical trials. JAMA. 1998;279:125–9.

Rebuck JA, Fish DN, Abraham E. Pharmacokinetics of intravenous and oral levofloxacin in critically ill adults in a medical intensive care unit. Pharmacotherapy. 2002;22:1216–25.

Sowinski KM, Lucksiri A, Kays MB, Stott MK, Mueller BA, Hamburger RJ. Levofloxacin pharmacokinetics in ESRD and removal by the cellulose acetate high performance-210 hemodialyzer. Am J Kidney Dis. 2003;42:342–9.

Traunmüller F, Thalhammer-Scherrer R, Locker GJ, et al. Single-dose pharmacokinetics of levofloxacin during continuous veno-venous haemofiltration in critically ill patients. J Antimicrob Chemother. 2001;47:229–31.

Tsaganos T, Kouki P, Digenis P, Giamarellou H, Giamarellos-Bourboulis EJ, Kanellakopoulou K. Pharmacokinetics of levofloxacin after single and multiple oral doses in patients undergoing intermittent haemodialysis. Int J Antimicrob Agents. 2008;32:46–9.

Tsuruoka S, Yokata N, Hayaaka T, Saito T, Yamagata K. Pharmacokinetics of multiple-dose levofloxacin in hemodialysis patients [letter]. Am J Kidney Dis. 2011;58(3):498–9. doi:10.1053/j.ajkd.2011.05.014.

Dosage Adjustment of Medications Eliminated by the Kidneys

Levofloxacin/Levaquin®   {Antibacterial; fluoroquinolone}

Usual initial dose:	500 mg enterally or IV
Usual maintenance dose:	250–750 mg enterally or IV every 24 h
Typical maximum dose:	750 mg/day
Proportion eliminated unchanged:	70 %

Adjustment for Kidney Disease

FDA-approved product labeling:

Levofloxacin dosage adjustment in adult patients with renal impairment (CrCL <50 mL/min)

Dosage in normal renal function	CrCL 20–49 mL/min	CrCL 10–19 mL/min	Hemodialysis or chronic ambulatory peritoneal dialysis (CAPD)
750 mg every 24 h	750 mg every 48 h	750 mg initial dose, then 500 mg every 48 h	750 mg initial dose, then 500 mg every 48 h
500 mg every 24 h	500 mg initial dose, then 250 mg every 24 h	500 mg initial dose, then 250 mg every 48 h	500 mg initial dose, then 250 mg every 48 h
250 mg every 24 h	No dosage adjustment required	250 mg every 48 h. If treating uncomplicated UTI, then no dosage adjustment is required	No information on dosing adjustment is available

No adjustment is necessary for patients with CrCL ≥50 mL/min

Alternative adjustment:	*GFR >50 mL/min*	*500–750 mg orally or IV once followed by 250–750 mg orally or IV every 24 h*
	GFR 10–50 mL/min	*500–750 mg orally or IV once followed by 250–750 mg orally or IV every 24–48 h*
	GFR <10 mL/min	*500–750 mg orally or IV once followed by 250–500 mg orally or IV every 48 h*
	Hemodialysis	*500–750 mg orally or IV once followed by 250–500 mg orally or IV every 48 h; administer after hemodialysis on dialysis days.*
	CAPD	*500–750 mg orally or IV once followed by 250–500 mg orally or IV every 48 h*
	CVVH	*500–750 mg IV once followed by 250 mg IV every 24 h*
	CVVHD	*500–750 mg IV once followed by 250–500 mg IV every 24 h*
	CVVHDF	*500–750 mg IV once followed by 250–750 mg IV every 24 h*

Dosage Adjustment of Medications Eliminated by the Kidneys

Lisinopril - Selected References

Agarwal R, Lewis R, Davis JL, Becker B. Lisinopril therapy for hemodialysis hypertension: hemodynamic and endocrine responses. Am J Kidney Dis. 2001;38:1245–50.

Aronoff GA, Bennett WM, Berns JS, et al. Drug prescribing in renal failure: dosing guidelines for adults and children. 5th ed. Philadelphia: American College of Physicians; 2007.

Åsberg A, Midtvedt K, Vassbotn T, Hartmann A. Better microvascular function on long-term treatment with lisinopril than with nifedipine in renal transplant recipients. Nephrol Dial Transplant. 2001;16:1465–70.

August P, Cody RJ, Sealey JE, Laragh JH. Hemodynamic responses to converting enzyme inhibition in patients with renal disease. Am J Hypertens. 1989;2:599–603.

Begg EJ, Bailey RR, Lynn KL, Robson RA, Frank GJ, Olson SC. The pharmacokinetics of angiotensin converting enzyme inhibitors in patients with renal impairment. J Hypertens. 1989;7(Suppl 5):S29–32.

Cannella G, PaolettiE, Delfino R, Peloso G, Rolla D, Molinari S. Prolonged therapy with ACE inhibitors induces a regression of left ventricular hypertrophy of dialyzed uremic patients independently from hypotensive effects. Am J Kidney Dis. 1997;30:659–64.

Cinotti GA, Zucchelli PC, Albertazzi A, et al. Effect of lisinopril on the progression of renal insufficiency in mild proteinuric non-diabetic nephropathies. Nephrol Dial Transplant. 2001;16:961–6.

Donohoe JF, Kelly J, Laher MS, Doyle GD. Lisinopril in the treatment of hypertensive patients with renal impairment. Am J Med. 1988;85(Suppl 3B):31–4.

Greenbaum R, Zucchelli P, Caspi A, et al. Comparison of the pharmacokinetics of fosinoprilat with enalaprilat and lisinopril in patients with congestive heart failure and chronic renal insufficiency. Br J Clin Pharmacol. 2000;49:23–31.

Hoyer J, Schulte K-L, Lenz T. Clinical pharmacokinetics of angiotensin converting enzyme (ACE) inhibitors in renal failure. Clin Pharmacokinet. 1993;24:230–54.

Jackson B, Cubela RB, Conway EL, Johnston CI. Lisinopril pharmacokinetics in renal failure. Br J Clin Pharmacol. 1988;25:719–24.

Karlberg BE, Rosenqvist U. Antihypertensive and hormonal effects of lisinopril , a new angiotensin converting enzyme (ACE) inhibitor in patients with renovascular hypertension. Acta Med Scand Suppl. 1986;714:33–42.

Kelly JG, Doyle GD, Carmody M, Glover DR, Cooper WD. Pharmacokinetics of lisinopril, enalapril and enalaprilat in renal failure: effects of haemodialysis. Br J Clin Pharmacol. 1988;26:781–6.

Küntziger HE, Pouthier D, Bellucci A. Treatment of hypertension with lisinopril in end-stage renal failure. J Cardiovasc Pharmacol. 1987;10(Suppl 7):S157–9.

Massie BM, Armstrong PW, Cleland JGF, et al. Toleration of high doses of angiotensin-converting enzyme inhibitors in patients with chronic heart failure: results from the ATLAS Trial. Arch Intern Med. 2001;161:165–71.

Mitchell HC, Smith RD, Cutler RE, et al. Racial differences in the renal response to blood pressure lowering during chronic angiotensin-converting enzyme inhibition: a prospective double-blind randomized comparison of fosinopril and lisinopril in older hypertensive patients with chronic renal insufficiency. Am J Kidney Dis. 1997;29:897–906.

Neubeck M, Fliser D, Pritsch M, et al. Pharmacokinetics and pharmacodynamics of lisinopril in advanced renal failure: consequence of dose adjustment. Eur J Clin Pharmacol. 1994;46:537–43.

Prinivil® tablet [package insert]. Whitehouse Station: Merck Sharp & Dohme Corp; 2010.

Schlanger LE, Haire HM, Zuckerman AM, Loscalzo CE, Mitch WE. Reversible renal failure in an elderly woman with renal artery stenosis. Am J Kidney Dis. 1994;23:123–6.

Shionoiri H, Minamisawa K, Ueda S, et al. Pharmacokinetics and antihypertensive effects of lisinopril in hypertensive patients with normal and impaired renal function. J Cardiovasc Pharmacol. 1990;16:594–600.

Tarnow L, Hansen BV, Rossing P, Parving H-H, Jensen C. Long-term renoprotective effect of nisoldipine and lisinopril in diabetic patients with diabetic nephropathy. Diabetes Care. 2000;23:1725–30.

Thomson AH, Kelly JG, Whiting B. Lisinopril population pharmacokinetics in elderly and renal disease patients with hypertension. Br J Clin Pharmacol. 1989;27:57–65.

van Schaik, Geyskes GG, van der Wouw PA, van Rooij HH, Porsius AJ. Pharmacokinetics of lisinopril in hypertensive patients with normal and impaired renal function. Eur J Clin Pharmacol. 1988;34:61–5.

Dosage Adjustment of Medications Eliminated by the Kidneys

<u>Lisinopril</u>/Prinivil®, Zestril®	{**Antihypertensive, vasodilator, angiotensin converting enzyme (ACE)/ renin inhibitor**}

Usual initial dose:	5–10 mg orally
Usual maintenance dose:	5–40 mg orally once daily
Typical maximum dose:	40 mg/day
Proportion eliminated unchanged:	85 %

Adjustment for Kidney Disease

FDA-approved product labeling:

Lisinopril dosage in renal function impairment

Renal status	CrCL (mL/min)	SCr (mg/dL)	Initial dose (mg/day)
Healthy renal function to mild impairment	>30	<3	10
Moderate to severe renal function impairment	≥10 ≤30	≥3.0	5
Dialysis patients	<10	–	2.5

No adjustment is necessary for patients with CrCL ≥30 mL/min

Alternative adjustment:

GFR >50 mL/min	5–10 mg initially followed by 5–40 mg/day
GFR 10–50 mL/min	2.5–5 mg initially followed by 5–20 mg/day (25–50 % decrease)
GFR <10 mL/min	2.5 mg initially followed by 2.50–20 mg/day (50–75 % decrease)
Hemodialysis	2.5 mg initially followed by 2.50–20 mg/day (50–75 % decrease)
CAPD	Data not available
CRRT	2.5–5 mg initially followed by 5–20 mg/day

Dosage Adjustment of Medications Eliminated by the Kidneys

Lithium - Selected References

Aronoff GA, Bennett WM, Berns JS, et al. Drug prescribing in renal failure: dosing guidelines for adults and children. 5th ed. Philadelphia: American College of Physicians; 2007.

Bjarnason NH, Munkner R, Kampmann JP, Tornoe CW, Ladefoged S, Dalhoff K. Optimizing lithium dosing in hemodialysis. Ther Drug Monit. 2006;28:262–6.

Clericetti N, Beretta-Piccoli C. Lithium clearance in patients with chronic renal diseases. Clin Nephrol. 1991;36:281–9.

Dias N, Hocken AG, Oliguric renal failure complicating lithium carbonate therapy. Nephron. 1972;10:246–9.

Donaldson IMacG, Cunningham J. Persisting neurologic sequelae of lithium carbonate therapy. Arch Neurol. 1983;40:747–51.

Eyer F, Pfab R, Felgenhauer N, et al. Lithium poisoning: pharmacokinetics and clearance during different therapeutic measures. J Clin Psychopharmacol. 2006;26:325–30.

Gelenberg AJ, Wojcik JD, Coggins CH, Rosenbaum JF, LaBrie RA. Renal function monitoring in patients receiving lithium carbonate. J Clin Psychiatry. 1981;42:428–31.

Goodnick PJ, Schorr-Cain CB. Lithium pharmacokinetics. Psychopharmacol Bull. 1991;27:475–91.

Grandjean EM, Aubry J-M. Lithium: updated human knowledge using an evidence-based approach. Part II: Clinical pharmacology and therapeutic monitoring. CNS Drugs. 2009;23:531–49.

Jefferson JW. Lithium: a therapeutic magic wand. J Clin Psychiatry. 1989;50:81–6.

Johnson GFS, Hunt GE. Pharmacokinetics of lithium preparations in patients. Prog Neuropsychopharmacol Biol Psychiatry. 1984;8:63–70.

Kim G-H, Choi NW, Jung J-Y, et al. Treating lithium-induced nephrogenic diabetes insipidus with a COX-2 inhibitor improves polyuria via upregulation of AQP2 and NKCC2. Am J Physiol Renal Physiol. 2008;294:F702–9.

Lavender S, Brown JN, Berrill WT. Acute renal failure and lithium intoxication. Postgrad Med J. 1973;49:277–9.

Levy NB. Psychopharmacology in patients with renal failure. Int J Psychiatry Med. 1990;20:325–34.

Lithium carbonate tablet, capsule gelatin coated, solution. Columbus: Roxane Laboratories Inc; 2009.

Lithobid® tablet extended release [package insert]. Miami: Noven Therapeutics LLC; 2009.

Mason RW, McQueen EG, Keary PJ, James NMcI. Pharmacokinetics of lithium: elimination half-time, renal clearance and apparent volume of distribution in schizophrenia. Clin Pharmacokinet. 1978;3:241–6.

Mitchell PB. Therapeutic monitoring of psychotropic medications. Br J Clin Pharmacol. 2001;52(Suppl 1):45S–54S.

Port FK, Kroll PD, Rosenqeig J. Lithium therapy during maintenance hemodialysis. Psychosomatics. 1979;20:130–2.

Prien RF, Caffey RM Jr, Klett CJ. Lithium carbonate: a survey of the history and current status of lithium in treating mood disorder. Dis Nerve Syst. 1971;32:521–31.

Ramsey TA, Mendels J, Stokes JW, Fitzgerald RG. Lithium carbonate and kidney function: a failure in renal concentrating ability. JAMA. 1972;219:1446–9.

Schou M. Serum lithium monitoring of prophylactic treatment: critical review and updated recommendations. Clin Pharmacokinet. 1988;15:283–6.

Thomsen K, Schou M. Renal lithium excretion in man. Am J Physiol. 1968;215:823–7.

Tredget J, Kirov A, Kirov G. Effects of chronic lithium treatment on renal function. J Affect Disord. 2010;126:436–40.

Uldall PR, Awad AG, McCormick WO, et al. Renal function in patients receiving long-term lithium therapy. Can Med Assoc J. 1981;124:1471–4.

Von Hartitzsch B, Hoenich NA, Leigh RJ, et al. Permanent neurological sequelae despite haemodialysis for lithium intoxication. Br Med J. 1972;4:757–9.

Wallin L, Alling C, Asrell M. Impairment of renal function in patients on long-term lithium treatment. Clin Nephrol. 1982;18:23–8.

Ward ME, Musci MN, Bailey L. Clinical pharmacokinetics of lithium. J Clin Pharmacol. 1994;34:280–5.

Yukawa E, Nomiyama N, Higuchi S, Aoyama T. Lithium population pharmacokinetics from routine clinical data: role of patient characteristics for estimating dosing regimens. Ther Drug Monit. 1993;15:75–82.

Dosage Adjustment of Medications Eliminated by the Kidneys

Lithium/Lithane®, Lithobid®	{Antimanic agent}
Usual initial dose:	600 mg orally
Usual maintenance dose:	900–2,400 mg/day in three or four divided doses or 900–1,800 mg/day in two divided doses (sustained release); dosage must be individualized according to serum levels and clinical response.
Typical maximum dose:	2,400 mg/day
Proportion eliminated unchanged:	95 %

Adjustment for Kidney Disease

FDA-approved product labeling: *When kidney function is assessed, for baseline data prior to starting lithium therapy or thereafter, routine urinalysis and other tests may be used to evaluate tubular function (e.g., urine specific gravity or osmolality following a period of water deprivation or 24-h urine volume) and glomerular function (e.g., SCr or CrCL). During lithium therapy, progressive or sudden changes in renal function, even within the normal range, indicate the need for reevaluation of treatment. Chronic lithium therapy may be associated with diminution of renal concentrating ability, occasionally presenting as nephrogenic diabetes insipidus with polyuria and polydipsia. Morphologic changes with glomerular and interstitial fibrosis and nephron atrophy have been reported. Lithium should generally not be given to patients with significant renal or cardiovascular disease, severe debilitation or dehydration or sodium depletion, and patients receiving diuretics, since the risk of lithium toxicity is very high in these patients.*

For acute mania, optimal response usually can be established with 1,800 mg/day.

For long-term control, desirable serum lithium concentrations usually can be achieved with 900–1,200 mg/day.

Alternative adjustment:	*GFR >50 mL/min*	*900–1,200 mg/day orally in divided doses*
	GFR 10–50 mL/min	*300–600 mg/day orally in divided doses (25–50 % decrease)*
	GFR <10 mL/min	*150–450 mg/day orally in divided doses (50–75 % decrease)*
	Hemodialysis	*150–450 mg/day orally in divided doses; dose after dialysis*
	CAPD	*150–450 mg/day orally in divided doses*
	CRRT	*300–600 mg/day enterally in divided doses*

Therapeutic Drug Monitoring

Therapeutic plasma levels: *0.6–1.2 mEq/L; draw sample 8–12 h after previous dose (just before next dose).*

Dosage Adjustment of Medications Eliminated by the Kidneys

Lomustine - Selected References

Aronoff GA, Bennett WM, Berns JS, et al. Drug prescribing in renal failure: dosing guidelines for adults and children. 5th ed. Philadelphia: American College of Physicians; 2007.

Borel AG, Abbott FS. Identification of carbamoylated thiol conjugates as metabolites of the antineoplastic 1-(2-chloroethyl)-3-cyclohexyl-1-nitrosourea, in rats and humans. Drug Metab Dispos. 1993;21:889–901.

CeeNU® capsule gelatin coated [package insert]. Princeton: Bristol-Myers Squibb Co; 2010.

Kastrissios H, Chao NJ, Blaschke TF. Pharmacokinetics of high-dose oral CCNU in bone marrow transplant recipients. Cancer Chemother Pharmacol. 1996;38:425–30.

Kramer RA, Boyd MR. Nephrotoxicity of 1-(2-chloroethyl)-3-(*trans*-4-methylcyclohexyl)-1-nitrosourea in the Fischer 344 rat. J Pharmacol Exp Ther. 1983;227:409–14.

Kramer RA, Boyd MR, Dees JH. Comparative nephrotoxicity of 1-(2-chloroethyl)-3-(*trans*-4-methylcyclohexyl)-1-nitrosourea (MeCCNU) and chlorozotocin: functional-structural correlations in the Fischer 344 rat. Toxicol Appl Pharmacol. 1986;82:540–50.

Kramer RA, McMenamin MG, Boyd MR. *In vivo* studies on the relationship between hepatic metabolism and the renal toxicity of 1-(2-chloroethyl)-3-(*trans*-4-methylcyclohexyl)-1-nitrosourea. Toxicol Appl Pharmacol. 1986;87:221–30.

Lee FYF, Workman P, Roberts JT, Bleehen NM. Clinical pharmacokinetics of oral CCNU (lomustine). Cancer Chemother Pharmacol. 1985;14:125–31.

Levin VA, Kabra PA, Freeman-Dove MA. Relationship of 1,3-bis(2-chloroethyl)-1-nitrosourea (BCNU) and 1-(2-chloroethyl)-3-cyclohexyl-1-nitrosourea (CCNU) pharmacokinetics of uptake, distribution, and tissue/plasma partitioning in rat organs and intracerebral tumors. Cancer Chemother Pharmacol. 1978;1:233–42.

Levin VA, Stearns J, Byrd A, Finn A, Weinkam RJ. The effect of phenobarbital pretreatment on the antitumor activity of 1,3-bis2-chloroethyl)-1-nitrosourea (BCNU), 1-(2-chloroethyl)-3-cyclohexyl-1-nitrosourea (CCNU), and 1-(2-chloroethyl)-3-(2,6-dioxo-3-piperidyl)-1-nitrosourea (PCNU), and on the plasma pharmacokinetics and biotransformation of BCNU. J Pharmacol Exp Ther 1979;208:1–6.

McIntyre CW, Owen PJ. Prescribing drugs in kidney disease. In: Brenner BM, editor. Brenner & Rector's the kidney. 8th ed. Philadelphia: Saunders/Elsevier; 2008. p. 1930–55.

Micetich KC, Jensen-Akula M, Mandard JC, Fisher RI. Nephrotoxicity of semustine (Methyl-CCNU) in patients with malignant melanoma receiving adjuvant chemotherapy. Am J Med. 1981;71:967–72.

Schacht RG, Feiner HD, Gallo GR, Lieberman A, Baldwin DS. Nephrotoxicity of nitrosoureas. Cancer. 1981;48:1328–34.

Wick W, Puduvalli VK, Chamberlain MC, et al. Phase III study of enzastaurin compared with lomustine in the treatment of recurrent intracranial glioblastoma. J Clin Oncol. 2010;28:1168–74.

Dosage Adjustment of Medications Eliminated by the Kidneys

<u>**Lomustine**</u>/CeeNU®   {**Antineoplastic; alkylating agent; nitrosourea**}

Usual initial dose:	130 mg/m^2 orally
Usual maintenance dose:	130 mg/m^2 as a single oral dose every 6 weeks
Typical maximum dose:	130 mg/m^2
Proportion eliminated unchanged:	50 %

Adjustment for Kidney Disease

FDA-approved product labeling: *Renal abnormalities consisting of progressive azotemia, decrease in kidney size, and renal failure have been reported in patients who received large cumulative doses after prolonged therapy with lomustine. Kidney damage has also been reported occasionally in patients receiving lower total doses.*

Alternative adjustment:

GFR >50 mL/min	*130 mg/m^2 as a single oral dose every 6 weeks*
GFR 10–50 mL/min	*65–100 mg/m^2 as a single oral dose every 6 weeks (25–50 % decrease)*
GFR <10 mL/min	*30–65 mg/m^2 as a single oral dose every 6 weeks (50–75 % decrease)*
Hemodialysis	*30–65 mg/m^2 as a single oral dose every 6 weeks; supplemental dose after dialysis not necessary*
CAPD	*30–65 mg/m^2 as a single oral dose every 6 weeks (50–75 % decrease)*
CRRT	*Data not available*

Note: Hematological and other considerations may suggest further dosage adjustments.

Loracarbef - Selected References

Amsden GW. Tables of antimicrobial agent pharmacology. In: Mandell GL, Bennett JE, Dolin R, editors. Mandell, Douglas, and Bennett's principles and practice of infectious diseases. Vol 1. 6th ed. Philadelphia: Elsevier; 2005. p. 634–700.

Aronoff GA, Bennett WM, Berns JS, et al. Drug prescribing in renal failure: dosing guidelines for adults and children. 5th ed. Philadelphia: American College of Physicians; 2007.

Biedenbach DJ, Jones RN. Predictive accuracy of disk diffusion test for *Proteus vulgaris* and *Providencia* species against five newer orally administered cephalosporins, cefdinir, cefetamet, cefprozil, cefuroxime, and loracarbef. Antimicrob Agents Chemother. 1994;32:559–62.

Brogden RN, McTavish D. Loracarbef: a review of its antimicrobial activity, pharmacokinetic properties and therapeutic efficacy. Drugs. 1993;45:716–36.

Cappelletty DM, Rybak MJ. Bactericidal activities of cefprozil, penicillin, cefaclor, cefixime, and loracarbef against penicillin-susceptible and –resistant *Streptococcus pneumoniae* in an in vitro pharmacodynamic infection model. Antimicrob Agents Chemother. 1996;40:1148–52.

Dantzig AH, Duckworth DC, Tabas LB. Transport mechanisms responsible for the absorption of loracarbef, cefixime, and cefuroxime axetil into human intestinal Caco-2 cells. Biochim Biophys Acta. 1994;1191:7–13.

DeSante KA, Zeckel ML. Pharmacokinetic profile of loracarbef. Am J Med. 1992;92(Suppl 6A):16–9S.

Fassbender M, Lode H, Schaberg T, Borner K, Koeppe P. Pharmacokinetics of new oral cephalosporins, including a new carbacephem. Clin Infect Dis. 1993;16:646–53.

Gwaltney JM Jr, Jones JG, Kennedy DW. Medical management of sinusitis: educational goals and management guidelines. The International Conference on Sinus Disease. Ann Otol Rhinol Laryngol Suppl. 1995;167:22–30.

Hill SL, Bilton D, Johnson MM, Pye A, Mitchell JL, Stockley RA. Sputum and serum pharmacokinetics of loracarbef (LY163892) in patients with chronic bronchial sepsis. J Antimicrob Chemother. 1994;33:129–36.

Hyslop DL. Efficacy and safety of loracarbef in the treatment of pneumonia. Am J Med. 1992;92(Suppl 6A):65–9S.

Lees AS, Andrews JM, Wise R. The pharmacokinetics, tissue penetration and in-vitro activity of loracarbef, a β-lactam antibiotic of the carbacephem class. J Antimicrob Chemother. 1993;32:853–9.

Lorabid® tablet [package insert]. Bristol: Monarch Pharmaceuticals Inc; 2002.

Müller O, Wettich K. Comparison of loracarbef (LY163892) versus amoxicillin in the treatment of bronchopneumonia and lobar pneumonia. Infection. 1992;20:176–82.

Pasini CE, Indelicato JM. Pharmaceutical properties of loracarbef: the remarkable solution stability of an oral 1-carba-1-dethiacephalosporin antibiotic. Pharm Res. 1992;9:250–4.

Rodman DP, McKnight JT, Anderson RL. A critical review of the new oral cephalosporins: considerations and place in therapy. Arch Fam Med. 1994;3:975–80.

Roller S, Lode H, Stelzer I, Deppermann KM, Boeckh M, Koeppe P. Pharmacokinetics of loracarbef and interaction with acetylcysteine. Eur J Clin Microbiol Infect Dis. 1992;11:851–5.

Sifaoui F, Kitzis M-D, Gutmann L. In vitro selection of one-step mutants of Streptococcus pneumoniae resistant to different oral β-lactam antibiotics is associated with alterations of PBP2x. Antimicrob Agents Chemother. 1996;40:152–6.

Sitar DS, Hoban DJ, Aoki FY. Pharmacokinetic disposition of loracarbef in healthy young men and women at steady state. J Clin Pharmacol. 1994;34:924–9.

Stenquist M, Olen L, Jannert M, Näslund L, Zeckel ML. Penetration of loracarbef into the maxillary sinus: a pharmacokinetic assessment. Clin Ther. 1996;18:273–84.

Therasse DG, Farlow DS, Davidson RL, et al. Effects of renal dysfunction on the pharmacokinetics of loracarbef. Clin Pharmacol Ther. 1993;54:311–6.

Tune BM, Hsu C-Y, Fravert D. Cephalosporin and carbacephem nephrotoxicity : roles of tubular cell uptake and acylating potential. Biochem Pharmacol. 1996;51:557–61.

Wenzel U, Thwaites DT, Daniel H. Stereoselective uptake of β-lactam antibiotics by the intestinal peptide transporter. Br J Pharmacol. 1995;116:3021–7.

Zeckel ML, Johns D, Masica DN, Farlow D. Twice-daily dosing of loracarbef 200 mg versus 400 mg in the treatment of patients with acute maxillary sinusitis. Clin Ther. 1995;17:214–30.

Dosage Adjustment of Medications Eliminated by the Kidneys

Loracarbef/Lorabid®   {**Antibacterial; second-generation cephalosporin**}

Usual initial dose:	400 mg orally
Usual maintenance dose:	200–400 mg orally every 12 h for 7–14 days
Typical maximum dose:	800 mg/day
Proportion eliminated unchanged:	85 %

Adjustment for Kidney Disease

FDA-approved product labeling:	*CrCL ≥50 mL/min*	*200–400 mg orally every 12 h*
	CrCL 10–49 mL/min	*200–400 mg every 24 h*
	CrCL <10 mL/min	*200–400 mg orally every 3–5 days*
	Hemodialysis	*200–400 mg orally every 3–5 days; administer supplemental dose following hemodialysis on dialysis days.*
Alternative adjustment:	*GFR >50 mL/min*	*200–400 mg orally every 12 h*
	GFR 10–50 mL/min	*200–400 mg orally every 24 h*
	GFR <10 mL/min	*200–400 mg orally every 3–5 days*
	Hemodialysis	*200–400 mg orally every 3–5 days; administer supplemental dose following hemodialysis on dialysis days.*
	CAPD	*200–400 mg orally every 3–5 days*
	CRRT	*Not applicable (consider an IV cephalosporin)*

Lurasidone - Selected References

Caccia S. Pharmacokinetics and metabolism update for some recent antipsychotics. Expert Opin Drug Metab Toxicol. 2011;7:829–46.

Harvey PD, Ogasa M, Cucchiaro J, Loebel A, Keefe RSE. Performance and interview-based assessments of cognitive change in a randomized, double-blind comparison of lurasidone vs. ziprasidone. Schizophr Res. 2011;127:188–94.

Ishibashi T, Horisawa T, Tokuda K, et al. Pharmacological profile of lurasidone, a novel antipsychotic agent with potent 5-hydroxytryptamine 7 5-HT$_7$) and 5-HT$_{1A}$ receptor activity. J Pharmacol Exp Ther. 2010;334:171–81.

Latuda® tablet [package insert]. Marlborough: Sunovion Pharmaceuticals Inc; 2010.

Lurasidone (*Latuda*) for schizophrenia. Med Lett Drugs Ther. 2011;53:13–4.

Meltzer HY, Cucchiaro J, Ogasa M, et al. Lurasidone in the treatment of schizophrenia: a randomized, double-blind, placebo- and olanzapine-controlled study. Am J Psychiatry. 2011;168:957–67. doi:10.1176/appi.ajp.2011.10060907.

Nakamura M, Ogasa M, Guarino J, et al. Lurasidone in the treatment of acute schizophrenia: a double-blind, placebo-controlled trial. J Clin Psychiatry. 2009;70:829–36.

Newman-Tancredi A, Sleven MS. Comparative pharmacology of antipsychotics possessing combined dopamine D$_2$ and serotonin 5-HT$_{1A}$ receptor properties. Psychopharmacology (Berl). 2011;216:451–73. doi:10.1007/s00213-011-2247-y.

Dosage Adjustment of Medications Eliminated by the Kidneys

Lurasidone/Latuda®   {Atypical antipsychotic}

Usual initial dose: 40 mg orally once daily

Usual maintenance dose: 40–80 mg orally once daily

Typical maximum dose: 80 mg/day

Proportion eliminated unchanged: 5 %

Adjustment for Kidney Disease

FDA-approved product labeling:	*CrCL ≥50 mL/min*	*40–80 mg orally once daily*
	CrCL ≥10 to <50 mL/min	*Do not exceed 40 mg orally once daily.*
Alternative adjustment:	*GFR <10 mL/min*	*Data not available; preferably avoid*
	Hemodialysis	*Data not available; preferably avoid*
	CAPD	*Data not available; preferably avoid*
	CRRT	*Data not available; preferably avoid*

M

L.K. Golightly et al. (eds.), *Renal Pharmacotherapy*,
DOI 10.1007/978-1-4614-5800-5_12, © Springer Science+Business Media New York 2013

Magnesium Citrate - Selected References

Fassler CA, Rodriguez RM, Badesch DB, Stone WJ, Marini JJ. Magnesium toxicity as a cause of hypotension and hypoventilation: occurrence in patients with normal renal function. Arch Intern Med. 1985;145:1604–6.

Lacy CF, Armstrong LL, Goldman MP, Lance LL, editors. Drug information handbook: a comprehensive source for all clinicians and healthcare professionals. 20th ed. Hudson: Lexi-Comp/American Pharmacists Association; 2011.

Magnesium Citrate Oral Solution [package insert]. Livonia: Major Pharmaceuticals; 2009.

Randall E Jr, Cohen MD, Spray CC Jr, Rossmeisl EC. Hypermagnesemia in renal failure: etiology and toxic manifestations. Ann Intern Med. 1964;61:73–88.

van Staden PD, Müller FO, van Heerden MA. Influence of long-term citro-soda ingestion on acid-base balance and blood gases. S Afr Med J. 1979;55:887–90.

Dosage Adjustment of Medications Eliminated by the Kidneys

<u>Magnesium Citrate</u>/Citroma®   {Saline laxative}

Usual initial dose:	195–300 mL orally (8.72–17.45 g)
Usual maintenance dose:	195–300 mL orally once daily
Typical maximum dose:	300 mL/day
Proportion eliminated unchanged:	Variable, unknown

Adjustment for Kidney Disease

FDA-approved product labeling:	*Kidney disease*	*Warning, ask a doctor before use.*
Alternative adjustment:	*GFR ≥50 mL/min*	*150–300 mL (4 mL/kg) orally once daily or PRN constipation*
	GFR 30–49 mL/min	*150 mL orally once daily or PRN constipation; monitor serum magnesium levels.*
	GFR <30 mL/min	*Preferably avoid due to potential toxicity from magnesium accumulation. Consider use of stool softener or bulk-forming or stimulant laxative.*

Magnesium Hydroxide - Selected References

Alfrey AC, Terman DS, Brettschneider L, Simpson KM, Ogden DA. Hypermagnesemia after renal homotransplantation. Ann Intern Med. 1970;73:367–71.

Goodwin FJ, Vince FP. Hypermagnesemic encephalopathy due to antacid ingestion occurring during regular dialysis treatment. Br J Urol. 1970;42:586–9.

Johannson G, Backman U, Danielson BG, Fellström B, Ljunghall S, Wikstöm B. Effects of magnesium hydroxide in renal stone disease. J Am Coll Nutr. 1982;1:179–85.

Krumlovsky F, Del Greco F. Use of antacids in patients on chronic dialysis [letter]. Lancet. 1970;2:150.

Lacy CF, Armstrong LL, Goldman MP, Lance LL, editors. Drug information handbook: a comprehensive resource for all clinicians and healthcare professionals. 20th ed. Hudson: Lexi-Comp/American Pharmacists Association; 2011.

Milk of Magnesia Original [package insert]. Minneapolis: Nash-Finch Co; 2009.

Randall E Jr, Cohen MD, Spray CC Jr, Rossmeisl EC. Hypermagnesemia in renal failure: etiology and toxic manifestations. Ann Intern Med. 1964;61:73–88.

<u>Magnesium Hydroxide (Milk of Magnesia)</u>   **{Laxative; antacid}**

Usual initial dose:	30 mL (2,400 mg) orally
Usual maintenance dose:	30–60 mL (2,400–4,800 mg) orally once daily at bedtime or in divided doses
Typical maximum dose:	60 mL (4,800 mg)
Proportion eliminated unchanged:	Variable, unknown

Adjustment for Kidney Disease

FDA-approved product labeling:	*Kidney disease*	*Warning, ask a doctor before use.*
Alternative adjustment:	*GFR ≥50 mL/min*	*30–60 mL orally at bedtime and/or in divided doses PRN constipation*
	GFR 30–49 mL/min	*30 mL orally at bedtime and/or PRN constipation; monitor serum magnesium levels.*
	GFR <30 mL/min	*Preferably avoid due to potential toxicity from magnesium accumulation. Consider use of stool softener or bulk-forming or stimulant laxative.*

Magnesium/Aluminum Hydroxide and Simethicone - Selected References

Alfrey AC Terman DS, Brettschneider L, Simpson KM, Ogden DA. Hypermagnesemia after renal homotransplantation. Ann Intern Med. 1970;73:367–71.

Drake D, Hollander D. Neutralizing capacity and cost effectiveness of antacids. Ann Intern Med. 1981;94:215–7.

Federman DG, Oster JR, Aviles AI, Singer I, Vaamonde CA. Effects of chronic magnesia-alumina antacid use on serum electrolyte levels. Hosp Pharm. 1994;29:1002, 1004–6, 1009, 1017.

Fordtran JS, Morawski SG, Richardson CT. In vivo and in vitro evaluation of liquid antacids. N Engl J Med. 1973;288:923–8.

Goodwin FJ, Vince FP. Hypermagnesaemic encephalopathy due to antacid ingestion occurring during regular dialysis treatment. Br J Urol. 1970;42:586–9.

Hastings PR, Skillman JJ, Bushnell LS, Silen W. Antacid titration in the prevention of acute gastrointestinal bleeding: a controlled, randomized trial in 100 critically ill patients. N Engl J Med. 1978;298;1041–5.

Hollander D, Harlan J. Antacids vs placebos in peptic ulcer therapy: a controlled double-blind investigation. JAMA. 1973;226:1181–5.

Krumlovsky F, Del Greco F. Use of antacids in patients on chronic dialysis [letter]. Lancet. 1970;2:150.

Littman A. Antacids and anticholinergic drugs. Ann Intern Med. 1975;82:544–51.

Maalox® Advanced Maximum Strength Antacid and Antigas suspension [package insert]. Parsippany: Novartis Consumer Health Inc; 2007.

Massarrat S, Eisenmann A. Factors affecting the healing rate of duodenal and pyloric ulcers with low-dose antacid treatment. Gut. 1981;22:97–102.

Morrissey JF, Barreras RF. Drug therapy: antacid therapy. N Engl J Med. 1974;290;550–4.

Mylanta® Maximum Strength Original liquid [package insert]. Modesto: Aaron Industries/Today's Health Inc; 2009.

Peterson WL, Sturdevant RAL, Frankl HD, et al. Healing of duodenal ulcer with an antacid regiment. N Engl J Med. 1977;297:341–5.

Randall RE Jr, Cohen MD, Spray CC Jr, Rossmeisl EC. Hypermagnesemia in renal failure: etiology and toxic manifestations. Ann Intern Med. 1964;61:73–88.

Rauch H, Fleischer F, Böhrer H, Jürs G, Wilhelm M, Krier C. Serum aluminum levels of intensive care patients treated with two different antacids for prevention of stress ulceration. Intensive Care Med. 1989;15:84–6.

Dosage Adjustment of Medications Eliminated by the Kidneys

Magnesium/Aluminum Hydroxide and Simethicone/Maalox®, Mylanta®   {Antacid; antiflatulent}

Usual initial dose:	15–60 mL orally
Usual maintenance dose:	10–20 mL between meals and at bedtime as needed or 60 mL 2 and 4 h after meals and at bedtime
Typical maximum dose:	300 mL/day
Proportion eliminated unchanged:	Variable, unknown

Adjustment for Kidney Disease

FDA-approved product labeling:	*Kidney disease*	*Warning, ask a doctor before use.*
Alternative adjustment:	*GFR > 50 mL/min*	*30 mL orally 1 and 3 h after each meal three times daily and at bedtime; or 30 mL enterally hourly as necessary to maintain gastric contents pH >3.5; or 30 mL orally PRN abdominal discomfort*
	GFR 30–49 mL/min	*30 mL orally every 4 h PRN abdominal discomfort; monitor serum magnesium levels.*
	GFR <30 mL/min	*Preferably avoid due to potential toxicity from magnesium accumulation. Consider use of proton pump inhibitor, dose-adjusted histamine H_2 antagonist, or sucralfate.*

Magnesium Sulfate - Selected References

Abraham AS, Rosenmann D, Kramer M, et al. Magnesium in the prevention of lethal arrhythmias in acute myocardial infarction. Arch Intern Med. 1987;147:753–5.

England MR, Gordon G, Salem M, Chernow B. Magnesium administration and dysrhythmias after cardiac surgery: a placebo-controlled, double-blind, randomized trial. JAMA. 1992;268:2395–402.

Hamill-Ruth RJ, McGory R. Magnesium repletion and its effect on potassium homeostasis in critically ill adults: results of a double-blind, randomized, controlled trial. Crit Care Med. 1996;24:38–45.

James MFM, Beer RE, Esser JD. Intravenous magnesium sulfate inhibits catecholamine release associated with tracheal intubation. Anesth Analg. 1989;66:772–6.

Koinig H, Wallner T, Marhofer P, Andel H, Hörauf K, Mayer N. Magnesium sulfate reduces intra- and postoperative analgesic requirements. Anesth Analg. 1998;87:206–10.

Kraft MD, Btaiche IF, Sacks GS, Kudsk KA. Treatment of electrolyte disorders in adult patients in the intensive care unit. Am J Health Syst Pharm. 2005;62:1663–82.

Magnesium sulfate injection. Lake Forest: Hospira Inc; 2007

McLean RM. Magnesium and its therapeutic uses. Am J Med. 1994;96:63–76.

Nadler JL, Rude RK. Disorders of magnesium metabolism. Endocrinol Metab Clin North Am. 1995;24:623–41.

Owen P, Monahan MF, MacLaren R. Implementing and assessing an evidence-based electrolyte dosing order form in the medical ICU. Intensive Crit Care Nurs. 2008;24(1):8–19.

Rasmussen HS, McNair P, Norregard P, Backer V, Lindeneg O, Balslev S. Intravenous magnesium in acute myocardial infarction. Lancet. 1986;1:234–5.

Reinhart RA. Magnesium metabolism: a review with special reference to the relationship between intracellular content and serum levels. Arch Intern Med. 1988;148:2415–20.

Rude RK. Physiology of magnesium metabolism and the important role of magnesium in potassium deficiency. Am J Cardiol. 1989;63:G31–4.

Sager PT, Widerhorn J, Petersen R, et al. Prospective evaluation of parenteral magnesium sulfate in the treatment of patients with reentrant AV supraventricular tachycardia. Am Heart J. 1990;119:308–16.

Salem M, Kasinski N, Munoz R, Chernow B. Progressive magnesium deficiency increases mortality from endotoxin challenge: protective effects of acute magnesium replacement therapy. Crit Care Med. 1995;23:108–18.

Schenck P, Vonbank K, Schnack B, Haber P, Lehr S, Smetana R. Intravenous magnesium sulfate for bronchial hyperreactivity: a randomized, controlled, double-blind study. Clin Pharmacol Ther. 2001;69:365–71.

Shechter M, Merz CNB, Paul-Labrador M, et al. Oral magnesium supplementation inhibits platelet-dependent thrombosis in patients with coronary heart disease. Am J Cardiol. 1999;84:152–6.

Smith LF, Heagerty AM, Bing RF, Barnett DB. Intravenous infusion of magnesium sulphate after acute myocardial infarction: effects on arrhythmias and mortality. Int J Cardiol. 1986;12:175–80.

Thel MC, Armstrong AL, McNulty SE, Califf RM, O'Connor CM. Randomised trial of magnesium in in-hospital cardiac arrest. Lancet. 1997;350:1272–6.

Tzivoni D, Banai S, Schuger C, et al. Treatment of torsade de pointes with magnesium sulfate. Circulation. 1988;77:392–7.

University of Colorado Hospital ICU Electrolyte Replacement Guideline, 2010.

University of Colorado Hospital Med-Surg Electrolyte Replacement Guideline, 2011.

Wesley RC Jr, Haines DE, Lerman BB, DiMarco JP, Crampton RS. Effect of magnesium sulfate on supraventricular tachycardia. Am J Cardiol. 1989;63:1129–31.

Whang R, Hampton EM, Whang DD. Magnesium homeostasis and clinical disorders of magnesium deficiency. Ann Pharmacother. 1994;28:220–6.

Woods KL, Fletcher S, Roffe C, Haider Y. Intravenous magnesium sulphate in suspected acute myocardial infarction: results of the second Leicester Intravenous Magnesium Intervention Trial (LIMIT-2). Lancet. 1992;339:1553–8.

Woods KL, Fletcher S. Long-term outcome after intravenous magnesium sulphate in suspected acute myocardial infarction: the second Leicester Intravenous Magnesium Intervention Trial (LIMIT-2). Lancet. 1994;343:816–9.

Magnesium Sulfate (IV),
Magnesium Gluconate/Uro-Mag®   {Electrolyte supplement; antispasmodic}

Usual initial dose: 1–4 g IV; 500–1,000 mg orally

Usual maintenance dose: 1–40 g daily IV; 500–1,000 mg orally twice daily

Typical maximum dose: 3 g/h IV; 4,000 mg/day orally

Proportion eliminated unchanged: ~95 %

Adjustment for Kidney Disease

FDA-approved product labeling: *Serious impairment of renal function Give very cautiously since it is excreted almost entirely by the kidneys.*

Alternative adjustment: *Magnesium dosage adjustment for (a) ICU patients and (b) Non-ICU patients (magnesium replacement)*

Serum/plasma magnesium level	Glomerular filtration rate (GFR in mL/min)		
	>50	*25–50*	*<25*
(a) *ICU patients*			
1.3–1.7 mEq/L	*Magnesium gluconate 1,000 mg via enteral route every 6 h × 4*	*Magnesium gluconate 1,000 mg via enteral route every 12 h × 2*	*Magnesium gluconate 1,000 mg via enteral route every 12 h × 2*
	If enteral route NOT available, magnesium sulfate 2 g IV × 2	*If enteral route NOT available, magnesium sulfate 2 g IV × 1*	*If enteral route NOT available, magnesium sulfate 1 g IV × 1*
0.6–1.2 mEq/L	*Magnesium sulfate 2 g IV × 4*	*Magnesium sulfate 2 g IV × 2*	*Magnesium sulfate 2 g IV × 1*
≤0.5 mEq/L	*Notify MD*	*Notify MD*	*Notify MD*
(b) *Non-ICU patients*			
1.3–1.7 mEq/L	*Magnesium gluconate 1,000 mg via enteral route every 6 h × 4*	*Magnesium gluconate 1,000 mg via enteral route every 12 h × 2*	*Magnesium gluconate 1,000 mg via enteral route every 12 h × 2*
	If enteral route NOT available, magnesium sulfate 2 g IV × 2	*If enteral route NOT available, magnesium sulfate 2 g IV × 1*	*If enteral route NOT available, magnesium sulfate 1 g IV × 1*
1.0–1.2 mEq/L	*Magnesium sulfate 2 g IV × 3*	*Magnesium sulfate 2 g IV × 2*	*Magnesium sulfate 2 g IV × 1*
<1.0 mEq/L or symptomatic patient	*Notify MD*	*Notify MD*	*Notify MD*

Note: Magnesium gluconate 500 mg tablet = 27 mg magnesium (approx = magnesium oxide 200 mg)
Preferred IV rate £1 g/h. Maximum rate: £4 g/h (emergency)
Maximum IV dose = 24 g in 24 h

Dosage Adjustment of Medications Eliminated by the Kidneys

<u>Mannitol</u> - Selected References

Barry KG. Post-traumatic renal shutdown in humans: its prevention and treatment by the intravenous infusion of mannitol. Milit Med. 1963;128:224–30.

Barry KG, Malloy JP. Oliguric renal failure: evaluation and therapy by the intravenous infusion of mannitol. JAMA. 1962;179:510–3.

Berger EY, Farber SJ, Earle DP Jr. Renal excretion of mannitol. Proc Soc Exp Biol Med. 1947;66:62–6.

Berry AJ, Peterson ML. Hyponatremia after mannitol administration in the presence of renal failure. Anesth Analg. 1981;60:165–7.

Borges HF, Hocks J, Kjellstrand CM. Mannitol intoxication in patients with renal failure. Arch Intern Med. 1982;142:63–6.

Brody MJ, Hook JB, Blatt AH, Williamson HE. Effect of several diuretics on autoregulation of renal blood flow. Arch Int Pharmacodyn Ther. 1969;180:114–20.

Cloyd JC, Snyder BD, Cleeremans B, Bundlie SR. Mannitol pharmacokinetics and serum osmolality in dogs and humans. J Pharmacol Exp Ther. 1986;236:301–6.

Doi K, Ogawa N, Suzuki E, Noiri E, Fujita T. Mannitol-induced acute renal failure. Am J Med. 2003;115:593–4.

Dorman HR, Sondheimer JH. Mannitol-induced acute renal failure. Medicine (Baltimore). 1990;69:153–9.

Dziedzic T, Szczudlik A, Klimkowicz A, Rog TM, Slowick A. Is mannitol safe for patients with intracerebral hemorrhages? Renal considerations. Clin Neurol Neurosurg. 2003;105:87–9.

Feldman BH, Kjellstrand CM, Fraley EE. Mannitol intoxication. J Urol. 1971;106:622–3.

Gondim Fde A, Aiyaqari V, Shackleford A, Diringer MN. Osmolality not predictive of mannitol-induced acute renal insufficiency. J Neurosurg. 2005;103:444–7.

Horgan KJ, Ottaviano YL, Watson AJ. Acute renal failure due to mannitol intoxication. Am J Nephrol. 1989;9:106–9.

Martinez-Maldonado M, Eknoyan G, Suki WN. Importance of aerobic and anaerobic metabolism in renal concentration and dilution. Am J Physiol. 1970;218:1076–81.

Mees EJD. Relation between maximal urine concentration, maximal water reabsorption capacity, and mannitol clearance in patients with renal disease. Br Med J. 1959;1(5130):1159–60.

O'Leary MJ, Bihari DJ. Preventing renal failure in the critically ill: there are no magic bullets – just high quality intensive care. BMJ. 2001;322:1437–9.

Osmitrol® injection [package insert]. Deerfield: Baxter Healthcare Corp; 2009.

Parry WI Schaefer JA, Mueller CB. Experimental studies of acute renal failure. I. The protective effect of mannitol. J Urol. 1963;89:1–5.

Pérez- Pérez AJ, Pazos B, Sobrado J, Gonzalez L, Gándara A. Acute renal failure following massive mannitol infusion. Am J Nephrol. 2002;22:573–5.

Powers SR Jr, Boba A, Hostnik W, Stein A. Prevention of renal failure with mannitol in 100 cases. Surgery. 1964;55:15–23.

Randall RE Jr, Singh R, Laster J, Belle C, Setter JG. Increased intracranial pressure from unsustained levels of mannitol during hemodialysis. J Lab Clin Med. 1967;70:129–37.

Reubi GC, Schreder HA, Futcher PH, Reubi C. A discrepancy between renal extraction and urinary excretion of various substances (para-aminohippurate, mannitol, creatinine, thiosulphate) in man. J Appl Physiol. 1950;3:63–76.

Sakemi T, Ikeda Y, Ohtsuka N, Ohtsuka Y, Tomiyoshi Y, Baba N. Acute renal failure associated with mannitol infusion and reversal with ultrafiltration and hemodialysis. Nephron. 1996;73:733–4.

Schwartz IL, Breed ES, Maxwell MH. Comparison of the volume of distribution, renal and extrarenal clearances of inulin and mannitol in man. J Clin Invest. 1950;29:517–20.

Seitzman DM, Mazze RI, Schwartz FD, Barry KG. Mannitol diuresis: a method of protection during surgery. J Urol. 1963;90:139–43.

Silber SJ, Thompson N. Mannitol induced central nervous system toxicity in renal failure. Invest Urol. 1972;9:310–2.

Swamy AP, Cestero RVM. Mannitol and maintenance hemodialysis. Artif Organs. 1979;3:116–9.

Visweswaran P, Massin EK, Dubose TD Jr. Mannitol-induced acute renal failure. J Am Soc Nephrol. 1997;8:1028–33.

Dosage Adjustment of Medications Eliminated by the Kidneys

<u>Mannitol</u>/Osmitrol® {**Osmotic diuretic; genitourinary irrigant**}

Usual initial dose: 12.5 g (200 mg/kg) IV over 5 min (test dose to assess renal function)

0.5–1.5 g/kg IV

Usual maintenance dose: 0.25–0.5 g/kg IV every 4–6 h

Typical maximum dose: 3 g/kg

Proportion eliminated unchanged: 90 %

Adjustment for Kidney Disease

FDA-approved product labeling:	*Well-established (not acute or impending) anuria due to severe renal disease*	*Contraindicated*
	Progressive renal damage or dysfunction after institution of mannitol, including increasing oliguria and azotemia	*Contraindicated*
Alternative adjustment:	*Data not available*	

Dosage Adjustment of Medications Eliminated by the Kidneys

Maraviroc - Selected References

Abel S, Davis JD, Ridgway CE, Hamlin JC, Vourvahis M. Pharmacokinetics, safety and tolerability of a single oral dose of maraviroc in HIV-negative subjects with mild and moderate hepatic impairment. Antivir Ther. 2009;14:831–7.

Abel S, Jenkins TM, Whitlock LA, Ridgway CE, Muirhead GJ. Effects of CYP3A4 inhibitors on the pharmacokinetics of maraviroc in healthy volunteers. Br J Clin Pharmacol. 2008;65(Suppl 1):38–46.

Abel S, van der Ryst E, Rosario MC, et al. Assessment of the pharmacokinetics, safety and tolerability of maraviroc, a novel CCR5 antagonist, in healthy volunteers. Br J Clin Pharmacol. 2008;65(Suppl 1):5–18.

Brown KC, Patterson KB, Malone SA, et al. Single and multiple dose pharmacokinetics of maraviroc in saliva, semen, and rectal tissue of healthy HIV-negative men. J Infect Dis. 2011;203:1484–90.

Calcagno A, Nozza S, Bonora S, et al. Pharmacokinetics of the raltegravir/maraviroc/etravirine combination [letter]. J Antimicrob Chemother. 2011;66:1932–4.

Chan PLS, Jacqmin P, Lavielle M McFadyen L, Weatherley B. The use of the SAEM algorithm in MONOLIX software for estimation of population pharmacokinetic-pharmacodynamic-viral dynamics parameters of maraviroc in asymptomatic HIV subjects. J Pharmacokinet Pharmacodyn. 2011;38:41–61.

Chan PLS, Weatherley B, McFadyen L. A population pharmacokinetic meta-analysis of maraviroc in healthy volunteer and symptomatic HIV-infected subjects. Br J Clin Pharmacol. 2008;65(Suppl 1):76–85.

Dorr P, Westby M, Dobbs S, et al. Maraviroc (UK-427,857), a potent, orally bioavailable, and selective small-molecule inhibitor of chemokine receptor CCR5 with broad-spectrum anti-human immunodeficiency virus type 1 activity. Antimicrob Agents Chemother. 2005;49:4721–32.

Hyland R, Dickins M, Collins C, Jones H, Jones B. Maraviroc: in vitro assessment of drug-drug interaction potential. Br J Clin Pharmacol. 2008;66:498–507.

Kakuda TN, Abel S, Davis J, et al. Pharmacokinetic interactions of maraviroc with darunavir-ritonavir , etravirine, and etravirine-darunavir-ritonavir in healthy volunteers: results of two drug interaction trials. Antimicrob Agents Chemother. 2011;55:2290–6.

Melica G, Canestri A, Peytavin G, et al. Maraviroc-containing regimen suppresses HIV replication in the cerebrospinal fluid of patients with neurological symptoms [letter]. AIDS. 2010;24:2130–3.

Pau AK, Boyd SD. Recognition and management of significant drug interactions in HIV patients: challenges in using available data to guide therapy. Clin Pharmacol Ther. 2010;88:712–9.

Pau AK, Penzak SR, Boyd SD, McLaughlin M, Morse CG. Impaired maraviroc and raltegravir clearance in a human immunodeficiency virus-infected patient with end-stage liver disease and renal impairment: a management dilemma. Pharmacotherapy. 2012;32:e1–6. doi:10.1002/PHAR.1003.

Perry CM. Maraviroc: a review of its use in the management of CCR5-tropic HIV-1 infection. Drugs. 2010;70:1189–213.

Pozniak AL, Boffito M, Russell Rridgway CE, Muirhead GJ. A novel probe drug interaction study to investigate the effect of selected antiretroviral combinations on the pharmacokinetics of a single oral dose of maraviroc in HIV-positive subjects Br J Clin Pharmacol. 2008;65(Suppl 1):54–9.

Rosario MC, Jacqmin P, Dorr P, et al. Population pharmacokinetic/pharmacodynamic analysis of CCR5 receptor occupancy by maraviroc in healthy subjects and HIV-positive patients. Br J Clin Pharmacol. 2008;65(Suppl 1):86–94.

Rosario MC, Poland B, Sullivan J, Westby M, van der Ryst E. A pharmacokinetic-pharmacodynamic model to optimize the phase IIa development program of maraviroc. J Acquir Immune Defic Syndr. 2006;42:183–91.

Selzentry® tablet film coated [package insert]. New York: Pfizer Inc; 2010.

Siccardi M, D'Avolio A, Nozza S, et al. Maraviroc is a substrate for OATP1B1 in vitro and maraviroc plasma concentrations are influenced by SLCO1B1 521 T>C polymorphism. Pharmacogenet Genom. 2010;20:759–65.

Soriano V, Perno C-F, Kaiser R, et al. When and how to use maraviroc in HIV-infected patients. AIDS. 2009;23:2377–85.

Walker DK, Abel S, Comby P, Muirhead GJ, Nedderman ANR, Smith DA. Species differences in the disposition of the CCR5 antagonist, UK-427,857, a new potential treatment for HIV. Drug Metab Dispos. 2005;33:587–95.

Walker DK, Bowers SJ, Mitchell RJ, Potchoiba MJ, Schroeder DM, Small HF. Preclinical assessment of the distribution of maraviroc to potential human immunodeficiency virus (HIV) sanctuary sites in the central nervous system (CNS) and gut-associated lymphoid tissue (GALT). Xenobiotica. 2008;38:1330–9.

Weatherley B, McFadyen L. Maraviroc modeling strategy: use of early phase 1 data to support a semi-mechanistic population pharmacokinetic model. Br J Clin Pharmacol. 2008;68:355–69.

Dosage Adjustment of Medications Eliminated by the Kidneys

<u>Maraviroc</u>/Selzentry® {Human CCR5 antagonist, HIV entry inhibitor antiretroviral}

Usual initial dose: 300 mg orally

Usual maintenance dose: 150–600 mg orally twice daily

Typical maximum dose: 1,200 mg/day

Proportion eliminated unchanged: 8 %

Adjustment for Kidney Disease

FDA-approved product labeling: *Maraviroc dose based on renal function*

Concomitant medications	Normal CrCL >80 mL/min	Mild CrCL 51–80 mL/min	Moderate CrCL 30–50 mL/min	Severe CrCL <30 mL/min	End-stage renal disease (ESRD) On regular hemodialysis
Potent CYP3A inhibitors (with or without a CYP3A inducer)[a]	150 mg twice daily	150 mg twice daily	150 mg twice daily	Not recommended	Not recommended
Other concomitant medications[b]	300 mg twice daily	300 mg twice daily	300 mg twice daily	300 mg twice daily	300 mg twice daily
Potent CYP3A inducers (without a potent CYP3A inhibitor)[c]	600 mg twice daily	600 mg twice daily	600 mg twice daily	Not recommended	Not recommended

Concomitant medications	Maraviroc dose for normal renal function
[a]Potent CYP3A inhibitors (with or without a potent CYP3A inducer) including: Protease inhibitors (except tipranavir/ritonavir) Delavirdine Ketoconazole, itraconazole, clarithromycin Other potent CYP3A inhibitors (e.g., nefazodone, telithromycin)	150 mg twice daily
[b]Other concomitant medications, including tipranavir/ritonavir, nevirapine, raltegravir, all nucleoside reverse-transcriptase inhibitors, and enfuvirtide	300 mg twice daily
[c]Potent CYP3A inducers (without a potent CYP3A inhibitor) including: Efavirenz Rifampin Etravirine Carbamazepine, phenobarbital, and phenytoin	600 mg twice daily

Alternative adjustment: *Data not available*

Dosage Adjustment of Medications Eliminated by the Kidneys

Mefenamic Acid - Selected References

Aronoff GA, Bennett WM, Berns JS, et al. Drug prescribing in renal failure: dosing guidelines for adults and children. 5th ed. Philadelphia: American College of Physicians; 2007.

Baker LRI, Cattell WR, Levison DA, Edelman JB. Mefenamic acid-induced interstitial nephritis and renal failure [letter]. Postgrad Med J. 1984;60:82–3.

Boletis J, Williams JR, Shortland JR, Brown CB. Irreversible renal failure following mefenamic acid. Nephron. 1989;51:575–6.

Brix AE. Renal papillary necrosis. Toxicol Pathol. 2002;30:672–4.

Champion de Crespigny PJ, Hewitson TD, Birchall I, Kincaid-Smith P. Caffeine potentiates the nephrotoxicity of mefenamic acid on the rat renal papilla. Am J Nephrol. 1990;10:311–15.

Gaganis P, Miners JO, Knights KM. Glucuronidation of fenamates: kinetic studies using human kidney cortical microsomes and recombinant UDP-glucuronosyltransferase (UGT) 1A9 and 2B7. Biochem Pharmacol. 2007;73:1683–91.

Hamaguchi T, Shinkuma D, Yamanaka Y, Mizuno N. Bioavailability of mefenamic acid: influence of food and water intake. J Pharm Sci. 1986;75:891–3.

Handa SI, Freestone S. Mefenamic acid-induced neutropenia and renal failure in elderly females with hypothyroidism. Postgrad Med J. 1990;66:557–7.

Hewitson TD, Champion de Crespigny PJ, Kincaid-Smith P. Caffeine potentiation of mefenamic acid-induced lesions in the rat renal medulla. J Pathol. 1991;165:343–7.

Itami N, Akutsu Y, Yasoshima K, Tochimaru H, Takekoshi Y, Matsumoto S. Progressive renal failure despite discontinuation of mefenamic acid. Nephron. 1990;54:281–2.

Jenkins DAS, Harrison DJ, MacDonald MK, Winney RJ. Mefenamic acid nephropathy: an interstitial and mesangial lesion. Nephrol Dial Transplant. 1988;2:217–20.

Mingatto FE, Santos AC, Uyemua SA, Jordani MC, Curti C. In vitro interaction of nonsteroidal anti-inflammatory drugs on oxidative phosphorylation of rat kidney mitochondria: respiration and ATP synthesis. Arch Biochem Biophys. 1996;334:303–8.

Ponstel® capsule [package insert]. Atlanta: Shionogi Pharma Inc; 2010.

Poulton S, Craft T, Severs M. Non-oliguric renal failure during treatment with mefenamic acid in elderly females [letter]. Br Med J (Clin Res Ed). 1985;291:1048.

Rawashdeh NM, Najib NM, Jalal IM. Comparative bioavailability of two capsule formulations of mefenamic acid. Int J Clin Pharmacol Ther. 1997;65:329–33.

Robertson CE, Ford MJ, Van Someren V, Dlugolecka M, Prescott LF. Mefenamic acid nephropathy. Lancet. 1980;2:232–3.

Sinniah R, Lye WC. Acute renal failure from hemoglobinuric and interstitial nephritis secondary to iodine and mefenamic acid. Clin Nephrol. 2001;55:254–8.

Taha A, Lenton RJ, Murdoch PS, Peden NR. Non-oliguric renal failure during treatment with mefenamic acid in elderly patients: a continuing problem. Br Med J (Clin Res Ed). 1985;291:661–2.

Turnbull AJ, Campbell P, Hughes JA. Mefenamic acid nephropathy—acute renal failure in overdose [letter]. Br Med J (Clin Res Ed). 1988;296:646.

Wang L-H, Lee CS, Marbury TC. Hemodialysis of mefenamic acid in uremic patients. Am J Hosp Pharm. 1980;37:956–8.

Whiting PH, Tisocki K, Hawksworth GM. Human renal medullary interstitial cells and analgesic nephropathy. Ren Fail. 1999;21:387–92.

Yokobori S, Yokota H, Yamamoto Y. Pediatric posterior reversible leukoencephalopathy syndrome NSAID-induced acute tubular interstitial nephritis. Pediatr Neurol. 2006;34:245–7.

Dosage Adjustment of Medications Eliminated by the Kidneys

Mefenamic Acid/Ponstel®   {Anti-inflammatory; nonsteroidal anti-inflammatory drug}

Usual initial dose:	500 mg orally
Usual maintenance dose:	250 mg orally every 6 h
Typical maximum dose:	1,500 mg/day
Proportion eliminated unchanged:	6 %

Adjustment for Kidney Disease

FDA-approved product labeling:	*Preexisting renal disease*	*Contraindicated*
Alternative adjustment:	*GFR >50 mL/min*	*250 mg orally every 6 h*
	GFR 10–50 mL/min	*Preferably avoid due to risk of gastrointestinal and renal toxicity.*
	GFR <10 mL/min	*Preferably avoid due to risk of gastrointestinal and renal toxicity.*
	Hemodialysis	*Preferably avoid due to risk of gastrointestinal and renal toxicity.*
	CRRT	*Not applicable; preferably avoid.*

Meloxicam - Selected References

Bae J-W, Choi C-I, Jang C-G, Lee S-Y. Effects of CYP2C9*1/*13 on the pharmacokinetics and pharmacodynamics of meloxicam. Br J Clin Pharmacol. 2011;71:550–5.

Busch U, Heinzel G, Narjes H. Effect of food on pharmacokinetics of meloxicam, a new non steroidal anti-inflammatory drug (NSAID). Agents Actions. 1991;32:52–3.

Busch U, Schmid J, Heinzel G, et al. Pharmacokinetics of meloxicam in animals and the relevance to humans. Drug Metab Dispos. 1998;26:576–84.

Carrasco-Portugal MdC, Aguilar-Carrasco JC, Luján M, et al. Further evidence for interethnic differences in the oral pharmacokinetics of meloxicam. Clin Drug Invest. 2005;25:307–13.

Davies NM, Skjodt NM. Clinical pharmacokinetics of meloxicam: a cyclo-oxygenase-2 preferential nonsteroidal anti-inflammatory drug. Clin Pharmacokinet. 1999;36:115–26.

Ghorab MM, Abdel-Salam HM, El-Sayad MA, Mekhel MM. Tablet formulation containing meloxicam and beta-cyclodextrin: mechanical characterization and bioavailability evaluation. AAPS PharmSci Tech. 2004;5:e59.

Harirforoosh S, Jamali F. Effect of inflammation on kidney function and pharmacokinetics of COX-2 selective nonsteroidal anti-inflammatory drugs rofecoxib and meloxicam. J Appl Toxicol. 2008;28:829–38.

Meineke I, Türck D. Population pharmacokinetic analysis of meloxicam in rheumatoid arthritis patients. Br J Clin Pharmacol. 2003;55:32–8.

Mobic® tablet and suspension [package insert]. Ridgefield: Boehringer Ingelheim Pharmaceuticals Inc; 2007.

Müller FO, Middle MV, Schall R, Terblanché J, Hundt HKL, Groenwoud G. An evaluation of the interaction of meloxicam with frusemide in patients with compensated chronic cardiac failure. Br J Clin Pharmacol. 1997;44:393–8.

Ogino K, Hatanaka K, Kawamura M, Katori M, Harada Y. Evaluation of pharmacological profile of meloxicam as an anti-inflammatory agent, with particular reference to its relative selectivity for cyclooxygenase-2 over cyclooxygenase-1. Pharmacology. 1997;55:44–53.

Schmid J, Busch U, Heinzel G, Bozler G, Kaschke S, Kummer M. Meloxicam: pharmacokinetics and metabolic pattern after intravenous infusion and oral administration to healthy patients. Drug Metab Dispos. 1995;23:1206–13.

Türck D, Roth W, Busch U. A review of the clinical pharmacokinetics of meloxicam. Br J Rheumatol. 1996;35(Suppl 1):13–6.

Türck D, Schwarz A, Höffler D, Narjes HH, Nehmiz G, Heinzel G. Pharmacokinetics of meloxicam in patients with end-stage renal failure on haemodialysis: a comparison with healthy volunteers. Eur J Clin Pharmacol. 1996;51:309–13.

Dosage Adjustment of Medications Eliminated by the Kidneys

Meloxicam/Mobic®	{Anti-inflammatory; nonsteroidal anti-inflammatory drug; selective cyclooxygenase (COX)-2 inhibitor}

Usual initial dose:	7.5 mg orally
Usual maintenance dose:	7.5–15 mg orally once daily
Typical maximum dose:	15 mg/day
Proportion eliminated unchanged:	1 %

Adjustment for Kidney Disease

FDA-approved product labeling:	*Preexisting mild to moderate kidney disease*	*Use with caution; no dose adjustment is necessary*
	Severe renal impairment (CrCL <15 mL/min)	*Not recommended; avoid*
Alternative adjustment:	*Hemodialysis*	*7.5 mg orally once daily*

Dosage Adjustment of Medications Eliminated by the Kidneys

Melphalan (IV) - Selected References

Alberts DS, Chang SY, Chen H-SG, et al. Kinetics of intravenous melphalan. Clin Pharmacol Ther. 1979;26:73–80.

Alkeran® injection [package insert]. Research Triangle Park: GlaxoSmithKline LLC; 2008.

Bronx L, Birkett L. Pharmacology of intravenous melphalan in patients with multiple myeloma. Cancer Treat Rev. 1979;6(Suppl):27–32.

Carlson K. Melphalan 200 mg/m^2 with blood stem cell support as first-line myeloma therapy: impact of glomerular filtration rate on engraftment, transplantation-related toxicity and survival. Bone Marrow Transplant. 2005;35:985–90.

Carlson K, Hjorth M, Knudsen LM. Toxicity in standard melphalan-prednisone therapy among myeloma patients with renal failure: a retrospective analysis and recommendations for dose adjustment. Br J Haematol. 2005;128:631–5.

Casserly LF, Fadia A Sanchorawala V, et al. High-dose intravenous melphalan with autologous stem cell transplantation in AL amyloidosis-associated end-stage renal disease. Kidney Int. 2003;63:1051–7.

Clark AD, Shetty A, Soutar R. Renal failure and multiple myeloma: pathogenesis and treatment of renal failure and management of underlying myeloma. Blood Rev. 1999;13:79–90.

Dimopoulos MA, Richardson PG, Schlag R, et al. VMP (bortezomib, melphalan, and prednisone) is active and well tolerated in newly diagnosed patients with multiple myeloma with moderately impaired renal function, and results in reversal of renal impairment: cohort analysis of the phase III VISTA study. J Clin Oncol. 2009;36:6086–93.

Kergueris MF, Milpied N, Moreau P, Harousseau JL, Larousse C. Pharmacokinetics of high-dose melphalan in adults: influence of renal function. Anticancer Res. 1994;14:2379–82.

Loos U, Musch E, Engel M, Hartlapp AJH, Hügl E, Dengler HJ. The pharmacokinetics of melphalan during intermittent therapy of multiple myeloma. Eur J Clin Pharmacol. 1988;35:187–93.

McElwain TJ, Hedley DW, Burton G, et al. Marrow autotransplantation accelerates haematological recovery in patients with malignant melanoma treated with high-dose melphalan. Br J Cancer. 1979;40:72–80.

Nath CE, Shaw PJ, Trotman J, et al. Population pharmacokinetics of melphalan in patients with multiple myeloma undergoing high dose therapy. Br J Clin Pharmacol. 2010;69:484–97.

Nath CE, Shaw PJ, Trotman J, Zeng L. Pharmacokinetics of melphalan in myeloma patients undergoing an autograft [letter]. Bone Marrow Transplant. 2007;40:707–8.

Pinguet F, Martel P, Fabbro M, et al. Pharmacokinetics of high-dose intravenous melphalan in patients undergoing peripheral blood hematopoietic progenitor-cell transplantation. Anticancer Res. 1997;17:605–12.

Rabb MS, Breitkreutz I, Hundemer M, et al. The outcome of autologous stem cell transplantation in patients with plasma cell disorders and dialysis-dependent renal failure. Haematologica. 2006;91:1555–8.

Reece PA, Hill HS, Green M, et al. Renal clearance and protein binding of melphalan in patients with cancer. Cancer Chemother Pharmacol. 1988;22:348–52.

Rosenweig M, Seldin DC, Remick DG, et al. Febrile reactions occurring with a second cycle of high-dose melphalan and SCT in patients with AL amyloidosis: a 'melphalan recall' reaction. Bone Marrow Transplant. 2010;45:21–4.

San Miguel JF, Lahuerta JJ, García-Sanz R, et al. Are myeloma patients with renal failure candidates for autologous stem cell transplantation? Hematol J. 2000;1:28–36.

Sanada S, Ookawara S, Karube H, et al. Marked recovery of severe renal lesions in POEMS syndrome with high-dose melphalan therapy supported by autologous blood stem cell transplantation. Am J Kidney Dis. 2006;47:672–9.

Sirohi B, Powles R, Kulkarni S, et al. Glomerular filtration rate prior to high-dose melphalan 200 mg/m^2 as a surrogate marker of outcome in patients with myeloma. Br J Cancer. 2001;85:325–32.

Tauro S, Clark FJ, Duncan N, Lipkin G, Richards N, Mahendra P. Recovery of renal function after autologous stem cell transplantation in myeloma patients with end-stage renal failure. Bone Marrow Transplant. 2002;30:471–3.

Tendas A, Cupelli L, Dentamoro T, et al. Feasibility of a dose-adjusted fludarabine-melphalan conditioning prior autologous stem cell transplantation in a dialysis-dependent patient with mantle cell lymphoma [letter]. Ann Hematol. 2009;88:285–6.

Tricot G, Alberts DS, Johnson C, et al. Safety of autotransplants with high-dose melphalan in renal failure: a pharmacokinetic and toxicity study. Clin Cancer Res. 1996;2:947–52.

Woodhouse KW, Hamilton P, Lennard A, Rawlins MD. The pharmacokinetics of melphalan in patients with multiple myeloma: an intravenous/oral study using a conventional dose regimen. Eur J Clin Pharmacol. 1983;24:283–5.

Dosage Adjustment of Medications Eliminated by the Kidneys

Melphalan (IV)/Alkeran® IV   {Antineoplastic; alkylating agent; nitrogen mustard}

Usual initial dose:	16 mg/m² IV
Usual maintenance dose:	16 mg/m² IV every 2 weeks times four doses then 16 mg/m² IV every 4 weeks
Typical maximum dose:	16 mg/m² IV
Proportion eliminated unchanged:	40 % (range 5–90 %)

Adjustment for Kidney Disease

FDA-approved product labeling:	*Renal insufficiency (BUN ≥30 mg/dL)*	*8 mg/m²/dose IV (50 % decrease)*
Alternative adjustment:	*GFR >50 mL/mi:*	*16 mg/m² IV every 2 weeks times four doses then 16 mg/m² IV every 4 weeks*
	GFR 10–50 mL/min	*12 mg/m² IV every 2 weeks times four doses then 12 mg/m² IV every 4 weeks (25 % decrease)*
	GFR <10 mL/min	*8 mg/m² IV every 2 weeks times four doses then 8 mg/m² IV every 4 weeks (50 % decrease)*
	Hemodialysis	*8 mg/m² IV every 2 weeks times four doses then 8 mg/m² IV every 4 weeks (50 % decrease)*
	CAPD	*8 mg/m² IV every 2 weeks times four doses then 8 mg/m² IV every 4 weeks (50 % decrease)*
	CRRT	*12 mg/m² IV every 2 weeks times four doses then 12 mg/m² IV every 4 weeks (50 % decrease)*

Note: Patients with multiple myeloma undergoing hematopoietic stem cell transplantation may be treated with conditioning high-dose IV melphalan. Although highly controversial due to wide individual variations in drug clearance, some authorities recommend decreasing the dose of IV melphalan from 140–200 to 100 mg/m² in patients with GFR <30 mL/min.

Note: Hematological and other considerations may suggest further dosage adjustments.

Melphalan (Oral) - Selected References

Adair CG, Bridges JM, Desai ZR. Renal function in the elimination of oral melphalan in patients with multiple myeloma. Cancer Chemother Pharmacol. 1986;17:185–8.

Alberts DS, Chang SY, Chen H-SG, Evans TL, Moon TE. Oral melphalan kinetics. Clin Pharmacol Ther. 1979;26:737–45.

Alkeran® tablet film coated [package insert]. Research Triangle Park: GlaxoSmithKline LLC; 2008.

Aronoff GA, Bennett WM, Berns JS, et al. Drug prescribing in renal failure: dosing guidelines for adults and children. 5th ed. Philadelphia: American College of Physicians; 2007.

Booth LJ, Minielly JA, Smith EKM. Acute renal failure in multiple myeloma. Can Med Assoc J. 1974;111:334–5.

Boros L, Peng Y-M, Alberts DA, et al. Pharmacokinetics of very high-dose oral melphalan in cancer patients. Am J Clin Oncol. 1990;13:19–22.

Bosanquet AG, Gilby ED. Pharmacokinetics of oral and intravenous melphalan during routine treatment of multiple myeloma. Eur J Cancer Clin Oncol. 1982;18:355–62.

Choi KE, Ratain MJ, Williams SF, et al. Plasma pharmacokinetics of high-dose oral melphalan in patients treated with trial-kalator chemotherapy and autologous bone marrow reinfusion. Cancer Res. 1989;49:1318–21.

Cornwell GG III, Pajak TF, McIntyre OR, Kochwa S, Dosik H. Influence of renal failure on myelosuppressive effects of melphalan: Cancer and Leukemia Group B experience. Cancer Treat Rep. 1982;66:475–81.

Loos U, Musch E, Engel M, Hartlapp AJH, Hügl E, Dengler HJ. The pharmacokinetics of melphalan during intermittent therapy of multiple myeloma. Eur J Clin Pharmacol. 1988;35:187–93.

McIntyre CW, Owen PJ. Prescribing drugs in kidney disease. In: Brenner BM, editor. Brenner & Rector's the kidney. 8th ed. Philadelphia: Saunders/Elsevier; 2008. p. 1930–55.

Österborg A, Ehrsson H, Eksborg S, Wallin I, Mellstedt H. Pharmacokinetics of oral melphalan in relation to renal function in multiple myeloma patients. Eur J Cancer Clin Oncol. 1989;25:899–903.

Penfield JG. Multiple myeloma in end-stage renal disease. Semin Dial. 2006;19:329–34.

Reese PA, Kotasek D, Morris RG, Dale BM, Sage RE. The effect of food on oral melphalan absorption. Cancer Chemother Pharmacol. 1986;16:194–7.

Woodhouse KW, Hamilton P, Lennard A, Rawlins MD. The pharmacokinetics of melphalan in patients with multiple myeloma: an intravenous/oral study using a conventional dose regimen. Eur J Clin Pharmacol. 1983;24:283–5.

Dosage Adjustment of Medications Eliminated by the Kidneys

Melphalan (Oral)/Alkeran®   {Antineoplastic; alkylating agent; nitrogen mustard}

Usual initial dose: 6 mg (3 tablets) orally once daily times 2–3 weeks

Usual maintenance dose: 6 mg (3 tablets) once daily times 2–3 weeks then discontinue times 4 weeks then 2 mg orally once daily

Typical maximum dose: 0.25 mg/kg/day

Proportion eliminated unchanged: 10–30 %

Adjustment for Kidney Disease

FDA-approved product labeling: *It may be prudent to use a reduced dose initially.*

Alternative adjustment:

GFR >50 mL/min	*6 mg (3 tablets) orally once daily times 2–3 weeks then discontinue times 4 weeks then 2 mg orally once daily*	
GFR 10–50 mL/ min	*4 mg (2 tablets) orally once daily times 2–3 weeks then discontinue times 4 weeks then 2 mg orally once daily (~25 % decrease)*	
GFR <10 mL/min	*3 mg (1.5 tablets) orally once daily times 2–3 weeks then discontinue times 4 weeks then 1 mg orally once daily (50 % decrease)*	
Hemodialysis	*3 mg (1.5 tablets) orally once daily times 2–3 weeks then discontinue times 4 weeks then 1 mg orally once daily (50 % decrease); dose after dialysis*	
CAPD	*3 mg (1.5 tablets) orally once daily times 2–3 weeks then discontinue times 4 weeks then 1 mg orally once daily (50 % decrease)*	
CRRT	*4 mg (2 tablets) orally once daily times 2–3 weeks then discontinue times 4 weeks then 2 mg orally once daily (~25 % decrease)*	

Note: Hematological and other considerations may suggest further dosage adjustments.

Memantine - Selected References

Freudenthaler S, Meineke I, Schreeb K-H, Boakye E, Gundert-Remy U, Gleiter CH. Influence of urine pH and urinary flow on the renal excretion of memantine. Br J Clin Pharmacol. 1998;46:541–6.

Gomolin IH, Smith C, Jeitner TM. Once-daily memantine: pharmacokinetic and clinical considerations [letter]. J Am Geriatr Soc. 2010;58:1812–3.

Hanlon JT, Aspinall SL, Semla TP, et al. Consensus guidelines for oral dosing of primarily renally cleared medications in older adults. J Am Geriatr Soc. 2009;57:335–40.

Kornhuber J, Kennepohl EM, Bleich S, et al. Memantine pharmacology: a naturalistic study using a population pharmacokinetic approach. Clin Pharmacokinet. 2007;46:599–612.

McKeage K. Memantine: a review of its use in moderate to severe Alzheimer's disease. CNS Drugs. 2009;23:881–97.

Namenda® [package insert]. St Louis: Forest Laboratories Inc; 2011.

Parsons CG, Danysz W, Quack G. Memantine is a clinically well tolerated N-methyl-D-aspartate (NMDA) receptor antagonist—a review of preclinical data. Neuropharmacology. 1999;38:735–67.

Periclou A, Ventura D, Rao N, Abramowitz W. Pharmacokinetic study of memantine in healthy and renally impaired subjects. Clin Pharmacol Ther. 2006;79:134–43.

Rao N, Chou T, Ventura D, Abramowitz W. Investigation of the pharmacokinetic and pharmacodynamic interactions between memantine and glyburide/metformin in healthy young subjects: a single-center, multiple-dose, open-label study. Clin Ther. 2005;27:1596–606.

Verbeeck RK, Masuamba FT. Pharmacokinetics and dosage adjustment in patients with renal dysfunction. Eur J Clin Pharmacol. 2009;65:757–73.

Videau O, Delaforge M, Levi M, et al. Biochemical and analytical development of the CIME cocktail for drug fate assessment in humans. Rapid Commun Mass Spectrom. 2010;24:2407–19.

Dosage Adjustment of Medications Eliminated by the Kidneys

Memantine/Namenda™   {N-**Methyl-D-aspartate (NMDA) antagonist;** ℞ **for Alzheimer's disease**}

Usual initial dose:	5 mg orally once daily
Usual maintenance dose:	10 mg orally twice daily
Typical maximum dose:	20 mg/day
Proportion eliminated unchanged:	50 %

Adjustment for Kidney Disease

FDA-approved product labeling:	*CrCL ≥30 mL/min*	*10 mg orally twice daily*
	CrCL 5–29 mL/min	*5 mg orally twice daily*
Alternative adjustment:	*Data not available*	

Dosage Adjustment of Medications Eliminated by the Kidneys

Meperidine - Selected References

Burgess KR, Burgess EE, Whitelaw WA. Impaired ventilatory response to carbon dioxide in patients with chronic renal failure: implications for the intensive care unit. Crit Care Med. 1994;22:413–9.

Chan K. Disposition of pethidine in man under acidic urinary pH. I. Plasma level and urinary elimination of pethidine and norpethidine. J Clin Hosp Pharm. 1981;6:107–16.

Chan K. The effects of physiochemical properties of pethidine and its basic metabolites on their buccal absorption and renal elimination. J Pharm Pharmacol. 1979;31:672–5.

Chan K, Tse J, Jennings F, Orme ML'E. Pharmacokinetics of low-dose intravenous pethidine in patients with renal dysfunction. J Clin Pharmacol. 1987;27:516–22.

Demerol® injection [package insert]. Lake Forest: Hospira Inc; 2005.

Demerol® tablets [package insert]. Bridgewater: Sanofi-Aventis US LLC; 2008.

Hagmeyer KO, Mauro LS, Mauro VF. Meperidine-related seizures associated with patient-controlled analgesia pumps. Ann Pharmacother. 1993;27:29–32.

Hanlon JT, Aspinall SL, Semla TP, et al. Consensus guidelines for oral dosing of primarily renally cleared medications in older adults. J Am Geriatr Soc. 2009;57:335–40.

Hochman MS. Meperidine-associated myoclonus and seizures in long-term hemodialysis patients [letter]. Ann Neurol. 1983;14:593.

Inturrisi CE. Disposition of narcotics in patients with renal disease. Am J Med. 1977;62:528–9.

Kaiko RF, Foley KM, Grabinski PY, et al. Central nervous system excitatory effects of meperidine in cancer patients. Ann Neurol. 1983;13:180–5.

Latta KS, Ginsberg B, Barkin RL. Meperidine: a critical review. Am J Ther. 2002;9:53–68.

Marinella MA. Meperidine-induced generalized seizures with normal renal function. South Med J. 1997;90:556–8.

Mather LE, Meffin PJ. Clinical pharmacokinetics pethidine. Clin Pharmacokinet. 1978;3:352–68.

Mauro VF, Bonfiglio MF, Spunt AL. Meperidine-induced seizure in a patient without renal dysfunction or sickle cell anemia. Clin Pharm. 1986;5:837–9.

McIntyre CW, Owen PJ. Prescribing drugs in kidney disease. In: Brenner BM, editor. Brenner & Rector's the kidney. 8th ed. Philadelphia: Saunders/Elsevier; 2008. p. 1930–55.

Odar Cederlöf I, Boréus LO, Bondesson U, Holmberg L, Heyner I. Comparison of renal excretion of pethidine (meperidine) and its metabolites in old and young patients. Eur J Clin Pharmacol. 1985;28:171–5.

Olyaei AJ, Bennett WM. Drug dosing in elderly patients with chronic kidney disease. Clin Geriatr Med. 2009;25:459–527.

Olyaei AJ, Bennett WM. Pharmacologic approach to renal insufficiency. In: Dale DC, Federman DD, Antman K, editors. ACP medicine, WebMD June 2007 update. Hamilton: BC Decker; 2007. Nephrology IX: Appendix A1–25.

Olyaei AJ, DeMattos AM, Bennett WM. Use of drugs in patients with renal failure. In: Schrier RW, editor. Diseases of the kidney and urinary tract. 8th ed. Philadelphia: Lippincott Williams & Wilkins; 2007. p. 2765–807.

Reutens DC, Stewart-Wynne EG. Norpethidine induced myoclonus in a patient with renal failure [letter]. J Neurol Neurosurg Psychiatry. 1989;52:1450–1.

Seifert CF, Kennedy S. Meperidine is alive and well in the new millennium: evaluation of meperidine usage patterns and frequency of adverse drug reactions. Pharmacotherapy. 2004;24:776–83.

Szeto HH, Inturrisi CE, Houde R, Saal S, Cheigh J, Reidenberg MM. Accumulation of normeperidine, an active metabolite of meperidine, in patients with renal failure or cancer. Ann Intern Med. 1977;86:738–41.

Verbeeck RK, Branch RA, Wilkinson GR. Drug metabolites in renal failure: pharmacokinetic and clinical implications. Clin Pharmacokinet. 1981;6:329–45.

Dosage Adjustment of Medications Eliminated by the Kidneys

Meperidine/Demerol®	{Analgesic, opioid μ-receptor agonist}
Usual initial dose:	50–150 mg PO, IM, or subcutaneously or 10–25 mg IV
Usual maintenance dose:	50–150 mg PO, IM, or subcutaneously or 10–25 mg IV every 3–4 h as necessary
Typical maximum dose:	600 mg/day
Proportion eliminated unchanged:	5 % (active metabolite normeperidine predominantly eliminated in urine)

Adjustment for Kidney Disease

FDA-approved product labeling:	*Severe renal impairment*	*Give with caution.*
Alternative adjustment:	*GFR >50 mL/min*	*50–150 mg PO, IM, or subcutaneously or 10–25 mg IV every 3 h as necessary*
	GFR 10–50 mL/min	*Avoid due to risk for neurotoxicity/seizures.*
	GFR <10 mL/mi	*Avoid due to risk for neurotoxicity/seizures.*
	Hemodialysis	*Avoid due to risk for neurotoxicity/seizures.*
	CAPD	*Avoid due to risk for neurotoxicity/seizures.*
	CRRT	*Avoid due to risk for neurotoxicity/seizures.*

Meprobamate - Selected References

Aronoff GA, Bennett WM, Berns JS, et al. Drug prescribing in renal failure: dosing guidelines for adults and children. 5th ed. Philadelphia: American College of Physicians; 2007.

Bruusgaard A. Suicide attempts with benzene derivatives. Dan Med Bull. 1963;10:142–4.

De Broe ME, Verpooten BA, Vanhaesebrouck B. Recent experience with prolonged hemoperfusion-hemodialysis treatment. Artif Organs. 1979;3:188–90.

Greene FE. Absence of a renal effect from two substituted propanediols: meprobamate and mebutamate. Proc Soc Exp Biol Med. 1963;114:165–8.

Jacobsen D, Wiik-Larsen E, Saltvedt E, Bredesen JE. Meprobamate kinetics during and after terminated hemoperfusion in acute intoxications. J Toxicol Clin Toxicol. 1987;25:317–31.

Lin J-L, Lim P-S, Lai B-C, Lin W-L. Continuous arteriovenous hemoperfusion in meprobamate poisoning. J Toxicol Clin Toxicol. 1993;31:645–52.

Littrell RA, Sage T, Miller W. Meprobamate dependence secondary to carisoprodol (Soma) use. Am J Drug Alcohol Abuse. 1993;19:133–4.

Lobo PI, Surratt P, Westervelt FB Jr. Use of hemodialysis in meprobamate overdosage. Clin Nephrol. 1977;7:73–5.

McIntyre CW, Owen PJ. Prescribing drugs in kidney disease. In: Brenner BM, editor. Brenner & Rector's the kidney. 8th ed. Philadelphia: Saunders/Elsevier; 2008. p. 1930–55.

Meprobamate tablets USP [package insert]: Corona: Watson Laboratories; 2004.

Meyer MC, Melikian AP, Straughn AB. Relative bioavailability of meprobamate tablets in humans. J Pharm Sci. 1978;67:1290–3.

Olyaei AJ, Bennett WM. Drug dosing in elderly patients with chronic kidney disease. Clin Geriatr Med. 2009;25:459–527.

Olyaei AJ, Bennett WM. Pharmacologic approach to renal insufficiency. In: Dale DC, Federman DD, Antman K, editors. ACP medicine, WebMD June 2007 update. Hamilton: BC Decker; 2007. Nephrology IX: Appendix A1–25.

Olyaei AJ, DeMattos AM, Bennett WM. Use of drugs in patients with renal failure. In: Schrier RW, editor. Diseases of the kidney and urinary tract. 8th ed. Philadelphia: Lippincott Williams & Wilkins; 2007. p. 2765–807.

Schwartz HS. Acute Meprobamate poisoning with gastrotomy and removal of a drug-containing mass. N Engl J Med. 1976;295:1177–8.

Dosage Adjustment of Medications Eliminated by the Kidneys

<u>Meprobamate</u>/Miltown® {Anxiolytic; carbamate derivative}

Usual initial dose:	400 mg orally
Usual maintenance dose:	1,200–1,600 mg/day orally in three or four divided doses
Typical maximum dose:	2,400 mg/day
Proportion eliminated unchanged:	10 %

Adjustment for Kidney Disease

FDA-approved product labeling:	*Compromised kidney function*	*Caution should be exercised.*
Alternative adjustment:	*GFR >50 mL/min*	*200–400 mg orally every 6 h*
	GFR 10–50 mL/min	*200–400 mg orally every 8–12 h*
	GFR <10 mL/min	*200–400 mg orally every 12–18 h*
	Hemodialysis	*Data not available*
	CAPD	*Data not available*
	CRRT	*Not applicable, preferably avoid*

Mercaptopurine - Selected References

Aronoff GA, Bennett WM, Berns JS, et al. Drug prescribing in renal failure: dosing guidelines for adults and children. 5th ed. Philadelphia: American College of Physicians; 2007.

Balis FM, Adamson PC. Application of pharmacogenetics to optimization of mercaptopurine dosing [editorial]. J Natl Cancer Inst. 1999;91:1983–5.

Bergan S, Rugstad HE, Bentdal Ø, Endresen L, Stokke O. Kinetics of Mercaptopurine and thioguanine nucleotides in renal transplant recipients during azathioprine treatment. Ther Drug Monit. 1994;16:13–20.

Chan GLC, Erdmann GR, Gruber SA, et al. Pharmacokinetics of 6-thiouric acid and 6-mercaptopurine in renal allograft recipients after oral administration of azathioprine. Eur J Clin Pharmacol. 1989;36:265–71.

Coffey JJ, White CA, Lesk AB, Rogers WI, Serpick AA. Effect of allopurinol on the pharmacokinetics of 6-mercaptopurine (NSC 755) in cancer patients. Cancer Res. 1972;32:1283–9.

Derijks LJJ, Gilssen LPL, Engels LGJB, et al. Pharmacokinetics of 6-mercaptopurine in patients with inflammatory bowel disease: implications for therapy. Ther Drug Monit. 2004;26:311–8.

Endresen L, Lie AO, Storm-Mathisen, Rugstad E, Stokke O. Pharmacokinetics of oral 6-mercaptopurine: relationship between plasma levels and urine excretion of parent drug. Ther Drug Monit. 1990;12:227–34.

Escousse A, Guedon F, Mounie J, Rifle G, Mousson C, D'Athis P. 6-Mercaptopurine pharmacokinetics after use of azathioprine in renal transplant recipients with intermediate or high thiopurine methyl transferase activity phenotype. J Pharm Pharmacol. 1998;50:1261–6.

Gardiner SJ, Gearry RB, Burt MJ, et al. Allopurinol might improve response to azathioprine and 6-mercaptopurine by correcting an unfavorable metabolite ratio. J Gastroenterol Hepatol. 2010;26:49–54.

Gearry RB, Day AS, Barclay ML, Leong RWL, Sparrow MP. Azathioprine and allopurinol: a two-edged interaction [editorial]. J Gastroenterol Hepatol. 2010;25:649–56.

Hindorf U, Lindqvist M, Peterson C, et al. Pharmacogenetics during standardised initiation of thiopurine treatment in inflammatory bowel disease. Gut. 2006;55:1423–31.

Huang RS, Ratain MJ. Pharmacogenetics and pharmacogenomics of anticancer agents. CA Cancer J Clin. 2009;42–55.

Lennard L. The clinical pharmacology of 6-mercaptopurine. Eur J Clin Pharmacol. 1992;43:329–39.

Papadakis KA. Optimizing the therapeutic potential of azathioprine/6-mercaptopurine in the treatment of inflammatory bowel disease [editorial]. J Clin Gastroenterol. 2003;36:379–85.

Purinethol® tablet [package insert]. Sellersville: Gate Pharmaceuticals division of Teva Pharmaceuticals USA; 2011.

Roberts RL, Gearry RB, Barclay ML. Allopurinol-thiopurine combination therapy in inflammatory bowel disease: are there genetic clues to this puzzle? [editorial]. Pharmacogenomics. 2010;11:1505–8.

Sahasranaman S, Howard D, Roy S. Clinical pharmacology and pharmacogenetics of thiopurines. Eur J Clin Pharmacol. 2008;64:753–67.

Tterlikkis L, Ortega E, Solomon R, Day JL. Pharmacokinetics of mercaptopurine. J Pharm Sci. 1977;66:14547.

Witte TN, Ginsberg AL. Use of allopurinol with low-dose 6-mercaptopurine in inflammatory bowel disease to achieve optimal active metabolite levels: a review of four cases and the literature. Can J Gastroenterol. 2008;22:181–5.

Zimm S, Johnson GE, Chabner BA, Poplack DG. Cellular pharmacokinetics of mercaptopurine in human neoplastic cells and cell lines. Cancer Res. 1985;45:4156–61.

Dosage Adjustment of Medications Eliminated by the Kidneys

<u>Mercaptopurine</u>/Purinethol®   **{Antineoplastic; antimetabolite; purine analog}**

Usual initial dose:	1.5–2.5 mg/kg
Usual maintenance dose:	1.5–2.5 mg/kg orally once daily
Typical maximum dose:	5 mg/kg/day
Proportion eliminated unchanged:	22 %

Adjustment for Kidney Disease

FDA-approved product labeling: *Impaired renal function*   *It is probably advisable to start with lower dosages.*

Alternative adjustment: *GFR <50 mL/min*   *1.5–2.5 mg/kg orally every 48 h*

Note: Most authorities suggest that mercaptopurine dosing may be optimized with pharmacogenetic therapeutic drug monitoring.

Dosage Adjustment of Medications Eliminated by the Kidneys

<u>Meropenem</u> - Selected References

Aronoff GA, Bennett WM, Berns JS, et al. Drug prescribing in renal failure: dosing guidelines for adults and children. 5th ed. Philadelphia: American College of Physicians; 2007.

Bilgrami I, Roberts JA, Wallis SC, et al. Meropenem dosing in critically ill patients with sepsis receiving high-volume continuous venovenous hemofiltration. Antimicrob Agents Chemother. 2010;54:3974–8.

Christensson BA, Nilsson-Ehle I, Hutchinson M, Haworth SJ, Öqvist B, Norrby SR. Pharmacokinetics of meropenem in subjects with various degrees of renal impairment. Antimicrob Agents Chemother. 1992;36:1532–7.

Dandekar PK, Maglio D, Sutherland CA, Nightingale CH, Nicolau DP. Pharmacokinetics of meropenem 0.5 and 2 g every 8 hours as a 3-hour infusion. Pharmacotherapy. 2003;23:988–91.

Giles LJ, Jennings AC, Thomson AH, Creed G, Beale RJ, McLuckie A. Pharmacokinetics of meropenem in intensive care unit patients receiving continuous veno-venous hemofiltration or hemodiafiltration. Crit Care Med. 2000;28:632–7.

Harrison MP, Haworth SJ, Moss SR, Wilkinson DM, Featherstone A. The disposition and metabolic fate of ^{14}C-meropenem in man. Xenobiotica. 1993;23:1311–23.

Harrison MP, Moss SR, Featherstone A, Gowkes AG, Sanders AM, Case DE. The disposition and metabolism of meropenem in laboratory animals and man. J Antimicrob Chemother. 1989;24(Suppl A):265–77.

Heintz BH, Matzke GR, Dager WF. Antimicrobial dosing concepts and recommendations for critically ill adult patients receiving continuous renal replacement therapy or intermittent hemodialysis. Pharmacotherapy. 2009;29:562–77.

Isla A, Rodríguez-Gascón A, Trocóniz IF, et al. Population pharmacokinetics of meropenem in critically ill patients undergoing continuous renal replacement therapy. Clin Pharmacokinet. 2008;47:175–80.

Kielstein JT, Czock D, Schöpke T, et al. Pharmacokinetics and total elimination of meropenem and vancomycin in intensive care patients undergoing extended daily dialysis. Crit Care Med. 2006;34:51–6.

Krueger WA, Bulitta J, Kinzig-Schippers M, et al. Evaluation by Monte Carlo simulation of the pharmacokinetics of two doses of meropenem administered intermittently or as a continuous infusion in healthy volunteers. Antimicrob Agents Chemother. 2005;49:1881–9.

Kuti JL, Nightingale CH, Knauft F, Nicolau DP. Pharmacokinetic properties and stability of continuous-infusion meropenem in adults with cystic fibrosis. Clin Ther. 2004;26:493–501.

Langgartner J, Vasold A, Glück T, Reng M, Kees F. Pharmacokinetics of meropenem during intermittent and continuous intravenous application in patients treated by continuous renal replacement therapy. Intensive Care Med. 2008;34:1091–6.

Lee C, Kuti JL, Nightingale CH, Nicolau DP. Population pharmacokinetic analysis and dosing regimen optimization of meropenem in adult patients. J Clin Pharmacol. 2006;46:1171–8.

Lee LS, Kinzig-Schippers M, Nafziger AN, et al. Comparison of 30-min and 3-h infusion regimens for imipenem/cilastatin and meropenem evaluated by Monte Carlo simulation. Diagn Microbiol Infect Dis. 2010;68:251–8.

Leroy A, Fillastre JP, Borsa-Lebas F, Etienne I, Humbert G. Pharmacokinetics of meropenem (ICI 194,660) and its metabolite (ICI 213,689) in healthy subjects and in patients with renal impairment. Antimicrob Agents Chemother. 1992;36:2794–8.

Lomaestro BM, Drusano GL. Pharmacodynamic evaluation of extending the administration time of meropenem using a Monte Carlo simulation. Antimicrob Agents Chemother. 2005;49:461–3.

Merrem® IV injection [package insert]. Wilmington: AstraZeneca Pharmaceuticals LP; 2010.

Mouton JW, van den Anker JN. Meropenem clinical pharmacokinetics. Clin Pharmacokinet. 1995;28:275–86.

Robatel C, Decosterd LA, Biollaz J, Eckert P, Schaller MD, Buclin T. Pharmacokinetics and dosage adaptation of meropenem during continuous venovenous hemodiafiltration n critically ill patients. J Clin Pharmacol. 2003;43:1329–40.

Thalhammer F, Hörl WH. Pharmacokinetics of meropenem in patients with renal failure and patients receiving renal replacement therapy. Clin Pharmacokinet. 2000;39:271–9.

Thalhammer F, Schenk P, Burgmann H, et al. Single-dose pharmacokinetics of meropenem during continuous venovenous hemofiltration. Antimicrob Agents Chemother. 1998;42:2417–20.

Trotman RL, Williamson JC, Shoemaker M, Salzer WL. Antibiotic dosing in critically ill adult patients receiving continuous renal replacement therapy. Clin Infect Dis. 2005;41:1159–66.

Valtonen M, Tiula E, Backman JT, Neuvonen PJ. Elimination of meropenem during continuous veno-venous haemofiltration and haemodiafiltration in patients with acute renal failure. J Antimicrob Chemother. 2000;45:701–4.

Watanabe A, Fujimura S, Kikuchi T, Gomi K, Fuse K, Nukiwa T. Evaluation of dosing designs of carbapenems for severe respiratory infection using Monte Carlo simulation. J Infect Chemother 2007;13:332–40.

Dosage Adjustment of Medications Eliminated by the Kidneys

Meropenem/Merrem® {**Carbapenem/thienamycin antibiotic**}

Usual initial dose: 500–2,000 mg IV

Usual maintenance dose: 1–2 g IV every 8 h

Typical maximum dose: 2,000 mg IV every 8 h

Proportion eliminated unchanged: 66–79 %

Adjustment for Kidney Disease

FDA-approved product labeling: *Meropenem dosing for adults with renal impairment*

CrCL (mL/min)	Dose (mg IV)	Dosing interval
≥51	500–1,000	Every 8 h
26–50	500–1,000	Every 12 h
10–25	250–500	Every 12 h
<10	500–1,000	Every 24 h

Alternative adjustment:

GFR >50 mL/min	500–2,000 mg IV over 30 min or 1–2 g IV over 1–3 h every 8 h or 2–6 g/24 h continuous IV infusion
GFR 10–50 mL/min	1 g IV every 12 h
GFR <10 mL/min	500–1,000 mg IV every 24 h
Hemodialysis	500–1,000 mg IV every 24 h; dose after hemodialysis on dialysis days
Extended daily dialysis	500–1,000 mg IV every 8 h
CAPD	500–1,000 mg IV every 24 h
CVVH	500–1,000 mg IV every 12 h
CVVHD or CVVHDF	750–1,000 mg IV every 8 h or 1,500 mg IV every 12 h or 2 g/24 h continuous IV infusion

Dosage Adjustment of Medications Eliminated by the Kidneys

Metaxalone - Selected References

Bruce RB, Turnbull L, Newman J, Pitts J. Metabolism of metaxalone. J Med Chem. 1966;9:286–8.

Chou R, Peterson K, Helfand M. Comparative efficacy and safety of skeletal muscle relaxants for spasticity and musculoskeletal conditions: a systematic review. J Pain Symptom Manage. 2004;28:140–75.

Dent RW Jr, Ervin DK. A study of metaxalone (Skelaxin) vs placebo in acute musculoskeletal disorders: a cooperative study. Curr Ther Res Clin Exp. 1975;18:433–40.

Diamond S. Double-blind study of metaxalone: use as a skeletal muscle relaxant. JAMA. 1966;195:479–80.

Fathie K. A second look at a skeletal muscle relaxant: a double-blind study of metaxalone. Curr Ther Res Clin Exp. 1964;6:677–83.

Gruszecki AC, Kloda S, Simmons GT, Daly TM, Hardy RW, Robinson CA. Polydrug fatality involving metaxalone. J Forensic Sci. 2003;48:432–4.

Pfeifer MA, Schumer MP, Ross DR, et al. A highly successful and novel model for treatment of chronic painful diabetic peripheral neuropathy. Diabetes Care. 1993;16:1103–15.

See S, Ginzburg R. Choosing a skeletal muscle relaxant. Am Fam Physician. 2008;78:365–70.

Skelaxin® tablet [package insert]. Bristol: King Pharmaceuticals Inc; 2007.

Toth PP, Urtis J. Commonly used muscle relaxant therapies for acute low back pain: a review of carisoprodol, cyclobenzaprine hydrochloride, and metaxalone. Clin Ther. 2004;26:1355–67.

Dosage Adjustment of Medications Eliminated by the Kidneys

<u>Metaxalone</u>/Skelaxin® {**Centrally acting skeletal muscle relaxant**}

Usual initial dose: 800 mg orally

Usual maintenance dose: 800 mg orally three to four times daily

Typical maximum dose: 3,200 mg/day

Proportion eliminated unchanged: 27 %

Adjustment for Kidney Disease

FDA-approved product labeling: *Renal impairment* *Use with caution.*

Significantly impaired renal function *Contraindicated*

Alternative adjustment: *Data not available*

Dosage Adjustment of Medications Eliminated by the Kidneys

Metformin - Selected References

Abe M, Okada K, Soma M. Antidiabetic agents in patients with chronic kidney disease and end-stage renal disease on dialysis: metabolism and clinical practice. Curr Drug Metab. 2011;12:57–69

Connolly V, Kesson CM. Metformin treatment in NIDDM patients with mild renal impairment. Postgrad Med J. 1996;72:352–4.

DeFronzo JA, Goodman AM, and the Multicenter Metformin Study Group. Efficacy of metformin in patients with non-insulin-dependent diabetes mellitus. N Engl J Med. 1995;333:541–9.

Dunn CJ, Peters DH, Metformin: a review of its pharmacological properties and therapeutic use in non-insulin-dependent diabetes mellitus. Drugs. 1995;49:727–49.

Glucophage® tablet, film coated; tablet, extended release [package insert]. Princeton: Bristol-Myers Squibb Co; 2009.

Goergen SK, Rumbold G, Compton G, Harris C. Systematic review of current guidelines, and their evidence base, on risk of lactic acidosis after administration of contrast medium for patients receiving metformin. Radiology. 2010;254:261–9.

Graham GG, Punt J, Arora M, et al. Clinical pharmacokinetics of metformin. Clin Pharmacokinet. 2011;50:81–98.

Gudmundsdottir H, Aksnes H, Heldal K, et al. Metformin and antihypertensive therapy with drugs blocking the renin angiotensin system, a cause of concern? Clin Nephrol. 2006;66:380–5.

Guo PYF, Storsley LJ, Finkle SN. Severe lactic acidosis treated with prolonged hemodialysis: recovery after massive overdoses of metformin. Semin Dial. 2006;19:80–3.

Holman RR, Cull CA, Fox C, et al. United Kingdom prospective diabetes study (UKPDS) 13: relative efficacy of randomly allocated diet, sulphonylurea, insulin, or metformin in patients with newly diagnosed non-insulin dependent diabetes followed for three years. BMJ. 1995;310:83–8.

Keller G, Cour M, Hernu R, Illinger J, Robert D, Argaud L. Management of metformin-associated lactic acidosis by continuous renal replacement therapy. PLoS One. 2011;6:e23200. doi:10.1371/journal.pone.0023200.

Lalau JD. Lactic acidosis induced by metformin: incidence, management and prevention. Drug Saf. 2010;33:727–43.

Lalau JD, Guérin Lacroix C, et al. Role of metformin accumulation in metformin-associated lactic acidosis. Diabetes Care. 1995;18:779–84.

Luft FC. Lactic acidosis update for critical care clinicians. J Am Soc Nephrol. 2001;12:S15–9.

Nye HJ, Herrington WG. Metformin: the safest hypoglycaemic agent in chronic kidney disease? Nephron Clin Pract. 2011;118:c380–3.

Pan LT, MacLaren G. Continuous venovenous haemodiafiltration for metformin-induced lactic acidosis. Anaesth Intensive Care. 2009;37:830–2.

Pentikäinen PJ, Neuvonen PJ, Pentilä A. Pharmacokinetics of metformin after intravenous and oral administration to man. Eur J Clin Pharmacol. 1979;16:195–202.

Pilmore HL. Metformin: potential benefits and use in chronic kidney disease. Nephrology (Carlton). 2010;15:412–8.

Rifkin SI, McFerren C, Juvvadi R, Weinstein SS. Prolonged hemodialysis for severe metformin intoxication. Ren Fail. 2011;33:459–61.

Salpeter SR, Greyber E, Pasternak GA, Salpeter EE. Risk of fatal and nonfatal lactic acidosis with metformin use in type 2 diabetes mellitus (review). Cochrane Database Syst Rev. 2010;(4):CD002967. doi:10.1002/14651858.CD002967.pub4.

Sambol NC, Chiang J, Lin ET, et al. Kidney function and age are both predictors of pharmacokinetics of metformin. J Clin Pharmacol. 1995;35:1094102.

Schmidt R, Horn E, Richards J, Stamatakis M. Survival after metformin-associated lactic acidosis in peritoneal dialysis-dependent renal failure. Am J Med. 1997;102:486–8.

Sirtori CR, Franceschini G, Galli-Kienle M, et al. Disposition of metformin (N,N-dimethylbiguanide) in man. Clin Pharmacol Ther. 1978;24:683–93.

Tucker GT, Casey C, Phillips PJ, Connor H, Ward JD, Woods HF. Metformin kinetics in healthy subjects and in patients with diabetes mellitus. Br J Clin Pharmacol. 1981;12:235–46.

van Berlo-van de Laar IRF, Vermeij CG, Doorenbos CJ. Metformin associated lactic acidosis: incidence and clinical correlation with metformin serum concentration measurements. J Clin Pharm Ther. 2011;36:376–82.

Warren RE, Strachan MWJ, Wild S, McKnight JA. Introducing estimated glomerular filtration rate (eGFR) into clinical practice in the UK: implications for the use of metformin. Diabet Med. 2007;24:494–7.

Dosage Adjustment of Medications Eliminated by the Kidneys

<u>Metformin</u>/Glucophage®	{Biguanide antidiabetic}	
Usual initial dose:	850 mg orally once daily with food or 500 mg orally twice daily with meals or 500 mg extended-release orally once daily with the evening meal	
Usual maintenance dose:	850–1,000 mg orally twice daily with meals or 1,000–2,000 mg extended-release orally once daily with the evening meal	
Typical maximum dose:	2,550 mg/day	
Proportion eliminated unchanged:	90 %	

Adjustment for Kidney Disease

FDA-approved product labeling:	*Kidney disease/abnormal CrCL (SCr ≥1.5 [males] or ≥1.4 [females]) and use in patients undergoing radiologic studies involving intra-vascular administration of iodinated contrast materials*	*Contraindicated*
Alternative adjustment:	*GFR >60 mL/min*	*500–1,000 mg orally twice daily with meals*
	GFR 41–60 mL/min	*250–750 mg orally twice daily with meals*
	GFR 10–40 mL/min	*Avoid due to risk for metabolic complications such as lactic acidosis.*
	GFR <10 mL/min	*Avoid due to risk for metabolic complications such as lactic acidosis.*
	Hemodialysis	*Avoid due to risk for metabolic complications such as lactic acidosis.*
	CAPD	*Avoid due to risk for metabolic complications such as lactic acidosis.*
	CVVH	*Not applicable; avoid due to risk for metabolic complications such as lactic acidosis.*
	CVVHD or CVVHDF	*Not applicable; avoid due to risk for metabolic complications such as lactic acidosis.*

Dosage Adjustment of Medications Eliminated by the Kidneys

Methadone - Selected References

Aronoff GA, Bennett WM, Berns JS, et al. Drug prescribing in renal failure: dosing guidelines for adults and children. 5th ed. Philadelphia: American College of Physicians; 2007.

Bellward GD, Warren PM, Howald W, Axelson JE, Abbott FS. Methadone maintenance: effect of urinary pH on renal clearance in chronic high and low doses. Clin Pharmacol Ther. 1977;22:92–9.

Chan GLC, Matzke GR. Effects of renal insufficiency on the pharmacokinetics and pharmacodynamics of opioid analgesics. Drug Intell Clin Pharm. 1987;21:773–83.

Davison SN. Pain in hemodialysis: prevalence, cause, severity, and management. Am J Kidney Dis. 2003;42:1239–47.

Dean M. Opioids in renal failure and dialysis patients. J Pain Symptom Manage. 2004;28:497–504.

Dolophine® tablet [package insert]. Columbus: Roxane Laboratories Inc; 2009.

Foster DJR, Somogyi AA, Dyer KR, White JM, Bochner F. Steady-state pharmacokinetics of (R)- and (S)-methadone in methadone maintenance patients. Br J Clin Pharmacol. 2000;50:427–40.

Furlan V, Hafi A, Dessalles M-C, Bouchez J, Charpentier B, Taburet A-M. Methadone is poorly removed by hemodialysis [letter]. Nephrol Dial Transplant. 1999;14:254.

Glazer WM, Cohn GL Methadone maintenance in a patient on chronic hemodialysis. Am J Psychiatry. 1977;134:931–2.

Inturrisi CE. Disposition of narcotics in patients with renal disease. Am J Med. 1977;62:528–9.

Inturrisi CE, Colburn WA, Kaiko RF, Houde RW, Foley KM. Pharmacokinetics and pharmacodynamics of methadone in patients with chronic pain. Clin Pharmacol Ther. 1987;41:392–401.

King S, Forbes K, Hanks GW, Ferro CJ, Chambers EJ. A systematic review of the use of medication for those with moderate to severe cancer pain and renal impairment: a European Palliative Care Research Collaborative opioid guidelines project. Palliat Med. 2011;25:525–52.

Leppert W. The role of methadone in cancer pain treatment: a review. Int J Clin Pract. 2009;63:1095–109.

Lugo RA, Satterfield KL, Kern SE. Pharmacokinetics of methadone. J Pain Palliat Care Pharmacother. 2005;19:13–24.

McIntyre CW, Owen PJ. Prescribing drugs in kidney disease. In: Brenner BM, editor. Brenner & Rector's the kidney. 8th ed. Philadelphia: Saunders/Elsevier; 2008. p. 1930–55.

Murphy EJ. Acute pain management pharmacology for the patient with concurrent renal or hepatic disease. Anaesth Intensive Care. 2005;33:311–23.

Murtagh FEM, Chai M-O, Donohoe P, Edmonds PM, Higginson IJ. The use of opioid analgesia in end-stage renal disease patients managed without dialysis: recommendations for practice. J Pain Palliat Care Pharmacother. 2007;21:5–16.

Nilsson JI, Meresaar U, Änggård E. Clinical pharmacokinetics of methadone. Acta Anaesth Scand Suppl. 1982;74:66–9.

Olyaei AJ, Bennett WM. Drug dosing in elderly patients with chronic kidney disease. Clin Geriatr Med. 2009;25:459–527.

Olyaei AJ, Bennett WM. Pharmacologic approach to renal insufficiency. In: Dale DC, Federman DD, Antman K, editors. ACP medicine, WebMD June 2007 update. Hamilton: BC Decker; 2007. NEPHROLOGY IX: Appendix A1–25.

Olyaei AJ, DeMattos AM, Bennett WM. Use of drugs in patients with renal failure. In: Schrier RW, editor. Diseases of the kidney and urinary tract. 8th ed. Philadelphia: Lippincott Williams & Wilkins; 2007. p. 2765–807.

Pergolizzi J, Böger RH, Budd K, et al. Opioids and the management of chronic severe pain in the elderly: consensus statement of an international expert panel with focus on the six clinically most often used World Health Organization step III opioids (buprenorphine, fentanyl, hydromorphone, methadone, morphine, oxycodone). Pain Pract. 2007;8:287–313.

Pollock AB, Tegeler ML, Morgan V, Baumrucker SJ. Morphine to methadone conversion: an interpretation of published data. Am J Hospice Palliat Med. 2011;28:135–40.

Weinberg DS, Inturrisi CE, Reidenberg B, et al. Sublingual absorption of selected opioid analgesics. Clin Pharmacol Ther. 1988;44:335–52.

Wolfert AI, Sica DA. Narcotic usage in renal failure [editorial]. Int J Artif Organs. 1988;11:411–5.

Yennurajalingam S, Peuckmann V, Bruera E. Recent developments in cancer pain assessment and management. Support Cancer Ther. 2004;1:97–110.

Dosage Adjustment of Medications Eliminated by the Kidneys

<u>Methadone</u>/Dolophine®   {Analgesic, opioid μ-receptor agonist}

Usual initial dose: 2.5–10 mg orally or IV

Usual maintenance dose: 2.5–10 mg orally or IV every 8–12 h

Typical maximum dose: 120 mg/day

Proportion eliminated unchanged: 20 %

Adjustment for Kidney Disease

FDA-approved product labeling: *Methadone has not been extensively evaluated in patients with renal insufficiency.*

Alternative adjustment:

GFR >50 mL/min	*2.5–10 mg orally or IV every 8–12 h*
GFR 10–50 mL/min	*2.5–10 mg orally or IV every 8–12 h*
GFR <10 mL/min	*1.25–5 mg orally or IV every 8–12 h (25–50 % decrease)*
Hemodialysis	*1.25–5 mg orally or IV every 8–12 h (25–50 % decrease)*
CAPD	*1.25–5 mg orally or IV every 8–12 h (25–50 % decrease)*
CRRT	*2.5–10 mg orally or IV every 8–12 h*

Note: Rate of urinary elimination and half-life of methadone vary according to urine pH; particular caution is advised in patients receiving urinary alkalinizers such as sodium bicarbonate.

Methenamine - Selected References

Abramowicz M, Zuccotti G, Pflomm J-M, et al., editors. Handbook of antimicrobial therapy. 19th ed. New Rochelle: The Medical Letter; 2011.

Aronoff GA, Bennett WM, Berns JS, et al. Drug prescribing in renal failure: dosing guidelines for adults and children. 5th ed. Philadelphia: American College of Physicians; 2007.

Freeman RB, Richardson JA, Thurm RH, Griep RJ. Long-term therapy for chronic bacteriuria in men: US Public Health Service Cooperative Study. Ann Intern Med. 1975;83:133–47.

Gollamudi R, Meyer MC, Straughn AB. Simultaneous determination of methenamine and formaldehyde in the urine of humans after methenamine administration. Biopharm Drug Dispos. 1979;1:27–36.

Gollamudi R, Straughn AB, Meyer MC. Urinary excretion of methenamine and formaldehyde: evaluation of 10 methenamine products in humans. J Pharm Sci. 1981;70:596–9.

Hiprex® [package insert]. Bridgewater: Sanofi-Aventis US LLC; 2006.

Kalowski S, Nandra RS, Friedman A, Radford N, Standish H, Kincaid-Smith P. Controlled trial comparing co-trimoxazole and methenamine hippurate in the prevention of recurrent urinary tract infections. Med J Aust. 1975;1:585–9.

Klinge E, Männistö P, Mäntylä R, Lamminivu U, Ottoila P. Pharmacokinetics of methenamine in healthy volunteers. J Antimicrob Chemother. 1982;9:209–16.

Lee BSB, SimpsonJM, Craig JC, Bhuta T. Methenamine hippurate for preventing urinary tract infections (review). Cochrane Database Syst Rev. 2010;(4):CD003265. doi:10.1002/14651858.CD003265.pub2.

McIntyre CW, Owen PJ. Prescribing drugs in kidney disease. In: Brenner BM, editor. Brenner & Rector's the kidney. 8th ed. Philadelphia: Saunders/Elsevier; 2008. p. 1930–55.

Nilsson S. Long-term treatment with methenamine hippurate in recurrent urinary tract infection. Acta Med Scand. 1975;198:81–5.

Scudi JV, Reinhard JF. Absorption, distribution, and renal excretion of Mandelamine (methenamine mandelate). J Lab Clin Med. 1948;33:1304–10.

Dosage Adjustment of Medications Eliminated by the Kidneys

<u>Methenamine</u>/Hiprex®, Mandelamine®   {**Antibacterial; urinary antiseptic**}

Usual initial dose:	1 g orally
Usual maintenance dose:	1 g orally twice daily after meals
Typical maximum dose:	4 g/day
Proportion eliminated unchanged:	80 %

Adjustment for Kidney Disease

FDA-approved product labeling:	*Renal insufficiency*	*Contraindicated*
Alternative adjustment:	*GFR >50 mL/min*	*1 g orally every twice daily after meals*
	GFR 10–50 mL/min	*Avoid due to risk for drug and/or formaldehyde accumulation.*
	GFR <10 mL/min	*Avoid due to risk for drug and/or formaldehyde accumulation.*
	Hemodialysis	*Avoid due to risk for drug and/or formaldehyde accumulation.*
	CAPD	*Avoid due to risk for drug and/or formaldehyde accumulation.*
	CRRT	*Not applicable; avoid.*

Methocarbamol (IV) - Selected References

Anah CO. Tetanus: conservative management made easier by combination of muscle relaxants. Am J Trop Med Hyg. 1974;23:930–4.

Dent RW, Ervin DK. Relief of musculoskeletal symptoms with intravenous methocarbamol (Robaxin® injectable): a placebo-controlled study. Curr Ther Res Clin Exp. 1976;20:661–5.

Ferslew KE, Hagardorn AN, McCormick WF. A fatal interaction of methocarbamol and ethanol in an accidental poisoning. J Forensic Sci. 1990;35:477–82.

Forist AA, Judy RW. Comparative pharmacokinetics of chlorphenesin carbamate and methocarbamol in man. J Pharm Sci. 1971;60:1686–8.

Kemal M, Imami R, Pollis A. A fatal methocarbamol intoxication. J Forensic Sci. 1982;27:217–22.

Key GF. A comparison of calcium gluconate and methocarbamol (Robaxin®) in the treatment of latrodectism (black widow spider envenomation). Am J Trop Med Hyg. 1981;30:273–7.

Luo X, Pietrobon R, Curtis LH, Hey LA. Prescription of nonsteroidal anti-inflammatory drugs and muscle relaxants for back pain in the United States. Spine. 2004;29:e531–7. doi:10.1097/01.brs.0000146453.76528.7c.

Preston KL, Guarino JJ, Kirk WT, Griffiths RR. Evaluation of the abuse potential of methocarbamol. J Pharmacol Exp Ther. 1989;248:1146–57.

Preston KL, Wolf B, Guarino JJ, Griffiths RR. Subjective and behavioral effects of diphenhydramine, lorazepam and methocarbamol: evaluation of abuse liability. J Pharmacol Exp Ther. 1992;262:707–20.

Robaxin® IV [package insert]. Deerfield: Baxter Healthcare Corp.; 2006.

Scott RB, Tisdale SA Jr, Cummings WB. Hemolytic potential of methocarbamol. Clin Pharmacol Ther. 1977;21:208–11.

Sica DA, Comstock TJ, Davis J, et al. Pharmacokinetics and protein binding of methocarbamol in renal insufficiency and normals. Eur J Clin Pharmacol. 1990;39:193–4.

Tisdale SA Jr, Ervin AK. A controlled study of methocarbamol (Robaxin®) in acute painful musculoskeletal conditions. Curr Ther Res Clin Exp. 1975;17:525–30.

Voci JM, Al-Hakim M, Dokko Y, Katirji MB. Intravenous methocarbamol in the treatment of stiff man syndrome [letter]. Muscle Nerve. 1993;16:434–5.

<u>**Methocarbamol (IV)**</u>/Robaxin® IV   {**Centrally acting skeletal muscle relaxant**}

Usual initial dose:	1,000 mg IV
Usual maintenance dose:	1,000 mg IV, repeated if necessary up to twice within 24 h
Typical maximum dose:	3,000 mg/day
Proportion eliminated unchanged:	<10 %

Adjustment for Kidney Disease

FDA-approved product labeling:	*Renal impairment*	*Contraindicated (due to excipient content [polyethylene glycol 300])*
Alternative adjustment:	*Data not available*	

Dosage Adjustment of Medications Eliminated by the Kidneys

<u>Methotrexate</u> - Selected References

Abelson HT, Fosburg MT, Beardsley GP, et al. Methotrexate-induced renal impairment: clinical studies and rescue from systemic toxicity with high-dose leucovorin and thymidine. J Clin Oncol. 1983;1:208–16.

Al-Hasani H, Roussou E. Methotrexate for rheumatoid arthritis patients who are on hemodialysis. Rheumatol Int. 2011;31:1545–7. doi:10.1007/s00296-011-2041-5.

Aronoff GA, Bennett WM, Berns JS, et al. Drug prescribing in renal failure: dosing guidelines for adults and children. 5th ed. Philadelphia: American College of Physicians; 2007.

Braun J. Optimal administration and dosage of methotrexate. Clin Exp Rheumatol. 2010;28(Suppl 61):S46–51.

Cheng KKT, Chow KM, Szeto CC, et al. Fatal pancytopenia in a hemodialysis patient after treatment with low-dose methotrexate. J Clin Rheumatol. 2009;15:177–80.

Darbhammula A, Bhal K, Lal S. Is routine monitoring of hepatic and renal function beneficial following single-dose methotrexate treatment for ectopic pregnancy? A 4-year review of experience from a teaching hospital. J Obstet Gynaecol. 2008;28:434–5.

Diskin CJ, Stokes TJ, Dansby LM, Radcliff L, Carter TB. Removal of methotrexate by peritoneal dialysis and hemodialysis in a sing patient with end-stage renal disease. Am J Med Sci. 2006;332:156–8.

Green MR, Chamberlain MC. Renal dysfunction during and after high-dose methotrexate. Cancer Chemother Pharmacol. 2009;63:599–604.

Hartmann B, Czock D, Keller F. Drug therapy in patients with chronic renal failure. Dtsch Ärztebl Int. 2010;107:647–55.

Holmboe L, Andersen AM, Mørkrid L, Slørdal L, Hall KS. High-dose methotrexate chemotherapy: pharmacokinetics, folate and toxicity in osteosarcoma patients. Br J Clin Pharmacol. 2012;73:106–14. doi:10.1111/1365-2125.2011.04054.x.

Jolivet J, Cowan KH, Curt GA, Clendeninn NJ, Chabner BA. The pharmacology and clinical use of methotrexate. N Engl J Med. 1983;309:1094–104.

Jundt JW, Browne BA, Fiocco GP, Steele AD, Mock D. A comparison of low dose methotrexate bioavailability: oral solution, oral tablet, subcutaneous and intramuscular dosing. J Rheumatol. 1993;20:1845–9.

Karie S, Gandjbakhch F, Janus N, et al. Kidney disease in RA patients: prevalence and implication on RA-related drugs management: the MATRIX study. Rheumatology. 2008;47:350–4.

Karstila KL, Rantalaiho VM, Mustonen JT, et al. Renal safety of initial combination versus single DMARD therapy in patients with early rheumatoid arthritis: an 11-year experience from the FIN-RACo trial. Clin Exp Rheumatol. 2010;28:73–8.

Lim AYN, Gaffney K, Scott DGI. Methotrexate-induced pancytopenia: serious and under-reported? Our experience of 25 cases in 5 years. Rheumatology. 2005;44:1051–5.

Matsumoto K. Pharmacokinetics of cisplatin and methotrexate after M-VAC chemotherapy for advanced urothelial cancer in hemodialysis patients [letter]. Int J Urol. 2008;15:949–50.

McKendry RJR, Dale P. Adverse effects of low dose methotrexate therapy in rheumatoid arthritis. J Rheumatol. 1993;20:1850–6.

Morgaceva O, Furst DE. Use of MTX in the elderly and in patients with compromised renal function. Clin Exp Rheumatol. 2010;28(Suppl 61):S85–94.

Murashima M, Adamski J, Milone MC, Shaw L, Tsai DE, Bloom RD. Methotrexate clearance by high-flux hemodialysis and peritoneal dialysis: a case report. Am J Kidney Dis. 2009;53:871–4.

Ory SJ, Villanueva AL, Sand PK, Tamura RK. Conservative treatment of ectopic pregnancy with methotrexate. Am J Obstet Gynecol. 1986;154:1299–306.

Soon C, Ilchyshyn A. Methotrexate toxicity induced by acute renal failure [letter]. J R Soc Med. 2005;98:83–4.

Trexall™ [package insert]. Pomona: Duramed Pharmaceuticals Inc, Subsidiary of Barr Pharmaceuticals Inc; 2005.

Widemann BC, Balis FM, Kim AR, et al. Glucarpidase, leucovorin, and thymidine for high-dose methotrexate-induced renal dysfunction: clinical and pharmacologic factors affecting outcome. J Clin Oncol. 2010;28:3979–86.

Wiland P, Wiela-Hojenska Glowska A, et al. Renal function in rheumatoid arthritis patients treated with methotrexate and infliximab. Clin Exp Rheumatol. 2004;22:469–72.

Dosage Adjustment of Medications Eliminated by the Kidneys

<u>Methotrexate</u>/Rheumatrex®, Trexall™   {Antineoplastic; antimetabolite; disease-modifying antirheumatic drug}

Usual initial dose:	7.5 mg orally
Usual maintenance dose:	5–15 mg orally once weekly
Typical maximum dose:	30 mg/week
Proportion eliminated unchanged:	85 %

Adjustment for Kidney Disease

FDA-approved product labeling: *Injection—Adequate renal function must be documented; SCr must be normal, and CrCL must be >60 mL/min before initiation of therapy.*

Oral—Patients with renal impairment require especially careful monitoring for toxicity and require dose reduction or, in some cases, discontinuation of methotrexate administration.

Alternative adjustment:

GFR >50 mL/min	*5–15 mg orally once weekly*
GFR 10–50 mL/min	*2.5–5 mg orally once weekly (50 % decrease; avoid high-dose therapy)*
GFR <10 mL/min	*Avoid unless no suitable alternative exists; if indeed necessary, 2.5–5 mg orally once weekly*
Hemodialysis	*2.5–5 mg orally once weekly (50 % decrease); avoid high-dose therapy.*
CAPD	*Minimal data available. Avoid unless no suitable alternative exists; if indeed necessary, 2.5–5 mg orally once weekly*
CRRT	*2.5–5 mg orally once weekly (50 % decrease); avoid high-dose therapy.*

Methyldopa (IV) - Selected References

Barnett AJ, Bobik A, Carson V, Korman JS, McLean AJ. Pharmacokinetics of methyldopa: plasma levels following single intravenous, oral and multiple oral dosage in normotensive and hypertensive subjects. Clin Exp Pharmacol Physiol. 1977;4:331–9.

Kwan KC, Foltz EL, Breault GO, Baer JE, Totaro JA. Pharmacokinetics of methyldopa in man. J Pharmacol Exp Ther. 1976;198:264–77.

Levine RJ, Strauch BS. Hypertensive responses to methyldopa. N Engl J Med. 1966;275:946–8.

Manolis AS, Varriale P, Nobile J. Short-term hemodynamic effects of intravenous methyldopa in patients with congestive heart failure. Pharmacotherapy. 1987;7:216–22.

Methyldopate injection [package insert]. Shirley: American Regent Laboratories Inc; 2006.

Myhre E, Brodwall EK, Stenbæk Ø, Hansen T. Conjugation of methyldopa in renal failure. Scand J Clin Lab Invest. 1972;29:195–9.

Myhre E, Brodwall EK, Stenbæk Ø, Hansen T. The renal excretion of methyldopa. Scand J Clin Lab Invest. 1972;29:201–4.

Myhre E, Rugstad HE, Hansen T. Clinical pharmacokinetics of methyldopa. Clin Pharmacokinet. 1982;7:221–33.

Robertson D, Tung C-S, Goldberg MR, Hollister AS, Gerkens JF, Oates JA. Antihypertensive metabolites of α-methyldopa. Hypertension. 1984;6(Supp II):45–50.

Saavedra JA, Reid JL, Jordan W, Rawlins MD, Dollery CT. Plasma concentration of α-methyldopa and sulphate conjugate after oral administration of methyldopa and intravenous administration of methyldopa and methyldopa hydrochloride ethyl ester. Eur J Clin Pharmacol. 1975;8:381–6.

Stenbæk Ø, Myhre E, Rugstad HE, Arnold E, Hansen T. Pharmacokinetics of methyldopa in man. Eur J Clin Pharmacol. 1977;12:117–23.

Dosage Adjustment of Medications Eliminated by the Kidneys

__Methyldopate__/Aldomet® IV   {Antihypertensive; α_2-adrenergic agonist}

Usual initial dose:	250–500 mg IV
Usual maintenance dose:	250–500 mg IV every 6 h as necessary
Typical maximum dose:	1,000 mg IV every 6 h
Proportion eliminated unchanged:	~50 %

Adjustment for Kidney Disease

FDA-approved product labeling:	*Patients with impaired renal function may respond to smaller doses.*	
Alternative adjustment:	*GFR >50 mL/min*	*250–500 mg IV every 8 h*
	GFR 10–50 mL/min	*250–500 mg IV every 8–12 h*
	GFR <10 mL/min	*250–500 mg IV every 12–24 h*
	Hemodialysis	*250–500 mg IV every 12–24 h; administer after hemodialysis on dialysis days.*
	CAPD	*250–500 mg IV every 12–24 h*
	CRRT	*250–500 mg IV every 8–12 h; titrate.*

Dosage Adjustment of Medications Eliminated by the Kidneys

Methylnaltrexone - Selected References

Amin HM, Sopchak AM, Foss JF, Esposito BF, Roizen MF, Camporesi EM. Efficacy of methylnaltrexone versus naloxone for reversal of morphine-induced depression of hypoxic ventilatory response. Anesth Analg. 1994;78:701–5.

Bader S, Jaroslawski K, Blum HE, Becker G. Opioid-induced constipation in advanced illness: safety and efficacy of methylnaltrexone bromide. Clin Med Insights Oncol. 2011;5:201–11.

Chamberlain BH, Cross K, Winston JL, et al. Methylnaltrexone treatment of opioid-induced constipation in patients with advanced illness. J Pain Symptom Manage. 2009;38:683–90.

Chandrasekaran A, Tong Z, Li H, et al. Metabolism of intravenous methylnaltrexone in mice, rats, dogs, and humans. Drug Metab Dispos. 2010;38:606–16.

Diego L, Atayee R, Helmons P, Hsiao G, von Gunten CF. Novel opioid antagonists for opioid-induced bowel dysfunction. Expert Opin Investig Drugs. 2011;20:1047–58.

Earnshaw SR, Klok RM, Iyer S, McCade C. Methylnaltrexone bromide for the treatment of opioid-induced constipation in patients with advanced illness—a cost-effectiveness analysis. Aliment Pharmacol Ther. 2010;31:911–21.

Foss JF, O'Connor MF, Yuan C-S, Murphy M, Moss J, Roizen MF. Safety and tolerance of methylnaltrexone in healthy humans: a randomized, placebo-controlled, intravenous, ascending dose, pharmacokinetics study. J Clin Pharmacol. 1997;37:25–30.

Iskedjian M, Iyer S, Librach SL, Wang M, Farah B, Berbari J. Methylnaltrexone in the treatment of opioid-induced constipation in cancer patients receiving palliative care: willingness-to-pay and cost-benefit analysis. J Pain Symptom Manage. 2011;41:104–115.

Lipman AG, Karver S, Cooney GA, Stambler N, Israel RJ. Methylnaltrexone for opioid-induced constipation in patients with advanced illness: a 3-month open-label treatment extension study. J Pain Palliat Care Pharmacother. 2011;25:436–45.

Michna E, Blonsky ER, Schulman S, et al. Subcutaneous methylnaltrexone for treatment of opioid-induced constipation in patients with chronic, nonmalignant pain: a randomized controlled study. J Pain. 2011;12:554–62.

Michna E, Weil AJ, Duerden M, et al. Efficacy of subcutaneous methylnaltrexone in the treatment of opioid-induced constipation: a responder post hoc analysis. Pain Med. 2011;12:1223–30.

Osinski J, Wang A, Wu JA, Foss JF, Yuan C-S. Determination of methylnaltrexone in clinical samples by solid-phase extraction and high-performance liquid chromatography for a pharmacokinetics study. J Chromatogr B Analyt Technol Biomed Life Sci. 2002;25:251–9.

Relistor® injection [package insert]. Philadelphia: Wyeth Pharmaceuticals Inc; 2010.

Rosow CE, Gomery P, Chen TY, Stefanovich P, Stamble N, Israel R. Reversal of opioid-induced bladder dysfunction by intravenous naloxone and methylnaltrexone. Clin Pharmacol Ther. 2007;82:48–53.

Rotshteyn Y, Boyd TA, Yuan C-S. Methylnaltrexone bromide: research update of pharmacokinetics following parenteral administration. Expert Opin Drug Metab Toxicol. 2011;7:227–35.

Singleton PA, Mambetsariev N, Lennon FE, et al. Methylnaltrexone potentiates the anti-angiogenic effects of mTOR inhibitors. J Angiogenes Res. 2010;19:5. doi:10.1186/2040-2384-2-5.

Slatkin N, Thomas J, Lipman AG, et al. Methylnaltrexone for treatment of opioid-induced constipation in advanced illness patients. J Support Oncol. 2009;7:39–46.

Tong Z, Chandrasekaran A, Li H, et al. In vitro metabolism and identification of human enzymes involved in the metabolism of methylnaltrexone. Drug Metab Dispos. 2010;38:801–7.

Wong BS, Rao AS, Camilleri M, et al. The effects of methylnaltrexone alone and in combination with acutely administered codeine on gastrointestinal and colonic transit in health. Aliment Pharmacol Ther. 2010;32:884–93.

Yu CS, Chun H-K, Stambler N, et al. Safety and efficacy of methylnaltrexone in shortening the duration of postoperative ileus following segmental colectomy: results of two randomized, placebo-controlled phase 3 trials. Dis Colon Rectum. 2011;54:570–8.

Yuan C-S, Foss JF, O'Connor M, et al. Methylnaltrexone for reversal of constipation due to chronic methadone use: a randomized controlled trial. JAMA. 2000;283:367–72.

Yuan C-S, Doshan H, Charney MR, et al. Tolerability, gut effects, and pharmacokinetics of methylnaltrexone following repeated intravenous administration in humans. J Clin Pharmacol. 2005;45:538–46.

Dosage Adjustment of Medications Eliminated by the Kidneys

<u>Methylnaltrexone</u>/Relistor®	{Peripherally acting opioid antagonist; ℞ for opioid-induced constipation}

Usual initial dose: 0.15 mg/kg (8 mg if 38–61 kg, 12 mg if 62–114 kg) subcutaneously

Usual maintenance dose: 0.15 mg/kg (8 mg if 38–61 kg, 12 mg if 62–114 kg) subcutaneously every other day

Typical maximum dose: 0.15 mg/kg every other day

Proportion eliminated unchanged: 60 %

Adjustment for Kidney Disease

FDA-approved product labeling:	*CrCL ≥30 mL/min*	*0.15 mg/kg (8 mg if 38–61 kg, 12 mg if 62–114 kg) subcutaneously every other day*
	CrCL <30 mL/min	*0.075 mg/kg (4 mg if 38–61 kg, 6 mg if 62–114 kg) subcutaneously every other day (50 % dose reduction)*
	End-stage renal disease/dialysis	*No data; avoid.*
Alternative Adjustment:	*Data not available*	

Dosage Adjustment of Medications Eliminated by the Kidneys

<u>Metoclopramide</u> - Selected References

Aronoff GA, Bennett WM, Berns JS, et al. Drug prescribing in renal failure: dosing guidelines for adults and children. 5th ed. Philadelphia: American College of Physicians; 2007.

Bateman DN. Clinical pharmacokinetics of metoclopramide. Clin Pharmacokinet. 1983;8:523–9.

Bateman DN, Gokal R, Dodd TRP, Blain PG. The pharmacokinetics of single doses of metoclopramide in renal failure. Eur J Clin Pharmacol. 1981;19:437–41.

Berardi RR, Cornish LA, Hyneck ML. Metoclopramide removal during continuous ambulatory peritoneal dialysis [letter]. Drug Intell Clin Pharm. 1986;20:154–5.

Brechot JM, Dupeyron JP, Delattre C, Chastang L, Laaban JP, Rochemaure J. Continuous infusion of high-dose metoclopramide: comparison of pharmacokinetically adjusted and standard doses for the control of cisplatin-induced acute emesis. Eur J Clin Pharmacol. 1991;40:283–6.

Bryson SM, McGovern EM, Kelman AW, White K, Addis GJ, Whiting B. The pharmacokinetics of high dose metoclopramide in patients with renal disease. Br J Clin Pharmacol. 1985;19:757–66.

Fujita Y, Yasukawa T, Mihira M, Sasaki T, Yokoya S. Metoclopramide in a patient with renal failure may be an increased risk of neuroleptic malignant syndrome [letter]. Intensive Care Med. 1996;22:717.

Gora ML, Visconti JA, Seth S, Shields B, Bay W. Pharmacokinetics of intraperitoneal metoclopramide in a patient with renal failure. Clin Pharm. 1992;11:174–6.

Grafner C, Lagerström P-O, Lundborg P, Rönn O. Pharmacokinetics of metoclopramide intravenously and orally determined by liquid chromatography. Br J Clin Pharmacol. 1979;8:469–74.

Grevel J, Whiting B, Kelman AW, Taylor WB, Bateman DN. Population analysis of the pharmacokinetic variability of high-dose metoclopramide in cancer patients. Clin Pharmacokinet. 1988;14:52–63.

Israel R, O'Mara V, Austin B Bellucci A, Meyer BR. Metoclopramide decreases renal plasma flow. Clin Pharmacol Ther. 1986;39:261–4.

Leroith D, Danovitz G, Trestan S, Spitz IM. Dissociation of prolactin response to thyrotropin-releasing hormone and metoclopramide in chronic renal failure. J Clin Endocrinol Metab. 1979;49:815–7.

Manara AR, Bolsin S, Monk CR, Hartnell G, Harris RA. Metoclopramide and renal vascular resistance. Br J Anaesth. 1991;66:129–30.

McGovern EM, Grevel J, Bryson SM. Pharmacokinetics of high-dose metoclopramide in cancer patients. Clin Pharmacokinet. 1986;11:415–24.

Munn J, Tooley M, Bolsin S, Hronek I, Lowson S, Willcox J. Effect of metoclopramide on renal vascular resistance index and renal function in patients receiving low-dose infusion of dopamine. Br J Anaesth. 1993;71:379–82.

O'Connell ME, Awni WM, Goodman M, et al. Bioavailability and disposition of metoclopramide after single- and multiple-dose administration in diabetic patients with gastroparesis. J Clin Pharmacol. 1987;27:610–4.

Regan LA, Hoffman RS, Nelson LS. Slower infusion of metoclopramide decreases the rate of akithisia. Am J Emerg Med. 2009;27:475–80.

Reglan® [package insert]. Marietta: Alaven Pharmaceutical LLC; 2009 and Deerfield: Baxter Healthcare Corp; 2010.

Ross-Lee LM, Eadie MJ, Hooper WD, Bochner F. Single-dose pharmacokinetics of metoclopramide. Eur J Clin Pharmacol. 1981;20:465–71.

Taylor WB, Bateman DN. Oral bioavailability of high-dose metoclopramide. Eur J Clin Pharmacol. 1986;31:41–4.

Taylor WB, Proctor SJ, Bateman DN. Pharmacokinetics and efficacy of high-dose metoclopramide given by continuous infusion for the control of cytotoxic drug-induced vomiting. Br J Clin Pharmacol. 1984;18:679–84.

Webb D, Buss DC, Fifield R, Bateman DN, Routledge PA. The plasma protein binding of metoclopramide in health and renal disease. Br J Clin Pharmacol. 1986;21:334–6.

Wright MR, Axelson JE, Rurak DW, et al. Effect of haemodialysis on metoclopramide kinetics in patients with severe renal failure. Br J Clin Pharmacol. 1988;469–73.

Wright MR, Axelson JE, Rurak DW, et al. Linearity of metoclopramide kinetics at doses of 5-20 mg. Br J Clin Pharmacol. 1988;26:469–73.

Wynne HA, Yelland C, Cope LH, Boddy A, Woodhouse KW, Bateman DN. The association of age and frailty with the pharmacokinetics and pharmacodynamics of metoclopramide. Age Aging. 1993;22:354–9.

Dosage Adjustment of Medications Eliminated by the Kidneys

<u>**Metoclopramide**</u>**/Reglan**®   {**Antiemetic; prokinetic; dopamine antagonist**}

Usual initial dose:	5–10 mg orally or IV
Usual maintenance dose:	10 mg orally or IV four times daily
Typical maximum dose:	10 mg/kg/day
Proportion eliminated unchanged:	20 %

Adjustment for Kidney Disease

FDA-approved product labeling:	*CrCL <40 mL/min*	*Initiate therapy at approximately one-half the recommended dosage.*
Alternative adjustment:	*GFR >50 mL/min*	*10 mg orally or IV four times daily or 2–10 mg/kg IV prior to administration of moderately or highly emetogenic chemotherapy agents*
	GFR 10–50 mL/min	*7.5 mg orally or IV four times daily (25 % decrease)*
	GFR <10 mL/min	*5 mg orally or IV four times daily (50 % decrease)*
	Hemodialysis	*5 mg orally or IV four times daily (no supplement after dialysis; 50 % decrease)*
	CAPD	*5 mg orally or IV four times daily (50 % decrease)*
	CRRT	*7.5 mg orally or IV four times daily (25 % decrease)*

Dosage Adjustment of Medications Eliminated by the Kidneys

Midodrine - Selected References

Alappan R, Cruz D, Abu-Alfa AK, Mahnensmith R, Perazella MA. Treatment of severe intradialytic hypotension with the addition of high dialysate calcium concentration to midodrine and/or cool dialysate. Am J Kidney Dis. 2001;37:294–9.

Alessandra C, Debernardi-Venon W, Carello M, Caretto S, Rizzetto M, Marzano A. Midodrine in the prevention of hepatorenal syndrome type 2 recurrence: a case-control study. Dig Liver Dis. 2009;41:298–302.

Anteli P, Volpin R, Raffaella G, et al. Reversal of type 1 hepatorenal syndrome with the administration of midodrine and octreotide. Hepatology. 1999;29:29:1690–7.

Aronoff GA, Bennett WM, Berns JS, et al. Drug prescribing in renal failure: dosing guidelines for adults and children. 5th ed. Philadelphia: American College of Physicians; 2007.

Blowey DL, Balfe JW, Gupta I, Gajaria MM, Koren G. Midodrine efficacy and pharmacokinetics in a patient with recurrent intradialytic hypotension. Am J Kidney Dis. 1996;28:132–6.

Caraceni P, Santi L, Mirici F, et al. Long-term treatment of hepatorenal syndrome as a bridge to liver transplantation. Dig Liver Dis. 2011;43:242–5.

Cruz DN, Mahnensmith RL, Brickel HM, Perazella MA. Midodrine and cool dialysate are effective therapies for symptomatic intradialytic hypotension. Am J Kidney Dis. 1999;33:920–6.

Cruz DN, Mahnensmith RL, Perazella MA. Intradialytic hypotension: is midodrine beneficial in symptomatic hemodialysis patients? Am J Kidney Dis. 1997;30:772–9.

Esrailian E, Pantangco ER, Kyulo NL, Ke-Qin H, Runyon BA. Octreotide/midodrine therapy significantly improves renal function and 30-day survival in patients with type 1 hepatorenal syndrome. Dig Dis Sci. 2007;52:742–8.

Fang J-T, Huang C-C. Midodrine hydrochloride in patients on hemodialysis with chronic hypotension. Ren Fail. 1996;18:253–60.

Fujisaki K, Kanai H, Hirakata H, et al. Midodrine hydrochloride and l-threo-3,4-dihydroxyphenylserine preserve cerebral blood flow in hemodialysis patients with orthostatic hypotension. Ther Apher Dial. 2007;11:49–55.

Grenon SM, Ziao X, Hurwitz S, et al. Why is orthostatic hypotension tolerance lower in women than men? Renal and cardiovascular responses to simulated microgravity and the role of midodrine. J Investig Med. 2006;54:180–90.

Izzedine H, Azar R, Zahiri K, Rottembourg J, Deray G. Haematological toxicity of midodrine n haemodialysis patients [letter]. Nephrol Dial Transplant. 2000;15:1715–6.

Khurana A, McCuskey C, Slavcheva EG. Orthostatic hypotension in kidney pancreas transplant patients and its relation to preexisting autonomic neuropathy. Exp Clin Transplant. 2008;6:127–31.

Lamarre-Cliché M, du Souich P, de Champlain J, Larochelle P. Pharmacokinetic and pharmacodynamic effects of midodrine on blood pressure, the autonomic nervous system, and plasma natriuretic peptides: a prospective, randomized, single-blind, two-period, crossover, placebo-controlled study. Clin Ther. 2009;30:1629–38.

Lin Y-F, Wang J-Y, Denq J-C, Lin S-H. Midodrine improves chronic hypotension in hemodialysis patients. Am J Med Sci. 2003;325:256–61.

Perazella MA. Pharmacologic options available to treat symptomatic intradialytic hypotension. Am J Kidney Dis. 2001;38(4 Suppl 4):S26–36.

Prakash S, Garg AX, Heidenheim AP, House AA. Midodrine appears to be safe and effective for dialysis-induced hypotension: a systematic review. Nephrol Dial Transplant. 2004;19:2553–8.

ProAmatine® tablet [package insert]. Newport: Shire US Inc; 2003.

Rubinstein S, Maimov M, Ross MJ. Midodrine-induced vascular ischemia in a hemodialysis patient: a case report and literature review. Ren Fail. 2008;30:808–12.

Skagen C, Einstein M, Lucey MR, Said A. Combination treatment with octreotide, midodrine, and albumin improves survival in patients with type 1 and type 2 hepatorenal syndrome. J Clin Gastroenterol. 2009;43:680–5.

Wong F, Pantea L, Sniderman K. Midodrine, octreotide, albumin, and TIPS in selected patients with cirrhosis and type 1 hepatorenal syndrome. Hepatology. 2004;40:55–64.

Wright RA, Kaufann HC, Perera R, et al. A double-blind, dose-response study of midodrine in neurogenic orthostatic hypotension. Neurology. 1998;51:120–4.

Yoshid H, Ohno Y, Yoshikuni K, Todoroki K, Nohta H, Yamaguchi M. Determination of midodrine n human plasma by high-performance liquid chromatography with fluorescence detection. Anal Sci. 2003;19:317–9.

Dosage Adjustment of Medications Eliminated by the Kidneys

Midodrine/ProAmatine®   {Vasopressor; α_1-agonist}

Usual initial dose: 10 mg orally

Usual maintenance dose: 10 mg orally three times daily while awake

Typical maximum dose: 45 mg/day

Proportion eliminated unchanged: 20 %

Adjustment for Kidney Disease

FDA-approved product labeling:	*Abnormal renal function*	*Because desglymidodrine is excreted renally, dosing in patients with abnormal renal function should be cautious; initiate treatment with 2.5 mg doses (three times daily).*
Alternative adjustment:	*GFR >50 mL/min*	*5–10 mg orally every 8 h*
	GFR 10–50 mL/min	*5–10 mg orally every 8 h*
	GFR <10 mL/min	*Data not available*
	Hemodialysis	*2.5 mg orally twice daily on dialysis days; 1.25 mg twice daily on non-dialysis days; titrate.*
	CAPD	*Data not available*
	CRRT	*5–10 mg orally every 8 h; titrate.*

Miglitol - Selected References

Abe M, Okada K, Soma M. Antidiabetic agents in patients with chronic kidney disease and end-stage renal disease on dialysis: metabolism and clinical practice. Curr Drug Metab. 2011;12:57–69

Aoki K, Kato H, Terauchi Y. Divided-dose administration of miglitol just before and 15 minutes after the start of a meal smoothes postprandial plasma glucose excursions and serum insulin responses in healthy men. Endocr J. 2007;54:1009–14.

Aoki K, Nakamura A, Ito S, et al. Administration of miglitol until 30 min after the start of a meal is effective in type 2 diabetic patients. Diabetes Res Clin Pract. 2007;78:30–3.

Charpentier G, Riveline JP, Varroud-Vial M. Management of drugs affecting blood glucose in diabetic patients with renal failure. Diabetes Metab. 2000;26:73–85.

Glyset® tablet [package insert]. New York: Pharmacia & Upjohn Division of Pfizer Inc; 2010.

Hans-Jürgen A, Boberg M, Brendel E, Krause HP, Steinke W. Pharmacokinetics of miglitol: Absorption, distribution, metabolism, and excretion following administration to rats, dogs, and man. Arzneimittelforschung. 1997;47:734–45.

Nirogi RVS, Kandikere VN, Shukla M, et al. Liquid chromatographic tandem mass spectrometry method for the quantification of miglitol in human plasma. Arzneimittelforschung. 2006;56:328–36.

Scott LJ, Spencer CM. Miglitol: a review of its therapeutic potential in type 2 diabetes mellitus. Drugs. 2000;59:521–49.

Sels JPJE, Nauta JJP, Menheere PPCA, Wolffenbuttel BHR, Niewenhuijzen Kruseman AC. Miglitol (Bay m 1099) has no extraintestinal effects on glucose control in healthy volunteers. Br J Clin Pharmacol. 1996;42:503–6.

Dosage Adjustment of Medications Eliminated by the Kidneys

Miglitol/Glyset®   {Antidiabetic; α-glucosidase inhibitor}

Usual initial dose:	25 mg orally three times daily with meals
Usual maintenance dose:	50 mg orally three times daily with meals
Typical maximum dose:	100 mg orally three times daily
Proportion eliminated unchanged:	95 %

Adjustment for Kidney Disease

    FDA-approved product labeling: *Significant renal dysfunction (SCr >2.0 mg/dL)   Use not recommended; avoid.*

    Alternative adjustment: *Data not available*

Dosage Adjustment of Medications Eliminated by the Kidneys

Miglustat - Selected References

Alfonso P, Pampin S, Estrada J, et al. Miglustat (NB-DNJ) works as a chaperone for mutated acid β-glucosidase in cells transfected with several Gaucher disease mutations. Blood Cells Mol Dis. 2005;35:268–76.

Belmatoug N, Burlina A, Giraldo P, et al. Gastrointestinal disturbances and their management in miglustat-treated patients. J Inherit Metab Dis. 2011;34:991–1001. doi:10.1007/s1045-011-9368-7.

Capablo JL, Franco R, Sáenz de Cabezón A, Alfonso P, Pocovi M, Giraldo P. Neurologic improvement in a type 3 Gaucher disease patient treated with imiglucerase/miglustat combination. Epilepsia. 2007;48:1406–8.

Chien Y-H, Lee N-C, Huang A-C, Peng S-F, Chen S-J, Hwu W-L. Treatment of Niemann-Pick disease type C in two children with miglustat: initial responses and maintenance of effects over 1 year. J Inherit Metab Dis. 2007;30:826.

Cox TM, Aerts JMFG, Beck AM, et al. The role of the iminosugar N-butyldeoxynojirimycin (miglustat) in the management of type 1 (non-neuropathic) Gaucher disease: a position statement. J Inherit Metab Dis. 2003;26:513–26.

Cox T, Lachmann R, Hollak C, et al. Novel oral treatment of Gaucher's disease with N-butyldeoxynojirimycin (OGT 918) to decrease substrate biosynthesis. Lancet. 2000;355:1481–5.

Elstein D, Dweck A, Attias D, et al. Oral maintenance clinical trial with miglustat for type 1 Gaucher disease: switch from or combination with intravenous enzyme replacement. Blood. 2007;110:2296–301.

Elstein D, Hollak C, Aerts JMFG, et al. Sustained therapeutic effects of oral miglustat (Zavesca, N-butyldeoxynojirimycin, OGT 918) in type 1 Gaucher disease. J Inherit Metab Dis. 2004;327:757–66.

Giraldo P, Alfonso P, Atutxa K, et al. Real-world experience with long-term miglustat maintenance therapy in type 1 Gaucher disease: the ZAGAL project. Haematologica. 2009;94:1771–5.

Giraldo P, Latre P, Alfonso P, et al. Short-term effect of miglustat in every day clinical use in treatment-naïve or previously treated patients with type 1 Gaucher's disease. Haematologica. 2006;91:703–6.

Guitton J, Coste S, Guffon-Fouilhous N, Cohen S, Manchon M, Guilaumont M. Rapid quantification of miglustat in human plasma and cerebrospinal fluid by liquid chromatography coupled with tandem mass spectrometry. J Chromatogr B Analyt Technol Biomed Life Sci. 2009;877:149–54.

Heitner R, Elstein D, Aerts J, van Weely S, Zimran A. Low-dose N-butyldeoxynojirimycin (OGT 918) for type 1 Gaucher disease. Blood Cells Mol Dis. 2002;28:127–33.

Hollack CEM, Hughes D, van Scaik IN, Schwierin B, Bembi B. Miglustat (Zavesca®) in type 1 Gaucher disease: 5-year results of a post-authorisation safety surveillance programme. Pharmacoepidemiol Drug Saf. 2009;18:770–7.

Maegawa FHB, van Giersbergen PLM, Yang S, et al. Pharmacokinetics, safety and tolerability of miglustat in the treatment of pediatric patients with GM2 gangliosidosis. Mol Genet Metab. 2009;97:284–91.

Marcus NY, Permutter DH. Glucosidase and mannosidase inhibitors mediate increased secretion of mutant α1 antitrypsin Z. J Biol Chem. 2000;275:1987–92.

McCormack PL, Goa KL. Miglustat. Drugs. 2003;63:2427–34.

Pastores GM, Barnett NL, Kolodny EH. An open-label, noncomparative study of miglustat in type 1 Gaucher disease: efficacy and tolerability over 24 months of treatment. Clin Ther. 2005;27:1215–27.

Pastores GM, Elstein D, Hrebícek M, Zimran A. Effect of miglustat on bone disease in adults with type 1 Gaucher disease: a pooled analysis of three multinational, open-label studies. Clin Ther. 2007;29:1645–54.

Patterson MC, Vecchio D, Prady H, Abel L, Wraith JE. Miglustat for treatment of Niemann-Pick C disease: a randomised controlled study. Lancet. 2007;6:765–72.

Pined M, Wraith JE, Sedel F, et al. Miglustat in patients with Niemann-Pick disease type C (NP-C): a multicenter observational retrospective study. Mol Genet Metab. 2009;98:2453–9.

Schiffmann R, FitzGibbon EJ, Harris C, et al. Randomized, controlled trial of miglustat in Gaucher's disease type 3. Ann Neurol. 2008;64:514–22.

Treiber A, Morand O, Clozel M, The pharmacokinetics and tissue distribution of the glucosylceramide synthetase inhibitor miglustat in the rat. Xenobiotica. 2007;37:298–314.

van Giersbergen PLM, Dingemanse J. Influence of food intake on the pharmacokinetics of miglustat, an inhibitor of glucosylceramide synthetase. J Clin Pharmacol. 2007;47:1277–82.

Zavesca® capsule [package insert]. South San Francisco: Actelion Pharmaceuticals Inc; 2010.

Dosage Adjustment of Medications Eliminated by the Kidneys

<u>Miglustat</u>/Zavesca® {**Enzyme (glucosylceramide synthetase) inhibitor; R for type 1 Gaucher disease**}

Usual initial dose:	100 mg orally
Usual maintenance dose:	100 mg orally three times daily
Typical maximum dose:	300 mg/day
Proportion eliminated unchanged:	~95 %

Adjustment for Kidney Disease

FDA-approved product labeling:	*CrCL >70 mL/min*	*100 mg orally three times daily*
	CrCL 50–70 mL/min	*100 mg orally twice daily*
	CrCL 30–50 mL/min	*100 mg orally once daily*
	CrCL <30 mL/min	*Use not recommended; avoid.*
Alternative adjustment:	*Data not available*	

Milnacipran - Selected References

Arai M. Parkinsonism associated with a serotonin and noradrenaline reuptake inhibitor, milnacipran [letter]. J Neurol Neurosurg Psychiatry. 2003;74:137–8.

Bonnaud B, Cousse H, Mouzin G, et al. 1-Aryl-2-(aminomethyl)cyclopropanecarboxylic acid derivatives: a new series of potential antidepressants. J Med Chem. 1987;30:318–25.

Branco JC, Cherin P, Mongagne A, Bouroubi A. Longterm therapeutic response to milnacipran treatment for fibromyalgia: a European 1-year extension study following a 3-month study. J Rheumatol. 2011;38:1403–12.

Choy E, Marshall D, Gabriel ZL, Mitchell SA, Gylee E, Dakin HA. A systematic review and mixed treatment comparison of the efficacy of pharmacological treatments for fibromyalgia. Semin Arthritis Rheum. 2011;41:335–45.e6. doi:10.1016/j.semarthrit.2011.06.003.

Goldenberg DL, Clauw DJ, Palmer RH, Mease P, Chen W, Gendreau M. Durability of therapeutic response to milnacipran treatment for fibromyalgia: results of a randomized, double-blind, monotherapy 6-month extension study. Pain Med. 2010.11:180–94.

Häuser W, Petzke F, Sommer C. Comparative efficacy and harms of duloxetine, milnacipran, and pregabalin in fibromyalgia syndrome. J Pain. 2010;11:505–21.

Häuser W, Petzke F, Üçeyler N, Sommer C. Comparative efficacy and acceptability of amitriptyline, duloxetine and milnacipran in fibromyalgia syndrome: a systematic review with meta-analysis. Rheumatology (Oxford). 2011;50:532–43.

Higuchi K, Yoshida K, Takahashi H, et al. Milnacipran plasma levels and antidepressant response in Japanese major depressive patients. Hum Psychopharmacol. 2003;18:255–9.

Hindmarch I, Rigney U, Stanley N, Briley M. Pharmacodynamics of milnacipran in young and elderly volunteers. Br J Clin Pharmacol. 2000;49:118–25.

Levine M, Truit CA, O'Connor AD. Cardiotoxicity and serotonin syndrome complicating a milnacipran overdose. J Med Toxicol. 2011;7:312–6. doi:10.1007/s13181-0011-0167-1.

Ormseth MJ, Eyler AE, Hammonds CL, Boomershine CS. Milnacipran for the management of fibromyalgia syndrome. J Pain Res. 2010;3:15–24.

Puozzo C, Filaquier C, Briley M. Plasma levels of F 2207, milnacipran, a novel antidepressant after single oral administration in volunteers [abstract]. Br J Clin Pharmacol. 1985;20:291–2P.

Puozzo C, Pozet N, Deprez D, Baille P, Ung HL, Zech P. Pharmacokinetics of milnacipran in renal impairment. Eur J Drug Metab Pharmacokinet. 1998;23:280–6.

Puozzo C, Panconi E, Deprez D. Pharmacology and pharmacokinetics of milnacipran. Int Clin Psychopharmacol. 2002;17(Suppl 1):S25–35.

Roskell NS, Beard SM, Zhao Y, Le TK. A meta-analysis of pain response in the treatment of fibromyalgia. Pain Pract. 2011;11:516–27. doi:10.1111/j.1533-2500.00441.x.

Rouillon F, Berdeaux G, Bisserbe JC, et al. Prevention of recurrent depressive episodes with milnacipran: consequences on quality of life. J Affect Disord. 2000;28:171–80.

Savella® tablet [package insert]. St Louis: Forest Pharmaceuticals Inc; 2009.

Serretti A, Chiesa A, Calati R, Perna G, Bellodi L, De Ronchi D. Novel antidepressants and panic disorder: evidence beyond current guidelines. Neuropsychobiology. 2011;63:1–7.

Song Z, Meyerson BA, Linderoth B. The interaction between antidepressant drugs and the pain-relieving effect of spinal cord stimulation in a rat model of neuropathy. Anesth Analg. 2011;113:1260–5. doi:10.1213/ANE.0b013e182288851.

Spencer CM, Wilde MI. Milnacipran: a review of its use in depression. Drugs. 1998;56:405–27.

Stenger A, Couzinier J-P, Briley M. Psychopharmacology of milnacipran, 1-phenyl-1-diethy-amino-carbonyl-2-aminomethylcyclopropane hydrochloride (F 2207), a new potential antidepressant. Psychopharmacology (Berl). 1987;91:147–53.

Tsai C-S, Wu C-L, Chou S-Y, Tsang H-Y, Hung T-H, Su A-A. Prevention of post-stroke depression with milnacipran in patients with acute ischemic stroke: a double-blind randomized placebo-controlled trial. Int Clin Psychopharmacol. 2011;26:263–7.

Yacoub HA, Johnson WG, Souayah N. Serotonin syndrome after administration of milnacipran for fibromyalgia. Neurology. 2010;74:699–700.

Dosage Adjustment of Medications Eliminated by the Kidneys

<u>Milnacipran</u>/Savella™   **{Antidepressant; serotonin and norepinephrine reuptake inhibitor (SNRI)}**

Usual initial dose:	12.5 mg once on day 1, 25 mg/day (12.5 mg twice daily) on days 2 and 3, 50 mg/day (25 mg twice daily) on days 4–7, and 100 mg/day (50 mg twice daily) after day 7
Usual maintenance dose:	50 mg orally twice daily
Typical maximum dose:	200 mg/day
Proportion eliminated unchanged:	55 % (renally eliminated metabolites are pharmacologically inactive)

Adjustment for Kidney Disease

FDA-approved product labeling:	*Moderate renal impairment (CrCL ≥30 mL/min)*	*50 mg orally twice daily; use with caution.*
	Severe renal impairment (CrCL 5–29 mL/min)	*25 mg orally twice daily (50 % decrease)*
	End-stage renal disease. (CrCL <5 mL/min)	*Not recommended; avoid.*
Alternative adjustment:	*Data not available*	

Dosage Adjustment of Medications Eliminated by the Kidneys

<u>Milrinone</u> - Selected References

Aronoff GA, Bennett WM, Berns JS, et al. Drug prescribing in renal failure: dosing guidelines for adults and children. 5th ed. Philadelphia: American College of Physicians; 2007.

Cody RJ, Kubo SH, Covit AB, et al. Regional blood flow and neurohormonal responses to milrinone in congestive heart failure. Clin Pharmacol Ther. 1986;39:128–35.

Cuffe MS, Califf RM, Adams KF Jr, et al. Short-term intravenous milrinone for acute exacerbation of chronic heart failure: a randomized controlled trial. JAMA. 2002;287:1541–7.

Heringlake M, Wernerus M, Grünefeld J, et al. The metabolic and renal effects of adrenaline and milrinone in patients with myocardial dysfunction after coronary artery bypass grafting. Crit Care. 2007;11:R51. doi:10.1186/cc5904.

Larsson R, Líedholm H, Andersson KE, Keane MA, Henry G. Pharmacokinetics and effects on blood pressure of a single oral dose of milrinone in healthy subjects and patients with renal impairment. Eur J Clin Pharmacol. 1986;29:549–53.

Mebazaa A, Pitsis AA, Rudiger A, et al. Critical review: practical recommendations on the management of perioperative heart failure in cardiac surgery. Crit Care. 2010;14:201. doi:10.1186/cc8153.

Primacor® injection [package insert]. Bridgewater: Sanofi-Aventis US LLC; 2007.

Saab G, Mindel G, Ewald G, Vijayan A. Acute renal failure secondary to milrinone in a patient with cardiac amyloidosis. Am J Kidney Dis. 2002;40:e7. doi:10.1053/ajkd.2002.34552.

Saltzman HE, Sharma K, Mather RJ, Rubin S, Adams S, Whellan DJ. Renal dysfunction in heart failure patients: what is the evidence? Heart Fail Rev. 2007;12:37–47.

Staffeld CG, Pastan SO. Cardiac disease in patients with end-stage renal disease. Cardiol Clin. 1995;13:209–23.

Stroshane RM, Koss RF, Biddlecome CE, Luczkowec C, Edelson J. Oral and intravenous pharmacokinetics of milrinone in human volunteers. J Pharm Sci. 1984;73:1438–41.

Taniguchi T, Shibata K, Saito S, Matsumoto H, Okeie K. Pharmacokinetics of milrinone in patients with congestive heart failure during continuous venovenous hemofiltration. Intensive Care Med. 2000;26:1089–93.

Woolfrey SG, Hegbrant J, Thysell H, et al. Dose regimen adjustment for milrinone in congestive heart failure patients with moderate and severe renal failure. J Pharm Pharmacol. 1995;47:651–5.

Dosage Adjustment of Medications Eliminated by the Kidneys

<u>Milrinone</u>/Primacor®   {**Inotropic agent; phosphodiesterase inhibitor**}

Usual initial dose:	50 mcg/kg; administer IV slowly over 10 min.
Usual maintenance dose:	0.375–0.75 mcg/kg/min IV
Typical maximum dose:	1.13 mg/kg/day
Proportion eliminated unchanged:	80 %

Adjustment for Kidney Disease

FDA-approved product labeling: *Milrinone dosage adjustment in renally impaired patients*

CrCL (mL/min)	Infusion rate (mcg/kg/min)
5	0.20
10	0.23
20	0.28
30	0.33
40	0.38
50	0.43

Alternative adjustment:

GFR >50 mL/min	*50 mcg/kg IV followed by 0.375 mcg/kg/min IV; titrate (max 0.75 mcg/kg/min).*
GFR 31–50 mL/min	*0.375 mcg/kg/min IV*
GFR 10–30 mL/min	*0.25 mcg/kg/min IV*
Hemodialysis	*Data not available*
CAPD	*Data not available*
CVVH	*0.2–0.25 mcg/kg/min IV*

Moexipril - Selected References

Aronoff GA, Bennett WM, Berns JS, et al. Drug prescribing in renal failure: dosing guidelines for adults and children. 5th ed. Philadelphia: American College of Physicians; 2007.

Brogden RN, Wiseman LR. Moexipril: a review of its use in the management of essential hypertension. Drugs. 1998;55:845–60.

Cawello W, Boekens H, Waitzinger J, Miller U. Moexipril show a long duration of action related to an extended pharmacokinetic half-life and prolonged ACE inhibition. Int J Clin Pharmacol Ther. 2002;40:9–17.

Chrysant SG, Chrysant GS. Pharmacological and clinical profile of moexipril: a concise review. J Clin Pharmacol. 2004;44:827–36.

Chrysant SG, Fox AAL, Stimpel M. Comparison of moexipril, a new ACE inhibitor, to Verapamil-SR as add on therapy to low dose hydrochlorothiazide in hypertensive patients. Am J Hypertens. 1995;8:418–21.

Dickstein K, Aarsland TY, Ferrari P, Todd M, Stimpel M. Comparison of the efficacy of three dose levels of moexipril versus placebo as add-on therapy to hydrochlorothiazide in patients with moderate hypertension. J Cardiovasc Pharmacol. 1994;24:247–55.

Froeje J. Ney P. Pharmacological and toxicological studies of the new angiotensin converting enzyme inhibitor moexipril hydrochloride. Arzneimittelforschung. 1997;47:132–44.

Kalász H, Petroianu G, Tekes K, Klebovich I, Ludányi K, Gulyás Z. Metabolism of moexipril to moexiprilat: determination of in vitro metabolism using HPLC-ES-MS. Med Chem. 2007;3:101–6.

Persson B, Stimpel M. Evaluation of the antihypertensive efficacy and tolerability of moexipril, a new ACE inhibitor, compared to hydrochlorothiazide in elderly patients. Eur J Clin Pharmacol. 1996;50:259–64.

Sayegh F, Topouchian J, Hlawaty M, Olzewska M, Asmar R. Regression of left ventricular hypertrophy with moexipril, an angiotensin-converting enzyme inhibitor, in hypertensive patients. Am J Ther. 2005;12:3–8.

Song JC, White CM. Clinical pharmacokinetics and selective pharmacodynamics of new angiotensin converting enzyme inhibitors: an update. Clin Pharmacokinet. 2002;41:207–24.

Špinar J, Vítovec J. MORE—MOexipril and REgression of left ventricle hypertrophy in combination therapy: a multicentric open label clinical trial. Int J Cardiol. 2005;100:199–206.

Univasc® [package insert]. Smyrna: Schwarz Pharma Inc; 2009.

White WB, Whelton A, Fox AAL, Stimpel M, Kaihlanen PM. Tricenter assessment of the efficacy of the ACE inhibitor, moexipril, by ambulatory blood pressure monitoring. J Clin Pharmacol. 1995;35:233–8.

Zannad F, Matzinger A, Larché J. Trough/peak ratios of once daily angiotensin converting enzyme inhibitors and calcium antagonists. Am J Hypertens. 1996;9:633–43.

Dosage Adjustment of Medications Eliminated by the Kidneys

<u>Moexipril</u>/Univasc®   {**Antihypertensive, vasodilator, angiotensin-converting enzyme (ACE)/renin inhibitor**}

Usual initial dose:	7.5 mg orally once daily taken 1 h before food
Usual maintenance dose:	7.5–30 mg orally in one or two divided doses taken 1 h before meals
Typical maximum dose:	60 mg/day
Proportion eliminated unchanged:	40 %

Adjustment for Kidney Disease

FDA-approved product labeling:	*CrCL ≤40 mL/min*	*3.75 mg once daily initially, titrated if necessary to a maximum daily dose of 15 mg*
Alternative adjustment:	*GFR >50 mL/min*	*7.5–30 mg orally in one or two divided doses taken 1 h before meals*
	GFR 10–50 mL/min	*3.75–15 mg orally in one or two divided doses taken 1 h before meals (50 % decrease)*
	GFR <10 mL/min	*3.75–15 mg orally in one or two divided doses taken 1 h before meals (50 % decrease)*
	Hemodialysis	*3.75–15 mg orally in one or two divided doses taken 1 h before meals*
	CAPD	*3.75–15 mg orally in one or two divided doses taken 1 h before meals*
	CRRT	*3.75–15 mg orally in one or two divided doses taken 1 h before meals (50 % decrease)*

Dosage Adjustment of Medications Eliminated by the Kidneys

<u>Morphine</u> - Selected References

Angst MS, Bührer M, Lötsch J, Insidious intoxication after morphine treatment in renal failure: delayed onset of morphine-6-glucuronide action. Anesthesiology. 2000;92:1473–6.

Aronoff GA, Bennett WM, Berns JS, et al. Drug prescribing in renal failure: dosing guidelines for adults and children. 5th ed. Philadelphia: American College of Physicians; 2007.

Ball M, McQuay HJ, Moore RA, Allen MC, Fisher A, Sear J. Renal failure and the use of morphine in intensive care. Lancet. 1985;1:784–6.

Bodd E, Jacobsen D, Lund E, Rípel Å, Mørland J, Wiik-Larsen E. Morphine-6-glucuronide might mediate the prolonged effect of morphine in acute renal failure. Hum Exp Toxicol. 1990;9:317–21.

Chauvin M, Sandouk P, Scherrmann JM, Farinotti R, Strumza P, Duvaldestin P. Morphine pharmacokinetics in renal failure. Anesthesiology. 1987;66:327–31.

D'Honneur G, Gilton A, Sandouk P, Scherrmann JM, Duvaldestin P. Plasma and cerebrospinal fluid concentrations of morphine and morphine glucuronides after oral morphine: the influence of renal failure. Anesthesiology. 1994;81:87–93.

Davison SN. Pain in hemodialysis: prevalence, cause, severity, and management. Am J Kidney Dis. 2003;42:1239–47.

Dean M. Opioids in renal failure and dialysis patients. J Pain Symptom Manage. 2004;28:497–504.

Embeda™ capsule extended release morphine and naltrexone [package insert]. Bristol: Alpharma Pharmaceuticals LLC Subsidiary of King Pharmaceuticals Inc; 2009.

Jamal JA, Joh J, Bastani B. Removal of morphine with the new high-efficiency and high-flux membranes during haemofiltration and haemodiafiltration. Nephrol Dial Transplant. 1998;13:1535–7.

Johnson FK, Ciric S, Boudriau S, Kisicki JC, Stauffer J. The relative bioavailability of morphine sulfate and naltrexone hydrochloride extended release capsules (Embeda®) and an extended release morphine sulfate capsule formulation (Kadian®) in healthy adults under fasting conditions. Am J Ther. 2011;18:2–8.

King S, Forbes K, Hanks GW, Ferro CJ, Chambers EJ. A systematic review of the use of medication for those with moderate to severe cancer pain and renal impairment: a European Palliative Care Research Collaborative opioid guidelines project. Palliat Med. 2011;25:525–52.

Lugo RA, Kern SE. Clinical pharmacokinetics of morphine. J Pain Palliat Care Pharmacother. 2002;16:5–18.

Morphine sulfate injection [package insert]. Lake Forest: Hospira Inc; 2006.

MS Contin® tablet film coated extended release [package insert]. Stamford: Purdue Pharma LP; 2006.

Murtagh FEM, Chai M-O, Donohoe P, Edmonds PM, Higginson IJ. The use of opioid analgesia in end-stage renal disease patients managed without dialysis: recommendations for practice. J Pain Palliat Care Pharmacother. 2007;21:5–16.

Osborne RJ, Joel SP, Slevin ML. Morphine intoxication in renal failure: the role of morphine-6-glucuronide. Br Med J (Clin Res Ed). 1986;292:1548–9.

Pauli-Magnus C, Hofmann U, Mikus G, Kuhlmann U, Mettang T. Pharmacokinetics of morphine and its glucuronides following intravenous administration of morphine in patients undergoing continuous ambulatory peritoneal dialysis. Nephrol Dial Transplant. 1999;14:903–9.

Pergolizzi J, Böger RH, Budd K, et al. Opioids and the management of chronic severe pain in the elderly: consensus statement of an international expert panel with focus on the six clinically most often used World Health Organization step III opioids (buprenorphine, fentanyl, hydromorphone, methadone, morphine, oxycodone). Pain Pract. 2007;8:287–313.

Portenoy RK, Foley KM, Stulman J, et al. Plasma morphine and morphine-6-glucuronide during chronic morphine therapy for cancer pain: plasma profiles, steady-state concentrations and the consequences of renal failure. Anesthesiology. 1991;47:13–9.

Portenoy RK, Thaler HT, Inturrisi CE, Friedlander-Klar H, Foley KM. The metabolite morphine-6-glucuronide contributes to the analgesia produced by morphine infusion in patients with pain and normal renal function. Clin Pharmacol Ther. 1992;51:422–31.

Säwe J, Odar-Cederlöf I. Kinetics of morphine in patients with renal failure. Eur J Clin Pharmacol. 1987;32:377–82.

Wolfert AI, Sica DA. Narcotic usage in renal failure [editorial]. Int J Artif Organs. 1988;11:411–5.

Wolff J, Bigler D, Christensen CB, Rasmussen SN, Andersen HB, Tønnesen KH. Influence of renal function on the elimination of morphine and morphine glucuronides. Eur J Clin Pharmacol. 1988;34:353–7.

Yennurajalingam S, Peuckmann V, Bruera E. Recent developments in cancer pain assessment and management. Support Cancer Ther. 2004;1:97–110.

Dosage Adjustment of Medications Eliminated by the Kidneys

<u>Morphine</u>/Embeda™,
Kadian®, MS Contin®   {Analgesic, opioid μ-receptor agonist}

Usual initial dose: 2–4 mg IV or 10 mg orally

Usual maintenance dose: 1–2 mg IV every 6–10 min (patient-controlled analgesia, PCA);

2–4 mg IV every 2–4 h PRN; 10–30 mg orally every 4 h PRN;

In opioid-tolerant patients, 30 mg orally every 12 h (escalating doses may be required)

Typical maximum dose: 80 mg/h (chronic pain in opioid-tolerant patient)

Proportion eliminated unchanged: 2–12 % (active metabolite [morphine-6-glucuronide] predominantly eliminated in urine)

Adjustment for Kidney Disease

FDA-approved product labeling: *Care should be exercised in administering morphine to patients with renal dysfunction, since high blood morphine levels, due to reduced clearance, may take several days to develop.*

Alternative adjustment:

GFR >50 mL/min	*100 % of usual dose*
GFR 10–50 mL/min	*75 % of usual dose*
GFR <10 mL/min	*Preferably avoid or 50 % of usual dose*
Hemodialysis	*Preferably avoid or 50 % of usual dose*
CAPD	*Preferably avoid or 50 % of usual dose*
CRRT	*75 % of usual dose; titrate.*

Dosage Adjustment of Medications Eliminated by the Kidneys

<u>Mycophenolate Mofetil</u> – Selected References

Akhlaghi F, Patel CG, Zuniga XP, Halilovic J, Preis IS, Gohh RY. Pharmacokinetics of mycophenolic acid and metabolites in diabetic kidney transplant recipients. Ther Drug Monit. 2006;28:95–101.

Behrend M. Mycophenolate mofetil: suggested guidelines for use in kidney transplantation. BioDrugs. 2001;15:37–53.

Budde K, Glander P, Krämer BK, et al. Conversion from mycophenolate mofetil to enteric-coated mycophenolate sodium in maintenance renal transplant recipients receiving tacrolimus: clinical, pharmacokinetic, and pharmacodynamic outcomes. Transplantation. 2007;83:417–24.

Budde K, Tedesco-Silva H, Arns W. Improved rejection prophylaxis with an initially intensified dosing regimen of enteric-coated mycophenolate sodium in de novo renal transplant recipients. Transplantation. 2011;92:321–7.

Bullingham R, Monroe S, Nicholls A, Hale M. Pharmacokinetics and bioavailability of mycophenolate mofetil in healthy subjects after single-dose oral and intravenous administration. J Clin Pharmacol. 1996;36:315–24.

CellCept® tablet [package insert]. South San Francisco: Genentech USA Inc; 2010.

González-Roncero FM, Gentil MA, et al. Pharmacokinetics of mycophenolate mofetil in kidney transplant patients with renal insufficiency. Transplant Proc. 2005;37:3749–51.

Johnson HJ, Swan SK, Heim-Duthoy KL, et al The pharmacokinetics of a single oral dose of mycophenolate mofetil in patients with varying degrees of renal function. Clin Pharmacol Ther. 1998;63:512–8.

Johnston A, He X, Holt DW. Bioequivalence of enteric-coated mycophenolate sodium and mycophenolate mofetil: a meta-analysis of three studies in stable renal transplant recipients. Transplantation. 2006;82:1413–8.

Kuypers DRJ, Vanrenterghem Y, Squifflet JP, et al. Twelve-month evaluation of the clinical pharmacokinetics of total and free mycophenolic acid and its glucuronide metabolites in renal allograft recipients on low dose tacrolimus in combination with mycophenolate mofetil. Ther Drug Monit. 2003;25:609–22.

Lloberas N, Torras J, Cruzado JM, et al. Influence of MRP2 on MPA pharmacokinetics in renal transplant recipients—results of the Pharmacogenomic Study within the Symphony Study. Nephrol Dial Transplant. 2011;26:3784–93. doi:10.1093/ndt/gfr130.

MacPhee IAM, Spreafico S, Bewick M, Pharmacokinetics of mycophenolate mofetil in patients with end-stage renal failure. Kidney Int. 2000;57:1164–8.

Maldonado AQ, Davies NM, Crow SA, Little C, Ojogho ON, Weeks DL. Effects of plasmapheresis on mycophenolic acid concentrations [letter]. Transplantation. 2011;91:e3–4.

Morgera S, Budde K, Lampe D, et al. Mycophenolate mofetil pharmacokinetics in renal transplant recipients on peritoneal dialysis. Tranpl Int. 1998;11:53–7.

Morgera S, Neumayer H-H, Fritsche L, et al. Pharmacokinetics of mycophenolate mofetil in renal transplant recipients on peritoneal dialysis. Int J Clin Pharmacol Ther. 1998;36:159–63.

Mourad M, Malaise J, Eddour DC, et al. Correlation of mycophenolic acid pharmacokinetic parameters with side effects in kidney transplant patients treated with mycophenolate mofetil. Clin Chem. 2001;47:88–94.

Myfortic® tablet delayed release [package insert]. East Hanover; Novartis Pharmaceuticals Inc; 2010.

Shaw LM, Mick R, Nowak I, Korecka M, Brayman KL. Pharmacokinetics of mycophenolic acid in renal transplant patients with delayed graft function. J Clin Pharmacol. 1998;38:268–75.

Smak Gregoor PJH, Hesse GJ, van Gelder T, et al. Relation of mycophenolic acid trough levels and adverse events in kidney allograft recipients. Transplant Proc. 1998;30:1192–3.

Sommerer C, Glander P, Arns W, et al. Safety and efficacy of intensified versus standard dosing regimens of enteric-coated mycophenolate sodium in de novo renal transplant patients. Transplantation. 2011;91:779–85.

Staatz CE, Tett SE. Clinical pharmacokinetics and pharmacodynamics of mycophenolate in solid organ transplant recipients. Clin Pharmacokinet. 2007;46:13–58.

Wakahashi K, Yamamori M, Minagawa K, et al. Pharmacokinetics-based optimal dose prediction of donor source-dependent response to mycophenolate mofetil in unrelated hematopoietic cell transplantation. Int J Hematol. 2011;94:193–202.

Weber LT, Shipkova M, Lamersdorf T, et al. Pharmacokinetics of mycophenolic acid (MPA) and determinants of MPA free fraction in pediatric and adult renal transplant recipients. J Am Soc Nephrol. 1998;9:1511–20.

Wollenberg K, Krumme B, Pisrski P, Schollmeyer P, Kriste G. Pharmacokinetics of mycophenolic acid in the early period after kidney transplantation. Transplant Proc. 1998;30:4090–1.

Dosage Adjustment of Medications Eliminated by the Kidneys

Mycophenolate Mofetil,
Mycophenolate Sodium/
CellCept®, Myfortic®   {Immunosuppressant; antirejection agent; inosine monophosphate dehydro-
                                         genase inhibitor}

Usual initial dose: 1,000 mg orally or IV (CellCept®), 720 mg orally (Myfortic®)

Usual maintenance dose: 1,000 mg (1,500 mg in hepatic transplant patients) orally or IV twice daily
                                         (CellCept®);

                                         720 mg orally at least 1 h before or 2 h after meals twice daily (Myfortic®)

Typical maximum dose: 3,000 mg/day (CellCept®), 2,880 mg/day (Myfortic®)

Proportion eliminated unchanged: 3 % (plus 60 % of absorbed dose as glucuronidated metabolite)

Adjustment for Kidney Disease

FDA-approved product labeling:	*Severe chronic renal impairment (GFR <25 mL/min) outside the immediate posttransplant period*	*Doses >1 g twice a day should be avoided. These patients should be carefully observed. No dose adjustments are needed in renal transplant patients experiencing delayed graft function postoperatively (CellCept®).*
	Severe chronic renal impairment (GFR <25 mL/min)outside the immediate posttransplant period	*These patients should be carefully followed for potential adverse reactions due to increase in free mycophenolic acid and mycophenolic acid glucuronide (inactive metabolite) concentrations (Myfortic®).*
Alternative adjustment:	*de novo renal transplant patients*	*1,440 mg orally at least twice daily for 2 weeks, followed by 1,080 mg orally twice daily for 4 weeks followed by 720 mg twice daily thereafter (Myfortic®; presently, only limited data support intensified posttransplant regimens)*
	Hemodialysis	*250–500 mg orally twice daily (CellCept®; monitor)*
	CAPD	*1,000 mg orally twice daily (CellCept®; monitor)*

N

L.K. Golightly et al. (eds.), *Renal Pharmacotherapy*,
DOI 10.1007/978-1-4614-5800-5_13, © Springer Science+Business Media New York 2013

Dosage Adjustment of Medications Eliminated by the Kidneys

Nabumetone - Selected References

Aronoff GA. Therapeutic implications associated with renal studies of nabumetone. J Rheumatol. 1992;19(Suppl 36):25–31.

Aronoff GA, Bennett WM, Berns JS, et al. Drug prescribing in renal failure: dosing guidelines for adults and children. 5th ed. Philadelphia: American College of Physicians; 2007.

Blackwell E, Loughlin K, Dumler F, Smythe M. Nabumetone-associated interstitial nephritis. Pharmacotherapy. 1995;15:669–72.

Bolaert JR, Jonnaert HA, Daneels RF, et al. Nabumetone pharmacokinetics in patients with varying degrees of renal impairment. Am J Med. 1987;82(Suppl 4B):107–9.

Brier ME, Sloan RS, Aronoff GA. Population pharmacokinetics of the active metabolite of nabumetone in renal dysfunction. Clin Pharmacol Ther. 1995;57:622–7.

Cangiano JL, Figueroa J, Palmer R. Renal hemodynamic effects of nabumetone, sulindac, and placebo in patients with osteoarthritis. Clin Ther. 1999;21:503–12.

Cipiolini F, Ganci A, Panara MR, et al. Effects of nabumetone on prostanoid biosynthesis in humans. Clin Pharmacol Ther. 1995;58:335–41.

Cook ME, Wallin JD, Thakur VD, et al. Comparative effects of nabumetone, sulindac, and ibuprofen on renal function. J Rheumatol. 1997;24:1137–44.

Davies NM. Clinical pharmacokinetics of nabumetone: the dawn of selective cyclo-oxygenase-2 inhibition? Clin Pharmacokinet. 1997;33:403–16.

De Caterina R, Giannessi D, Lazzerini G, et al. Effect of nabumetone on metabolism of renal arachidonate in humans. J Rheumatol. 1992;19(Suppl 36):80.

Fleischmann RM. Clinical efficacy and safety of nabumetone in rheumatoid arthritis and osteoarthritis. J Rheumatol. 1992;19(Suppl 36):32–40.

Freed MI, Audet PR, Zarifa N, et al. Comparative effects of nabumetone, sulindac, and indomethacin on urinary prostaglandin excretion and platelet function in volunteers. J Clin Pharmacol. 1994;34:1098–108.

Freston JW. Rationalizing cyclooxygenase (COX) inhibition for maximal efficacy and minimal adverse events. Am J Med. 1999;107(Suppl 6A):78–89S.

Friedel HA, Langtry HD, Buckley MM. Nabumetone: a reappraisal of its pharmacology and therapeutic use in rheumatic diseases. Drugs. 1993;45:131–56.

Giannessi D, Lazzerini G, Filiponi P, et al. Effects of nabumetone, a new non-steroidal anti-inflammatory drug, on urinary prostaglandin excretion in man. Pharmacol Res. 1993;28:229–41.

Hedner T, Samulesson O, Währborg P, Wadenvik H, Ung K-A, Ekbom A. Nabumetone: therapeutic use and safety profile in the management of osteoarthritis and rheumatoid arthritis. Drugs. 2004;64:2315–43.

Hynek ML. An overview of the clinical pharmacokinetics of nabumetone. J Rheumatol. 1992;19(Suppl 36):20–4.

Kendall MJ, Chellingsworth MC, Jubb R, Thawley AR, Undre NA, Kill DC. A pharmacokinetic study of the active metabolite of nabumetone in young healthy subjects and older arthritis patients. Eur J Clin Pharmacol. 1989;36:299–305.

Mangan FR, Flack JD, Jackson D. Preclinical overview of nabumetone: pharmacology, bioavailability, metabolism, and toxicology. Am J Med. 1987;82(Suppl 4B):6–10.

McMahon FG, Vargas R, Ryan JR, Fitts DA. Nabumetone kinetics in the young and elderly. Am J Med. 1987;82(Suppl 4B):92–5.

Miehlke RK, Schneider S, Sörgel F, et al. Penetration of the active metabolite of nabumetone into synovial fluid and adherent tissue of patients undergoing knee joint surgery. Drugs. 1990;40(Suppl 5):57–61.

Morgan GJ, Poland M, DeLapp RE. Efficacy and safety of nabumetone versus diclofenac, naproxen, ibuprofen, and piroxicam in the elderly. Am J Med. 1993;95(Suppl 2A):19–27S.

Pal B, Hutchinson A, Bhattacharya A, Ralston A. Cardiac arrest due to severe hyperkalemia in patient taking nabumetone and low salt diet. BMJ. 1995;311:1486–7.

Radford MG, Holley KE, Grande JP, et al. Reversible membranous nephropathy associated with the use of nonsteroidal anti-inflammatory drugs. JAMA. 1996;276:466–9.

Relafen® tablet film coated [package insert]. Research Triangle Park: GlaxoSmithKline; 2006.

Dosage Adjustment of Medications Eliminated by the Kidneys

Nabumetone/Relafen®   **{Anti-inflammatory; nonsteroidal anti-inflammatory drug}**

Usual initial dose:	1,000 mg orally
Usual maintenance dose:	1,000 mg orally once daily
Typical maximum dose:	2,000 mg/day
Proportion eliminated unchanged:	30 % (as primary active metabolite)

Adjustment for Kidney Disease

FDA-approved product labeling:	*CrCL ≥50 mL/min*	*1,000 mg orally once daily*
	CrCL 30–49 mL/min	*750 mg orally once daily; max 1,500 mg/day*
	CrCL <30 mL/min	*500 mg orally once daily; max 1,000 mg/day*
Alternative adjustment:	*GFR >50 mL/min*	*1,000 mg orally once daily*
	GFR 10–50 mL/min	*500–1,000 mg once daily (0–50 % decrease)*
	GFR <10 mL/min	*500–1,000 mg once daily (0–50 % decrease)*
	Hemodialysis	*1,000 mg orally once daily*
	CAPD	*Data not available*
	CRRT	*Not applicable; preferably avoid*

Dosage Adjustment of Medications Eliminated by the Kidneys

Nadolol - Selected References

Beaufils M. Alterations in renal hemodynamics during chronic and acute beta-blockade in humans. Am J Hypertens. 1989;2(2 Suppl):233–6S.

Borchard U. Pharmacokinetics of beta-adrenoceptor blocking agents: clinical significance of hepatic and/or renal clearance. Clin Physiol Biochem. 1990;8(Suppl 2):28–34.

Buice RG, Subramanian VS, Duchin KL, Uko-Nne S. Bioequivalence of a high variable drug: an experience with nadolol. Pharm Res. 1996;13:1109–15.

Corgard® tablet [package insert]. Bristol: King Pharmaceuticals Inc; 2011.

Dreyfuss J, Griffith DL, Singhvi SM, et al. Pharmacokinetics of nadolol, a beta-receptor antagonist: administration of therapeutic single- and multiple-dosage regimens to hypertensive patients. J Clin Pharmacol. 1979;19:712–20.

Dupont AG, Vandrniepen P, Bossuyt AM, Jonckheer MH, Six RO. Nadolol in essential hypertension: effect on ambulatory blood pressure, renal haemodynamics and cardiac function. Br J Clin Pharmacol. 1985;20:93–9.

Fallo F, Gregianin M, Bui F, Macri C, Folino P, Mantero F. Comparison of the antihypertensive and renal effects of tertatolol and nadolol in hypertensive patients with mild renal impairment. Eur J Clin Pharmacol. 1991;40:309–11.

Frolich ED, Messerli FH, Deslinski GR. Long-term renal hemodynamic effects of nadolol in patients with essential hypertension. Am Heart J. 1984;108:1141–3.

Herrera J, Vukovich RA, Griffith DL. Elimination of nadolol by patients with renal impairment. Br J Clin Pharmacol. 1979;7(Suppl 2):227–31S.

Hollenberg NK. The kidney and strategies for the treatment of hypertension. Am J Med. 1984;77(Suppl 4A):60–3.

Kostis JB, Lacy CR, Krieger SD, Cosgrove NM. Atenolol, nadolol, and pindolol in angina pectoris on effort: effect on pharmacokinetics. Am Heart J. 1984;108:1131–6.

Krukemyer JJ, Boudoulas H, Binkley PF, Lima JJ. Comparison of single-dose and steady-state nadolol plasma concentrations. Pharm Res. 1990;7:953–6.

Mancia G, Ferrari A, Pomidossi G, et al. Twenty-four-hour blood pressure profile and blood pressure variability in untreated hypertension and during antihypertensive treatment by once-a-day nadolol. Am Heart J. 1984;108:1078–83.

Michaels RS, Duchin KL, Akbar S, Meister J, Levin NW. Nadolol in hypertensive patients maintained on long-term hemodialysis. Am Heart J. 1984;108:1091–4.

Mitenko PA, McKenzie JK, Sitar DS, Penner SB. Nadolol antihypertensive effect and disposition in young and elderly adults with mild to moderate hypertension. Clin Pharmacol Ther. 1989;46:56–62.

Nowicki M, Miszczak-Kuban J. Nonselective beta-adrenergic blockade augments fasting hyperkalemia in hemodialysis patients. Nephron. 2002;91:222–7.

O'Callaghan WG, Laher MS, McGarry K, O'Brien E, O'Malley K. Antihypertensive and renal haemodynamic effect of atenolol and nadolol in elderly hypertensive patients. Br J Clin Pharmacol. 1983;16:417–21.

O'Connor DT, Barg AP, Duchin KL. Preserved renal perfusion during treatment of essential hypertension with the beta blocker nadolol. J Clin Pharmacol. 1982;22:187–95.

Pun KK, Yeung CK, Chan MK. Effects of nadolol and propranolol on renal function n hypertensive patients with moderately impaired renal function. Br J Clin Pharmacol. 1985;20:401–4.

Schäfer-Korting M, Bach N, Knauf H, Mutschler E. Pharmacokinetics of nadolol in healthy subjects. Eur J Clin Pharmacol. 1984;26:125–7.

Textor SC, Fouad FM, Bravo EL, Tarazi RC, Vidt DG, Gifford RW Jr. Redistribution of cardiac output to the kidneys during oral nadolol administration. N Engl J Med. 1982;307:601–5.

Valvo E, Gammaro L, Bedogna V, et al. Effects of Nadolol on systemic and renal renoparenchymal hypertension and various degrees of renal function. Int J Clin Pharmacol Ther Toxicol. 1986;24:202–6.

van Zyl A, Jennings AA, Byrne MJ, Opie LH. Effects of therapy on renal impairment in essential hypertension. S Afr Med J. 1992;82:407–10.

Waal-Manning HJ, Hobson CH. Renal function in patients with essential hypertension receiving nadolol. Br Med J. 1980;281:423–4.

Wood AJJ. Pharmacologic differences between beta blockers. Am Heart J. 1984;108:1070–9.

Dosage Adjustment of Medications Eliminated by the Kidneys

Nadolol/Corgard®	{Antihypertensive, vasodilator, angiotensin-converting enzyme (ACE)/renin inhibitor}

Usual initial dose:	40 mg orally
Usual maintenance dose:	40–120 mg orally once daily
Typical maximum dose:	320 mg/day
Proportion eliminated unchanged:	95 %

Adjustment for Kidney Disease

FDA-approved product labeling: *Nadolol dosage adjustment in renal failure*

CrCL (mL/min)	Dosage interval (h)
>50	24
31–50	24–36
10–30	24–48
<10	40–60

Alternative adjustment:

GFR >50 mL/min	40–240 mg orally once daily
GFR 10–50 mL/min	20–80 mg orally every 24 h (50 % decrease)
GFR <10 mL/min	10–40 mg orally every 24 h (~75 % decrease)
Hemodialysis	10–40 mg orally three times weekly after dialysis
CAPD	Data not available
CRRT	20–120 mg orally every 24 h (50 % decrease)

Dosage Adjustment of Medications Eliminated by the Kidneys

Nalidixic Acid - Selected References

Adam WR, Dawborn JK. Plasma levels and urinary excretion of nalidixic acid in patients with renal failure. Aust NZ J Med. 1971;2:126–31.

Alessio L, Morselli G. Occupational exposure to nalidixic acid [letter]. Br Med J. 1972;4:110–1.

Aronoff GA, Bennett WM, Berns JS, et al. Drug prescribing in renal failure: dosing guidelines for adults and children. 5th ed. Philadelphia: American College of Physicians; 2007.

Barbeau G, Belanger P-M. Pharmacokinetics of nalidixic acid in old and young volunteers. J Clin Pharmacol. 1982;22:490–6.

Bilsland D, Douglas WS. Sunbed pseudoporphyria induced by nalidixic acid [letter]. Br J Dermatol. 1990;123:547.

Boisvert A, Barbeau G. Nalidixic acid-induced photodermatitis after minimal sun exposure. Drug Intell Clin Pharm. 1981;15:126–7.

Boréus LO, Sundström B. Intracranial hypertension in a child during treatment with nalidixic acid. Br Med J. 1967;2:744–5.

Cuisinaud G, Ferry N, Pozet N, Zech PY, Sassard J. Nalidixic acid kinetics in renal insufficiency. Br J Clin Pharmacol. 1982;14:489–93.

Dan M, Aderka D, Topilsky M, Livni E, Levo Y. Hypersensitivity pneumonitis induced by nalidixic acid. Arch Intern Med. 1986;146:1423–4.

Dash H, Mills J. Severe metabolic acidosis associated with nalidixic acid overdose [letter]. Ann Intern Med. 1976;84:570–1.

Eijadi-Mood N, Gheshlagi F. Nalidixic acid overdose and metabolic acidosis [letter]. Can J Emerg Med. 2006;8:78.

Ferry N, Bernard N, Pozet N, et al. The effect of infinitesimal drug dilutions on the pharmacokinetics of nalidixic acid and atenolol. Br J Clin Pharmacol. 1991;32:39–44.

Fraser AG, Harrower ADB. Convulsions and hyperglycaemia associated with nalidixic acid. Br Med J. 1977;2:1518.

Garrett MH. "Negram" and photosensitivity reactions [letter]. Med J Aust. 1969;1:83.

Gedroyc W, Shorvon SD. Acute intracranial hypertension and nalidixic acid therapy. Neurology. 1982;32:212–5.

Goff JB, Schlegel JU, O'Dell RM. Urinary excretion of nalidixic acid, sulfamethoxazole and nitrofurantoin in patients with reduced renal function. J Urol. 1968;99:371–5.

Kremer L, Walton M, Wardle EN. Nalidixic acid and intracranial hypertension [letter]. Br Med J. 1967;4:488.

Jo M, Tachi N, Shinoda M. Convulsions from excessive dosage of nalidixic acid: a case report. Brain Dev. 1979;1:327–9.

Kilpatrick C, Ebeling P. Intracranial hypertension in nalidixic acid therapy [letter]. Med J Aust. 1982;1:252.

Leslie PJA, Cregeen RJ, Proudfoot AT. Lactic acidosis, hyperglycaemia and convulsions following nalidixic acid overdosage. Hum Toxicol. 1984;3:239–43.

Mandal BK, Stevenson J. Hæmolytic crisis produced by nalidixic acid [letter]. Lancet. 1970;1:614.

NegGram® tablet [package insert]. Bridgewater: Sanofi-Aventis US LLC; 2008.

Nogué S, Bertrán A, Mas A, Nadal P, Anguita A, Millá J. Metabolic acidosis and coma due to an overdose of nalidixic acid. Intensive Care Med. 1979;5:141–2.

Nomeir AA, Markham P, Rurka LT, Griffin RJ, Ghanayem BI. Species differences in the disposition and metabolism of nalidixic acid. J Pharmacol Exp Ther. 1996;279:222–30.

Palmer JM. Differential antibiotic excretion in unilateral structural pyelonephritis. West J Med. 1974;120:363–8.

Phillips PJ, Need AG, Thomas DW, Conyers RAJ, Edwards JB, Lehmann D. Nalidixic acid and lactic acidosis. Aust NZ J Med. 1979;9:694–6.

Poe TE, Marioni GS, Jackson DS. Seizures due to nalidixic acid therapy [letter]. South Med J. 1984;77:539–40.

Ramavat LG. Nalidixic acid (Negram) toxicity. Indian Pediatr. 1976;13:325.

Rubinstein A. LE-like disease caused by nalidixic acid [letter]. N Engl J Med. 1979;301:1288.

Suganthi AR, Ramanan AS, Pandit N, Yashwanth M. Severe metabolic acidosis in nalidixic acid overdosage. Indian Pediatr. 1993;30:1025–6.

Tafani O, Mazzoli M, Landini G, Alterini B. Fatal acute immune haemolytic anaemia caused by nalidixic acid. Br Med J (Clin Res Ed). 1982;285:936–7.

Vree TB, Hekster YA, Anderson PG. Contribution of the human kidney to the metabolic clearance of drugs. Ann Pharmacother. 1992;26:1421–8.

Dosage Adjustment of Medications Eliminated by the Kidneys

<u>Nalidixic Acid</u>/NegGram®   {Antibacterial; urinary antiseptic}

Usual initial dose: 1 g orally

Usual maintenance dose: 1 g orally four times daily

Typical maximum dose: 4 g/day

Proportion eliminated unchanged: 95 % (as parent drug, fully pharmacologically active hydroxylated and, in lesser proportions, inactive carboxylated metabolites)

Adjustment for Kidney Disease

FDA-approved product labeling: *This drug is known to be excreted by the kidney, and the risk of toxic reactions to this drug may be greater in patients with impaired renal function.*

SCr <300 μmol/L (3.6 mg/dL) or CrCL >20 mL/min	*1 g orally four times daily*
SCr ≥300 μmol/L (3.6 mg/dL) or CrCL ≤20 mL/min	*500 mg orally four times daily*

Alternative adjustment:

GFR >50 mL/min	*1 g orally four times daily*
GFR 10–50 mL/min	*Avoid due to risk of acute neurological and/or metabolic complications*
GFR <10 mL/min	*Avoid due to risk of acute neurological and/or metabolic complications*
Hemodialysis	*Avoid due to risk of acute neurological and/or metabolic complications*
CAPD	*Avoid due to risk of acute neurological and/or metabolic complications*
CRRT	*Not applicable; avoid*

Dosage Adjustment of Medications Eliminated by the Kidneys

Naproxen - Selected References

Aarbakke J, Gadeholt G, Høylandskjær A. Pharmacokinetics of naproxen after oral administration of two tablet formulations in healthy volunteers. Int J Clin Pharmacol Ther Toxicol. 1983;21:281–3.

Antilla M, Haataja M, Kasanen A. Pharmacokinetics of naproxen in subjects with normal and impaired renal function. Eur J Clin Pharmacol. 1980;18:263–8.

Bruno R, Iliadis A, Jullien I, et al. Naproxen kinetics in synovial fluid of patients with osteoarthritis. Br J Clin Pharmacol. 1988;26:41–4.

Calvo MV, Dominguez-Gil A, Muriel C. Pharmacokinetics of naproxen in patients with hypoprothrombinemia. Int J Clin Pharmacol Ther Toxicol. 1981;19:326–30.

Cohen A, Basch C. Steady state pharmacokinetics of naproxen in young and elderly healthy volunteers. Semin Arthritis Rheum. 1988;17(Suppl 2):7–11.

Dahl H. Naproxen (Naprosyn®) pharmacokinetics: therapeutical relevance and tolerance profile. Cephalgia. 1986;6(Suppl 4):69–75.

Elsinghorst PW, Kinzig M, Rodamer M, Holzgrabe U, Sörgel F. An LC-MS/MS procedure for the quantification of naproxen in human plasma: development, validation, comparison with other methods, and application to a pharmacokinetic study. J Chromatogr B Analyt Technol Biomed Life Sci. 2011;879:1686–96.

Franssen JJAM, Tan Y, van de Putte LBA, van Ginneken CAM, Gribnau FWJ. Pharmacokinetics of naproxen at two dosage regimens in healthy volunteers. Int J Clin Pharmacol Ther Toxicol. 1986;24:139–2.

Gøtzsche PC, Andreasen F, Egsmose C, Lund B. Steady state pharmacokinetics of naproxen in elderly rheumatics compared with young volunteers. Scand J Rheumatol. 1988;17:11–6.

Martinez R, Smith DW, Frankel LR. Severe metabolic acidosis after acute naproxen sodium ingestion. Ann Emerg Med. 1989;18:1102–4.

McVerry RM, Lethbridge J, Martin N, et al. Pharmacokinetics of naproxen in elderly patients. Eur J Clin Pharmacol. 1986;31:463–8.

Morris ME, Freer JP, Watson WA. Sulfate homeostasis. III. Effect of chronic naproxen or sulindac treatment on inorganic sulfate disposition in arthritic patients with renal impairment. Pharm Res. 1991;8:242–6.

Moyer S. Pharmacokinetics of naproxen sodium. Cephalgia. 1986;6(Suppl 4):77–80.

Naprosyn® tablet [package insert]. South San Francisco: Genentech USA Inc; 2010.

Runkel R, Chaplin MD, Sevelius H, Ortega E, Segre E. Pharmacokinetics of naproxen overdoses. Clin Pharmacol Ther. 1976;20:269–77.

Segre EJ. Naproxen metabolism in man. J Clin Pharmacol. 1975;15:316–23.

Sevelius H, Runkel R, Segre E, Bloomfield SS. Bioavailability of naproxen sodium and its relationship to clinical analgesic effects. Br J Clin Pharmacol. 1980;10:259–63.

Todd PA, Clissold SP. Naproxen: a reappraisal of its pharmacology and therapeutic use in rheumatic diseases and pain states. Drugs. 1990;40:91–137.

Upton RA, Buskin JN, Williams RL, Holford NH, Riegleman S. Negligible excretion of unchanged ketoprofen, naproxen, and probenecid in urine. J Pharm Sci. 1980;69:1254–7.

Upton RA, Williams RL, Kelly J, Jones RM. Naproxen pharmacokinetics in the elderly. Br J Clin Pharmacol. 1984;18:207–14.

van den Ouweland FA, Franssen MJAM, van de Putte LBA, Tan Y, van Ginneken CAM, Gribnau FWJ. Naproxen pharmacokinetics during active polyarticular inflammation. Br J Clin Pharmacol. 1987;23:189–93.

van den Ouweland FA, Jansen PAF, Tan Y, van de Putte LBA, van Ginneken CAM, Gribnau FWJ. Pharmacokinetics of high-dosage naproxen in elderly patients. Int J Clin Pharmacol Ther Toxicol. 1988;26:143–7.

Wang-Smith L, Fort J, Zhang Y, Sostek M. Pharmacokinetics and relative bioavailability of a fixed-dose combination of enteric-coated naproxen and non-enteric coated esomeprazole magnesium. J Clin Pharmacol. 2012;52:670–80. doi:10.1177/0091270011405500.

Watson WA, Freer JP, Katz RS, Basch C. Kidney function during naproxen therapy in patients at risk for renal insufficiency. Semin Arthritis Rheum. 1988;17(Suppl 2):12–6.

Dosage Adjustment of Medications Eliminated by the Kidneys

Naproxen/Aleve®, Naprosyn®   {**Anti-inflammatory; nonsteroidal anti-inflammatory drug**}

Usual initial dose: 500 mg

Usual maintenance dose: 250–500 mg orally twice daily

Typical maximum dose: 1,250 mg/day

Proportion eliminated unchanged: 1 % (~95 % of a dose is eliminated in urine as demethylated and glucuronidated conjugates)

Adjustment for Kidney Disease

    FDA-approved product labeling: *CrCL <30 mL/min*   *Not recommended*

    Alternative adjustment: *GFR 30–50 mL/min*   *125–250 mg orally twice daily, titrate carefully (50 % decrease)*

                                                       GFR <30 mL/min   *Limited data; preferably avoid due to risk for gastrointestinal and renal toxicity*

Dosage Adjustment of Medications Eliminated by the Kidneys

Naratriptan - Selected References

Amerge® tablet film coated. Research Triangle Park: GlaxoSmithKline LLC; 2010.

Bomhof MAM, Heywood J, Pradalier A, et al. Tolerability and efficacy of naratriptan tablets with long-term treatment (6 months). Cephalgia. 1998;18:33–7.

Christensen ML, Eades SK, Fuseau E, Kempsford RD, Phelps SJ, Hak LJ. Pharmacokinetics of naratriptan in adolescent subjects with a history of migraine. J Clin Pharmacol. 2001;41:170–5.

Connor HE, Feniuk W, Beattie DT, et al. Naratriptan: biological profile in animal models relevant to migraine. Cephalgia. 1997;17:145–52.

Ferrari MJ, Goadsby PJ, Roon KI, Lipton RB. Triptans (serotonin, 5-HT$_{1B/1D}$ agonists) in migraine: detailed results and methods of a meta-analysis of 53 trials. Cephalgia. 2002;22:633–58.

Fuseau E, Baille P, Kempsford RD. A study to determine the absolute bioavailability naratriptan [abstract]. Cephalgia. 1997;17:417.

Fuseau E, Webster C, Asgharnejad M, Huffman C. Factors affecting oral naratriptan pharmacokinetics in migraine subjects [abstract]. J Neurol Sci. 1997;150(Suppl):S33.

Fuseau E, Webster C, Asgharnejad M, Huffman C. Naratriptan oral pharmacokinetics in migraine subjects [abstract]. J Neurol Sci. 1997;150(Suppl):S33.

Gawel MJ, Worthington I, Maggisano A. A systematic review of the use of triptans in acute migraine. Can J Neurol Sci. 2001;28:30–41.

Gueorguieva I, Nestorov IA, Aarons L, Rowland M. Uncertainty analysis in pharmacokinetics and pharmacodynamics: application to naratriptan. Pharm Res. 2005;22:1614–26.

Haag G, Diener H-C, May A, et al. Self-medication of migraine and tension-type headache: summary of the evidence-based recommendations of the Deutsche Migräne und Kopfschmerzgesellschaft (DMKG), the Deutsche Gesellschaft für Neurologie (DGN), the Österreichische Kopfschmerzgesellschaft (ÖKSG) and the Schweizerische Kopfwehgesellschaft (SKG). J Headache Pain. 2011;12:201–17.

Jhee SS, Shiovitz T, Crawford AW, Cutler NR. Pharmacokinetics and pharmacodynamics of the triptan antimigraine agents: a comparative review. Clin Pharmacokinet. 2001;40:189–205.

Kempsford RD, Hoke JF, Huffman CS. The safety, tolerability and pharmacokinetics of oral naratriptan in healthy subjects [abstract]. Cephalgia. 1997;17:416–7.

Kempsford RD, Nicholls B, Lam R, Wintermute S. A study to investigate the potential interaction of naratriptan and dihydroergotamine [abstract]. Cephalgia. 1997;17:416.

Kempsford RD, Nicholls B, Lam R, Wintermute S. A study to investigate the potential interaction of naratriptan and ergotamine [abstract]. Cephalgia. 1997;17:416.

Klassen A, Elkind A, Ssgharnejad M, et al. Naratriptan is effective and well tolerated in the acute treatment of migraine. Results of a double-blind, placebo-controlled, parallel-group study. Headache. 1997;37:640–5.

Lambert GA. Preclinical neuropharmacology of naratriptan. CNS Drug Rev. 2005;11:289–316.

Maas HJ, Danhof M, Della Pasqua O. A model-based approach to treatment comparison in acute migraine. Br J Clin Pharmacol. 2006;62:591–600.

Mathew NT, Asgharnejad M, Peykamian M, et al. Naratriptan is effective and well tolerated in the acute treatment of migraine: results of a double-blind, placebo-controlled, crossover study. Neurology. 1997;49:1485–90.

Tfelt-Hansen P. Parenteral vs oral sumatriptan and naratriptan: plasma levels and efficacy in migraine. A comment. J Headache Pain. 2007;8:273–6.

Williams P, Kempsford R, Fuseau E, Dow J, Smith J. Absence of significant pharmacodynamic or pharmacokinetic interaction with naratriptan and sumatriptan co-administration [abstract]. Cephalgia. 1997;17:417.

Dosage Adjustment of Medications Eliminated by the Kidneys

Naratriptan/Amerge®   {**Anti-migraine; serotonin 5-HT$_3$ receptor antagonist**}

Usual initial dose:	2.5 mg orally taken with fluid
Usual maintenance dose:	2.5 mg orally taken with fluid. If the headache returns or if the patient has only partial response, the dose may be repeated once after 4 h.
Typical maximum dose:	5 mg/24 h
Proportion eliminated unchanged:	50 %

Adjustment for Kidney Disease

FDA-approved product labeling:	*Mild to moderate renal impairment*	*A lower starting dose should be considered; maximum daily dose should not exceed 2.5 mg/24 h.*
	CrCL <15 mL/min	*Contraindicated*
Alternative adjustment:	*Data not available*	

Nebivolol - Selected References

Ambrosio G, Flather MD, Böhm M, et al. β-Blockade with nebivolol for prevention of acute ischaemic events in elderly patients with heart failure. Heart. 2011;97:209–14.

Bystolic™ tablet [package insert]. St Louis: Forrest Laboratories Inc; 2010.

Cheng JWM. Nebivolol: a third-generation β-blocker for hypertension. Clin Ther. 2009;31:447–62.

Cheymol G, Poirier J-M, Carrupt P-A, et al. Pharmacokinetics of β-adrenoceptor blockers in obese and normal volunteers. Br J Clin Pharmacol. 1997;43:563–70.

Cheymol G, Woestenborghs R, Snoeck E, et al. Pharmacokinetic study and cardiovascular monitoring of nebivolol in normal and obese subjects. Eur J Clin Pharmacol. 1997;51:493–8.

Cohen-Solal A, Kotefcha D, van Veldhuisen DJ, et al. Efficacy and safety of nebivolol in elderly heart failure patients with impaired renal function: insights from the SENIORS trial. Eur J Heart Fail. 2009;11:872–80.

Duranay M, Kanbay M, Akay H, et al. Nebivolol improves renal function in patients who underwent angioplasty due to renal artery stenosis: a pilot study. Nephron Clin Pract. 2010;114:c213–7.

Georgescu A, Pluteanu F, Flonta M-L, Badila E, Dorobantu M, Popov D. The cellular mechanisms involved in the vasodilator effect of nebivolol on the renal artery. Eur J Pharmacol. 2005;508:159–66.

Himmelmann A, Hedner T, Snoeck E, Lundgren B, Hedner J. Haemodynamic effects and pharmacokinetics of oral *d*- and *l*-nebivolol in hypertensive patients. Eur J Clin Pharmacol. 1996;51:259–64.

Kalinowski L, Dobrucki LW, Szczepanska-Konkel M, et al. Third-generation β-blockers stimulate nitric oxide release from endothelial cells through ATP efflux: a novel mechanism for antihypertensive action. Circulation. 2003;107:2747–52.

Lefebvre J, Poirier L, Poirier P, Turgeon J, Lacourciere Y. The influence of CYP2D6 phenotype on the clinical response of nebivolol in patients with essential hypertension. Br J Clin Pharmacol. 2007;63:575–82.

McNeely W, Goa K. Nebivolol in the management of essential hypertension: a review. Drugs. 1999;57:633–51.

Toprak O, Cirit M, Tanrisev M, et al. Preventive effect of nebivolol on contrast-induced nephropathy in rats. Nephrol Dial Transplant. 2008;23:853–9.

Dosage Adjustment of Medications Eliminated by the Kidneys

Nebivolol/Bystolic™	{Antihypertensive; antianginal; β-adrenergic receptor blocker}

Usual initial dose:	5 mg orally
Usual maintenance dose:	5–20 mg orally once daily
Typical maximum dose:	40 mg/day
Proportion eliminated unchanged:	Nil (38–67 % of absorbed dose appears in urine as glucuronide metabolites in extensive and poor metabolizers, respectively)

Adjustment for Kidney Disease

FDA-approved product labeling:	*Severe renal impairment (CrCL <30 mL/min)*	*Initial dose 2.5 mg once daily; upward titration should be performed cautiously if needed.*
	Hemodialysis	*No data*
Alternative adjustment:	*Elderly patients*	*No dose adjustment needed*
	Hemodialysis	*Data not available*
	CRRT	*Data not available*

Dosage Adjustment of Medications Eliminated by the Kidneys

Neomycin - Selected References

Aguilera A, Gonzalez-Espinoza L, Codoceo R, et al. Bowel bacterial overgrowth as another cause of malnutrition, inflammation, and atherosclerosis syndrome in peritoneal dialysis patients. Adv Perit Dial. 2010;26:130–6.

Benjamin JB, Volz RG, Efficacy of a topical antibiotic irrigant in decreasing or eliminating bacterial contamination in surgical wounds. Clin Orthop Relat Res. 1984;184:114–7.

Bennett WM, Plamp CE, Parker RA, Gilbert DN, Houghton DC, Porter GA. Renal transport of organic acids and bases in aminoglycoside nephrotoxicity. Antimicrob Agents Chemother. 1979;16:231–3.

Davia JE, Siemsen AW, Anderson RW. Uremia, deafness, and paralysis due to antibiotic irrigating solutions. Arch Intern Med. 1970;125:135–9.

de Jong TPVM, Donckerwolcke RAMG, Boemers TM. Neomycin toxicity in bladder irrigation. J Urol. 1993;150:1199.

DiPiro JT, Patrias JM, Townsend RJ, et al. Oral neomycin and erythromycin base before colon surgery: a comparison of serum and tissue concentrations. Pharmacotherapy. 1985;5:91–4.

Ericsson CD, Duke JH Jr, Pickering LK. Clinical pharmacology of intravenous and intraperitoneal aminoglycoside antibiotics in prevention of wound infections. Ann Surg. 1978;188:66–70.

Förström L, Pirilä V. Cross-sensitivity with the neomycin group of antibiotics. Contact Dermatitis. 1978;4:312.

Garrison LW, Dutro MP. Ototoxicity from topical neomycin [letter]. Clin Pharm. 1982;1:301.

Gelman ML, Frazier CH, Chandler HP. Acute renal failure after total hip replacement. J Bone Joint Surg Am. 1979;61:657–60.

Gerharz EW, Weingartner K, Varga MS, Feiber H, Riedmiller H. Neomycin-induced perception deafness following bladder irrigation in patients with end-stage renal disease. Br J Urol. 1995;76:479–81.

Gilbert TB, Jacobs SC, Quaddoura AA. Deafness and prolonged neuromuscular blockade following single-dose peritoneal irrigation. Can J Anaesth. 1998;45:568–70.

Golightly LK, Branigan TA. Surgical antibiotic irrigations. Hosp Pharm. 1989;24:167–70.

Gruhl VR. Renal failure, deafness, and brain lesions following irrigation of the mediastinum with neomycin. Ann Thorac Surg. 1971;11:376–9.

Johnson CA. Hearing loss following the application of topical neomycin. J Burn Care Rehabil. 1988;9:162–4.

Kavanagh KT, McCabe BF. Ototoxicity of neomycin and vancomycin. Laryngoscope. 1983;93:649–53.

Kelly DR, Nilo ER, Berggren RB. Deafness after topical neomycin irrigation. N Engl J Med. 1969;280:1338–9.

Kunin CM, Chalmers TC, Leevy CM, Sebastyen SC, Lieber CS, Finland M. Absorption of orally administered neomycin and kanamycin with special reference to patients with severe hepatic and renal disease. N Engl J Med. 1960;262:380–5.

Manuel MA, Kurtz I, Saiphoo CS, Nedzelski JM. Nephrotoxicity and ototoxicity following irrigations of wounds with neomycin. Can J Surg. 1979;22:274–7.

Masur H, Whelton PK, Whelton A. Neomycin toxicity revisited. Arch Surg. 1976;111:822–5.

Matz GJ. Aminoglycoside cochlear toxicity. Otolaryngol Clin North Am. 1993;26:705–12.

Meakins JL, Allard J. Neomycin absorption following Clagett procedure for postpneumonectomy empyema. Ann Thorac Surg. 1980;29:32–5.

Nachamie BA, Siffert RS, Bryer MS. A study of neomycin instillation into orthopedic surgical wounds. JAMA. 1968;204:139–41.

Neo-Fradin® oral solution. Big Flats: X-Gen Pharmaceuticals; 2005.

Neomycin sulfate tablet [package insert]. Sellersville: Teva Pharmaceuticals USA; 2007.

Phongsamran PV, Kim JW, Abbott JC, Rosenblatt A. Pharmacotherapy for hepatic encephalopathy. Drugs. 2010;70:1131–48.

Pittinger CB, Eryasa Y, Adamson R. Antibiotic-induced paralysis. Anesth Analg. 1970;49:487–501.

Sharma BK, Smith EC, Rodriguez H, Pillay VKG, Gandhi VC, Dunea G. Trial of oral neomycin during peritoneal dialysis. Am J Med Sci. 1971;262:175–8.

Topical antiseptics and antibiotics. Med Lett Drugs Ther. 1977;19:83–4.

Waisbren BA, Spink WW. A clinical appraisal of neomycin. Ann Intern Med. 1950;33:1099–119.

Watson D. Pharmacist liability for injury resulting from use of neomycin irrigation [letter]. Am J Hosp Pharm. 1988;45:73–4.

Weinstein AJ, McHenry MC, Gavan TL. Systemic absorption of neomycin irrigating solution. JAMA. 1977;238:152–3.

Yao F-S, Seidman SF, Artusio JF Jr. Disturbance of consciousness and hypocalcemia after neomycin irrigation, and reversal by calcium and physostigmine. Anesthesiology. 1980;53:69–71.

Dosage Adjustment of Medications Eliminated by the Kidneys

<u>Neomycin</u>/Mycifradin®, Neo-Fradin®   {**Antibacterial; aminoglycoside**}

Usual initial dose:	500–1,000 mg orally
Usual maintenance dose:	500–1,000 mg orally four times daily
Typical maximum dose:	12 g/day
Proportion eliminated unchanged:	95 % (oral bioavailability ~4 % with normal gastrointestinal function; substantial systemic assimilation occurs from irrigation of open or enclosed wounds)

Adjustment for Kidney Disease

FDA-approved product labeling: *Systemic absorption of neomycin occurs following oral administration, and toxic reactions may occur. Patients treated with neomycin should be under close clinical observation because of the potential toxicity associated with use. Neurotoxicity (including ototoxicity) and nephrotoxicity following oral use of neomycin have been reported, even when used in recommended doses. The potential for nephrotoxicity, permanent bilateral auditory ototoxicity, and sometimes vestibular toxicity is present in patients with normal renal function when treated with higher doses of neomycin and/or for longer periods than recommended. Serial, vestibular, and audiometric tests, as well as tests of renal function, should be performed (especially in high-risk patients). The risk of nephrotoxicity and ototoxicity is greater in patients with impaired renal function.*

Alternative adjustment:

GFR >50 mL/min	*500 mg enterally every 6 h*
GFR ≤50	*Avoid (all routes of administration including oral) due to risk for oto- and nephrotoxicity*
Hemodialysis	*Avoid (all routes of administration including oral) due to risk for oto- and nephrotoxicity*
CAPD	*Avoid (all routes of administration including oral) due to risk for oto- and nephrotoxicity*
CRRT	*Avoid (all routes of administration including oral) due to risk for oto- and nephrotoxicity*

Dosage Adjustment of Medications Eliminated by the Kidneys

Neostigmine - Selected References

Aquilonius S-M, Hartvig P. Clinical pharmacokinetics of cholinesterase inhibitors. Clin Pharmacokinet. 1986;11:236–49.

Aronoff GA, Bennett WM, Berns JS, et al. Drug prescribing in renal failure: dosing guidelines for adults and children. 5th ed. Philadelphia: American College of Physicians; 2007.

Barber HE, Bourne GR. The pharmacokinetics of neostigmine and 3-hydroxyphenyltrimethylammonium in the rat: dose-dependent effects after portal vein administration. Br J Pharmacol. 1974;52:567–77.

Barber HE, Calvey TN, Muir KT. The relationship between the pharmacokinetics, cholinesterase inhibition and facilitation of twitch tension of the quaternary ammonium anticholinesterase drugs, neostigmine, pyridostigmine, edrophonium, and 3-hydroxyphenyltrimethylammonium. Br J Pharmacol. 1979;66:525–30.

Breen PJ, Doherty WG, Donati F, Bevan DR. The potencies of edrophonium and neostigmine as antagonists of pancuronium. Anaesthesia. 1985;40:844–7.

Burdfield PA, Calvey TN. Plasma clearance of neostigmine and pyridostigmine in rats with ligated renal pedicles. Eur J Pharmacol. 1973;24:252–5.

Calvey T, Wareing M, Williams NE, Chan K. Pharmacokinetics and pharmacological effects of neostigmine in man. Br J Clin Pharmacol. 1979;7:149–55.

Chan PCK, Tam SCF, Cheng IKP. Oral neostigmine and lymphatic absorption in a myasthenia gravis patient on continuous ambulatory peritoneal dialysis (CAPD). Perit Dial Int. 1990;10:93–6.

Clark RB, Brown MA, Lattin DL. Neostigmine, atropine, and glycopyrrolate: does neostigmine cross the placenta: Anesthesiology. 1996;84:450–2.

Cronnelly R, Stanski DR, Miller RD, Sheiner LB, Sohn YJ. Renal function and the pharmacokinetics of neostigmine in anesthetized man. Anesthesiology. 1979;51:222–6.

Di Costanzo A, Toriello A, Mannara C, Benvenuti C, Tadeschi G. Intranasal versus intravenous neostigmine in myasthenia gravis: assessment by computer analysis of saccadic eye movements. Clin Neuropharmacol. 1993;16:511–7.

Gencarelli PJ, Miller RD. Antagonism of ORG NC45 (vecuronium) and pancuronium neuromuscular blockade by neostigmine. Br J Anaesth. 1982;54:53–6.

Heier T, Clough D, Wright PMC, Sharma ML, Sessler DI, Caldwell JE. The influence of mild hypothermia on the pharmacokinetics and time course of action of neostigmine in anesthetized volunteers. Anesthesiology. 2002;97:90–5.

Husain MA, Roberts JB, Thomas BH, Wilson A. Metabolism and excretion of 3-hydroxyphenyltrimethylammonium and neostigmine. Br J Pharmacol. 1969;35:344–50.

Miller RD, Cullen DJ. Renal failure and postoperative respiratory failure: recurarization? Br J Anaesth. 1976;48:253–6.

Morris RB, Cronnelly R, Miller RD, Stanski DR, Fahey MR. Pharmacokinetics of edrophonium and neostigmine when antagonizing d-tubocurarine neuromuscular blockade in man. Anesthesiology. 1981;54:399–402.

Neostigmine methylsulfate injection [package insert]. Shirley: American Regent Inc; 2009.

Varin F, Couture J, Gao H. Determination of neostigmine in human plasma and cerebrospinal fluid by high-performance liquid chromatography with ultraviolet detection. J Chromatogr B Biomed Sci Appl. 1999;723:319–23.

Wilhite AO. Atropine facilitates neostigmine reversal of vecuronium-induced neuromuscular blockade [letter]. Anesthesiology. 1993;78:793.

Yeh M-K. Degradation kinetics of neostigmine in solution. Drug Dev Ind Pharm. 2000;26:1221–6.

Dosage Adjustment of Medications Eliminated by the Kidneys

Neostigmine/Prostigmin®	{Cholinergic muscle stimulant; acetylcholinesterase inhibitor}

Usual initial dose:	0.5–2 mg slow IV injection
Usual maintenance dose:	0.5–2 mg slow IV injection, repeated as necessary for reversal of nondepolarizing neuromuscular blockade
Typical maximum dose:	5 mg
Proportion eliminated unchanged:	50 %

Adjustment for Kidney Disease

FDA-approved product labeling:	*Mechanical obstruction of the urinary tract*	*Contraindicated*
Alternative adjustment:	*GFR >50 mL/min*	*0.5–2 mg slow IV injection*
	GFR 10–50 mL/min	*0.25–1 mg slow IV injection (50 % decrease)*
	GFR <10 mL/min	*0.125–0.5 mg slow IV injection (75 % decrease)*
	Hemodialysis	*0.125–0.5 mg slow IV injection (75 % decrease)*
	CAPD	*0.125–0.5 mg slow IV injection (75 % decrease)*
	CRRT	*0.25–1 mg slow IV injection (50 % decrease)*

Dosage Adjustment of Medications Eliminated by the Kidneys

Nitrofurantoin - Selected References

Abramowicz M, Zuccotti G, Pflomm J-M, et al. Handbook of antimicrobial therapy. 19th ed. New Rochelle: The Medical Letter; 2011.

Anderson J, Kopko F, Nohle EG, Siedler AJ. Intracellular accumulation of nitrofurantoin by rabbit renal cortical slices. Am J Physiol. 1969;217:1435–40.

Boileau MA, Corriere JN Jr, Liss RH. Visualization of bactericidal concentrations of nitrofurantoin macrocrystals in primate and human urinary tract tissue. J Urol. 1983;130:1010–2.

Bräunlich H, Bono A, Schröter S. Age-dependence of renal tubular reabsorption of nitrofurantoin. Arch Int Pharmacodyn Ther. 1978;232:92–101.

Buzard JA, Bender RC, Nohle EG, Humphrey DT, Paul MF. Renal tubular transport of nitrofurantoin. Am J Physiol. 1962;202:1136–8.

Drayer DE. Pharmacologically active drug metabolites: therapeutic and toxic activities, plasma and urine data in man, accumulation in renal failure. Clin Pharmacokinet. 1976;1:426–43.

Felts JH, Hayes Dm Gergen JA, Toole JF. Neural, hematologic and bacteriologic effects of nitrofurantoin in renal insufficiency. Am J Med. 1971;51:331–9.

Freeman RB, Richardson JA, Thurm RH, Griep RJ. Long-term therapy for chronic bacteriuria in men: US Public Health Service Cooperative Study. Ann Intern Med. 1975;83:133–47.

Furadantin® suspension [package insert]. Atlanta: Shionogi Pharma Inc; 2010.

Gilbert DN. Urinary tract infections in patients with chronic renal insufficiency. Clin J Am Soc Nephrol. 2006;1:327–331.

Goff JB, Schlegel JU, O'Dell RM. Urinary excretion of nalidixic acid, sulfamethoxazole and nitrofurantoin in patients with reduced renal function. J Urol. 1968;99:371–5.

Gong X-S. Transient acute renal failure due to nitrofurantoin poisoning. Pediatr Nephrol. 1999;13:936–7.

Hanlon JT, Aspinall SL, Semla TP, et al. Consensus guidelines for oral dosing of primarily renally cleared medications in older adults. J Am Geriatr Soc. 2009;57:335–40.

Hoener B-A, Patterson SE. Nitrofurantoin disposition. Clin Pharmacol Ther. 1981;29:808–16.

Kunin CM. Inappropriate medication use in older adults: does nitrofurantoin belong on the list for the reasons stated? [letter]. Arch Intern Med. 2004;164:1701.

Macrodantin® capsule [package insert]. Cincinnati: Procter & Gamble Pharmaceuticals Inc; 2009.

McGeown MG. Nitrofurantoin in chronic urinary tract infection associated with renal calculi. Br Med J. 1956;2:274–6.

Meyer MM, Meyer RJ. Nitrofurantoin-induced pulmonary hemorrhage in a renal transplant recipient receiving immunosuppressive therapy: a case report and review of the literature. J Urol. 1994;152:938–40.

Miller T. Scarring as a factor affecting the eradication of microorganisms from the kidney in pyelonephritis. Antimicrob Agents Chemother. 1983;23:500–2.

Miller T, Phillips S. Effects of physiological manipulations on the chemotherapy of experimentally induced renal infection. Antimicrob Agents Chemother. 1983;23:422–8.

Namagondlu G, Low SE, Seneviratne R, Banerjee A. Acute renal failure from nitrofurantoin-induced acute granulomatous interstitial nephritis. Q J Med. 2010;103:49–52.

Paul MF, Bender RC, Nohle E. Renal excretion of nitrofurantoin (Furadantin). Am J Physiol. 1959;197:580–4.

Sachs J, Geer T, Noell P, Kunin CM. Effect of renal function on urinary recovery of orally administered nitrofurantoin. N Engl J Med. 1968;278:1032–5.

Shah RR, Wade G. Reappraisal of the risk/benefit of nitrofurantoin: review of toxicity and efficacy. Adverse Drug React Acute Poisoning Rev. 1989;8:183–201.

Sullivan JW Bueschen AJ, Schlegel JU. Nitrofurantoin, sulfamethoxazole and cephalexin urinary concentration in unequally functioning pyelonephritic kidneys. J Urol. 1975;114:343–7.

White WT, Harrison L, Duman J II. Nitrofurantoin unmasking peripheral neuropathy in a type 2 diabetic patient. Arch Intern Med. 1984;144:821.

Woodruff MW, Malvin RL, Thompson IM. The renal transport of nitrofurantoin: effect of acid-base balance upon its excretion. JAMA. 1961;175:1132–5.

Zalmanovici Trestioreanu A, Green H, Paul M, Yaphe J, Leibovici L. Antimicrobial agents for treating uncomplicated urinary tract infection in women (review). Cochrane Database Syst Rev. 2010;(10):CD007182. doi:10.1002/14651858.CD007182.pub2.

Dosage Adjustment of Medications Eliminated by the Kidneys

<u>**Nitrofurantoin**</u>**/Macrodantin®, Macrobid®**   **{Antibacterial; urinary antiseptic}**

Usual initial dose:	100 mg orally
Usual maintenance dose:	50–100 mg orally every 6 h or 100 mg twice daily (long-acting monohydrate)
Typical maximum dose:	400 mg/day
Proportion eliminated unchanged:	47 %

Adjustment for Kidney Disease

FDA-approved product labeling:	*Anuria, oliguria, significant impairment of renal function (CrCL <60 mL/min or clinically significant elevated SCr)*	*Contraindicated*
Alternative adjustment:	*GFR ≥60 mL/min*	*50–100 mg orally every 6 h or 100 mg twice daily (long-acting monohydrate)*
	GFR 10–59 mL/min	*Usually ineffective; avoid*
	GFR <10 mL/min	*Ineffective; avoid*
	Hemodialysis	*Ineffective; avoid*
	CAPD	*Ineffective; avoid*
	CRRT	*Not applicable; avoid*

Dosage Adjustment of Medications Eliminated by the Kidneys

Nizatidine - Selected References

Abdel-Rahman SM, Johnson FK, Connor JD, et al. Developmental pharmacokinetics and pharmacodynamics of nizatidine. J Pediatr Gastroenterol Nutr. 2004;38:442–51.

Aronoff GA, Bennett WM, Berns JS, et al. Drug prescribing in renal failure: dosing guidelines for adults and children. 5th ed. Philadelphia: American College of Physicians; 2007.

Aronoff GA, Bergstrom RF, Bopp RJ, Sloan RS, Callaghan JT. Nizatidine disposition in subjects with normal and impaired renal function. Clin Pharmacol Ther. 1988;43:688–95.

Battaglia G, Di Mario F, Vigneri S, et al. Peptic ulcer in the elderly—a double-blind, short-term study comparing nizatidine 300 mg with ranitidine 300 mg. Aliment Pharmacol Ther. 1993;7:643–8.

Callaghan JT, Bergstrom RF, Rubin A, et al. A pharmacokinetic profile of nizatidine in man. Scand J Gastroenterol. 1987;22(Suppl 136):9–17.

Callaghan JT, Rubin A, Knadler MP, Bergstrom RF. Nizatidine, an H_2-receptor antagonist: disposition and safety in the elderly. J Clin Pharmacol. 1987;27:618–24.

Dammann HG, Gottlieb WR, Walter TA, Müller P, Simon B, Keohane P. The 24-hour acid suppression profile of nizatidine. Scand J Gastroenterol. 1987;22(Suppl 136):56–60.

Danziger L, Furmaga KM, Rodvold KA, Bombeck CT, Fischer JH. Nizatidine suppression of basal gastric acid output: a comparison of two intravenous dosage regimens. J Clin Pharmacol.1989;29:946–52.

Duroux P, Emde C, Bauerfeind P, Biollaz J, Arnstrong D, Blum L-L. Early evening nizatidine intake with a meal optimizes the antisecretory effect. Aliment Pharmacol Ther. 1993;7:47–54.

García Rodríguez LA, Wallander M-A, Johanson S, Björck S. Renal disease and acid-suppressing drugs. Pharmacoepidemiol Drug Saf. 1997;6:247–51.

Gladziwa U, Klotz U. Pharmacokinetics and pharmacodynamics of H2-receptor antagonists in patients with renal insufficiency. Clin Pharmacokinet. 1993;24:319–32.

Jamali F, Thomson ABR, Kirdeikis P, et al. Diurnal variation in the pharmacokinetics of nizatidine in healthy volunteers and in patients with peptic ulcer disease. J Clin Pharmacol.1995;35:1071–5.

Kovacs TOG, van Deventer GM, Maxwell V, Sytnik B, Walsh JH. The effect of an oral evening dose of nizatidine on nocturnal and peptone-stimulated gastric acid and gastrin secretion. Scand J Gastroenterol. 1987;22(Suppl 136):41–6.

Lackner TE, Heard T, Glunz S, Gann N, Babington M, Malone DC. Gastrointestinal disease control after histamine₂-receptor antagonist dose modification for renal impairment in frail chronically ill elderly patients. J Am Geriatr Soc. 2003;51:650–6.

Lin JH. Pharmacokinetic and pharmacodynamic properties of histamine H_2-receptor antagonists: relationship between intrinsic potency and effective plasma concentrations. Clin Pharmacokinet. 1991;20:218–36.

Nakano T, Kuroiwa T, Tsumita Y, et al. Aplastic anemia associated with initiation of nizatidine therapy in a hemodialysis patient. Clin Exp Nephrol. 2004;8:160–2.

Nizatidine capsule. Princeton: Sandoz Inc; 2011.

Pasanen M, Arvela P, Pelkonen O, Sotaniemi E, Klotz U. Effect of five structurally diverse H_2-receptor antagonists on drug metabolism. Biochem Pharmacol. 1986;35:4457–61.

Price AH, Brogden RN. Nizatidine: a preliminary review of its pharmacodynamic and pharmacokinetic properties, and its therapeutic use in peptic ulcer disease. Drugs. 1988;36:521–39.

Saima S, Echizen H, Yoshimoto K, Ishizaki T. Hemofiltrability of histamine H_2-receptor antagonist, nizatidine, and its metabolites in patients with renal failure. J Clin Pharmacol. 1993;33:324–9.

Sasaki M, Sudoh T, Fujimura A. Pharmacokinetics of ranitidine and nizatidine in very elderly patients. Am J Ther. 2005;12:223–5.

Schneck DW, Callaghan JT, Bergstrom RF, Obermeyer BD, Offen WW. Relationship between steady-state plasma nizatidine concentrations and inhibition of basal and stimulated gastric acid secretion. Clin Pharmacol Ther. 1990;47:499–503.

Simon B, Cremer M, Dammann HG, et al. 300 Mg nizatidine at night versus 300 mg ranitidine at night in patients with duodenal ulcer. Scand J Gastroenterol. 1987;22(Suppl 136):61–70.

Vargas R, Ryan J, McMahon FG, Regel G, Offen WW, Matsumoto C. Pharmacokinetics and pharmacodynamics of oral nizatidine. J Clin Pharmacol. 1988;28:71–5.

Dosage Adjustment of Medications Eliminated by the Kidneys

Nizatidine/Axid®   {Antacid; histamine H$_2$ receptor antagonist}

Usual initial dose: 300 mg orally

Usual maintenance dose: 150 mg orally twice daily or 300 mg orally at bedtime

Typical maximum dose: 300 mg/day

Proportion eliminated unchanged: 60 %

Adjustment for Kidney Disease

FDA-approved product labeling: *Nizatidine dosage in renal function impairment*

CrCL (mL/min)	Dosage	
	Active duodenal ulcer, GERD, benign gastric ulcer	Maintenance therapy
20–50	150 mg daily	150 mg every other day
<20	150 mg every other day	150 mg every 3 days

Alternative adjustment:

GFR >50 mL/min	150–300 mg orally at bedtime
GFR 10–50 mL/min	150 mg orally every 24–48 h
GFR <10 mL/min	150 mg orally every 48–72 h
Hemodialysis	150 mg orally every 48–72 h
CAPD	150 mg orally every 48–72 h
CRRT	Not applicable (consider IV histamine H$_2$ blocker)

Dosage Adjustment of Medications Eliminated by the Kidneys

Norfloxacin - Selected References

Alestig K. The pharmacokinetics of oral quinolones (norfloxacin, ciprofloxacin, ofloxacin). Scand J Infect Dis Suppl. 1990;68:19–22.

Aronoff GA, Bennett WM, Berns JS, et al. Drug prescribing in renal failure: dosing guidelines for adults and children. 5th ed. Philadelphia: American College of Physicians; 2007.

Arrigo G, Cavaliere G, D'Amico G, Passarella E, Broccali G. Pharmacokinetics of norfloxacin in chronic renal failure. Int J Clin Pharmacol Ther Toxicol. 1985;23:491–6.

Bergeron MG, Thabet M, Roy R, Lessard C, Foucault P. Norfloxacin penetration into human renal and prostatic tissues. Antimicrob Agents Chemother. 1985;28:349–50.

Boelaert J, de Jaegere PP, Daneels R, Schurgers M, Gordts B, van Landuyt HW. Case report of renal failure during norfloxacin therapy [letter]. Clin Nephrol. 1986;25:272.

Eandi M, Viano I, DiNola F, Leone L, Genazzani E. Pharmacokinetics of norfloxacin in healthy volunteers and patients with renal and hepatic damage. Eur J Clin Microbiol. 1983;2:253–9.

Eliopoulos GM. New quinolones: pharmacology, pharmacokinetics, and dosing in patients with renal insufficiency. Rev Infect Dis. 1988;10(Suppl 1):S102–5.

Fillastre JP, Hannedouche T, Leroy A, Humbert G. Pharmacokinetics of norfloxacin in renal failure [letter]. J Antimicrob Chemother. 1984;14:439.

Fillastre JP, Leroy A, Moulin B, Dhib M, Borsa-Lebas F, Humbert G. Pharmacokinetics of quinolones in renal insufficiency. J Antimicrob Chemother. 1990;26(Suppl B):51–60.

Hadimeri H, Almroth G, Cederbrant K, Eneström S, Hultman P, Lindell Å. Allergic nephropathy associated with norfloxacin and ciprofloxacin therapy. Scand J Urol Nephrol. 1997;31:481–5.

Hernandez Poblete G, Morales JM, Prieto C, Andrés A Ortuño T, Rodicio JL. Usefulness of norfloxacine prophylaxis in late recurrent urinary tract infection after renal transplantation [letter]. Nephron. 1990;54:193–4.

Holmes B, Brogden RN, Richards DM. Norfloxacin: a review of its antibacterial activity, pharmacokinetic properties and therapeutic use. Drugs. 1985;30:482–513.

Hughes PJ, Webb DB, Asscher AW. Pharmacokinetics of norfloxacin (MK 366) in patients with impaired kidney function—some preliminary results. J Antimicrob Chemother. 1984;13(Suppl B):55–7.

Kelly JG, Deaney NB, Lavan J, Noel J. Chronic dose urinary and serum pharmacokinetics of norfloxacin in the elderly. Br J Clin Pharmacol. 1988;26:787–90.

Lau AH, Fitzloff J, Jain R. Hemodialysis removal of norfloxacin. Chemotherapy. 1994;40:369–73.

Lomaestro BM. Fluoroquinolone-induced renal failure. Drug Saf. 2000;22:479–85.

MacGowan AP, Greig MA, Clarke EA, White LO, Reeves DS. The pharmacokinetics of norfloxacin in the aged. J Antimicrob Chemother. 1988;22:721–7.

Mandel L, Bergeron M, Marrie T, Scheifele D, Shafran S. Norfloxacin: a new quinolone. CMAJ. 1988;139:305–7.

Neuman M. Clinical pharmacokinetics of the newer antibacterial 4-quinolones. Clin Pharmacokinet. 1988;14:96–121.

Noroxin® tablet film coated [package insert]. Whitehouse Station: Merck Sharp & Dohme Corp; 2011.

Norrby SR, Ljungberg B. Pharmacokinetics of fluorinated 4-quinolones in the aged. Rev Infect Dis. 11(Suppl 5):S1102–6.

Ohta K-Y, Imamura Y, Okudaira N, Atsumi R, Inoue K, Yuasa H. Functional characterization of multidrug and toxin extrusion protein 1 as a facultative transporter for fluoroquinolones. J Pharmacol Exp Ther. 2009;328:628–34.

Renneberg J, Walder M. Postantibiotic effects of imipenem, norfloxacin, and amikacin in vitro and in vivo. Antimicrob Agents Chemother. 1989;33:1714–20.

Shimada J, Yamui T, Ueda Y, Uchida H, Kasajima H, Irikura T. Mechanism of renal excretion of AM-715, a new quinolonecarboxylic acid derivative, in rabbits, dogs, and humans. Antimicrob Agents Chemother. 1983;23:1–7.

Sörgel F, Kinzig M. Pharmacokinetics of gyrase inhibitors, part 2: renal and hepatic elimination pathways and drug interactions. Am J Med. 1993;94(Suppl 3A):56–69S.

Swanson BN, Boppana VK, Vlasses PH, Rotmensch HH, Ferguson RK. Norfloxacin disposition after sequentially increasing oral doses. Antimicrob Agents Chemother. 1983;23:284–8.

Dosage Adjustment of Medications Eliminated by the Kidneys

Norfloxacin/Noroxin®   {**Antibacterial; fluoroquinolone**}

Usual initial dose:	400 mg orally
Usual maintenance dose:	400 mg orally every 12 h
Typical maximum dose:	800 mg/day
Proportion eliminated unchanged:	30 %

Adjustment for Kidney Disease

FDA-approved product labeling:	*CrCL ≤30 mL/min*	*400 mg orally once daily*
Alternative adjustment:	*GFR >50 mL/min*	*400 mg orally every 12 h*
	GFR 10–50 mL/min	*400 mg orally every 12–24 h*
	GFR <10 mL/min	*400 mg orally every 24 h*
	Hemodialysis	*400 mg orally every 24 h*
	CAPD	*400 mg orally every 24 h*
	CRRT	*Not applicable (consider IV fluoroquinolone)*

O

L.K. Golightly et al. (eds.), *Renal Pharmacotherapy*,
DOI 10.1007/978-1-4614-5800-5_14, © Springer Science+Business Media New York 2013

Dosage Adjustment of Medications Eliminated by the Kidneys

Ofloxacin - Selected References

Bagon JA. Neuropsychiatric complications following quinolone overdose in renal failure [letter]. Nephrol Dial Transplant. 1999;14:1337.

De Bleecker JL, Vervaet VL, De Sarro A. Reversible orofacial dyskinesia after ofloxacin treatment. Mov Disord. 2004;19:731–2.

Dörfler A, Schulz W, Burkhardt F, Zichner M. Pharmacokinetics of ofloxacin in patients on haemodialysis treatment. Drugs. 1987;34(Suppl 1):62–70.

Fillastre JP, Leroy A, Humbert G. Ofloxacin pharmacokinetics in renal failure. Antimicrob Agents Chemother. 1987;31:156–60.

Flor S, Guay D, Opsahl J, Tack K, Matzke G. Pharmacokinetics of ofloxacin in healthy subjects and patients with varying degrees of renal impairment. Int J Clin Pharmacol Res. 1991;11:115–21.

Fuhrmann V, Schenk P, Mittermayer C, El Menyawi I, Ratheiser K, Thalhammer F. Single-dose pharmacokinetics of ofloxacin during continuous venovenous hemofiltration in critical care patients. Am J Kidney Dis. 2003;42:310–4.

Gilbert DN, Moellering RC Jr, Eliopoulos GM, Chambers HF, Saag MS. The sanford guide to antimicrobial therapy. 41st ed. Sperryville: Antimicrobial Therapy Inc; 2011.

Gusek A, Bren AF, Lindic J, Hergouth V, Mlinsek D. Is monotherapy with cefazolin or ofloxacin an adequate treatment for peritonitis in CAPD patients? Perit Dial Int. 1994;10:144–6.

Höffler D, Koeppe P. Pharmacokinetics of ofloxacin in healthy patients and patients with impaired renal function. Drugs. 1987;34(Suppl 1):51–5.

Kampf D, Borner K, Pustelnik A. Pharmacokinetics of ofloxacin and adequacy of maintenance dose for patients on haemodialysis. J Antimicrob Chemother. 1990;26(Suppl D):61–8.

Kampf D, Borner K, Pustelnik A. Multiple dose kinetics of ofloxacin and ofloxacin metabolites in haemodialysis patients. Eur J Clin Pharmacol. 1992;42:95–9.

Lameire N, Rosenkranz B, Malerczyk V, Lehr K-H, Veys N, Ringoir S. Ofloxacin pharmacokinetics in chronic renal failure and dialysis. Clin Pharmacokinet. 1991;21:357–71.

Lamp KC, Bailey EM, Rybak MJ. Ofloxacin clinical pharmacokinetics. Clin Pharmacokinet. 1992;22:32–46.

McMullin CM, Brown NM, Brown IM, et al. The pharmacokinetics of once-daily oral 400 mg ofloxacin in patients with peritonitis complicating continuous ambulatory peritoneal dialysis. J Antimicrob Chemother. 1997;39:829–31.

Molinaro M, Villani P, Regazzi MB, Rondanelli R, Doveri G. Pharmacokinetics of ofloxacin in elderly and in healthy young subjects. Eur J Clin Pharmacol. 1992;43:105–7.

Naber KG, Adam D, Kees F. *In vitro* activity and concentrations in serum, urine, prostatic secretion and adenoma tissue of ofloxacin in urological patients. Drugs. 1987;34(Suppl 1):44–50.

Ofloxacin tablet film coated [package insert]. Sellersville: Teva Pharmaceuticals USA; 2011.

Passlick J, Wonner R, Keller E, Essers L, Grabensee B. Single and multiple-dose kinetics of ofloxacin in patients on continuous ambulatory peritoneal dialysis. Perit Dial Int. 1989;9:267–72.

Rafat C, Vimont S, Ancel PY, et al. Ofloxacin: new applications for the prevention of urinary tract infections in renal graft recipients. Transplant Infect Dis. 2011;13:344–52.

Sanchez Navarro A, Martinez Lanao J, Sanchez Recio MM, et al. Effect of renal impairment on distribution of ofloxacin. Antimicrob Agents Chemother. 1990;34:455–9.

Thalhammer F, Kletzmayr I, Kovarik J, et al. Ofloxacin clearance during hemodialysis: a comparison of polysulfone and cellulose acetate hemodialyzers. Am J Kidney Dis. 1998;32:642–5.

Thomas RJ, Reagan DR. Association of a Tourette-like syndrome with ofloxacin. Ann Pharmacother. 1996;30:138–41.

Traeger SM, Bonfiglio MF, Wilson JA, Martin B, Nackes NA. Seizures associated with ofloxacin therapy. Clin Infect Dis. 1995;21:1504–6.

Vogt P, Schorn T, Frei U. Ofloxacin in the treatment of urinary tract infections in renal transplant recipients. Infection. 1988;16:175–8.

Walton GD, Hon JK, Mulpur TG. Ofloxacin-induced seizure. Ann Pharmacother. 1997;31:1475–7.

White LO, MacGowan AP, Lovering AM, Reeves DS, Mackay IG. A preliminary report on the pharmacokinetics of ofloxacin, desmethyl ofloxacin and ofloxacin N-oxide in patients with chronic renal failure. Drugs. 1987;34(Suppl 1):56–61.

White LO, MacGowan AP, Mackay IG, Reeves DS. The pharmacokinetics of ofloxacin, desmethyl ofloxacin and ofloxacin N-oxide in haemodialysis patients with end-stage renal failure. J Antimicrob Chemother. 1988;22(Suppl C):65–72.

Dosage Adjustment of Medications Eliminated by the Kidneys

<u>Ofloxacin</u>/Floxin®　　　　　{**Antibacterial; fluoroquinolone**}

Usual initial dose:	400 mg orally
Usual maintenance dose:	200–400 mg orally every 12 h
Typical maximum dose:	800 mg/day
Proportion eliminated unchanged:	80 %

Adjustment for Kidney Disease

FDA-approved product labeling:	*CrCL 20–50 mL/min*	*200–400 mg orally every 24 h*
	CrCL <20 mL/min	*100–200 mg orally every 24 h (half the usual recommended unit dose)*
Alternative adjustment:	*GFR >50 mL/min*	*200–400 mg orally every 12 h*
	GFR 10–50 mL/min	*200–400 mg orally every 12–24 h*
	GFR <10 mL/min	*200 mg orally every 24 h*
	Hemodialysis	*400 mg orally followed by 200–400 mg orally every 24 h; administer after hemodialysis on dialysis days.*
	CAPD	*400 mg orally followed by 200 mg orally once daily*
	CVVH	*400 mg orally every 8 h*

Dosage Adjustment of Medications Eliminated by the Kidneys

<u>Oprelvekin</u> - Selected References

Ault P, Kantarjian H, Welch MA, Giles F, Rios MB, Cortes J. Interleukin 11 may improve thrombocytopenia associated with imatinib mesylate therapy in chronic myelogenous leukemia. Leuk Res. 2004;28:613–8.

Berl T, Schwertschlag U. Preclinical pharmacologic basis for clinical use of rhIL-11 as an effective platelet-support agent. Oncology (Williston Park). 2000;14(Suppl 8):12–20.

Borbolla JR, López-Hernádez MA, DeDiego J, González-Avante M, Trueba E, Collados MT. Use of interleukin-11 after autologous stem cell transplant: report of three cases and a very brief review of the literature [letter]. Haematologica. 2001;86:891–2.

Bussel JB, Mukherjee R, Stone AJ. Pilot study of rhuIL-11 treatment of refractory ITP. Am J Hematol. 2001;66:172–7.

Cantor SB, Elting LS, Hudson DV Jr, Rubenstein EB. Pharmacoeconomic analysis of oprelvekin (recombinant human interleukin-11) for secondary prophylaxis of thrombocytopenia in solid tumor patients receiving chemotherapy. Cancer. 2003;97:3099–106.

Cotreau MM, Stonis L, Strahs A, Schwertschlag US. A multiple-dose, safety, tolerability, pharmacokinetics and pharmaco-dynamic study of oral recombinant human interleukin-11 (oprelvekin). Biopharm Drug Dispos. 2004;25:291–6.

Dykstra KH, Rogge H, Stone A, Loewy J, Keith JC Jr, Schwertschlag US. Mechanism and amelioration of recombinant human interleukin-11 (rhIL-11)-induced anemia in healthy subjects. J Clin Pharmacol. 2000;40:880–8.

Ellis M, Zwaan F, Hedström U, et al. Recombinant human interleukin 11 and bacterial infection n patients with haematological malignant disease undergoing chemotherapy: a double-blind placebo-controlled randomised trial. Lancet. 2003;361:275–80.

Ferrari S, Danova M, Porta C, et al. Recombinant human interleukin-11 (Neumega, rhIL-11) reduces thrombocytopenia in breast cancer patients receiving tandem autologous circulating progenitor cell transplantation. Ann Hematol. 2002;81:354–6.

Gordon MS, McCaskill-Stevens WJ, Battiato LA, et al. A phase I trial of recombinant human interleukin-11 (Neumega, rhIL-11 growth factor) in women with breast cancer receiving chemotherapy. Blood. 1996;87:3615–24.

Herlinger KR, Witthoeft T, Raedler A, et al. Randomized, double-blind controlled trial of subcutaneous recombinant human interleukin-11 versus prednisolone in active Crohn's disease. Am J Gastroenterol. 2006;101:793–7.

Isaacs C, Robert NJ, Bailery FA, et al. Randomized placebo-controlled study of recombinant human interleukin-11 to prevent chemotherapy-induced thrombocytopenia in patients with breast cancer receiving dose-intensive cyclophosphamide and doxorubicin. J Clin Oncol. 1997;15:3368–77.

Jung Y, Ahn H, Kim D-S, et al. Improvement of biological and pharmacokinetic features of human interleukin-11 by site-directed mutagenesis. Biochem Biophys Res Comm. 2011;405:399–404.

Montero AJ, Estrov Z, Freireich EJ, Hkouri IF, Koller CA, Kurzrock R. Phase II study of low-dose interleukin-11 in patients with myelodysplastic syndrome. Leuk Lymphoma. 2006;47:2049–54.

Neumega® injection [package insert]. Philadelphia: Wyeth Pharmaceuticals Inc subsidiary of Pfizer Inc; 2011.

Ong JP, Younossi ZM. Managing the hematologic side effects of antiviral therapy for chronic hepatitis C: anemia, neutropenia, and thrombocytopenia. Cleve Clin J Med. 2004;71(Suppl 3):S17–21.

Orazi A, Cooper RJ, Tong J, et al. Effects of recombinant human interleukin-11 (Neumega™ rhIL-11 growth factor) on megakaryocytopoiesis in human bone marrow. Exp Hematol. 1996;24:1289–97.

Trepicchio WL, Wang LL, Bozza M, Dorner AJ. IL-11 regulates macrophage effector function through the inhibition of nuclear factor-κB. J Immunol. 1997;159:5661–70.

Zondor SD, George JN, Medina PJ. Treatment of drug-induced thrombocytopenia. Expert Opin Drug Saf. 2002;1:173–80.

Dosage Adjustment of Medications Eliminated by the Kidneys

Oprelvekin/Neumega®	{**Thrombopoiesis stimulator; recombinant human interleukin 11; ℞ for severe thrombocytopenia**}

Usual initial dose:	50 mcg/kg subcutaneously
Usual maintenance dose:	50 mcg/kg subcutaneously once daily
Typical maximum dose:	100 mcg/kg/day
Proportion eliminated unchanged:	Low (metabolites predominantly excreted in urine; patients with severe renal impairment [CrCL ≤30 mL/min] attain blood levels two to three times greater and show clearance values less than half of those in normal subjects)

Adjustment for Kidney Disease

FDA-approved product labeling:	*CrCL <30 mL/min*	*25 mcg/kg subcutaneously once daily*
Alternative adjustment:	*Data not available*	

Dosage Adjustment of Medications Eliminated by the Kidneys

Oseltamivir - Selected References

Abdulkader RCRM, Ho YL, de Sousa Santos S, Caires R, Arantes MF, Andrade L. Characteristics of acute kidney injury in patients infected with the 2009 influenza A (H1N1) virus. Clin J Am Soc Nephrol. 2010;5:1916–21.

Abe M, Smith J, Urae A, Barrett J, Kinoshita H, Rayner CR. Pharmacokinetics of oseltamivir in young and very elderly subjects. Ann Pharmacother. 2006;40:1724–30.

Ariano RE, Sitar DS, Zelenitsky SA, et al. Enteric absorption and pharmacokinetics of oseltamivir in critically ill patients with pandemic (H1N1) influenza. CMAJ. 2010;182:357–63.

Callen EC, Kessler TL, Peace JF. Possible oseltamivir-induced angioedema in a patient with chronic renal failure. Hosp Pharm. 2011;46:591–5.

Choo D, Hossain M, Liew P, Chowdhury S, Tan J. Side effects of oseltamivir in end-stage renal failure patients. Nephrol Dial Transplant. 2011;26:2339–44.

Davies BE. Pharmacokinetics of oseltamivir: an oral antiviral for the treatment and prophylaxis of influenza in diverse populations. J Antimicrob Chemother. 2010;65(Suppl 2):ii2–10.

Dolley-Hitze T, Verdier M-C, Tribut O, Le Tulzo Y, Marqué S. Oseltamivir dose adjustment in an H1N1 patient requiring haemodialysis [letter]. Intensive Care Med. 2010;36:1618–9.

Eschenauer GA, Lam SW. Supratherapeutic oseltamivir levels during continuous dialysis: an expected risk [letter]. Intensive Care Med. 2011;37:371.

Gilbert DN, Moellering RC Jr, Eliopoulos GM, Chambers HF, Saag MS. The sanford guide to antimicrobial therapy. 41st ed. Sperryville: Antimicrobial Therapy Inc; 2011.

He G, Massarella J, Ward P. Clinical pharmacokinetics of the prodrug oseltamivir and its active metabolite Ro 64–0802. Clin Pharmacokinet. 1999;33:471–84.

Hill G, Cihlar T, Oo C, et al. The anti-influenza drug oseltamivir exhibits low potential to induce pharmacokinetic drug interactions vial renal secretion—correlation of in vivo and in vitro studies. Drug Metab Dispos. 2002;30:13–9.

Karkar A, Abdelrahman M, Jasim MR, Aloyouni W. H1N1 in dialysis units: prevention and management. Saudi J Kidney Dis Transplant. 2011;21:715–9.

Kute VB, Godara SM, Goplani KR, et al. High mortality in critically ill patients infected with 2009 pandemic influenza A (H1N1) with pneumonia and acute kidney injury. Saudi J Kidney Dis Transplant. 2011;22:83–9.

Li H, Wang S-X. Clinical features of 2009 pandemic influenza A (H1N1) virus infection in chronic hemodialysis patients. Blood Purif. 2010;30:172–7.

Marcelli D, Marelli C, Richards N. Influenza A (H1N1)v pandemic in the dialysis population : first wave results from an international survey. Nephrol Dial Transplant. 2009;24:3566–72.

Marfo K, Chapochnick-Friedmann J, Akalin E, Lu A. Postexposure prophylaxis of H1N1 with oseltamivir in a newly transplanted kidney recipient receiving intense immunosuppressive therapy. Transplant Proc. 2009;41:4411–3.

Rayner CR, Chanu P, Gieschke R, Boak LM, Jonsson EN. Population pharmacokinetics of oseltamivir when coadministered with probenecid. J Clin Pharmacol. 2008;48:935–47.

Rello J, Rodríguez A, Ibañenz P, et al. Intensive care adult patients with severe respiratory failure caused by influenza A (H1N1)v in Spain. Crit Care. 2009;13:R48. doi:10.1186/cc8044.

Robson R, Buttimore A, Lynn K, Brewster M, Ward P. The pharmacokinetics and tolerability of oseltamivir suspension in patients on haemodialysis and continuous ambulatory peritoneal dialysis. Nephrol Dial Transplant. 2006;21:2556–62.

Tamiflu® capsule and powder for suspension [package insert]. South San Francisco: Genentech USA Inc; 2011.

Veras de Sandes Freitas T, Ono G, Corréa L, et al. Clinical manifestations and evolution of infection by influenza A (HN) in kidney transplant recipients. J Bras Nefrol. 2011;33:136–41.

Watdharananan SP, Suwatanapongched T, Wacharawanichkul P, Chantratitaya W, Mavichak V, Mossad SB. Influenza A/H1N1 in kidney transplant recipients: characteristics and outcomes following high-dose oseltamivir exposure. Transpl Infect Dis. 2010;12:127–31.

Wattanagoon Y, Stepniewska K, Lindegårdh N, et al. Pharmacokinetics of high-dose oseltamivir in healthy volunteers. Antimicrob Agents Chemother. 2009;53:945–52.

Wiebe C, Reslerova M, Komenda P, Bueti J, Rigatto C, Sood MM. Atypical clinical presentation of H1N1 influenza in a dialysis patient. Lancet. 2009;374:1300.

Xi X, Xu Y, Jiang L, et al. Hospitalized adult patients with 2009 influenza A (H1N1) in Beijing, China: risk factors for hospital mortality. BMC Infect Dis. 2010;10:256. doi:10.1186/1471-2334-10-256.

Dosage Adjustment of Medications Eliminated by the Kidneys

<u>Oseltamivir</u>/Tamiflu®	{Antiviral; neuraminidase inhibitor; ℞ for influenza}		
Usual initial dose:	*75 mg orally*		
Usual maintenance dose:	*Influenza treatment*	75 mg orally every 12 h for 5 days	
	Influenza prophylaxis	75 mg orally once daily for ≥10 days	
Typical maximum dose:	*150 mg/day*		
Proportion eliminated unchanged:	10 % (as parent prodrug; 70 % of active de-esterified metabolite is excreted in urine)		

Adjustment for Kidney Disease

FDA-approved product labeling:	*CrCL 10–30 mL/min*	*Influenza treatment*	*75 mg orally once daily for 5 days*
	CrCL 10–30 mL/min	*Influenza prophylaxis*	*75 mg orally every other day or 30 mg every day*
	End-stage renal disease, hemodialysis, or peritoneal dialysis		*No recommended dosing recommendations available*
Alternative adjustment:	*GFR >50 mL/min*	*Influenza treatment*	*75 mg orally every 12 h (doses as high as 150 mg every 12 h have been tried in critically ill patients with influenza A/H1N1)*
		Influenza prophylaxis	*75 mg orally once daily*
	GFR 10–50 mL/min	*Influenza treatment*	*75 mg orally once daily*
		Influenza prophylaxis	*75 mg orally every other day*
	GFR <10 mL/min	*Data not available*	
	Hemodialysis	*Influenza treatment*	*30 mg orally daily on non-dialysis days or 75 mg after each dialysis (doses as high as 75 mg once or twice daily have been tried in critically ill patients with influenza A/H1N1)*
		Influenza prophylaxis	*75 mg orally every 5 days or 30 mg orally after each alternate dialysis session (limited data)*
	CAPD	*Influenza treatment*	*30 mg orally once or twice weekly*
		Influenza prophylaxis	*75 mg orally every 5 days (limited data)*
	CRRT	*Influenza treatment*	*75 mg enterally every 12 h (doses as high as 150 mg every 12 h have been tried in critically ill patients with influenza A/H1N1)*
		Influenza prophylaxis	*75 mg enterally once daily*

Oxacillin - Selected References

Abramowicz M, Zuccotti G, Pflomm J-M, et al. editors. Handbook of antimicrobial therapy. 19th ed. New Rochelle: The Medical Letter; 2011.

Aronoff GA, Bennett WM, Berns JS, et al. Drug prescribing in renal failure: dosing guidelines for adults and children. 5th ed. Philadelphia: American College of Physicians; 2007.

Baltch AL, Ritz WJ, Bopp, Michelsen PB, Smith RP. Antimicrobial activities of daptomycin, vancomycin, and oxacillin in human monocytes and of daptomycin in combination with gentamicin and/or rifampin in human monocytes and in broth against *Staphylococcus aureus*. Antimicrob Agents Chemother. 2007;51:1559–62.

Barza M, Kane A, Baum J. Ocular penetration of subconjunctival oxacillin, methicillin, and cefazolin in rabbits with staphylococcal endophthalmitis. J Infect Dis. 1982;145:899–903.

Barza M, Weinstock L. Pharmacokinetics of penicillins in man. Clin Pharmacokinet. 1976;1:297–308.

Fighali S, Strickman NE, Hall RJ. Congestive cardiomyopathy presumably secondary to oxacillin. Texas Heart Inst J. 1983;10:421–3.

Kampf D. Effects of mezlocillin on the pharmacokinetics of oxacillin and dicloxacillin. J Antimicrob Chemother. 1983;11(Suppl C):25–32.

Oxacillin injection [package insert]. Deerfield: Baxter Healthcare Corp; 2010.

Ruedy J. The effects of peritoneal dialysis on the physiological disposition of oxacillin, ampicillin and tetracycline in patients with renal disease. Can Med Assoc J. 1966;94:257–61.

Thijssen HHW, Mattie H. Active metabolites of isoxazolylpenicillins in humans. Antimicrob Agents Chemother. 1976;10:441–6.

Trotman RL, Williamson JC, Shoemaker M, Salzer WL. Antibiotic dosing in critically ill adult patients receiving continuous renal replacement therapy. Clin Infect Dis. 2005;41:1159–66.

Valentine RJ, Simon HJ, Rantz LA. Renal clearance of oxacillin. Proc Soc Exp Biol Med. 1964;115:1151–3.

Dosage Adjustment of Medications Eliminated by the Kidneys

Oxacillin/Prostaphlin® {Antibacterial; isoxazolyl penicillin}

Usual initial dose: 2 g IV

Usual maintenance dose: 500–2,000 mg IV every 4–6 h

Typical maximum dose: 12 g/day

Proportion eliminated unchanged: 45 %

Adjustment for Kidney Disease

FDA-approved product labeling: *Impaired renal function* *This drug is known to be excreted by the kidney, and the risk of toxic reactions to this drug may be greater in patients with impaired renal function. Because elderly patients are more likely to have decreased renal function, care should be taken in dose selection, and it may be useful to monitor renal function.*

Alternative adjustment: *GFR 5 to >50 mL/min* *500–2,000 mg IV every 4 h (no change)*

Hemodialysis *500–2,000 mg IV every 4 h (no change)*

CAPD *500–2,000 mg IV every 4 h (no change)*

CVVHD or CVVHDF *2 g IV every 4–6 h*

Oxaprozin - Selected References

Aronoff GA, Bennett WM, Berns JS, et al. Drug prescribing in renal failure: dosing guidelines for adults and children. 5th ed. Philadelphia: American College of Physicians; 2007.

Audet PR, Knowles JA, Troy SM, Walker BR, Morrison G. Effect of chronic renal failure on oxaprozin multiple-dose pharmacokinetics. Clin Pharmacol Ther. 1988;44:303–9.

Chiang ST, Knowles JA, Hubsher JA, Ruelius HW, Walker BR. Effects of food on oxaprozin bioavailability. J Clin Pharmacol. 1984;24:381–5.

Chiang ST, Morrison G, Knowles JA, Ruelius HW, Walker BR. Oxaprozin disposition in renal disease. Clin Pharmacol Ther. 1982;31:509–15.

Davies NM. Clinical pharmacokinetics of oxaprozin. Clin Pharmacokinet. 1998;35:425–36.

Daypro® caplet [package insert]. New York: GD Searle Division of Pfizer Inc; 2009.

Greenblatt DJ, Matlis R, Scavone JM, Blyden GT, Harmatz JS, Shader RI. Oxaprozin pharmacokinetics in the elderly. Br J Clin Pharmacol. 1985;19:373–8.

Hale VG, Bashaw ED. Pharmacokinetics of oxaprozin [letter]. Clin Pharm. 1993;12:255–6.

Janssen FW, Jusko WJ, Chiang ST, et al. Metabolism and kinetics of oxaprozin in normal subjects. Clin Pharmacol Ther. 1980;27:352–62.

Karim A. Inverse nonlinear pharmacokinetics of total and unbound drug (oxaprozin): clinical and pharmacokinetic implications. J Clin Pharmacol. 1996;36:985–97.

Karim A, Noveck R, McMahon G, et al. Oxaprozin and piroxicam, nonsteroidal antiinflammatory drugs with long half-lives: effect or protein-binding differences on steady-state pharmacokinetics. J Clin Pharmacol. 1987;37:267–78.

Kean WF. Oxaprozin: kinetic and dynamic profile in the treatment of pain. Curr Med Res Opin. 2004;20:1275–7.

Mitnik PD, Greenberg A, DeOreo PB, et al. Effects of two nonsteroidal anti-inflammatory drugs, indomethacin and oxaprozin, on the kidney. Clin Pharmacol Ther. 1980;28:680–9.

Todd PA, Brogden RN. Oxaprozin: a preliminary review of its pharmacodynamic and pharmacokinetic properties, and therapeutic efficacy. Drugs. 1986;32:291–312.

Dosage Adjustment of Medications Eliminated by the Kidneys

Oxaprozin/Daypro®   {Anti-inflammatory; nonsteroidal anti-inflammatory drug}

Usual initial dose: 600 mg orally

Usual maintenance dose: 1,200 mg orally once daily

Typical maximum dose: 1,800 mg/day

Proportion eliminated unchanged: 5 % (60 % of each dose as glucuronide metabolites)

Adjustment for Kidney Disease

FDA-approved product labeling:	*Renal function impairment*	*600 mg orally once daily; if there is insufficient relief of symptoms, the dose may be cautiously increased to 1,200 mg but only with close monitoring.*
	Hemodialysis	*600 mg orally once daily; if there is insufficient relief of symptoms, the dose may be cautiously increased to 1,200 mg but only with close monitoring.*
Alternative adjustment:	*GFR >50 mL/min*	*1,200 mg orally every 24 h*
	GFR 10–50 mL/min	*1,200 mg orally every 24 h*
	GFR <10 mL/min	*600 mg orally every 24 h (50 % decrease)*
	Hemodialysis	*600 mg orally every 24 h (50 % decrease)*
	CAPD	*Data not available*
	CRRT	*600 mg orally every 24 h*

Dosage Adjustment of Medications Eliminated by the Kidneys

Oxcarbazepine - Selected References

Andreasen A-H, Brøsen K, Damkier P. A comparative pharmacokinetic study in healthy volunteers of the effect of carbamazepine and oxcarbazepine on CYP3A4. Epilepsia. 2007;48:490–6.

Aronoff GA, Bennett WM, Berns JS, et al. Drug prescribing in renal failure: dosing guidelines for adults and children. 5th ed. Philadelphia: American College of Physicians; 2007.

Baruzzi A, Albani G, Riva R. Oxcarbazepine: pharmacokinetic interactions and their clinical significance. Epilepsia. 1994;35(Suppl 3):14–9.

Bring P, Ensom MHH. Does oxcarbazepine warrant therapeutic drug monitoring? A critical review. Clin Pharmacokinet. 2008;47:767–78.

Clinckers R, Smolders I, Meurs A, Ebinger G, Michotte Y. Quantitative in vivo microdialysis study on the influence of multidrug transporters on the blood-brain barrier passage of oxcarbazepine: concomitant use of hippocampal monoamines as pharmacodynamic markers for the anticonvulsant activity. J Pharmacol Exp Ther. 2005;314:725–31.

Dickinson RG, Hooper WD, Dunstan PR, Eadie MJ. First dose and steady-state pharmacokinetics of oxcarbazepine and its 10-hyroxymetabolite. Eur J Clin Pharmacol. 1989;37:68–74.

Flesch G, Czendlik C, Renard D, Lloyd P. Pharmacokinetics of the monohydroxy derivative of oxcarbazepine and its enantiomers after a single intravenous dose given as racemate compared to a single oral dose of oxcarbazepine. Drug Metab Dispos. 2011;39:1103–10.

French JA, Kanner AM, Bautista J, et al. Efficacy and tolerability of the new antiepileptic drugs. I: Treatment of new onset epilepsy: report of the Therapeutics and Technology Assessment Subcommittee and Quality Standards Subcommittee of the American Academy of Neurology and the American Epilepsy Society. Neurology. 2004;62:1252–60.

Lacerda G, Krummel T, Sabourdy C, Ryvlin P, Hirsch E. Optimizing therapy of seizures in patients with renal or hepatic dysfunction. Neurology. 2006;67(Suppl 4):S28–33.

Lloyd P, Flesch G, Dieterle W. Clinical pharmacology and pharmacokinetics of oxcarbazepine. Epilepsia 1994;35(Suppl 3):S10–3.

May TW, Korn-Merker E, Rambeck B. Clinical pharmacokinetics of oxcarbazepine. Clin Pharmacokinet. 2003;42:1023–42.

McKee PJW, Blacklaw J, Forrest G, et al. A double-blind, placebo-controlled interaction study between oxcarbazepine and carbamazepine, sodium valproate and phenytoin in epileptic patients. Br J Clin Pharmacol. 1994;37:27–32.

Pendlebury SC, Moses DK, Eadie MJ. Hyponatremia during oxcarbazepine therapy. Hum Toxicol. 1989;8:337–44.

Rouen MX, Lucaillion JB, Godbillon G, et al. The effect of renal impairment on the pharmacokinetics of oxcarbazepine and its metabolism and its metabolites . Eur J Clin Pharmacol. 1984;47:161–7

Sachdeo RC, Wasserstein A, Mesenbrink PJ, D'Souza J. Effects of oxcarbazepine on sodium concentration and water handling. Ann Neurol. 2002;51:613–20.

Tartara A, Galimberti CA, Manni R, et al. The pharmacokinetics of oxcarbazepine and its active metabolite 10-hydroxy-carbazepine in healthy subjects and epileptic patients treated with phenobarbitone or valproic acid. Br J Clin Pharmacol. 1993;36:366–8.

Theisohn M, Heimann G. Disposition of the antiepileptic oxcarbazepine and its metabolites in healthy volunteers. Eur J Clin Pharmacol. 1982;22:545–51.

Trileptal® tablet film coated and suspension [package insert]. East Hanover: Novartis Pharmaceutical Corp; 2011.

Van Amelswoort T, Bakshi R, Devaux CB, Schwabe S, Hyponatremia associated with carbamazepine and oxcarbazepine: a review. Epilepsia 1994;35(Suppl 3):S181–8a

van Heiningen PNM, Malcomlm DE, Ooserhuis B, et al. The influence of age on the pharmacokinetics of the antiepileptic agent oxcarbazepine. Clin Pharmacol Ther. 1991;50:410–9.

Volosov A, Xiaodong S, Perucca E, Yagen B, Sintov A, Bialer M. Enantioselective pharmacokinetics of 10-hydroxycarbazepine after oral administration of oxcarbazepine to healthy Chinese subjects. Clin Pharmacol Ther. 1999;66:547–53.

Wellington K, Goa KL. Oxcarbazepine: an update of its efficacy in the management of epilepsy. CNS Drugs. 2001;15:137–63.

Dosage Adjustment of Medications Eliminated by the Kidneys

__Oxcarbazepine__/Trileptal®	{__Antiepileptic; adjunctive analgesic; ℞ for bipolar disorder__}
__Usual initial dose:__	300 mg orally
__Usual maintenance dose:__	600 mg orally twice daily
__Typical maximum dose:__	2,400 mg/day
__Proportion eliminated unchanged:__	2–8 % (27 % of each dose is excreted in urine as 10-hydroxycarbazepine [MHD], the active monohydroxylated metabolite of oxcarbazepine)

Adjustment for Kidney Disease

__FDA-approved product labeling:__	*CrCL <30 mL/min*	*Initiate therapy with150 mg orally twice daily (300 mg/ day, half the usual dose) and increase slowly to achieve the desired clinical response.*
__Alternative adjustment:__	*GFR >50 mL/min*	*600 mg orally every 12 h*
	GFR 10–50 mL/min	*300–600 mg orally every 12 h (0–25 % decrease); monitor drug levels.[a]*
	GFR <10 mL/min	*300 mg orally every 12 h (50 % decrease); monitor drug levels.[a]*
	Hemodialysis	*300 mg orally every 12 h (50 % decrease); monitor drug levels.[a]*
	CAPD	*300 mg orally every 12 h (50 % decrease); monitor drug levels.[a]*
	CRRT	*300 mg orally every 12 h (50 % decrease); monitor drug levels.[a]*

[a]*__Therapeutic Drug Monitoring__*

__Therapeutic plasma levels:__	*Trough: 12–30 mg/L*

P

L.K. Golightly et al. (eds.), *Renal Pharmacotherapy*,
DOI 10.1007/978-1-4614-5800-5_15, © Springer Science+Business Media New York 2013

Dosage Adjustment of Medications Eliminated by the Kidneys

<u>Paliperidone</u> - Selected References

Arakawa R, Ito H, Takano A, et al. Dose-finding study of paliperidone ER based on striatal and extrastriatal dopamine D_2 receptor occupancy in patients with schizophrenia. Psychopharmacology (Berl). 2008;197:229–35.

Berecz R, Llerena A, de la Rubia A, et al. Relationship between risperidone and 9-hydroxyrisperidone plasma concentrations and CYP2D6 enzyme activity in psychiatric patients. Pharmacopsychiatry. 2002;35:231–4.

Boom S, Talluri K, Janssens L, et al. Single- and multiple-dose pharmacokinetics and dose proportionality of the psychotropic agent paliperidone extended release. J Clin Pharmacol. 2009;49:1318–30.

Caccia S. Biotransformation of post-clozapine antipsychotics: pharmacological implications. Clin Pharmacokinet. 2000;38:393–414.

Chwieduk CM, Keating GM. Paliperidone extended release: a review of its use in the management of schizophrenia. Drugs. 2010;70:1295–317.

de Leon J, Wynn G, Sandson NB. The pharmacokinetics of paliperidone versus risperidone. Psychosomatics. 2010;51:80–8.

Gahr M, Kölle MA, Schönfeldt-Lecuona C, Lepping P, Freudenmann RW. Paliperidone extended-release: does it have a place in antipsychotic therapy? Drug Des Devel Ther. 2011;5:125–46.

Gopal S, Gassmann-Mayer C, Samtani MN, Shiwach R, Alphs L. Practical guidance for dosing and switching paliperidone palmitate treatment in patients with schizophrenia. Curr Med Res Opin. 2010;26:377–87.

Invega® extended release tablet [package insert]. Titusville: Janssen Pharmaceuticals Inc; 2011.

Invega® Sustenna® injection [package insert]. Titusville: Janssen Division of Ortho-McNeil-Pharmaceuticals Inc; 2011.

Mannens G, Huang M-L, Meuldermans W, Hendrickx J, Woestenborghs, Heykants J. Absorption, metabolism, and excretion of risperidone in humans. Drug Metab Dispos. 1993;21:1134–41.

Mathot F, van Beijsterveldt L, Préat V, Brewster M, Ariën A. Intestinal uptake and biodistribution of novel polymeric micelles after oral administration. J Control Release. 2006;111:47–55.

Maxwell RA, Sweet RA, Mulsant BH, et al. Risperidone and 9-hydroxyrisperidone concentrations are not dependent on age or creatinine clearance among elderly subjects. J Geriatr Psychiatry Neurol. 2002;15:77–81.

Nazirizadeh Y, Vogel F, Bader W, et al. Serum concentrations of paliperidone versus risperidone and clinical effects. Eur J Clin Pharmacol. 2010;66:797–803.

Railton CJ, Kapur B, Koren G. Subtherapeutic risperidone serum concentrations in an adolescent during hemodialysis: a pharmacological puzzle. Ther Drug Monit. 2005;27:558–61.

Samtani MN, Vermeulen A, Stuyckens K. Population pharmacokinetics of intramuscular paliperidone palmitate in patients with schizophrenia: a novel once-monthly, long-acting formulation of an atypical antipsychotic. Clin Pharmacokinet. 2009;48:585–600.

Sheehan JJ, Sliwa JK, Amatniek JC, Grinspan A, Canuso CM. Atypical antipsychotic metabolism and excretion. Curr Drug Metab. 2010;11:516–25.

Tianmei S, Liang S, Yi L, Yun'Ai S, Chunmei G, Hongyan Z. Single-dose pharmacokinetics of paliperidone extended-release tablets in healthy Chinese subjects. Hum Psychopharmacol. 2010;25:404–9.

Varmeir M, Naessens I, Remmerie B, et al. Absorption, metabolism, and excretion of paliperidone, a new monoaminergic antagonist, in humans. Drug Metab Dispos. 2008;36:769–79.

Vermeulen A, Piotrovsky V, Ludwig EA. Population pharmacokinetics of risperidone and 9-hydroxyrisperidone in patients with acute episodes associated with bipolar I disorder. J Pharmacokinet Biopharm. 2006;34:183–206.

Zhu H-J, Wang J-S, Markowitz JS, Donovan JL, Gibson BB, DeVane CL. Risperidone and paliperidone inhibit P-glycoprotein activity in vitro. Neuropsychopharmacology. 2007;32:757–64.

Dosage Adjustment of Medications Eliminated by the Kidneys

<u>Paliperidone</u>/Invega®   {Atypical antipsychotic; benzisoxazole derivative}

Usual initial dose: 3 mg orally or 234 mg intramuscularly (extended-release intramuscular suspension) followed by 156 mg intramuscularly 1 week later

Usual maintenance dose: 6 mg orally once daily or 117 mg intramuscularly (extended-release intramuscular suspension) once monthly

Typical maximum dose: 12 mg/day orally

Proportion eliminated unchanged: 59 %

Adjustment for Kidney Disease

    FDA-approved product labeling: *Dosing must be individualized according to the patient's individual renal function status.*

CrCL ≥50–<80 mL/min	*3 mg orally once daily initially; max 6 mg daily or 156 mg intramuscularly on treatment day 1 followed by 117 mg intramuscularly 1 week later, then 78 mg intramuscularly once monthly.*
CrCL ≥10–<50 mL/min	*1.5 mg orally once daily initially; max 3 mg daily. Intramuscular use is not recommended.*
CrCL <10 mL/min	*Use not recommended.*

    Alternative adjustment: *Data not available.*

Dosage Adjustment of Medications Eliminated by the Kidneys

Pamidronate - Selected References

Aredia® injection [package insert]. East Hanover: Novartis Pharmaceuticals Corp; 2011.

Berenson JR, Lichtenstein A, Porter L, et al. Efficacy of pamidronate in reducing skeletal events in patients with advanced multiple myeloma. N Engl J Med. 1996;334:488–93.

Berenson JR, Rosen L, Vescio R, et al. Pharmacokinetics of pamidronate disodium in patients with cancer with normal or impaired renal function. J Clin Pharmacol. 1997;37:285–90.

Buttazzoni M, Rosa Diez GJK, Jager V, Crucelegui MS, Algranati SL, Plantalech L. Elimination and clearance of pamidronate by haemodialysis. Nephrology (Carlton). 2006;11:197–200.

Coco M, Glicklich D, Faugere MC, et al. Prevention of bone loss in renal transplant recipients: a prospective, randomized trial of intravenous pamidronate. J Am Soc Nephrol. 2003;14:2669–76.

Cremers S, Sparidans R, den Hartigh J, Hamdy N, Vermeij P, Papapoulos S. A pharmacokinetic and pharmacodynamic model for intravenous bisphosphonate (pamidronate) in osteoporosis. Eur J Clin Pharmacol. 2002;57:883–90.

Czosnowski LM, Hudson JQ, Canada RB. Hypercalcemia associated with tertiary hyperparathyroidism managed conservatively with pamidronate in a hemodialysis patient. Am J Med Sci. 2009;337:300–1.

Davenport A, Goel S, Mackenzie JC. Treatment of hypercalcaemia with pamidronate in patients with end stage renal failure. Scand J Urol Nephrol. 1993;27:447–51.

Fan SL-S, Kumar S, Cunningham J. Long-term effects on bone mineral density of pamidronate given at the time of renal transplantation. Kidney Int. 2003;63:2275–9.

Fenton AJ, Gutteridge DH, Kent GN, et al. Intravenous aminobisphosphonate in Paget's disease: clinical, biochemical, histomorphometric and radiological responses. Clin Endocrinol (Oxf). 1991;34:197–204.

Gimsing P, Carlson K, Turesson I, et al. Effect of pamidronate 30 mg versus 90 mg on physical function in patients with newly diagnosed multiple myeloma (Nordic Myeloma Study Group): a double-blind, randomised controlled trial. Lancet Oncol. 2010;11:973–82.

Henley D, Kaye J, Walsh J, Cull G. Symptomatic hypocalcemia and renal impairment associated with bisphosphonate treatment in patients with multiple myeloma. Intern Med J. 2005;35:726–8.

Kyle RA, Yee GC, Somerfield MR, et al. American Society of Clinical Oncology 2007 Clinical Practice Guideline update the role of bisphosphonates in multiple myeloma. J Clin Oncol. 2007;25:2464–72.

Lomashvili KA, Monier-Faugere M-C, Wang X, Malluche HH, O'Neill WC. Effect of bisphosphonates on vascular calcification and bone metabolism in experimental renal failure. Kidney Int. 2009;75:617–25.

Machado CE, Flombaum CD. Safety of pamidronate in patients with renal failure and hypercalcemia. Clin Nephrol. 1996;45:175–9.

Mhaskar R, Redzepovic J, Wheatley K, et al. Bisphosphonates in multiple myeloma (review). Cochrane Database Syst Rev. 2010;(3):CD003188. doi:10.1002/14651858.CD003188.pub2.

Nagahama M, Sica DA. Pamidronate-induced kidney injury in a patient with metastatic breast cancer. Am J Med Sci. 2009;338:225–8.

Smetana S, Michlin A, Rosenman E, Biro A, Boaz M, Katzir Z. Pamidronate-induced nephrotoxic tubular necrosis—a case report. Clin Nephrol. 2004;61:63–7.

Tanvetyanon T, Stiff PJ. Management of the adverse effects associated with intravenous bisphosphonates. Ann Oncol. 2006;17:897–907.

Terpos E, Moulopoulos LA, Dimopoulos MA. Advances in imaging and the management of myeloma bone disease. J Clin Oncol. 2011;29:1907–15.

Terpos E, Sezer O, Croucher PI, et al. The use of bisphosphonates in multiple myeloma: recommendations of an expert panel on behalf of the European Myeloma Network. Ann Oncol. 2009;20:1303–17.

Torregrosa J-V, Fuster D, Monegal A, et al. Efficacy of low doses of pamidronate in osteopenic patients administered in the early post-renal transplant. Osteoporos Int. 2011;22:281–7.

Trimarchi H, Lombi F, Forrester M, et al. Disodium pamidronate for treating severe hypercalcemia n a hemodialysis patient. Nat Clin Pract Nephrol. 2006;2:459–63.

Yap AS, Hockings GI, Khafagi FA. Use of aminohydroxypropylidene bisphosphonate (AHPrBP, "APD") for the treatment of hypercalcemia in patients with renal impairment. Clin Nephrol. 1990;34:225–9.

Dosage Adjustment of Medications Eliminated by the Kidneys

Pamidronate/Aredia®	{Hypocalcemic agent; bisphosphonate}	
Usual initial dose:	60–90 mg IV over 2–24 h or (for Paget's disease) 30 mg IV over 4 h daily times 3 days	
Usual maintenance dose:	After a minimum 7-day recovery, the dose may be repeated once as 60–90 mg IV over 2–24 h or (for Paget's disease) 30 mg IV daily times 3 days. For osteolytic bone lesions of cancer, the recommended maintenance dose is 90 mg IV over 2–4 h every 3–4 weeks	
Typical maximum dose:	90 mg	
Proportion eliminated unchanged:	30–60 %	

Adjustment for Kidney Disease

FDA-approved product labeling:	*SCr >3.0 mg/dL or CrCL < 30 mL/min*	*Use not recommended*
	Following treatment, if SCr increases by >0.5 mg/dL if previously normal or >1.0 mg/dL if previously abnormal	*Withhold re-treatment until SCr has returned to within 10 % of the baseline value*
Alternative adjustment:	*eCrCL ≥ 30 mL/min*	*30–90 mg IV over 2–4 h or (for Paget's disease) 30 mg IV over 4 h daily times 3 days; recent long-term prospective trials have demonstrated generally better biochemical and clinical outcomes when doses are limited to 30 mg IV over 2–4 h once monthly for up to 2 years in patients with multiple myeloma or 30 mg IV over 2 h approximately monthly for 2–4 doses in osteopenic patients following renal transplantation*
	eCrCL <30 mL/min	*In extraordinary cases of acute hypercalcemia, discretionary administration of modest doses (e.g., 30 mg) of IV pamidronate in carefully selected and closely monitored patients has been successfully employed; nephrotoxicity has been reported as an infrequent but potentially serious complication*

Dosage Adjustment of Medications Eliminated by the Kidneys

Pancuronium - Selected References

Abrams RE, Hornbein TF. Inability to reverse pancuronium blockade in a patient with renal failure and hepatic disease. Anesthesiology. 1975;42:362–4.

Aronoff GA, Bennett WM, Berns JS, et al. Drug prescribing in renal failure: dosing guidelines for adults and children. 5th ed. Philadelphia: American College of Physicians; 2007.

Bennett MJ, Hahn JF. Potentiation of the combination of pancuronium and metocurine by halothane and isoflurane in humans with and without renal failure. Anesthesiology. 1985;62:759–64.

Berntman L, Rosberg B, Shweikh I, Yousef H. Atracurium and pancuronium in renal insufficiency. Acta Anaesthesiol Scand. 1989;33:48–52.

D'Hollander AA, Camu F, Sanders M. Comparative evaluation of neuro-muscular blockade after pancuronium administration in patients with and without renal failure. Acta Anaesthesiol Scand. 1978;22:21–6.

de Lemos JM, Carr RR, Shalandsky KF, Bevan DR, Ronco JJ. Paralysis in the critically ill: intermittent bolus pancuronium compared with continuous infusion. Crit Care Med. 1999;27:2648–55.

Duvaldestin P, Demetriou M, D'Hollander A. Pharmacokinetics of pancuronium in man: a linear system. Eur J Clin Pharmacol. 1982;23:369–72.

Duvaldestin P, Saada J, Berger JL, D'Hollander A, Desmonts JM. Pharmacokinetics, pharmacodynamics, and dose–response relationships of pancuronium in control and elderly patients. Anesthesiology. 1982;56:36–40.

Geha DG, Blitt CD, Moon BJ. Prolonged neuromuscular blockade with pancuronium in the presence of acute renal failure: a case report. Anesth Analg. 1976;55:343–5.

Gramstad L. Atracurium, vecuronium, and pancuronium in end-stage renal failure: dose–response properties and interaction with azathioprine. Br J Anaesth. 1987;59:995–1003.

Havill JH, Mee AD, Wallace MR, Chin LS, Rothwell RPG. Prolonged curarisation in the presence of renal impairment. Anaesth Intensive Care. 1978;6:234–8.

Kamvyssi-Dea S, Papadimitriou K, Dousaitou P. The use of pancuronium bromide in operations for renal insufficiency: case reports. Br J Anaesth. 1972;44:1217–8.

McLeod K, Watson MJ, Rawlins MD. Pharmacokinetics of pancuronium in patients with normal and impaired renal function. Br J Anaesth. 1976;48:341–5.

Miller RD, Agoston S, Booij LHDJ, Kersten UW, Crul JF, Ham J. The comparative potency and pharmacokinetics of pancuronium and its metabolites in anesthetized man. J Pharmacol Exp Ther. 1978;207:539–43.

Miller RD, Eger EI II. Early and late relative potencies of pancuronium and d-tubocurarine in man. Anesthesiology. 1976;44:297–300.

Miller RD, Stevens WC, Way WL. The effect of renal failure and hyperkalemia on the duration of pancuronium neuromuscular blockade in man. Anesth Analg. 1973;52:661–6.

Pancuronium bromide injection. Lake Forest: Hospira Inc; 2101.

Ramzan MI, Somogyi AA, Walker JS, Shanks CA, Triggs EJ. Clinical pharmacokinetics of the non-depolarizing muscle relaxants. Clin Pharmacokinet. 1981;6:25–60.

Rouse JM, Galley RLA, Bevan DR. Prolonged curarisation following renal transplantation: a retrospective study. Anaesthesia. 1977;32:247–51.

Rupp SM, Castagnoli KP, Fisher DM, Miller RD. Pancuronium and vecuronium pharmacokinetics and pharmacodynamics in younger and elderly patients. Anesthesiology. 1987;67:45–9.

Sinclair ME, Suter PM. Detection of overdosage of sedation in a patient with renal failure by the absence of lower oesophageal motility. Intensive Care Med. 1988;14:69–71.

Sirotzky L, Lewis EJ. Anesthesia related muscle paralysis in renal failure. Clin Nephrol. 1978;10:38–42.

Somogyi AA, Shanks CA, Triggs EJ. Clinical pharmacokinetics of pancuronium bromide. Eur J Clin Pharmacol. 1976;10:367–72.

Somogyi AA, Shanks CA, Triggs EJ. The effect of renal failure on the disposition and neuromuscular blocking action of pancuronium bromide. Eur J Clin Pharmacol. 1977;12:23–9.

Wood M, Stone WJ, Wood AJJ. Plasma binding of pancuronium: effects of age, sex, and disease. Anesth Analg. 1983;62:29–32.

Dosage Adjustment of Medications Eliminated by the Kidneys

<u>Pancuronium</u>/Pavulon®	{**Nondepolarizing neuromuscular blocker; paralyzing agent**}
Usual initial dose:	0.04–0.1 mg/kg
Usual maintenance dose:	0.01 mg/kg IV every 25–60 min or 0.2–0.6 mcg/kg/min continuous IV infusion; monitoring of muscle twitch response to a peripheral nerve stimulator is advised
Typical maximum dose:	0.15 mg/kg IV
Proportion eliminated unchanged:	40 %

Adjustment for Kidney Disease

FDA-approved product labeling: *The elimination half-life is doubled, and the plasma clearance is reduced by approximately 60 % in patients with renal failure. The volume of distribution is variable, and in some cases elevated. The rate of recovery of neuromuscular blockade, as determined by peripheral nerve stimulation, is variable and sometimes very much slower than normal. This information should be taken into consideration if pancuronium is selected, for other reasons, to be used in a patient with renal failure. To obtain maximum clinical benefits of pancuronium and to minimize the possibility of overdosage, the monitoring of muscle twitch response to a peripheral nerve stimulator is advised*

Alternative adjustment:

GFR >50 mL/min	*0.04–0.1 mg/kg IV every 25–60 min*
GFR 10–50 mL/min	*0.02–0.05 mg/kg IV every 25–60 min (50 % decrease)*
GFR <10 mL/min	*Preferably avoid due to risk for excessively prolonged neuromuscular blockade and paralysis*
Hemodialysis	*Preferably avoid due to risk for excessively prolonged neuromuscular blockade and paralysis*
CAPD	*Preferably avoid due to risk for excessively prolonged neuromuscular blockade and paralysis*
CRRT	*0.02–0.05 mg/kg IV every 25–60 min (50 % decrease)*

Dosage Adjustment of Medications Eliminated by the Kidneys

Paroxetine - Selected References

Aronoff GA, Bennett WM, Berns JS, et al. Drug prescribing in renal failure: dosing guidelines for adults and children. 5th ed. Philadelphia: American College of Physicians; 2007.

Bayer AJ, Roberts NA, Allen EA, et al. The pharmacokinetics of paroxetine in the elderly. Acta Psychiatr Scand Suppl. 1989;350:85–8.

Catterson ML, Preskorn SH. Pharmacokinetics of selective serotonin reuptake inhibitors: clinical relevance. Pharmacol Toxicol. 1996;87:203–8.

Chen W-C, Huang C-C, Huang C-J, et al. Mechanism of paroxetine-induced cell death in renal tubular cells. Basic Clin Pharmacol Toxicol. 2008;103:407–13.

Crowe CC, Gabriel GM. Treatment of anxiety and depression in transplant patients: pharmacokinetic considerations. Clin Pharmacokinet. 2004;43:361–94.

Dechant KL, Clissold SP. Paroxetine: a review of its pharmacodynamic and pharmacokinetic properties, and therapeutic potential in depressive illness. Drugs. 1993;41:225–53.

DeVane CL. Pharmacokinetics of the selective serotonin reuptake inhibitors. J Clin Psychiatry. 1992;53(2 Suppl):13–20.

Doyle GD, Laher M, Kelly JG, Byrne MM, Clarkson A, Zussman BD. The pharmacokinetics of paroxetine in renal impairment. Acta Psychiatr Scand Suppl. 1989;350:89–90.

Feng Y, Pollock BG, Ferrell RE, et al. Paroxetine: population pharmacokinetic analysis in late-life depression using sparse concentration sampling. Br J Clin Pharmacol. 2006;61:558–69.

Ghose K. The pharmacokinetics of paroxetine in elderly depressed patients. Acta Psychiatr Scand Suppl. 1989;350:87–8.

Haddock RE, Johnson AM, Langley DR, et al. Metabolic pathway of paroxetine in animals and man and the comparative pharmacological properties of its metabolites. Acta Psychiatr Scand Suppl. 1989;350:24–6.

Kaye CM, Haddock RE, Langley PF, et al. A review of the metabolism and pharmacokinetics of paroxetine in man. Acta Psychiatr Scand Suppl. 1989;350:60–75.

Koo J-R, Yoon J-Y, Joo M-H, et al. Treatment of depression and effect of antidepression treatment on nutritional status in chronic hemodialysis patients. Am J Med Sci. 2004;329:1–5.

Lawrence KM, De Paermentier F, Lowther S, Crompton MR, Kalona CLE, Horton RW. Brain 5-hydroxytryptamine sites labeled with [3H]paroxetine in antidepressant drug-treated depressed suicide victims and controls. J Psychiatry Neurosci. 1997;22:185–91.

Lundmark J, Thomsen IS, Fjord-Larsen T, et al. Paroxetine: pharmacokinetic and antidepressant effect in the elderly. Acta Psychiatr Scand Suppl. 1989;350:76–80.

McIntyre CW, Owen PJ. Prescribing drugs in kidney disease. In: Brenner BM. Brenner & Rector's the kidney. 8th ed. Philadelphia: Saunders/Elsevier; 2008. p. 1930–55.

Paxil® tablet film coated and suspension [package insert]. Research Triangle Park: GlaxoSmithKline; 2011.

Reis M, Åberg-Wistedt A, Ågren H, Höglund P, Åkerblad A-C, Bengtsson F. Serum disposition of sertraline, N-desmethylsertraline and paroxetine: a pharmacokinetic evaluation of repeated drug concentration measurements during 6 months of treatment for major depression. Hum Psychopharmacol. 2004;19:283–91.

Sindrup SH, Brøsen K, Gram LF. Pharmacokinetics of the selective serotonin reuptake inhibitor paroxetine: nonlinearity and relation to the sparteine oxidation polymorphism. Clin Pharmacol Ther. 1992;51:288–95.

Sindrup SH, Brøsen K, Gram LF, et al. The relation between paroxetine and the sparteine oxidation polymorphism. Clin Pharmacol Ther. 1992;51:278–87.

Sindrup SH, Grodum E, Gram LF, Beck-Nielsen H. Concentration-response relationship in paroxetine treatment of diabetic neuropathy symptoms: a patient-blinded dose-escalation study. Ther Drug Monit. 1991;13:408–14.

Tasker TCG, Kaye CM, Zussman BD, Link CGG. Paroxetine plasma levels: lack of correlation with efficacy or adverse events. Acta Psychiatr Scand Suppl. 1989;350:152–5.

Tsurutra T, Tanaka K, Ishikawa K, et al. Dialysis-associated increase in the saliva level of paroxetine [letter]. J Clin Psychopharmacol. 2009;29:19–20.

Tulloch IF, Johnson AM. The pharmacologic profile of paroxetine, a new selective serotonin reuptake inhibitor. J Clin Psychiatry. 1992;53(2 Suppl):7–12.

Dosage Adjustment of Medications Eliminated by the Kidneys

<u>Paroxetine</u>/Paxil®	{Antidepressant; selective serotonin reuptake inhibitor (SSRI)}

Usual initial dose: 20 mg orally

Usual maintenance dose: 20–40 mg orally once daily

Typical maximum dose: 60 mg/day

Proportion eliminated unchanged: 2 % (60 % of each dose is eliminated in urine as metabolites; metabolites that are not considered to contribute to clinical response vary in pharmacologic activity from similar to parent paroxetine [minor sulfate metabolite] to essentially inactive [the majority of glucuronidated metabolites])

Adjustment for Kidney Disease

FDA-approved product labeling: *Severe renal impairment—initial dose is 10 mg/day; increases may be made if indicated; dosage should not exceed 40 mg/day*

Alternative adjustment:

GFR >50 mL/min	*20–40 mg orally once daily*
GFR 10–50 mL/min	*10–30 mg/day orally (25–50 % decrease)*
GFR <10 mL/min	*10–20 mg/day orally (50 % decrease)*
Hemodialysis	*10–20 mg/day orally (50 % decrease)*
CAPD	*10–20 mg/day orally (50 % decrease)*
CRRT	*10–30 mg/day orally (25–50 % decrease)*

Dosage Adjustment of Medications Eliminated by the Kidneys

Peginterferon Alfa-2a - Selected References

Barril G, Quiroga JA, Sanz P, Rodriguez-Salvanés P, Selgas R, Carreño V. Pegylated interferon α2a kinetics during experimental haemodialysis: impact of permeability and pore size of dialyzers. Aliment Pharmacol Ther. 2004;20:37–44.

Berenguer M. Treatment of chronic hepatitis C in hemodialysis patients. Hepatology. 2008;48:1690–9.

Breilh D, Djabarouti S, Trimoulet P, et al. Ribavirin plasma concentration predicts sustained virological response to peginterferon alfa 2a plus ribavirin in previously treated HCV-HIV-coinfected patients [letter]. J Acquir Immune Defic Syndr. 2009;52:428–30.

Bressler B, Wang K, Grippo JF, Heathcote J. Pharmacokinetics and response of obese patients with chronic hepatitis C treated with different doses of PEG-IFN α2a (40KD) (PEGASYS®). Br J Clin Pharmacol. 2009;67:280–7.

Bruno R, Sacchi P, Ciappina V, et al. Viral dynamics and pharmacokinetics of peginterferon alpha-2a and peginterferon alpha-2b in naïve patients with chronic hepatitis C: a randomized, controlled study. Antivir Ther. 2004;9:491–7.

Bruno R, Sacchi P, Scagnolari C, et al. Pharmacodynamics of peginterferon alfa-2a and peginterferon alfa-2b in interferon-naïve patients with chronic hepatitis C: a randomized, controlled study. Aliment Pharmacol Ther. 2007;26:369–76.

Diago M, Crespo J, Pérez R, et al. Clinical trial: pharmacodynamics and pharmacokinetics of re-treatment with fixed-dose induction of peginterferon α-2a in hepatitis C virus genotype 1 true non-responder patients. Aliment Pharmacol Ther. 2007;26:1131–8.

Espinoza M, Arena MD, Aumente MD, et al. Anemia associated with pegylated interferon-α_{2a} and α_{2b} therapy in hemodialysis patients. Clin Nephrol. 2007;67:366–73.

Forestier N, Reesink HW, Weegink CJ, et al. Antiviral activity of telaprevir (VX-950) and peginterferon alfa-2a in patients with hepatitis C. Hepatology. 2007;46:640–8.

Ghany MG, Strader DB, Thomas DL, Seeff LB. American Association for the Study of Liver Diseases Practice Guidelines. Diagnosis, management, and treatment of hepatitis C: an update. Hepatology. 2009;49:1335–74.

Keating GM, Curran MP. Peginterferon-α-2a (40kD) plus ribavirin: a review of its use in the management of chronic hepatitis C. Drugs. 2003;63:701–30.

Lamb MW, Martin NE. Weight-based versus fixed-dosing of peginterferon (40kDA) alfa-2a. Ann Pharmacother. 2002;36:933–5.

Lawitz E, Rodriguez-Torres M, Muir AJ, et al. Antiviral effects and safety of telaprevir, peginterferon alfa-2a, and ribavirin for 28 days in hepatitis C patients. J Hepatol. 2008;49:163–9.

Motzer RJ, Rakhit A, Ginsberg M, et al. Phase I trial of 40-kd branched pegylated interferon alfa-2a for patients with advanced renal cell carcinoma. J Clin Oncol. 2001;19:1312–9.

Pegasys® injection [package insert]. South San Francisco: Genentech Inc; 2011.

Perry CM, Jarvis B. Peginterferon-α-2a (40kD): a review of its use in the management of chronic hepatitis C. Drugs. 2001;61:2263–88.

Reddy KR. Development and pharmacokinetics and pharmacodynamics of pegylated interferon alfa-2a (40 kD). Semin Liver Dis. 2004;24(Suppl 2):33–8.

Sulkowski MS, Shiffman ML, Afdhal NH, et al. Hepatitis C virus treatment-related anemia is associated with higher sustained virologic response rate. Gastroenterology. 2010;139:1602–11.

Yeong WJ, Youn YS, Lee HS, et al. Long-acting interferon-α 2a modified with a trimer-structured polyethylene glycol: preparation, in vitro bioavailability, in vivo stability and pharmacokinetics. Int J Pharm. 2006;309:87–93.

Zeuzern S, Heathcote JE, Marin N, Nieforth K, Modi M. Peginterferon alfa-2a (40 kDa) monotherapy: a novel agent for chronic hepatitis C therapy. Expert Opin Investig Drugs. 2001;10:2201–13.

Dosage Adjustment of Medications Eliminated by the Kidneys

Peginterferon Alfa-2a/Pegasys®   {Antiviral; interferon; ℞ for hepatitis C}

Usual initial dose: 180 mcg (1.0-mL vial or 0.5-mL prefilled syringe) subcutaneously

Usual maintenance dose: 180 mcg (1.0-mL vial or 0.5-mL prefilled syringe) once weekly for 48 weeks by subcutaneous administration in the abdomen or thigh or 800–1,200 mg administered orally in two divided doses

Typical maximum dose: 180 mcg/day subcutaneously or 1,200 mg/day orally

Proportion eliminated unchanged:

Adjustment for Kidney Disease

FDA-approved product labeling: *CrCL <50 mL/min*   *Use with caution; monitor for toxicity.*

End-stage renal disease requiring hemodialysis   *Dose reduction to 135 μg subcutaneously once weekly is recommended; monitor for toxicity.*

Note: Do not administer ribavirin to patients with CrCL <50 mL/min.

Alternative adjustment: *Hemodialysis*   *135 μg subcutaneously once weekly (with reduced dose ribavirin 200 mg orally once daily)*

Dosage Adjustment of Medications Eliminated by the Kidneys

Peginterferon Alfa-2b - Selected References

Berenguer M. Treatment of chronic hepatitis C in hemodialysis patients. Hepatology. 2008;48:1690–9.

Bonetti A, Kim S. Pharmacokinetics of an extended-release human interferon alpha-2b formulation. Cancer Chemother Pharmacol. 1993;33:258–61.

Bruchfeld A, Lindahl K, Reichard O, Carlsson T, Schvarcz R. Pegylated interferon and ribavirin for hepatitis C in haemodialysis patients. J Viral Hepat. 2006;13:316–21.

Bukowski R, Ernstaff MS, Gore ME, et al. Pegylated interferon alfa-2b treatment for patients with solid tumors: a phase I/II study. J Clin Oncol. 2002;20:3841–9.

Daud AI, Xu C, Hwu W-J, et al. Pharmacokinetic/pharmacodynamic analysis of adjuvant pegylated interferon α-2b in patients with resected high-risk melanoma. Cancer Chemother Pharmacol. 2011;67:657–66.

Di Bisceglie AM, Stoddard AM, Dienstag JL, et al. Excess mortality in patients with advanced chronic hepatitis C treated with long-term peginterferon. Hepatology. 2011;53:1100–8.

Dimova RB, Talal AH. Pharmacokinetic and pharmacodynamic modeling of pegylated-interferon alfa [editorial]. J Hepatol. 2010;53:418–20.

Espinoza M, Arena MD, Aumente MD, et al. Anemia associated with pegylated interferon-α_{2a} and α_{2b} therapy in hemodialysis patients. Clin Nephrol. 2007;67:366–73.

François C, Descamps V, Brochot E, et al. Relationship between the hepatitis C viral load and the serum interferon concentration during the first week of peginterferon-alpha-2b-ribavirin combination therapy. J Med Virol. 2010;82:1640–6.

García-García I, González-Delgado CA, Valenzuela-Silva CM, et al. Pharmacokinetic and pharmacodynamic comparison of two "pegylated" interferon alpha-2 formulations in healthy male volunteers: a randomized, crossover, double-blind study. BMC Pharmacol. 2010;10:15. doi:10.1186/1471-2210/10/15.

Ghany MG, Strader DB, Thomas DL, Seeff LB. American Association for the Study of Liver Diseases Practice Guidelines. Diagnosis, management, and treatment of hepatitis C: an update. Hepatology. 2009;49:1335–74.

Gupta SK, Pittenger AL, Swan SK, et al. Single-dose pharmacokinetics and safety of pegylated interferon-α2b n patients with chronic renal dysfunction. J Clin Pharmacol. 2002;42:1109–15.

Hashemi N, Rossi S, Navarro VJ, Herrine SK. Safety of peginterferon in the treatment of chronic hepatitis C. Expert Opin Drug Saf. 2008;7:771–81.

Jen JF, Glue P, Ezzet F, et al. Population pharmacokinetic analysis of pegylated interferon alfa-2b and interferon alfa-2b in patients with chronic hepatitis B. Clin Pharmacol Ther. 2001;69:407–21.

Noureddin M, Ghany MG. Pharmacokinetics and pharmacodynamics of peginterferon and ribavirin: implications for clinical efficacy in the treatment of chronic hepatitis C. Gastroenterol Clin North Am. 2010;39:649–58.

Pegintron® injection [package insert]. Whitehouse Station: Schering Corp subsidiary of Merck & Co; 2010.

Rostaing L, Chatelut E, Payen J-L, et al. Pharmacokinetics of αIFN-2b in chronic hepatitis C virus patients undergoing chronic hemodialysis or with normal renal function: clinical implications. J Am Soc Nephrol. 1998;9:2344–8.

Scott LJ, Perry CM. Interferon-α-2b plus ribavirin: a review of its use in the management of chronic hepatitis C. Drugs. 2002;62:507–56.

Shudo E, Ribiero RM, Perelson AS. Modelling hepatitis C virus kinetics during treatment with pegylated interferon α-2b: errors in the estimation of viral kinetic parameters. J Viral Hepat. 2008;15:357–62.

Shudo E, Ribiero RM, Perelson AS. Modelling the kinetics of hepatitis C virus RNA decline over 4 weeks of treatment with pegylated interferon α-2b. J Viral Hepat. 2008;15:379–82.

Sulkowski MS, Shiffman ML, Afdhal NH, et al. Hepatitis C virus treatment-related anemia is associated with higher sustained virologic response rate. Gastroenterology. 2010;139:1602–11.

Sylatron™ [package insert]. Kenilworth: Schering Corp; 2011.

Tsubota A, Hirose Y, Izumi N, Kumada H. Pharmacokinetics of ribavirin in combined interferon-alpha 2b and ribavirin therapy for chronic hepatitis C infection. Br J Clin Pharmacol. 2003;55:360–7.

Peginterferon Alfa-2b/
PEG-Intron®, Sylatron™   {Antiviral; interferon}

Usual initial dose:	Melanoma, 6 mcg/kg subcutaneously; Hepatitis C, 1 mcg/kg subcutaneously
Usual maintenance dose:	Melanoma: 6 mcg/kg subcutaneously once weekly for 8 doses followed by 3 mcg/kg subcutaneously once weekly for up to 3 years

Hepatitis C monotherapy for patients with compensated liver disease previously untreated with interferon alpha who are significantly intolerant of ribavirin or in whom contraindications exist (e.g., CrCL <50 mL/min): 1 mcg/kg subcutaneously once weekly for 52 weeks

Hepatitis C combination therapy: 1.5 mcg/kg subcutaneously once weekly with oral ribavirin given according to body weight for 48 weeks in patients with hepatitis C genotype 1 or who fail to achieve loss of hepatitis C RNA at 24 weeks or have previously failed therapy and 24 weeks in patients with hepatitis C genotypes 2 and 3

Typical maximum dose:	1.5 mcg/kg/week
Proportion eliminated unchanged:	Nil

Adjustment for Kidney Disease

FDA-approved product labeling: *Melanoma*

CrCL 30–50 mL/min	*4.5 mcg/kg subcutaneously once weekly (25 % decrease)*
CrCL 10–29 mL/min	*3 mcg/kg subcutaneously once weekly (50 % decrease)*

Hepatitis C

CrCL 30–50 mL/min	*1.125 mcg/kg subcutaneously once weekly (25 % decrease)*
CrCL 10–29 mL/min	*0.75 mcg/kg subcutaneously once weekly (50 % decrease)*

Note: Do not administer ribavirin to patients with CrCL <50 mL/min.

Alternative adjustment: *Hepatitis C*

Hemodialysis	*1 mcg/kg subcutaneously once weekly (with ribavirin 200 mg orally once daily)*

Dosage Adjustment of Medications Eliminated by the Kidneys

Pemetrexed - Selected References

Alimta® injection [package insert]. Indianapolis: Eli Lilly and Co; 2004.

Baldwin CM, Perry CM. Pemetrexed: a review of its use in the management of advanced non-squamous non-small cell lung cancer. Drugs. 2009;69:2279–302.

Burris HA III, Infante JR, Jewell RC, et al. A phase I study of weekly topotecan in combination with pemetrexed in patients with advanced malignancies. Oncologist. 2010;15:954–60.

Clarke SJ, Boyer MJ, Millward M, et al. A phase I/II study of pemetrexed and vinorelbine in patients with non-small cell lung cancer. Lung Cancer. 2005;49:401–12.

Dai H, Chen Y, Elmquist WF. Distribution of the novel antifolates pemetrexed to the brain. J Pharmacol Exp Ther. 2005;315:222–9.

Dickgreber NJ, Sorensen JB, Paz-Ares LG, et al. Pemetrexed safety and pharmacokinetics in patients with third-space fluid. Clin Cancer Res. 2010;16:2872–80.

Dy GK, Suri A, Reid JM, et al. A phase IB study of the pharmacokinetics of gemcitabine and pemetrexed, when administered in rapid sequence to patients with advanced solid tumors. Cancer Chemother Pharmacol. 2005;55:522–30.

Latz JF, Chaudhary A, Ghosh Johnson RD. Population pharmacokinetic analysis of ten phase II clinical trials of pemetrexed in cancer patients. Cancer Chemother Pharmacol. 2006;57:401–11.

McDonald AC, Vasey PA, Adams L, et al. A phase I and pharmacokinetic study of LY231514, the multitargeted antifolates. Clin Cancer Res. 1998;4:605–10.

Misset JL, Gamelin E, Campone M, et al. Phase I and pharmacokinetic study of the multitargeted antifolates pemetrexed in combination with oxaliplatin in patients with advanced solid tumors. Ann Oncol. 2004;15:1123–9.

Mita AC, Sweeney CJ, Baker SD, et al. Phase I and pharmacokinetic study of pemetrexed administered every 3 weeks to advanced cancer patients with normal and impaired renal function. J Clin Oncol. 2006;24:552–62.

Okamoto I, Takeda K, Daga H, et al. Dose-escalation study of pemetrexed in combination with carboplatin followed by pemetrexed maintenance therapy for advanced non-small cell lung cancer. Lung Cancer. 2010;70:168–73.

Oullet D, Periclou AP, Johnson RD, Woodworth JR, Lalonde RL. Population pharmacokinetics of pemetrexed (Alimta) in patients with cancer. Cancer Chemother Pharmacol. 2000;46:227–34.

Paridaens R, Dirix L, Dumez H, et al. Phase I/II pharmacokinetic study of pemetrexed and epirubicin in patients with locally advanced or metastatic breast cancer. Clin Breast Cancer. 2007;7:861–6.

Ranson M, Reck M, Anthoney A, et al. Erlotinib in combination with pemetrexed for patients with advanced non-small-cell lung cancer (NSCLC): a phase I dose-finding study. Ann Oncol. 2010;21:2233–39.

Rinaldi DA, Burris HA, Dorr FA, et al. Initial phase I evaluation of the novel thymidylate synthetase inhibitor, LY231514, using the modified continual reassessment method for dose escalation. J Clin Oncol. 1995;13:2842–50.

Rowinsky EK, Beeram M, Hammond LA, et al. A phase I and pharmacokinetic study of pemetrexed plus irinotecan in patients with advanced solid malignancies. Clin Cancer Res. 2007;13:532–9.

Sørensen JB. Pharmacokinetic evaluation of pemetrexed. Expert Opin Drug Metab Toxicol. 2011;7:919–28.

Spigel DR, Hainsworth JD, Shipley DL, et al. A randomized phase II trial of pemetrexed/gemcitabine/bevacizumab or pemetrexed/carboplatin/bevacizumab in first-line treatment for elderly patients with advanced non-small cell lung cancer. J Thorac Oncol. 2012;7:196–202. doi:10.1097/JTO.0b013e3182307efe.

Thödtmann BR, Depenbrock H, Dumez H, et al. Clinical and pharmacokinetic phase I study of multitargeted antifolates (LY231514) in combination with cisplatin. J Clin Oncol. 1999;17:3009–16.

Zhang G-Z, Jiao S-C, Meng Z-T. Pemetrexed plus cisplatin/carboplatin in previously treated locally advanced or metastatic non-small cell lung cancer patients. J Exp Clin Cancer Res. 2010;29:38. doi:10.1186/1756-9966-29-38.

Zhao R, Babani S, Gao F, Liu L, Goldman ID. The mechanism of transport of the multitargeted antifolates (MTA) and its cross-resistance pattern in cells with markedly impaired transport of methotrexate. Clin Cancer Res. 2000;6:3687–95.

Dosage Adjustment of Medications Eliminated by the Kidneys

Pemetrexed/Alimta®   {**Antineoplastic; antimetabolite; antifolate**}

Usual initial dose:	500 mg/m^2 IV over 10 min
Usual maintenance dose:	500 mg/m^2 IV over 10 min on day 1 of each 21-day cycle
Typical maximum dose:	500 mg/m^2 IV
Proportion eliminated unchanged:	70–90 %

Adjustment for Kidney Disease

FDA-approved product labeling: *Decreased renal function will result in reduced clearance and greater exposure compared with patients with normal renal function.*

CrCL 45–79 mL/min   No dosage adjustment is needed; use with caution.

CrCL <45 mL/min   Do not administer; avoid.

Alternative adjustment: *Data not available; interindividual drug clearance varies widely, and available clinical data presently are not sufficient to recommend adequate and safe dose amounts in patients with impaired excretory kidney function.*

Note: Hematological and other considerations may suggest further dosage adjustments.

Penicillamine - Selected References

Clements PJ, Furst DE, Wong W-K, et al. High-dose versus low-dose d-penicillamine in early diffuse systemic sclerosis: analysis of a two-year, double-blind, randomized, controlled clinical trial. Arthritis Rheum. 1999;42:1194–203.

Cramer K, Goyer RA, Jagenburg R, Wilson MH. Renal ultrastructure, renal function, and parameters of lead toxicity in workers with different periods of lead exposure. Br J Ind Med. 1974;31:113–7.

Crawhall JC. Proteinuria in D-penicillamine-treated rheumatoid arthritis. J Rheumatol. 1981;8(Suppl 7):161–3.

Cuprimine® capsule [package insert]. Whitehouse Station: Merck & Co; 2004.

Davis P, Jayson MIV. Renal involvement in progressive systemic sclerosis. Proc R Soc Med. 1975;68:544–5.

Davison AM, Day AT, Golding JR, Thomson D. Effect of penicillamine on the kidney. Proc R Soc Med. 1977;70 (Suppl 3):109–13.

DeMarco PJ, Weisman MH, Seibold JR, et al. Predictors and outcomes of scleroderma renal crisis: the high-dose versus low-dose D-penicillamine in early diffuse systemic sclerosis trial. Arthritis Rheum. 2002;46:2983–9.

Dische FE, Swinson DR, Hamilton EBD, Parsons V. Immunopathology of penicillamine-induced glomerular disease. J Rheumatol. 1976;3:145–54.

Elsas LJ, Hayslett JP, Spargo BH, Durant JL. Wilson's disease with reversible renal tubular dysfunction: correlation with proximal tubular ultrastructure. Ann Intern Med. 1971;75:427–33.

Falck HM, Törnroth T, Kock B, Wegelius O. Fatal renal vasculitis and minimal change glomerulonephritis complicating treatment with penicillamine: report of two cases. Acta Med Scand. 1979;205:133–8.

Friedman R, Gallo GR, Buxbaum JN. Renal disease in rheumatoid arthritis [letter]. Arthritis Rheum. 1980;23:781–3.

Hall CL, Jawad S, Harrison PR, et al. Natural course of penicillamine nephropathy: a long term study of 33 patients. Br Med J. 1988;296:1083–6.

Hamlyn AN, Gollan J, Douglas AP, Sherlock S. Fulminant Wilson's disease with haemolysis and renal failure: copper studies and assessment of dialysis regimens. Br Med J. 1977;2:660–3.

Leeson PM, Fourman P. A disorder of copper metabolism treated with penicillamine in a patient with primary biliary cirrhosis and renal tubular acidosis. Am J Med. 1967;43:620–35.

Leu ML, Strickland GT, Gutman RA. Renal function in Wilson's disease: response to penicillamine therapy. Am J Med Sci. 1970;260:381–98.

Monro P. Effect of treatment on renal function in severe osteomalacia due to Wilson's disease. J Clin Pathol. 1970;23: 487–91.

Netter P, Bannwarth B, Péré P, Nicolas A. Clinical pharmacokinetics of penicillamine. Clin Pharmacokinet. 1987;13: 317–33.

Ross JH, McGinty F, Brewer DG. Penicillamine nephropathy. Nephron. 1980;26:184–6.

Seppälä E, Lehtinen K, Isomäki H, et al. Effects of long-term aurothiomalate and D-penicillamine treatments on renal function and urinary excretion of prostanoids in patients with rheumatoid arthritis. Int J Clin Pharmacol Res. 1988;8:149–56.

Suarez-Almazor ME, Belseck E, Spooner C. Penicillamine for treating rheumatoid arthritis (review). Cochrane Database Syst Rev. 2000;(4):CD001460. doi:10.1002/14651858.CD001460.

Walshe JM. Effect of penicillamine on failure of renal acidification in Wilson's disease. Lancet. 1968;1:775–8.

Williams AJ, Fordham JN, Barnes CG, Goodwin FJ. Progressive Proliferative glomerulonephritis in a patient with rheumatoid arthritis treated with D-penicillamine. Ann Rheum Dis. 1986;45:82–4.

Dosage Adjustment of Medications Eliminated by the Kidneys

Penicillamine/Cuprimine®, Depen®	{**Chelating agent; antirheumatic; R for Wilson's disease**}

Usual initial dose:	250 mg orally
Usual maintenance dose:	500–750 mg orally once daily 1 h before or 2 h after meals (rheumatoid arthritis)
	750–1,500 mg/day or as determined by measurement of urinary copper excretion (Wilson's disease)
	2,000 mg/day in divided doses (cystinuria)
Typical maximum dose:	1,500 mg/day (4,000 mg/day for cystinuria)
Proportion eliminated unchanged:	40–50 %

Adjustment for Kidney Disease

FDA-approved product labeling:	*Renal insufficiency*	*Contraindicated*
Alternative adjustment:	*GFR >50 mL/min*	*500–1,000 mg orally every 24 h 1 h before or 2 h after meals*
		125 mg orally every other day (early diffuse systemic sclerosis)
	GFR 10–50 mL/min	*Avoid due to risk of nephrotoxicity.*
	GFR <10 mL/min	*Avoid due to risk of nephrotoxicity.*
	Hemodialysis	*250–500 mg orally every 24 h (50 % decrease)*
	CAPD	*Data not available; avoid due to risk of nephrotoxicity.*
	CRRT	*Data not available*

Dosage Adjustment of Medications Eliminated by the Kidneys

Penicillin G - Selected References

Aronoff GA, Bennett WM, Berns JS, et al. Drug prescribing in renal failure: dosing guidelines for adults and children. 5th ed. Philadelphia: American College of Physicians; 2007.

Bergan T, Øydvin B. Cross-over study of penicillin pharmacokinetics after intravenous infusions. Chemotherapy. 1974;20:263–79.

Bins JW, Mattie H. The tubular excretion of benzylpenicillin in patients with cystic fibrosis. Br J Clin Pharmacol. 1989;27:291–4.

Bond JT, Bailie MD, Hook JB. Maturation of renal organic acid transport *in vivo*: substrate stimulation by penicillin. J Pharmacol Exp Ther. 1976;199:25–31.

Browning MC, Tune BM. Reactivity and binding of β-lactam antibiotics in rabbit renal cortex. J Pharmacol Exp Ther. 1983;226:640–4.

Bryan CS, Stone WJ. "Comparably massive" penicillin G therapy in renal failure. Ann Intern Med. 1975;82:189–95.

Bryan CS, Talwani R, Stinson MS. Penicillin dosing for pneumococcal pneumonia. Chest. 1997;112:1657–64.

Buchanan N, Robinson R, Koornhof HJ, Eyberg C. Penicillin pharmacokinetics in kwashiorkor. Am J Clin Nutr. 1979;32:2233–6.

Eagle H, Fleischman R, Levy M. "Continuous" vs "discontinuous" therapy with penicillin: the effect of the interval between injections on therapeutic efficacy. N Engl J Med. 1953;248:481–8.

Eagle H, Fleischman R, Musselman AD. The bactericidal action of penicillin in vivo: the participation of the host, and the slow recovery of the surviving organisms. Ann Intern Med. 1950;33:544–71.

Heintz BH, Matzke GR, Dager WF. Antimicrobial dosing concepts and recommendations for critically ill adult patients receiving continuous renal replacement therapy or intermittent hemodialysis. Pharmacotherapy. 2009;29:562–77.

Jariyawat S, Sekine T, Takeda M, et al. The interaction and transport of β-lactam antibiotics with the cloned rat renal organic anion transporter 1. J Pharmacol Exp Ther. 1999;290:672–77.

Johnson JR, Colombo DF, Gardner D, Cho E, Fan-Havard P, Shellhaas CS. Optimal dosing of penicillin G in the third trimester of pregnancy for prophylaxis against group B *Streptococcus*. Am J Obstet Gynecol. 2001;185:850–3.

Joos B, Schmidli M, Keusch G. Pharmacokinetics of antimicrobial agents in anuric patients during continuous venovenous haemofiltration. Nephrol Dial Transplant. 1996;11:1582–5.

Nierenberg DW. Drug inhibition of penicillin tubular secretion: concordance between *in vitro* and clinical findings. J Pharmacol Exp Ther. 1987;240:712–6.

Overbosch D, van Gulpen C, Hermans J, Mattie H. The effect of probenecid on the renal tubular excretion of benzylpenicillin. Br J Clin Pharmacol. 1988;25:51–8.

Pfizerpen® buffered penicillin G potassium injection [package insert]. New York: Roerig Division of Pfizer Inc; 2008.

Raichle ME, Kutt H, Louis S, McDowell F. Neurotoxicity of intravenously administered penicillin G. Arch Neurol. 1971;25:232–9.

Schliamser SE, Bolander H, Broholm K-A, Gerdes U, Kourtopoulos H, Norrby SR. Neurotoxicity of benzylpenicillin in experimental renal failure and *Enterobacter cloacae* meningitis. J Antimicrob Chemother. 1989;24:215–25.

Smith H, Lerner PI, Weinstein L. Neurotoxicity and "massive" intravenous therapy with penicillin: a study of possible predisposing factors. Arch Intern Med. 1967;120:47–53.

Toma Y, Ishiki T, Nagahama K, et al. Penicillin G-induced hemorrhagic cystitis with hydronephrosis. Intern Med. 2009;48:1667–9.

VanWert AL, Bailey RM, Sweet DH. Organic anion transporter 3 (Oat3/Slc22a8) knockout mice exhibit altered clearance and distribution of penicillin G. Am J Physiol Renal Physiol. 2007;293:F1332–41.

Visser IG, Arnouts P, van Furth R, Mattie H, van den Broek PJ. Clinical pharmacokinetics of continuous intravenous administration of penicillins. Clin Infect Dis. 1993;17:491–5.

Walker AE, Johnson HC, Kollros JJ. Penicillin convulsions: the convulsive effects of penicillin applied to the cerebral cortex of monkey and man. Surg Gynecol Obstet. 1945;81:692–701.

Wickerts CJ, Asaba H, Gunnarsson B, Bygdeman S, Bergström J. Combined carbon haemoperfusion and haemodialysis in treatment of penicillin intoxication. Br Med J. 1980;280:1254–5.

Dosage Adjustment of Medications Eliminated by the Kidneys

Penicillin G Potassium (Benzylpenicillin)/Pfizerpen®	{Antibacterial; prototypical β-lactam}	
Usual initial dose:	2–5 million units IV	
Usual maintenance dose:	5–30 million units/day in 4–12 divided doses or continuous IV infusion of 20–30 million units/day	
Typical maximum dose:	30 million units/day	
Proportion eliminated unchanged:	79 %	

Adjustment for Kidney Disease

FDA-approved product labeling:	*Impaired renal function*	*If impairment of function is suspected or known to exist, a reduction in the total dosage should be considered; frequent evaluation of electrolyte balance and renal and hematopoietic function is recommended when high doses are used.*
	CrCL ≥10 mL/min	*Administer a full loading dose followed by one-half of the loading dose every 4 h.*
	CrCL <10 mL/min	*Administer a full loading dose followed by one-half of the loading dose every 8 h.*
Alternative adjustment:	*GFR >50 mL/min*	*2.5–5 million units IV every 4–6 h or 20–30 million units/day continuous infusion*
	GFR 10–50 mL/min	*1–4 million units IV every 4–6 h (25 % decrease)*
	GFR <10 mL/min	*1–2.5 million units IV every 6 h (50–80 % decrease)*
	Hemodialysis	*1–2.5 million units IV every 4–6 h, dose after dialysis (50–80 % decrease)*
	CAPD	*0.2–2.5 million units IV every 4–6 h*
	CVVH	*4 million units IV once followed by 2 million units IV every 4–6 h*
	CVVHD	*4 million units IV once followed by 2–3 million units IV every 4–6 h*
	CVVHDF	*4 million units IV once followed by 2–4 million units IV every 4–6 h*

Note: Penicillin G is the antibiotic of first choice for every infection that is sensitive to it.

Dosage Adjustment of Medications Eliminated by the Kidneys

Pentamidine (IV) - Selected References

Abramowicz M, Zuccotti G, Pflomm J-M, et al., editors. Handbook of antimicrobial therapy. 19th ed. New Rochelle: The Medical Letter; 2011.

Aronoff GA, Bennett WM, Berns JS, et al. Drug prescribing in renal failure: dosing guidelines for adults and children. 5th ed. Philadelphia: American College of Physicians; 2007.

Briceland LL, Bailie GR. Pentamidine-associated nephrotoxicity and hyperkalemia in patients with AIDS. DICP Ann Pharmacother. 1991;25:1171–4.

Buff DD, Aboal AA. Pentamidine-associated renal dysfunction and hyperkalemia [letter]. Am J Med. 1990;88:552.

Comtois R, Pouliot J, Vinet B, Gervais A, Lemieux C. Higher pentamidine levels in AIDS patients with hypoglycemia and azotemia during treatment of *Pneumocystis carinii* pneumonia. Am Rev Respir Dis. 1992;146:740–4.

Conte JE Jr. Pharmacokinetics of intravenous pentamidine in patients with normal renal function or receiving hemodialysis. J Infect Dis. 1991;163:169–75.

Conte JE Jr, Chernoff D, Feigal DW Jr, Joseph P, McDonald C, Golden JA. Intravenous or inhaled pentamidine for treating *Pneumocystis carinii* pneumonia in AIDS: a randomized trial. Ann Intern Med. 1990;113:203–9.

Conte JE Jr, Hollander H, Golden JA. Inhaled or reduced-dose pentamidine for *Pneumocystis carinii* pneumonia: a pilot study. Ann Intern Med. 1987;107:495–8.

Conte JE Jr, Upton RA, Liu E-T. Pentamidine pharmacokinetics in patients with AIDS with impaired renal function. J Infect Dis. 1987;156:885–90.

Conte JE Jr, Upton RA, Phelps RT, Wofsy CB, Zurlinden E, Liu ET. Use of a sensitive assay to determine pentamidine pharmacokinetics in patients with AIDS. J Infect Dis. 1986;154:923–9.

Donnelly H, Bernard EM, Rothkotter H, Gold JWM, Armstrong D. Distribution of pentamidine in patients with AIDS. J Infect Dis. 1988;157:985–9.

EBPG Expert Group on Renal Transplantation. European Best Practice Guidelines for renal transplantation. Section IV: Long-term management of the transplant recipient. IV.7.1 late infections: *Pneumocystis carinii* pneumonia. Nephrol Dial Transplant. 2002;17(Suppl 4):36–9.

Fitzsimmons WE, Luskin SS. Pentamidine therapy in renal failure: case report and review of the literature. Drug Intell Clin Pharm. 1988;22:25–8.

Gradon JD, Fricchione L, Sekowitz D. Severe hypomagnesemia associated with pentamidine therapy. Rev Infect Dis. 1991;13:511–2.

Kuller J, First MR, D'Archiadi R, Munda R. *Pneumocystis carinii* pneumonia in renal transplant recipients. Am J Nephrol. 1982;2:312–5.

Lachaal M, Venuto RC. Nephrotoxicity and hyperkalemia in patients with acquired immunodeficiency syndrome treated with pentamidine. Am J Med. 1989;87:260–3.

Lidman C, Bronner U, Gstafsson LL, Rombo L. Plasma pentamidine concentrations vary between individuals with *Pneumocystis carinii* pneumonia and the drug is actively secreted by the kidney. J Antimicrob Chemother. 1994;33:803–10.

O'Brien JG, Dong BJ, Coleman RL, Gee L, Balano KB. A 5-year review of adverse drug reactions and their risk factors in human immunodeficiency virus-infected patients who were receiving intravenous pentamidine therapy for *Pneumocystis carinii* pneumonia. Clin Infect Dis. 1997;24:854–9.

Pentam® 300 injection [package insert]. Schaumburg: APP Pharmaceuticals LLC; 2008.

Sattler FR, Cowan R, Nielsen DM, Ruskin J. Trimethoprim-sulfamethoxazole compared with pentamidine for treatment of *Pneumocystis carinii* pneumonia in the acquired immunodeficiency syndrome: a prospective, noncrossover study. Ann Intern Med. 1989;109:280–7.

Soo Hoo GW, Mohsenifar Z, Meyer RD. Inhaled or intravenous pentamidine therapy for *Pneumocystis carinii* pneumonia in AIDS: a randomized trial. Ann Intern Med. 1990;113:195–202.

Sterhr-Green JK, Helmick CG. Pentamidine and renal toxicity [letter]. N Engl J Med. 1985;313:694–5.

Dosage Adjustment of Medications Eliminated by the Kidneys

Pentamidine (IV)/Pentam® 300   **{Antiprotozoal; antiparasitic}**

Usual initial dose:	4 mg/kg IV
Usual maintenance dose:	4 mg/kg IV once daily for 14–21 days
Typical maximum dose:	4 mg/kg/day
Proportion eliminated unchanged:	2–12 %

Adjustment for Kidney Disease

FDA-approved product labeling: *The efficacy or safety of alternative dosing protocols has not been established for patients with impaired renal function.*

Alternative adjustment:

GFR >35 mL/min	*3–4 mg/kg IV every 24 h*
GFR 10–35 mL/min	*4 mg/kg IV every 24–48 h*
GFR <10 mL/min	*4 mg/kg IV every 48 h*
Hemodialysis	*4 mg/kg IV every 24–36 h; supplement 0.75 mg/kg IV after hemodialysis on dialysis days.*
CAPD	*4 mg/kg IV every 48 h*
CRRT	*4 mg/kg IV every 24 h*

Dosage Adjustment of Medications Eliminated by the Kidneys

Pentazocine - Selected References

Aronoff GA, Bennett WM, Berns JS, et al. Drug prescribing in renal failure: dosing guidelines for adults and children. 5th ed. Philadelphia: American College of Physicians; 2007.

Berkowitz B. Pharmacokinetics and neurochemical effects of pentazocine and its optical isomers. Adv Biochem Psychopharmacol. 1974;8:495–501.

Brogden RN, Speight TM, Avery GS. Pentazocine: a review of its pharmacological properties, therapeutic efficacy and dependence liability. Drugs. 1973;5:6–91.

Bullingham RES, McQuay HJ, Moore RA. Clinical pharmacokinetic of narcotic agonist–antagonist drugs. Clin Pharmacokinet. 1983;8:332–43.

Carrano RA, Kimura KK, Landes RC, McCurdy DH. General pharmacology of a new analgesic—AP-237. Arch Int Pharmacodyn Ther. 1975;213:28–40.

Carter HS, Watson WA. IV pentazocine/methylphenidate abuse—the clinical toxicity of another Ts and Blues combination. J Toxicol Clin Toxicol. 1994;32:541–7.

Challoner KR, McCarron MM, Newton EJ. Pentazocine (Talwin®) intoxication: report of 57 cases. J Emerg Med. 1990;8:67–74.

Ehrnebo M, Boréus LO, Lönroth U. Single-dose kinetics and bioavailability of pentazocine. Acta Anaesth Scand Suppl. 1982;74:70–1.

Fritz AK, Benzier DP, Peterson JE, Park B, Edelson J. Relative bioavailability and pharmacokinetics: a combination of pentazocine and acetaminophen. J Pharm Sci. 1984;73:326–31.

Hunter JAA, Davison AM. Toxic epidermal necrolysis associated with pentazocine therapy and severe reversible renal failure. Br J Dermatol. 1973;88:287–90.

Kawamura K, Kobayashi T, Matsuno K, Ishiwata K. Different brain kinetics of two sigma1 receptor ligands, [^{3}H](+)-pentazocine and [^{11}C]SA4503, by P-glycoprotein modulation. Synapse. 2003;48:80–6.

Kornhuber J, Schoppmeyer K, Bendig C, Riederer P. Characterization of [3H]pentazocine binding sites in post-mortem human frontal cortex. J Neural Transm. 1996;103:45–53.

Meador KH, Sharon Z, Lewis EJ. Renal amyloidosis and subcutaneous drug abuse. Ann Intern Med. 1979;91:565–7.

Moeller N, Dietzel K, Nuernberg B, Geisslinger G, Brune K. High-performance liquid chromatographic determination of pentazocine in plasma. J Chromatogr. 1990;530:200–5.

Mostert JW, Evers JL, Hobika GH, Moore RH, Murphy GP. Circulatory effects of analgesic and neuroleptic drugs in patients with chronic renal failure undergoing maintenance dialysis. Br J Anaesth. 1970;42:501–13.

Muhalwas KK, Shah GM, Winer RL. Renal papillary necrosis caused by long-term ingestion of pentazocine and aspirin. JAMA. 1981;248:867–8.

Sigman EM, Elwood CM. Effect of intramuscular pentazocine on renal hemodynamics in normal human subjects. Anesth Analg. 1967;46:57–60.

Talwin™ injection [package insert]. Lake Forest: Hospira Inc; 2010.

Thompson EB, Bhargav HN. Cardiovascular responses to pentazocine and tripelennamine in anesthetized rats. Gen Pharmacol. 1980;11:543–9.

Yamashiro H. Effect of pentazocine on renal blood flow. Br J Anaesth. 1978;50:1337.

Dosage Adjustment of Medications Eliminated by the Kidneys

Pentazocine/Talwin™   {**Analgesic; opioid μ-receptor partial agonist**}

Usual initial dose:	30 mg IV, IM, or subcutaneously
Usual maintenance dose:	30 mg IV, IM, or subcutaneously every 3–4 h
Typical maximum dose:	30 mg/dose IV, 60 mg/dose IM or subcutaneously, or 360 mg/day
Proportion eliminated unchanged:	<13 %

Adjustment for Kidney Disease

FDA-approved product labeling: *Administer with caution; the effects of this drug may be greater than expected in patients with impaired renal function.*

Alternative adjustment:

GFR >50 mL/min	*30 mg IV every 4 h as necessary*
GFR 10–50 mL/min	*20 mg IV every 4 h as necessary (25 % decrease)*
GFR <10 mL/min	*15 mg IV every 4 h as necessary (50 % decrease)*
Hemodialysis	*15 mg IV every 4 h as necessary (50 % decrease)*
CAPD	*Data not available; preferably avoid.*
CRRT	*Data not available; preferably avoid.*

Dosage Adjustment of Medications Eliminated by the Kidneys

Pentostatin - Selected References

Aronoff GA, Bennett WM, Berns JS, et al. Drug prescribing in renal failure: dosing guidelines for adults and children. 5th ed. Philadelphia: American College of Physicians; 2007.

Brogden RN, Sorkin EM. Pentostatin: a review of its pharmacodynamic and pharmacokinetic properties, and therapeutic potential in lymphoproliferative disorders. Drugs. 1993;46:652–77.

Dearden CE, Matutes E, Catovsky D. Clinical overview of pentostatin (Nipent) use in lymphoid malignancies. Semin Oncol. 2000;27(Suppl 5):22–6.

Grever MR, Bisaccia E, Scarborough DA, Metz EN, Neidhart JA. An investigation of 2'-deoxycoformycin in the treatment of cutaneous T-cell lymphoma. Blood. 1983;61:279–82.

Grever MR, Siaw MFE, Jacob WF, et al. The biochemical and clinical consequences of 2'-deoxycoformycin in refractory lymphoproliferative disorders. Blood. 1981;57:406–17.

Higman M, Vogelsang GB, Chen A. Pentostatin—pharmacology, immunology, and clinical effects in graft-versus-host disease. Expert Opin Pharmacother. 2004;5:2605–13.

Ho AD, Suciu S, Stryckmans P, et al. Pentostatin (Nipent) in T-cell malignancies. Semin Oncol. 2000;27(Suppl 5):52–7.

Ho AD, Suciu S, Stryckmans P, et al. Pentostatin in T-cell malignancies—a phase II trial of the EORTC. Ann Oncol. 1999;10:1493–8.

Johnston B, Eisenhauer E, Wainman N, Corbett WEN, Zaentz SD, Daenick PJ. Long-term outcome following treatment of hairy cell leukemia with pentostatin (Nipent): a National Cancer Institute of Canada study. Semin Oncol. 2000;27(Suppl 5):32–6.

Kuttesch JF Jr, Nelson JA. Renal handling of 2'-deoxycoformycin and adenosine in humans and mice. Cancer Chemother Pharmacol. 1982;8:221–9.

Lathia C, Fleming GF, Meyer M, Ratain MJ, Whitfield L. Pentostatin pharmacokinetics and dosing recommendations in patients with mild renal impairment. Cancer Chemother Pharmacol. 2002;50:121–6.

Nipent® injection [package insert]. Lake Forest: Hospira Inc; 2009.

O'Dwyer PJ, Wagner B, Leyland-Jones B, Wittes RE, Cheson BD, Hoth DF. 2'-Deoxycoformycin (pentostatin) for lymphoid malignancies: rational development of an active new drug. Ann Intern Med. 1988;108:733–44.

Oken MM, Lee S, Kay NE, Knospe W, Cassileth PA. Pentostatin, chlorambucil and prednisone therapy for B-chronic lymphocytic leukemia: a phase I/II study for the Eastern Cooperative Oncology Group Study E1488. Leuk Lymphoma. 2004;45:79–84.

Prentice HG, Russell NH, Lee N, et al. Therapeutic selectivity of and prediction of response to 2'-deoxycoformycin in acute leukaemia. Lancet. 1981;2:1250–4.

Sakai C, Takagi T, Wakatsuki S, Matsuzaki O. Hemolytic-uremic syndrome due to deoxycoformycin: a report of the second case. Intern Med. 1995;34:593–6.

Sauter C, Lamanna N, Weiss MA. Pentostatin in chronic lymphocytic leukemia. Expert Opin Drug Metab Toxicol. 2008;4:1217–22.

Shanafelt TD, Lin T, Geyer SM, et al. Pentostatin, cyclophosphamide, and rituximab regimen in older patients with chronic lymphocytic leukemia. Cancer. 2007;109:2291–8.

Siaw MFE, Mitchell BS, Koller CA, Coleman MS, Hutton JJ. ATP depletion as a consequence of adenosine deaminase inhibition in man. Proc Natl Acad Sci. 1980;77:6157–61.

Singhal D, Morgan ME, Anderson BD. Role of altered metabolism in dideoxynucleoside pharmacokinetics: studies of 2'-β-fluoro-2'-3'-dideoxyinosine and 2'-β-fluoro-2'-3'-dideoxyadenosine in rats. Drug Metab Dispos. 1996;24:1155–61.

Singhal D, Morgan ME, Anderson BD. Role of brain tissue localized purine metabolizing enzymes in the central nervous system delivery of anti-HIV agents 2'-β-fluoro-2'-3'-dideoxyinosine and 2'-β-fluoro-2'-3'-dideoxyadenosine in rats. Pharm Res. 1997;14:789–92.

Tallman MS, Hakimian D. Purine nucleoside analogs: emerging roles in indolent lymphoproliferative disorders. Blood. 1995;86:2463–74.

Dosage Adjustment of Medications Eliminated by the Kidneys

<u>**Pentostatin**</u>/Nipent®   {Antineoplastic; antimetabolite; purine analog}

Usual initial dose:	4 mg/m² IV
Usual maintenance dose:	4 mg/m² IV every other week
Typical maximum dose:	4 mg/m²
Proportion eliminated unchanged:	90 %

Adjustment for Kidney Disease

FDA-approved product labeling: *Patients with impaired renal function should be treated only when the potential benefit justifies the potential risk. Two patients with impaired renal function (CrCL 50–60 mL/min) achieved complete response without unusual adverse events when treated with 2 mg/m².*

CrCL >60 mL/min	*4 mg/m² IV every other week*
CrCL 50–60 mL/min	*2 mg/m² IV every other week*
CrCL <50 mL/min	*Minimal data; avoid*

Alternative adjustment:

eCrCL >60 mL/min	*4 mg/m² IV every other week*
eCrCL 41–40 mL/min	*3 mg/m² IV every other week*
eCrCL 21–40 mL/min	*2 mg/m² IV every other week*
eCrCL ≤20 mL/min	*Data not available*

Note: Hematological and other considerations may suggest further dosage adjustments.

Dosage Adjustment of Medications Eliminated by the Kidneys

Pentoxifylline - Selected References

Beerman B, Ings R, Månsby J, Chamberlain J, McDonald A. Kinetics of intravenous and oral pentoxifylline in healthy subjects. Clin Pharmacol Ther. 1985;37:25–8.

Bianco JA, Almgren J, Kern DL, et al. Evidence that oral pentoxifylline reverses acute renal dysfunction in bone marrow transplant recipients receiving amphotericin B and cyclosporine: results of a pilot study. Transplantation. 1991;51:925–7.

Boldt J, Brosch C, Piper SN, Suttner S, Lehmann A, Werling C. Influence of prophylactic use of pentoxifylline on postoperative organ function in elderly cardiac surgery patients. Crit Care Med. 2001;29:952–8.

Bryce TA, Chamberlain J, Hillbeck D, Macdonald CM. Metabolism and pharmacokinetics of ^{14}C-pentoxifylline in healthy volunteers. Arzneimittelforschung. 1989;39:512–7.

Chen Y-M, Lin S-L, Chiang W-C, Wu K-D, Tsai T-J. Pentoxifylline ameliorates proteinuria through suppression of renal monocyte chemoattractant protein-1 in patients with proteinuric primary glomerular diseases. Kidney Int. 2006;69:1410–5.

Demir E, Paydas S, Balal M, Kurt C, Sertdemir Y, Erken U. Effects of pentoxifylline on the cytokines that may play a role in rejection and resistive index in renal transplant recipients. Transplant Proc. 2006;38:2883–6.

Eden G, Busch M, Kühn-Velten WN, Schneider A, Kielstein JT. Successful treatment of life-threatening pentoxifylline intoxication by high-flux hemodialysis. Clin Nephrol. 2011;75:171–3.

Guerrero-Romero F, Rodríguez-Morán M, Paniagua-Siera JR, García-Bulnes, Salas-Ramírez M Amato D. Pentoxifylline reduces proteinuria in insulin-dependent and non insulin-dependent diabetic patients. Clin Nephrol. 1995;;43:116–21.

Lin S-L, Che Y-M, Wu K-D, Tsai T-J. Effect of pentoxifylline in addition to losartan on proteinuria and GFR in CKD: a 12-month randomized trial. Am J Kidney Dis. 2008;52:464–74.

Mauro VF, Mauro LS, Hageman JH. Comparison of pentoxifylline pharmacokinetics between smokers and nonsmokers. J Clin Pharmacol. 1992;32:1054–8.

Navarro JF, Mora C, García J, et al. Effects of pentoxifylline on the haematologic status in anaemic patients with advanced renal failure. Scand J Urol Nephrol. 1999;33:121–5.

Navarro-González JF, Muros M, Mora-Fernández C, Herrera H, Meneses B, García J. Pentoxifylline for renoprotection in diabetic nephropathy: the PREDIAN study: rationale and basal results. J Diabetes Complications. 2011;25:314–9.

Nicklasson M, Björkman S, Roth B, Jönsson M, Höglund P. Stereoselective metabolism of pentoxifylline in vitro and in vivo in humans. Chirality. 2002;14:643–52.

Pap CM, Simpson KS, Horton MW, Schaefer KL, Lassman HB, Sack MR. Multiple-dose pharmacokinetics of pentoxifylline and its metabolites during renal insufficiency. Ann Pharmacother. 1996;30:724–9.

Rames A, Poirier J-M, LeCoz F, et al. Pharmacokinetics of intravenous and oral pentoxifylline in healthy volunteers and in cirrhotic patients. Clin Pharmacol Ther. 1990;47:354–9.

Shu K-H, Wu M-J, Chen C-H, Cheng C-H, Lian J-D, Lu Y-S. Effect of pentoxifylline on graft function of renal transplant recipients complicated with chronic allograft nephropathy. Clin Nephrol. 2007;67:157–6.

Smith RV, Waler E, Dolusio JT, et al. Pharmacokinetics of orally administered pentoxifylline in humans. J Pharm Sci. 1986;75:47–52.

Srinivasu P, Rambhau D, Rao BR, Rao YM. Pharmacokinetics of pentoxifylline after oral administration of a sustained release tablet at two different times of the day. Arzneimittelforschung. 1999;49:750–3.

Stojiljkovic N, Veljkovic S, Mihailovic D, et al. Protective effects of pentoxifylline treatment on gentamicin-induced nephrotoxicity in rats. Ren Fail. 2009;31:54–61.

Trental® tablet film coated [package insert]. Bridgewater: Sanofi-Aventis US LLC; 2007.

Tyagi P, Sharma P, Sharma BC, Puri AS, Kumar A, Sarin SK. Prevention of hepatorenal syndrome in patients with cirrhosis and ascites: a pilot randomized control trial between pentoxifylline and placebo. Eur J Gastroenterol Hepatol. 2011;23:210–7.

Vadiei K, Brunner LJ, Luke DR. Effects of pentoxifylline in experimental acute renal failure. Kidney Int. 1989;36:466–70.

Wang W, Zolty E, Falk S, Basava V, Reznilov L, Schrier R. Pentoxifylline protects against endotoxin-induced acute renal failure in mice. Am J Physiol Renal Physiol. 2006;291:F1090–5.

Ward A, Clissold SP. Pentoxifylline: a review of its pharmacodynamic and pharmacokinetic properties, and its therapeutic efficacy. Drugs. 1987;34:50–97.

Wasan KM, Vadiei K, Lopez-Berestein G, Verani RR, Luke DR. Pentoxifylline in amphotericin B toxicity in a rat model. Antimicrob Agents Chemother. 1990;34:241–4.

Dosage Adjustment of Medications Eliminated by the Kidneys

<u>Pentoxifylline</u>/Trental®	{Rheologic agent; blood viscosity reducer agent}

Usual initial dose:	400 mg orally
Usual maintenance dose:	400 mg orally three times daily with meals
Typical maximum dose:	1,200 mg/day
Proportion eliminated unchanged:	4 % (plus 50–80 % of each dose as active metabolite)

Adjustment for Kidney Disease

FDA-approved product labeling:	*The risk of toxic reactions to this drug may be greater in patients with impaired renal function.*	
Alternative adjustment:	*GFR >50 mL/min*	*400 mg orally every 8–12 h*
	GFR 10–50 mL/min	*400 mg orally every 12–24 h*
	GFR <10 mL/min	*400 mg orally every 24 h*
	Hemodialysis	*400 mg orally every 24 h (no supplemental post-dialysis dose)*
	CAPD	*400 mg orally every 24 h*
	CRRT	*Data not available*

Dosage Adjustment of Medications Eliminated by the Kidneys

Peramivir - Selected References

Atiee G, Lasseter K, Baughman S, et al. Absence of pharmacokinetic interaction between intravenous peramivir and oral oseltamivir or rimantadine in humans. J Clin Pharmacol. 2012;52:1410-9.

Bazan JA, Bauer KA, Hollister AS, et al. Peramivir pharmacokinetics in two critically ill adults with 2009 H1N1 influenza A concurrently receiving continuous renal replacement therapy. Pharmacotherapy. 2010;30:1016–20.

Birnkrant D, Cox E. The Emergency Use Authorization of peramivir for treatment of 2009 H1N1 influenza. N Engl J Med. 2009;361:2204–7.

Campbell AP, Jacob ST, Kuypers J, et al. Respiratory failure caused by 2009 novel influenza A/H1N1 in a hematopoietic stem-cell transplant recipient: detection of extrapulmonary N1N1 RNA and use of intravenous peramivir. Ann Intern Med. 2010;152:619–20.

Centers for Disease Control and Prevention. Emergency use authorization of peramivir IV fact sheet for health care providers. Available at: http://doc-00-94-docsviewer.googleusercontent.com/viewer/securedownload/dsn1aovipa7l846lsfcf94ned-j8q2p4u/qkukegav9tkab9mie6mpkohon6p229me/1318001400000/Ymw=/AGZ5hq8BgbJY1gwaOYx83cPOdNw6/QURHRUVTalF2UnRFSkFMUVBSWU1EMGdVUjZVMjRUNkxNMGRMS0NaZmE4ODlwOFBFeHIwSTNnVm1nTElvOXhBWXFFOcV9ibFhYLTgybS05aFliU1BvXy1iWEpJTE5DRnl4N3cxZ3daaWFFFzLWZPVGtqQ0RvWjdtM2xppekZEQ3dnb0c4cUlQwcFBkel83YTk=?docid=5748d3525f19d6c521cdd428005f87ad&chan=EgAAAHVgOoUv2Q92%2BIzKZD9CzLtVbWWuEIUfcgXaRS5uuqlz&sec=AHSqidaSNMKHIpxQXmM_5gkNzyTNtdSgMCw2GtkO8Pa6kcebSOsYlD6CTtpzfuXrfMauZ9A70v78&a=gp&filename=ucm187811.pdf&nonce=mh3numudl8b4i&user=AGZ5hq8BgbJY1gwaOYx83cPOdNw6&hash=2vfovop5a1b3vpnu5m3jol0ob34gv47r. Accessed 7 Oct 2011.

Centers for Disease Control and Prevention. Questions and answers for hospitals and healthcare professionals regarding termination of the emergency use authorization for peramivir IV. Available at: http://www.cdc.gov/H1N1flu/EUA/pdf/Peramivir_Attachment_22Jun2010.pdf. Accessed 7 Oct 2011.

Centers for Disease Control and Prevention. Termination of the emergency use authorization (EUA) of medical products and devices: peramivir IV. Available at: http://www.cdc.gov/h1n1flu/eua/. Accessed 7 Oct 2011.

Drusano GL, Preston SL, Smee D, Bush K, Bailey K, Sidwell RW. Pharmacodynamic evaluation of RWJ-270201, a novel neuraminidase inhibitor, in a lethal murine model of influenza predicts efficacy for once-daily dosing. Antimicrob Agents Chemother. 2001;45:2115–8.

Fry AM, Pérez A, Finelli L. Use of intravenous neuraminidase inhibitors during the 2009 pandemic: results from population-based surveillance [letter]. JAMA. 2011;306:160–2.

Hernandez JE, Adiga R, Armstrong R, et al. Clinical experience in adults and children treated with intravenous peramivir for 2009 influenza A (H1N1) under an emergency IND program in the United States. Clin Infect Dis. 2011;52:695–706.

Hollister AS, Sheridan WP. The emergency use authorization of peramivir IV: a view from the manufacturer. Clin Pharmacol Ther. 2011;89:172–4.

Iyer GR, Liao S, Massarella J. Population analysis of the pharmacokinetics and pharmacodynamics of RWJ-270201 (BCX-1812) in treating experimental influenza A and B virus in healthy volunteers. AAPS PharmSci. 2002;4(4):22. doi:10.1208/ps040422. Available at http://www.aapsj.org/articles/ps0404/ps040422/ps040422.pdf. Accessed 7 Oct 2011.

Kohno S, Kida H, Mizuguchi M, et al. Efficacy and safety of intravenous peramivir for treatment of seasonal influenza virus infection. Antimicrob Agents Chemother. 2010;54:4568–74.

Kohno S, Yen M-Y, Cheong H-J, et al. Phase III randomized, double-blind study comparing single-dose intravenous peramivir with oral oseltamivir in patients with seasonal influenza virus infection. Antimicrob Agents Chemother. 2011;55:5267–76.

Kohno S, Kida H, Mizuguchi M, et al. Intravenous peramivir for treatment of influenza A and B virus infection in high-risk patients. Antimicrob Agents Chemother. 2011;55:2803–12.

Lee BY, Tai JHY, Bailey RR, et al. Economic model for emergency use authorization of intravenous peramivir. Am J Manage Care. 2011;17:e1–9.

Mancuso CE, Gabay MP, Steinke LM, Van Osdol SJ. Peramivir: an intravenous neuraminidase inhibitor for the treatment of 2009 N1N1 influenza. Ann Pharmacother. 2010;44:1240–9.

Nasu T, Ogawa D, Wada J, Makino H. Peramivir for severe influenza infection in a patient with diabetic nephropathy [letter]. Am J Respir Crit Care Med. 2010;182:1209–10.

Thomas B, Hollister AS, Muczynski KA. Peramivir clearance in continuous renal replacement therapy [letter]. Hemodial Int. 2010;14:339–40.

Dosage Adjustment of Medications Eliminated by the Kidneys

Peramivir   **{Antiviral}**

Usual initial dose: 600 mg IV over 30 min

Usual maintenance dose: 600 mg IV over 30 min once daily for 5–10 days

Typical maximum dose: 600 mg IV

Proportion eliminated unchanged: 90 %

Adjustment for Kidney Disease

FDA-approved product labeling: *Peramivir adult renal function impairment dosage recommendations*

Creatinine clearance	Dose (IV)
Mild renal impairment (CrCL 50–80 mL/min)	600 mg daily
Moderate renal impairment (CrCL 31–49 mL/min)	150 mg daily
Severe renal impairment (CrCL 10–30 mL/min)	100 mg daily
End-stage renal impairment (CrCL <10 mL/min not on dialysis or renal replacement therapy)	100 mg on day, then 15 mg daily thereafter
End-stage renal disease on intermittent hemodialysis	100 mg on day 1, then 100 mg over 2 h after each hemodialysis session on dialysis days only

Dose modifications should be made, as appropriate for changes in patient renal function, changes to ultrafiltrate flow rate, or initiation, discontinuation, or changes to continuous renal replacement therapy (CRRT)

For renally impaired patients receiving CRRT, the peramivir dose should be selected according to the table above but using the CRRT clearance (Cl_{CRRT}) as outlined below instead of CrCL. If the patient has residual renal function while on CRRT, an estimate of the patient's renal clearance should be added to Cl_{CRRT} in order to estimate total clearance before using the table

Calculation of Cl_{CRRT} where Q_f = ultrafiltration rate (mL/min) and Q_d = dialysate flow rate (mL/min):

For slow continuous ultrafiltration (SCUP) or continuous arteriovenous hemofiltration (CAVH) or continuous venovenous hemofiltration (CVVH): $Cl_{CRRT} = Q_f$

For continuous arteriovenous hemodialysis (CAVHD) or continuous venovenous hemodialysis (CVVHD): $Cl_{CRRT} = Q_d$

For continuous arteriovenous hemodiafiltration (CAVHDF) and continuous venovenous hemodiafiltration (CVVHDF): $Cl_{CRRT} = Q_f + Q_d$

Alternative adjustment:

CRRT	*600 mg IV daily*
Slow low-efficiency hemodialysis	*600 mg IV daily*

Dosage Adjustment of Medications Eliminated by the Kidneys

Perindopril - Selected References

Aceon® tablet [package insert]. North Chicago: Abbott Laboratories Inc; 2011.

Aronoff GA, Bennett WM, Berns JS, et al. Drug prescribing in renal failure: dosing guidelines for adults and children. 5th ed. Philadelphia: American College of Physicians; 2007.

Bellissant E, Guidicelli J-F. Pharmacokinetic-pharmacodynamic model for perindoprilat regional haemodynamic effects in healthy volunteers and in congestive heart failure patients. Br J Clin Pharmacol. 2001;52:25–33.

Chaignon M, Barrou Z, Ayad M, et al. Effects of perindopril on renal haemodynamics and natriuresis in essential hypertension. J Hypertens. 1988;6(Suppl 3):S61–4.

de Galan BE, Perkovic V, Ninomiya T, et al. Lowering blood pressure reduces renal events in type 2 diabetes. J Am Soc Nephrol. 2009;20:883–93.

Guérin A, Resplandy G, Marchais S, Taillard F, London G. The effect of haemodialysis on the pharmacokinetics of perindoprilat after long-term perindopril. Eur J Clin Pharmacol. 1993;44:183–7.

Heerspink HJL, Ninomiya T, Perkovic V, et al. Effects of a fixed combination of perindopril and indapamide in patients with type 2 diabetes and chronic kidney disease. Eur Heart J. 2010;31:2888–96.

Hurst M, Jarvis B. Perindopril: an updated review of its use in hypertension. Drugs. 2001;61:867–96.

Lecocq B, Funck-Brentano C, Lecocq V, et al. Influence of food on the pharmacokinetics of perindopril and the time course of angiotensin-converting enzyme inhibition in serum. Clin Pharmacol Ther. 1990;47:397–402.

Lees KR, Green ST, Reid JL. Influence of age on the pharmacokinetics and pharmacodynamics of perindopril. Clin Pharmacol Ther. 1988;44:418–25.

Lees KR, Hughes DM, McNeill CA, Reid JL. Pharmacokinetics of perindopril: therapeutic consequences. Clin Exp Hypertens A. 1989;11(Suppl 2):499–506.

Louis WJ, Workman BS, Conway EL, et al. Single-dose and steady-state pharmacokinetics and pharmacodynamics of perindopril in hypertensive subjects. J Cardiovasc Pharmacol. 1992;20:505–11.

Meyrier A, Dratwa M, Sennesael J, Lachaud-Pettiti V. Fixed low-dose perindopril-indapamide combination in hypertensive patients with chronic renal failure. Am J Hypertens. 1998;11:1087–92.

Parker E, Aarons L, Rowland M, Resplandy G. The pharmacokinetics of perindoprilat in normal volunteers and patients: influence of age and disease state. Eur J Pharm Sci. 2005;26:104–13.

Resplandy G, Genissel P. Pharmacokinetics of perindopril in high-risk populations. J Cardiovasc Pharmacol 1991;18(Suppl 7): S9–18.

Sica DA. Dosage considerations with perindopril for systemic hypertension. Am J Cardiol. 2001;88(Suppl 7A):13–8.

Verpooten GA, Genissel PM, Thomas JR, De Broe ME. Single dose pharmacokinetics of perindopril and its metabolites in hypertensive patients with various degrees of renal insufficiency. Br J Clin Pharmacol. 1991;32:187–92.

Zoungas S, Marre M, de Galan BE, et al. Combined effects of routine blood pressure lowering and intensive glucose control on macrovascular and microvascular outcomes in patients with type 2 diabetes. Diabetes Care. 2009;32:2068–74.

Dosage Adjustment of Medications Eliminated by the Kidneys

__Perindopril__/Aceon®   **{Antihypertensive, vasodilator, angiotensin-converting enzyme (ACE)/ renin inhibitor}**

Usual initial dose:	4 mg orally
Usual maintenance dose:	4–8 mg orally once daily
Typical maximum dose:	16 mg/day
Proportion eliminated unchanged:	90 % (as perindopril and perindoprilat)

Adjustment for Kidney Disease: 1 h before or at least 2 h after meals

FDA-approved product labeling:	*CrCL ≥30 mL/min*	*4 mg orally once daily; usual max 8 mg/day*
	CrCL <30 mL/min	*Safety not established; use not recommended*
	Hemodialysis	*2 mg orally once daily; max 8 mg/day*
		Caution: As a consequence of inhibiting the renin-angiotensin system, changes in renal function may be anticipated in susceptible individuals. Renal function should be monitored periodically.
		In patients who are elderly, volume-depleted (including those on diuretic therapy), or with compromised renal function, coadministration of nonsteroidal anti-inflammatory drugs (NSAIDs), including selective cyclooxygenase (COX-2) inhibitors, with angiotensin-converting enzyme (ACE) inhibitors, including perindopril, may result in deterioration of renal function, including possible acute renal failure. These effects are usually reversible. Monitor renal function periodically in patients receiving perindopril and NSAID therapy. The antihypertensive effect of ACE inhibitors, including perindopril, may be attenuated by NSAIDs, including selective COX-2 inhibitors.
Alternative adjustment:	*GFR >50 mL/min*	*4 mg orally every 24 h 1 h before or at least 2 h after meals*
	GFR 10–50 mL/min	*2 mg orally every 24–48 h 1 h before or at least 2 h after meals*
	GFR <10 mL/min	*2 mg orally every 48 h 1 h before or at least 2 h after meals*
	Hemodialysis	*2 mg orally every 48 h 1 h before or at least 2 h after meals (no supplemental post-dialysis dose)*
	CAPD	*2 mg orally every 48 h 1 h before or at least 2 h after meals*
	CRRT	*2 mg orally every 24–48 h*

Phenazopyridine - Selected References

Alano FA Jr, Webster GD Jr. Acute renal failure and pigmentation due to phenazopyridine (Pyridium®). Ann Intern Med. 1970;72:89–91.

Cahan DH. Phenazopyridine overdose and renal failure [letter]. JAMA. 1979;241:2785.

Engle JE, Schoolwerth AC. Additive nephrotoxicity from roentgenographic contrast media: its occurrence in phenazopyridine-induced acute renal failure. Arch Intern Med. 1981;141:784–6.

Eybel CE, Armbruster KFW, Ing TS. Skin pigmentation and acute renal failure in a patient receiving phenazopyridine therapy. JAMA. 1974;228:1027–8.

Feinfeld DA, Ranieri R, Lipner HI, Avram MM. Renal failure in phenazopyridine overdose. JAMA. 1978;240:2661.

Fincher ME, Campbell HT. Methemoglobinemia and hemolytic anemia after phenazopyridine hydrochloride (Pyridium) administration in end-stage renal disease. South Med J. 1989;82:372–4.

Nathan DM, Siegel AJ, Bunn HF. Acute methemoglobinemia and hemolytic anemia with phenazopyridine. Arch Intern Med. 1977;137:1636–8.

Onder AM, Espinoza V, Berho ME, Chandar J, Zilleruelo G, Abitbol C. Acute renal failure due to phenazopyridine (Pyridium®) overdose: case report and review of the literature. Pediatr Nephrol. 2006;21:1760–4.

Phenazopyridine tablet [package insert]. Boca Raton: Breckinridge Pharmaceutical Inc; 2008.

Qureshi N, Hedger RW. Phenazopyridine (Pyridium®) and acute renal failure [letter]. Ann Intern Med. 1979;90:443.

Rule KA, Biggs AW. Transient renal failure following phenazopyridine overdose. Urology. 1984;24:178–9.

Shang E, Xiang B, Liu G, Xie S, Wei W, Lu J, Determination of phenazopyridine in human plasma via LC-MS and subsequent development of a pharmacokinetic model. Anal Bioanal Chem. 2005;382:216–22.

Tomlinson B, Cohen SL, Smith MR, Fisher C. Nephrotoxicity of phenazopyridine. Hum Toxicol. 1983;3:539–43.

Dosage Adjustment of Medications Eliminated by the Kidneys

__Phenazopyridine__/**Pyridium**®	**{Interstitial cystitis analgesic}**
Usual initial dose:	200 mg orally
Usual maintenance dose:	100–200 mg orally three times daily
Typical Maximum Dose:	800 mg/day
Proportion eliminated unchanged:	65 %

Adjustment for Kidney Disease

FDA-approved product labeling:	*Impaired renal function, uremia*	*Contraindicated*
Alternative adjustment:	*eCrCL ≥50 mL/min*	*100–200 mg orally every 8–12 h*
	eCrCL <50 mL/min	*Avoid due to risk for nephrotoxicity and possible methemoglobinemia and hemolytic anemia.*

Dosage Adjustment of Medications Eliminated by the Kidneys

Phenobarbital - Selected References

Abdel-Hameed I, Ebid M, Abdel-Rahman HM. Pharmacokinetics of phenobarbital during enhanced elimination modalities to evaluate their clinical efficacy in management of drug overdose. Ther Drug Monit. 2001;23:209–16.

Alvarez N, Hartford E, Cavalleri E. Low blood levels of phenobarbital due to poor gastrointestinal solubility of phenobarbital tablets [letter]. Ann Neurol. 1981;9:309–10.

Aronoff GA, Bennett WM, Berns JS, et al. Drug prescribing in renal failure: dosing guidelines for adults and children. 5th ed. Philadelphia: American College of Physicians; 2007.

Chow-Tung E, Lau AH, Vidyasagar D, John EG. Effect of peritoneal dialysis on serum concentrations of three drugs commonly used in pediatric patients. Dev Pharmacol Ther. 1985;8:85–95.

Clark JG, Suerling MD. Muscle necrosis and calcification in acute renal failure due to barbiturate intoxication. Br Med J. 1966;2:214–5.

Dodson WE, DeLorenzo RJ, Pedley TA, et al. Treatment of convulsive status epilepticus: recommendations of the Epilepsy Foundation of America's Working Group on Status Epilepticus. JAMA. 1993;270:854–9.

Kälviäinen R, Eriksson K, Parviainen I. Refractory generalised convulsive status epilepticus: a guide to treatment. CNS Drugs. 2005;19:759–68.

Meierkord H, Boon P, Engelsen B, et al. EFNS (European Federation of Neurological Societies) guideline on the management of status epilepticus in adults. Eur J Neurol. 2010;17:348–55.

Meyer MC, Straughn AB, Raghow G, Scary WL, Rotenberg KS. Absorption of phenobarbital from tablets and elixir. J Pharm Sci. 1984;73:485–8.

Nelson E, Powell JR, Conrad K, et al. Phenobarbital pharmacokinetics and bioavailability in adults. J Clin Pharmacol. 1982;22:141–8.

Ohnhaus EE, Siegl H. Changes in renal function following chronic phenobarbitone administration [abstract]. Br J Pharmacol. 1974;52:141P.

Ohnhaus EE, Siegl H. Glomerular filtration rate and effective renal plasma flow following treatment with phenobarbital. Arch Int Pharmacodyn Ther. 1976;223:107–13.

Palmer BF. Effectiveness of hemodialysis in the extracorporeal therapy of phenobarbital overdose. Am J Kidney Dis. 2000;36:640–3.

Phenobarbital liquid [package insert]. Buffalo Grove: Pack Pharmaceuticals LLC; 2011.

Phenobarbital sodium injection [package insert]. Eatontown: West-Ward Pharmaceuticals; 2011.

Phenobarbital tablet [package insert]. Rockford: UDL Laboratories Inc; 2010.

Pierides AM, Ellis HA, Ward M, et al. Barbiturate and anticonvulsant treatment in relation to osteomalacia with haemodialysis and renal transplantation. Br Med J. 1976;1:190–3.

Roberts DM, Buckley NA. Enhanced elimination in acute barbiturate poisoning—a systematic review. Clin Toxicol (Phila). 2011;49:2–12.

Sagraves R, Bradberry JC. The effects of exchange transfusion on the pharmacokinetics of phenobarbital. Drug Intell Clin Pharm. 1983;17:901–3.

Sedman AJ, Molitoris BA, Nakata LM, Gal J. Therapeutic drug monitoring in patients with chronic renal failure: evaluation of the Abbott TDx™ drug assay system. Am J Nephrol. 1986;6:132–4.

Thomson AH, Brodie MJ. Pharmacokinetic optimization of anticonvulsant therapy. Clin Pharmacokinet. 1992;23:216–30.

Turck JW, Ladenson JH. Phenytoin and phenobarbital concentrations in renal insufficiency [letter]. Ann Intern Med. 1984;101:568–9.

Viswanathan CT, Booker HE, Welling PG. Bioavailability of oral and intramuscular phenobarbital. J Clin Pharmacol. 1978;18:100–5.

Viswanathan CT, Booker HE, Welling PG. Pharmacokinetics of phenobarbital following single and repeated doses. J Clin Pharmacol. 1979;19:282–9.

Wilensky AJ, Friel PN, Levy RH, Comfort CP, Kaluzny SP. Kinetics of phenobarbital in normal subjects and epileptic patients. Eur J Clin Pharmacol. 1982;23:87–92.

Dosage Adjustment of Medications Eliminated by the Kidneys

<u>**Phenobarbital**</u>/**Luminal**®   {Antiepileptic; sedative}

Usual initial dose:	30–800 mg (20 mg/kg IV loading dose for refractory status epilepticus or [dose {mg/kg} = desired increase in plasma level {mg/L} ÷ 0.5 {V_d, volume of distribution in L/kg}] with good supportive care) PO, IV, or IM
Usual maintenance dose:	60–100 mg orally two to three times daily PO, IM, or IV (1–3 mg/kg/day)[a]
Typical maximum dose:	2,000 mg
Proportion eliminated unchanged:	16 % (plus 21 % of each dose as hydroxylated metabolite; urine pH dependent)

Adjustment for Kidney Disease

FDA-approved product labeling: *Not available*

Alternative adjustment:	*GFR >50 mL/min*	*30–100 mg orally every 8–12 h[a]*
	GFR 10–50 mL/min	*30–100 mg orally every 8–12 h[a]*
	GFR <10 mL/min	*30–100 mg orally every 12–16 h[a]*
	Hemodialysis	*30–100 mg orally every 12–16 h (administer supplemental dose before hemodialysis plus one-half usual dose amount after hemodialysis on dialysis days)[a]*
	CAPD	*15–60 mg orally every 12–16 h (approx 50 % decrease)[a]*
	CRRT	*30–100 mg orally every 8–12 h[a]*

[a]**Therapeutic Drug Monitoring**

    Therapeutic plasma levels: *Trough: 15–40 mg/L*

Dosage Adjustment of Medications Eliminated by the Kidneys

<u>Phenytoin</u> - Selected References

American College of Emergency Physicians Clinical Policy Committee. Critical issues in the evaluation and management of adult patients presenting to the emergency department with seizures. Ann Emerg Med. 2004;43:605–25.

Aronoff GA, Bennett WM, Berns JS, et al. Drug prescribing in renal failure: dosing guidelines for adults and children. 5th ed. Philadelphia: American College of Physicians; 2007.

Aweeka FT, Gottwald MD, Gambertoglio JG, et al. Pharmacokinetics of fosphenytoin in patients with hepatic or renal disease. Epilepsia. 1999;40:777–82.

Brown-Molnar CS, Bauer LA, Horn JR. Phenytoin removal by plasmapheresis in renal insufficiency. Am J Nephrol. 1986;6:302–6.

Dager WE, Inciardi JF, Howe TL. Estimating phenytoin concentrations by the Sheiner-Tozer method in adults with pronounced hypoalbuminemia. Ann Pharmacother. 1995;29:667–70.

Dilantin® extended phenytoin sodium capsule. New York: Parke-Davis Division of Pfizer Inc; 2011.

Dodson WE, DeLorenzo RJ, Pedley TA, et al. Treatment of convulsive status epilepticus: recommendations of the Epilepsy Foundation of America's Working Group on Status Epilepticus. JAMA. 1993;270:854–9.

Eadie MJ, Tyrer JH, Bochner F, Hooper WD. The elimination of phenytoin in man. Clin Exp Pharmacol Physiol. 1976;3:217–24.

Houghton GW, Richens A, Leighton M. Effect of age, height, weight and sex on serum phenytoin concentration in epileptic patients. Br J Clin Pharmacol. 1975;2:251–6.

Kälviäinen R, Eriksson K, Parviainen I. Refractory generalised convulsive status epilepticus: a guide to treatment. CNS Drugs. 2005;19:759–68.

Liponi DF, Winter ME, Tozer TN. Renal function and therapeutic concentrations of phenytoin. Neurology. 1984;34:395–7.

Martin E, Gambertoglio JG, Adler DS, Tozer TN, Roman LA. Graisz H. Removal of phenytoin by hemodialysis in uremic patients. JAMA. 1977;238:1750–3.

Martin E, Tozer TN, Sheiner LB, Riegelman S. The clinical pharmacokinetics of phenytoin. J Pharmacokinet Biopharm. 1977;5:579–96.

Meierkord H, Boon P, Engelsen B, et al. EFNS (European Federation of Neurological Societies) guideline on the management of status epilepticus in adults. Eur J Neurol. 2010;17:348–55.

Peterson GM, Khoo BHC, von Witt RJ. Clinical response in epilepsy in relation to total and free serum levels of phenytoin. Ther Drug Monit. 1991;13:415–9.

Phenytoin sodium injection. Lake Forest: Hospira Inc; 2010.

Reynolds F, Ziroyanis PN, Jones NF, Smith SE. Salivary phenytoin concentrations in epilepsy and in chronic renal failure. Lancet. 1976;2:384–6.

Richens A. Clinical pharmacokinetics of phenytoin. Clin Pharmacokinet. 1979;4:153–69.

Richens A, Dunlop A. Serum phenytoin levels in management of epilepsy. Lancet. 1975;2:247–8.

Rimmer EM, Buss DC, Routeledge PA, Richens A. Should we routinely measure free plasma phenytoin concentration? Br J Clin Pharmacol. 1984;17:99–102.

Schmidt D, Einicke I, Haenel F. The influence of seizure type on the efficacy of plasma concentrations of phenytoin, phenobarbital, and carbamazepine. Arch Neurol. 1986;263–5.

Surman OS, Parker SW. Complex partial seizures and psychiatric disturbance in end-stage renal disease. Psychosomatics. 1981;22:1077–80.

Treiman DM, Meyers PD, Walton NY, et al. A comparison of four treatments for generalized convulsive status epilepticus. N Engl J Med. 1998;339:792–8.

von Winckelmann SL, Spriet I, Willems L. Therapeutic drug monitoring of phenytoin in critically ill patients. Pharmacotherapy. 2008;28:1391–400.

Vožeh S, Uematsu T, Aarons L, Maitre P, Landolt H, Gratzl O. Intravenous phenytoin loading in patients after neurosurgery and in status epilepticus: a population pharmacokinetic study. Clin Pharmacokinet. 1988;14:122–8.

Zielmann S, Mielck F, Kahl R, et al. A rational basis for the measurement of free phenytoin concentration in critically ill trauma patients. Ther Drug Monit. 1994;16:139–44.

Dosage Adjustment of Medications Eliminated by the Kidneys

Phenytoin/Dilantin®	**{Antiepileptic}**
Usual initial dose:	50–200 mg PO or IV (750–1,500 mg [18–20 mg/kg] IV loading dose for status epilepticus or [dose {mg/kg} = desired increase in plasma level {mg/L} ÷ 0.75 {V_d, volume of distribution in L/kg}] with good supportive care)
Usual maintenance dose:	100 mg IV or orally three times daily
Typical maximum dose:	1,000 mg/day
Proportion eliminated unchanged:	5 % (protein binding markedly decreased in uremia)

Adjustment for Kidney Disease

FDA-approved product labeling: *Data not available*

Alternative adjustment:

GFR >50 mL/min	*100 mg IV or orally every 8 h[a]*
GFR 10–50 mL/min	*100 mg IV or orally every 8 h[a]*
GFR <10 mL/min	*50–100 mg IV or orally every 8–12 h[a]*
Hemodialysis	*50–100 mg IV or orally every 8–12 h (no supplemental post-dialysis dose)[a]*
CAPD	*50–100 mg IV or orally every 8–12 h[a]*
CRRT	*50–100 mg IV or orally every 8–12 h[a]*

[a]**Therapeutic Drug Monitoring**

Therapeutic plasma levels:	*Trough:*	*Phenytoin total: 10–20 mg/L*
		Phenytoin free: 8–10 % of total

Note: In severely uremic (CrCL <10 mg/dL) and/or hypoalbuminemic patients, measure free phenytoin levels or determine corrected total phenytoin levels using the following equation:

$$C_{corrected} = \frac{C_{observed}}{0.2 \times \text{albumin} \left(g / dL \right) + 0.1}$$

where

$C_{observed}$ = measured total serum phenytoin concentration

$C_{corrected}$ = serum phenytoin concentration corrected for altered protein binding in uremic patients

Dosage Adjustment of Medications Eliminated by the Kidneys

Phosphate - Selected References

Alaniz C, Rice TL. Evaluation of intravenous phosphate replacement in a university hospital. Hosp Pharm. 1993;28:385, 388, 391–2.

Bohannon NJV. Large phosphate shifts with treatment for hyperglycemia. Arch Intern Med. 1989;149:1423–5.

Chonchol M, Dale R, Schrier RW, Estacio R. Serum phosphorus and cardiovascular mortality in type 2 diabetes. Am J Med. 2009;122:380–6.

Hemstreet BA, Stolpman N, Badesch DB, May SK, McCollum M. Potassium and phosphorus repletion in hospitalized patients: implications for clinical practice and the potential use of healthcare information technology to improve prescribing and patient safety. Curr Med Res Opin. 2006;22:2449–55.

Kraft MD, Btaiche IF, Sacks GS, Kudsk KA. Treatment of electrolyte disorders in adult patients in the intensive care unit. Am J Health Syst Pharm. 2005;62:1663–82.

Laaban J-P, Waked M, Laromiguiere M, Vuong T-K, Rochemaure J. Hypophosphatemia complicating management of acute severe asthma. Ann Intern Med. 1990;112:68–9.

Lentz RD, Brown DN, Kjellstrand CM. Treatment of severe hypophosphatemia. Ann Intern Med. 1978;89:941–4.

Lloyd CW, Johnson CE. Management of hypophosphatemia. Clin Pharm. 1988;7:123–8.

Owen P, Monahan MF, MacLaren R. Implementing and assessing an evidence-based electrolyte dosing order form in the medical ICU. Intensive Crit Care Nurs. 2008;24(1):8–19.

Perreault MN, Ostrop NJ, Tierney MG. Efficacy and safety of intravenous phosphate replacement in critically ill patients. Ann Pharmacother. 1997;31:683–8.

Potassium phosphates injection USP [package insert]. Shirley: American Regent Inc; 2005.

Sedlacek M, Schoolwerth AC, Remillard BD. Electrolyte disturbances in the intensive care unit. Semin Dial. 2006;19:496–501.

Subramanian R, Khardori R. Severe hypophosphatemia: pathophysiologic implications, clinical presentations, and treatment. Medicine (Baltimore). 2000;79:1–8.

University of Colorado Hospital ICU Electrolyte Replacement Guideline, 2010.

University of Colorado Hospital Med-Surg Electrolyte Replacement Draft Guideline, 2011.

Yu GC, Lee DBN. Clinical disorders of phosphorus metabolism. West J Med. 1987;147:569–76.

Dosage Adjustment of Medications Eliminated by the Kidneys

<u>Phosphate, Sodium or Potassium (IV);</u>
<u>Sodium-Potassium Phosphate</u>/KPhos Neutral®   {Electrolyte}

Usual initial dose:	0.08 mmol/kg IV
Usual maintenance dose:	–
Typical maximum dose:	1 mmol/kg/day IV or potassium phosphate 1,000 mg orally four times daily
Proportion eliminated unchanged:	90 %

Adjustment for Kidney Disease

FDA-approved product labeling:	*The dose and rate of administration are dependent upon the needs of the patient*
Alternative adjustment:	*Phosphate dosage in (a) ICU patients and (b) non-ICU patients (phosphate replacement)*

(a) ICU patients

	Glomerular filtration rate (GFR in mL/min)		
Serum/plasma [PO$_4$]	*>50*	*25–50*	*<25*
2.1–3.0 mg/dL	*Sodium-potassium phosphate (KPhos Neutral®) 1,000 mg via enteral route every 6 h × 4.*	*Sodium-potassium phosphate (KPhos Neutral®) 1,000 mg via enteral route every 12 h × 2.*	*Sodium-potassium phosphate (KPhos Neutral®) 500 mg via enteral route every 12 h × 2.*
	If enteral route NOT available, sodium phosphate 45 mmol IV × 1	*If enteral route NOT available, sodium phosphate 22.5 mmol IV × 1*	*If enteral route NOT available, sodium phosphate 15 mmol IV × 1*
1.1–2.0 mg/dL	*Sodium phosphate 60 mmol IV × 1*	*Sodium phosphate 45 mmol IV × 1*	*Sodium phosphate 22.5 mmol IV × 1*
≤1.0 mg/dL	*Notify MD*	*Notify MD*	*Notify MD*

Note: Sodium-potassium phosphate (KPhos Neutral®) 250 mg tablet = 8 mmol phosphate, 13 mEq sodium, 1.1 mEq potassium. Every 7.5 mmol sodium phosphate contains 10 mEq sodium

Phosphate preferred IV rate ≤5 mmol/h; Maximum rate: ≤7.5 mmol/h (emergency)

Phosphate maximum IV dose = 135 mmol in 24 h

In renal impairment, IV sodium phosphate usually is preferred over IV potassium phosphate due to potassium content

(b) Non-ICU patients

	Mild depletion [PO$_4$] 2.1–2.4 mg/dL	Moderate depletion [PO$_4$] 1.0–2.0 mg/dL	Severe depletion [PO$_4$] <1.0 mg/dL
Initial treatment	*No treatment or sodium-potassium phosphate (KPhos Neutral®) 500 mg orally TID*	*Sodium phosphate 5–10 mmol (0.1 mmol/kg) IV over 2 h*	*Sodium phosphate 10–20 mmol (0.2 mmol/kg) IV over 4 h*

Note: Sodium-potassium phosphate (KPhos Neutral®) 250 mg tablet = 8 mmol phosphate, 13 mEq sodium, 1.1 mEq potassium. Every 7.5 mmol sodium phosphate contains 10 mEq sodium

Phosphate preferred IV rate ≤5 mmol/h. Maximum rate: ≤7.5 mmol/h (emergency)

Phosphate maximum IV dose = 135 mmol in 24 h

Unless sodium restricted, IV sodium phosphate usually is preferred over IV potassium phosphate due to potassium content and risk of resultant hyperkalemia, especially in patients with renal impairment. Potassium phosphate may be considered in the presence of hypokalemia—caution, every 1 mmol of potassium phosphate contains 1.5 mEq potassium

Replacement should be given with careful clinical monitoring, including post-dose confirmation of trends toward normalization of serum electrolyte values. Levels usually should be measured 2–4 h after oral therapy or at completion of IV infusion. Treatment should be repeated or continued until the patient is asymptomatic or levels are within acceptable ranges

Dosage Adjustment of Medications Eliminated by the Kidneys

Piperacillin and Tazobactam - Selected References

Arzuaga A, Maynar J, Gascón AR, et al. Influence of renal function on the pharmacokinetics and pharmacodynamics of piperacillin/tazobactam in intensive care unit patients during continuous venovenous hemofiltration. J Clin Pharmacol. 2005;45:168–76.

Buck C, Bertram N, Ackermann T, Sauerbruch T, Derendorf H, Paar WD. Pharmacokinetics of piperacillin-tazobactam: intermittent dosing versus continuous infusion. Int J Antimicrob Agents. 2005;25:62–7.

Bullita JB, Kinzig M, Jakob V, Holzgrabe U, Sörgel F, Holford NHG. Nonlinear pharmacokinetics of piperacillin in healthy volunteers—implications for optimal dosage regimens. Br J Clin Pharmacol. 2010;70:682–93.

Capellier G, Cornette C, Boillot A, et al. Removal of piperacillin in critically ill patients undergoing continuous venovenous hemofiltration. Crit Care Med. 1998;26:88–91.

Conil J-M, Georges B, Mimoz O, et al. Influence of renal function on trough serum concentrations of piperacillin in intensive care unit patients. Intensive Care Med. 2006;32:2063–66.

Connor MJ Jr, Salem C, Bauer SR, et al. Therapeutic drug monitoring of piperacillin-tazobactam using spent dialysate effluent in patients receiving continuous venovenous hemodialysis. Antimicrob Agents Chemother. 2011;55:557–60.

Debruyne D, Ryckelynck JP, Hurault De Ligny B, Moulin M. Pharmacokinetics of piperacillin in patients on peritoneal dialysis with and without peritonitis. J Pharm Sci. 1990;79:99–102.

Giron JA, Meyers BR, Hirschman SZ, Srulevitch E. Pharmacokinetics of piperacillin in patients with moderate renal failure and in patients undergoing hemodialysis. Antimicrob Agents Chemother. 1981;19:279–83.

Heim-Duthoy KL, Halstenson CE, Abraham PA, Matzke GR. The effect of hemodialysis on piperacillin pharmacokinetics. Int J Clin Pharmacol Ther Toxicol. 1986;24:680–4.

Koomanachai P, Bulik CC, Kuti JL, Nicolau DP. Pharmacodynamic modeling of intravenous antibiotics against gram-negative bacteria collected in the United States. Clin Ther. 2010;32:766–79.

Lau WK, Mercer D, Itani KM, et al. Randomized, open-label, comparative study of piperacillin-tazobactam administered by continuous infusion versus intermittent infusion for treatment of hospitalized patients with complicated intra-abdominal infection. Antimicrob Agents Chemother. 2006;50:6556–61.

Lin C-S, Cheng C-J, Chou C-H, Lin S-H. Piperacillin-tazobactam-induced seizure rapidly reversed by high flux hemodialysis in a patient on peritoneal dialysis. Am J Med Sci. 2007;333:181–4.

Lorente L, Jiménez A, Martín MM, Iribarren JL, Jiménez JJ, Mora ML. Clinical cure of ventilator-associated pneumonia treated with piperacillin-tazobactam administered by continuous or intermittent infusion. Int J Antimicrob Agents. 2009;33:464–8.

Manley HJ, Bailie GR, Frye R, McGoldrick MD. Intermittent intravenous piperacillin pharmacokinetics in automated peritoneal dialysis patients. Perit Dial Int. 2000;20:686–93.

Meyer B, Guttmann C, Dittrich E, Schmaldienst S, Thalhammer F. Intermittent administration of betalactam-antibiotics for treatment of severe infection in hemodialysis patients. Eur J Med Res. 2005;10:140–4.

Moriyama B, Henning SA, Neuhauser M, Danner RL, Walsh TJ. Continuous-infusion β-lactam antibiotics during continuous venovenous hemofiltration for the treatment of resistant gram-negative bacteria. Ann Pharmacother. 2009;43:1324–37.

Mueller SC, Majcher-Peszynska J, Hickstein H, et al. Pharmacokinetics of piperacillin-tazobactam in anuric intensive care patients during continuous venovenous hemodialysis. Antimicrob Agents Chemother. 2002;46:1557–60.

Patel N, Scheetz MH, Drusano GL, Lodise TP. Identification of optimal renal dosage adjustments for traditional and extended-infusion piperacillin-tazobactam dosing regimens in hospitalized patients. Antimicrob Agents Chemother. 2010;54:460–5.

Piperacillin and tazobactam injection [package insert]. Lake Forest: Hospira Worldwide Inc; 2009.

Seyler L, Cotton F, Taccone FS, et al. Recommended β-lactam regimens are inadequate in septic patients treated with continuous renal replacement therapy. Crit Care. 2011;15:R137. doi:10.1186/cc10257.

Thompson MIB, Russo ME, Matsen JM, Atkin-Thor E. Piperacillin pharmacokinetics in subjects with chronic renal failure. Antimicrob Agents Chemother. 1981;19:450–3.

van der Werf TS, Mulder POM, Zijlsta JG, Uges DRA, Stegeman CA. Pharmacokinetics of piperacillin and tazobactam in critically ill patients with renal failure, treated with continuous veno-venous hemofiltration (CVVH). Intensive Care Med. 1997;23:873–77.

Welling PG, Craig WA, Bundtzen RW, Kwok FW, Gerber AU, Madsen PO. Pharmacokinetics of piperacillin in subjects with various degrees of renal function. Antimicrob Agents Chemother. 1983;23:881–7.

Dosage Adjustment of Medications Eliminated by the Kidneys

Piperacillin and Tazobactam/Zosyn®   {Antibacterial; extended-spectrum penicillin/ β-lactamase inhibitor}

Usual initial dose:	4.5 g IV
Usual maintenance dose:	3.375 g IV over 30 min every 6 h or 13.5 g/24 h continuous IV infusion
Typical maximum dose:	18 g (piperacillin)/day
Proportion eliminated unchanged:	68 %/80 %

Adjustment for Kidney Disease

FDA-approved product labeling:

Piperacillin/tazobactam dosage recommendations for adults with renal function impairment

CrCL (mL/min)	All indications (except nosocomial pneumonia)	Nosocomial pneumonia
>40	3.375 g every 6 h	4.5 g every 6 h
20–40	2.25 g every 6 h	3.375 g every 6 h
<20	2.25 g every 8 h	2.25 g every 6 h
Hemodialysis[a]	2.25 g every 12 h	2.25 g every 8 h
CAPD	2.25 g every 12 h	2.25 g every 8 h

[a]Administer supplemental 0.75 g following each dialysis

Alternative adjustment:

GFR >40 mL/min	4.5 g IV over 30 min every 6 h or 3.375 g IV over 4 h every 8 h or 10.125–18 g/24 h IV continuous infusion
GFR 20–40 mL/min	3.375 g IV over 30 min every 6 h or 3.375 g IV over 4 h every 8 h
GFR <20 mL/min	2.25 g IV over 30 min every 6 h or 3.375 g IV over 4 h every 12 h
Hemodialysis	2.25 g IV over 30 min every 8 h; administer 2.25 g IV supplemental dose after dialysis.
CAPD	2.25 g IV over 30 min every 8 h
CVVH	2.25–3.375 g IV over 30 min every 6–8 h
CVVHD	3.375–4.5 g IV over 30 min every 6 h
CVVHDF	3.375–4.5 g IV over 30 min every 6 h

Note: GFR-based dosage recommendations are primarily based on treatment of nosocomial pneumonia or other serious infections caused by gram-negative bacteria with intermediate sensitivity to piperacillin-tazobactam.

Dosage Adjustment of Medications Eliminated by the Kidneys

Piroxicam - Selected References

Darragh A, Gordon AJ, O'Byrne H, Hobbs D, Casey E. Single-dose and steady-state pharmacokinetics of piroxicam n elderly vs young adults. Eur J Clin Pharmacol. 1985;28:305–9.

Feldene® capsule [package insert]. New York: Pfizer Inc; 2010.

Frais MA, Burgess ED, Mitchell LB. Piroxicam-induced renal failure and hyperkalemia [letter]. Ann Intern Med. 1988;99:129–30.

Henry D, McGettigan P. Epidemiology overview of gastrointestinal and renal toxicity of NSAIDs. Int J Clin Pract Suppl. 2003;135:43–9.

Hobbs DC. Piroxicam pharmacokinetics: recent clinical results relating kinetics and plasma levels to age, sex, and adverse effects. Am J Med. 1986;81(Suppl 5B):22–8..

Hobbs DC, Twomey TM. Piroxicam pharmacokinetics in man: aspirin and antacid interaction studies. J Clin Pharmacol. 1979;19:270–81.

Ishizaki T, Nomura T, Abe T. Pharmacokinetics of piroxicam, a new nonsteroidal anti-inflammatory agent, under fasting and postprandial states in man. J Pharmacokinet Biopharm. 1979;7:369–81.

Loeffler M, Hanson G, Philp T. Piroxicam-induced renal failure following relief of chronic retention. Br J Urol. 1989;63:438–9.

Mavrikakis ME, Georgilis KA, Ziroyannis PN, Kehayoglou KA, Moulopoulos SD. Piroxicam-induced acute renal failure (anuria) [letter]. Ann Rheum Dis. 1985;44:356–8.

McIntyre CW, Owen PJ. Prescribing drugs in kidney disease. In: Brenner BM, editor. Brenner & Rector's the kidney. 8th ed. Philadelphia: Saunders/Elsevier; 2008. p. 1930–55.

Mitnick PD, Klein WJ Jr. Piroxicam-induced renal disease. Arch Intern Med. 1984;144:63–4.

Olkkola KT, Brunetto AV, Mattila MJ. Pharmacokinetics of oxicam nonsteroidal anti-inflammatory agents. Clin Pharmacokinet. 1994;26:107–20.

Palma-Aguirre JA, Lopez-Gamboa M, Cariño L, Burke-Fraga V, González-de la Parra M. Relative bioavailability of two oral formulations of piroxicam 20 mg: a single-dose, randomized-sequence, open-label, two-period crossover comparison in healthy Mexican adult volunteers. Clin Ther. 2010;32:357–64.

Rudy AC, Figueroa NL, Hall SD, Brater DC. The pharmacokinetics of piroxicam in elderly persons with and without renal impairment. Br J Clin Pharmacol. 1994;37:1–5.

Sarma PSA. Fatal acute renal failure after piroxicam [letter]. Clin Nephrol. 1989;31:54.

Tilstone WJ, Lawson DH, Omara F, Cunningham F. The steady-state pharmacokinetics of piroxicam: effect of food and iron. Eur J Rheumatol Inflamm. 1981;4:309–13.

Whelton A, Stout RL, Spilman PS, Klassen DK. Renal effects of ibuprofen, piroxicam, and sulindac in patients with asymptomatic renal failure: a prospective, randomized, crossover comparison. Ann Intern Med. 1990;112:568–76.

Dosage Adjustment of Medications Eliminated by the Kidneys

<u>Piroxicam</u>/Feldene®   **{Anti-inflammatory; nonsteroidal anti-inflammatory drug}**

Usual initial dose:	20 mg orally
Usual maintenance dose:	20 mg orally once daily
Typical maximum dose:	40 mg/day
Proportion eliminated unchanged:	10 %

Adjustment for Kidney Disease

FDA-approved product labeling:	*Mild to moderate renal insufficiency*	*No adjustment necessary*
	Advanced renal disease	*No data, not recommended*
	Severe renal failure	*Contraindicated*
Alternative adjustment:	*GFR >50 mL/min*	*20 mg orally once daily*
	GFR 10–50 mL/min	*20 mg orally once daily*
	GFR <10 mL/min	*Preferably avoid due to risk for gastrointestinal and renal toxicity.*
	Hemodialysis	*Data not available; preferably avoid.*
	CAPD	*Data not available; preferably avoid.*
	CRRT	*Not applicable; preferably avoid.*

Dosage Adjustment of Medications Eliminated by the Kidneys

<u>Pitavastatin</u> - Selected References

Cheng XW, Kuzuya M, Sasaki T, et al. Inhibition of mineralocorticoid receptor is a renoprotective effect of 3-hydroxy-3-methylglutaryl coenzyme A reductase inhibitor pitavastatin. J Hypertens. 2011;29:542–52.

Corsini A, Ceska R. Drug-drug interactions with statins: will pitavastatin overcome the statins' Achilles' heel? Curr Med Res Opin. 2011;27:1551–62.

Eriksson M, Budinski D, Hounslow N. Comparative efficacy of pitavastatin and simvastatin in high-risk patients: a randomized controlled trial. Adv Ther. 2011;28:811–23.

Eriksson M, Budinski D, Hounslow N. Long-term efficacy of pitavastatin versus simvastatin. Adv Ther. 2011;28:799–810.

Hirano M, Maeda K, Shitara Y, Sugiyama Y. Contribution of OATP2 (OATP1B1) and OATP8 (OATP1B3) to the hepatic uptake of pitavastatin in humans. J Pharmacol Exp Ther. 2004;311:139–46.

Igel M, Sudhop T, von Bergmann K. Pharmacology of 3-hydroxy-3-methylglutaryl coenzyme A reductase inhibitors (statins), including rosuvastatin and pitavastatin. J Clin Pharmacol. 2002;42:835–45.

Kawai Y, Sato-Ishida R, Motoyama A, Kajinami K. Place of pitavastatin in the statin armamentarium: promising evidence for a role in diabetes mellitus. Drug Des Devel Ther. 2011;5:283–97.

Kimura K, Shimano H, Yokote K, Urashima M, Teramoto T. Effects of pitavastatin (Livalo tablet) on the estimated glomerular filtration rate (eGFR) in hypercholesterolemic patients with chronic kidney disease: sub-analysis of the Livalo Effectiveness and Safety (LIVES) study. J Atheroscler Thromb. 2010;17:601–9.

Livalo® tablet film coated [package insert]. Montgomery: Kowa Pharmaceuticals America Inc; 2009.

Malik S, Kumar A, Bharti S, et al. In vivo cardioprotection by pitavastatin from ischemic-reperfusion injury through suppression of IKK/NF-κB and upregulation of pAkt-e-NOS. J Cardiovasc Pharmacol. 2011;58:199–206.

Maruyama T, Takada M, Nishibori Y, et al. Comparison of preventive effect on cardiovascular events with different statins: the CIRCLE study. Circ J. 2011;75:1951–9.

Nakamura T, Sato E, Fujiwara N, et al. Co-administration of ezetimibe enhances proteinuria-lowering effects of pitavastatin in chronic kidney disease patients partly via a cholesterol-independent manner. Pharmacol Res. 2010;61:58–61.

Nakamura T, Sugaya T, Kawagoe Y, Suzuki T, Inoue T, Node K. Effect of pitavastatin on urinary liver-type fatty acid-binding protein levels in patients with nondiabetic mild chronic kidney disease. Am J Nephrol. 2006;26:82–6.

Nakamura T, Ueda Y, Sugaya T, Osada S, Kawagoe Y, Koide H. Effect of pitavastatin on urinary liver-type fatty acid-binding protein levels in patients with early diabetic nephropathy. Diabetes Care. 2005;28:2728–32.

Poolsup N, Suksomboon N, Wongyaowarat K, Rungkanchananon B, Niyomrat P, Kongsuwan S. Meta-analysis of the comparative efficacy and safety of pitavastatin in patients with dyslipidemia. J Clin Pharm Ther. 2012;37:166–72. doi:10.1111/j.1365-2710.2011.01274.x.

Saito Y, Yamada N, Teramoto T, et al. Clinical efficacy of pitavastatin, a new 3-hydroxy-3-methylglutaryl coenzyme A reductase inhibitor, in patients with hyperlipidemia : dose-finding study using the double-blind, three-group parallel comparison. Arzneimittelforschung. 2002;52:251–5.

Saku K, Zhang B, Noda K, et al. Randomized head-to-head comparison of pitavastatin, atorvastatin, and rosuvastatin for safety and efficacy (quantity and quality of LDL) : the PATROL trial. Circ J. 2011;75:1493–505.

Suh SY, Rha S-W, Ahn TH, et al. Long-term safety and efficacy of pitavastatin in patients with acute myocardial infarction (from the Livalo Acute Myocardial Infarction Study [LAMIS]). Am J Cardiol. 2011;108:1530–5. doi:10.1016/j.amjcard.2011.07.009.

Yagi S, Aihara K, Ikeda Y, et al. Pitavastatin, an HMG-CoA reductase inhibitor, exerts eNOS-independent protective actions against angiotensin II-induced cardiovascular remodeling and renal insufficiency. Circ Res. 2008;102:68–76.

Yagi S, Akaike M, Aihara K-I, et al. Effect of low-dose (1 mg/day) pitavastatin on left ventricular diastolic function and albuminuria in patients with hyperlipidemia. Am J Cardiol. 2011;107:1644–9.

Yamada I, Fujino H, Shimada S, Kojima J. Metabolic fate of pitavastatin, a new inhibitor of HMG-CoA reductase: similarities and difference in the metabolism of pitavastatin in monkeys and humans. Xenobiotica. 2003;33:789–903.

Yee LL, Wright EA. Pitavastatin calcium: clinical review of a new antihyperlipidemic medication. Clin Ther. 2011;33:1023–42.

Dosage Adjustment of Medications Eliminated by the Kidneys

Pitavastatin/Livalo®   {Antihypercholesterolemic agent; hydroxymethylglutaryl-coenzyme A (HMG-CoA) reductase inhibitor}

Usual initial dose: 2 mg orally once daily

Usual maintenance dose: 1–4 mg orally once daily

Typical maximum dose: 4 mg/day

Proportion eliminated unchanged: 15 %

Adjustment for Kidney Disease

FDA-approved product labeling: *Pitavastatin dosage in patients with renal impairment*

Renal function	Initial dose	Maximum dose
eGFR ≥60 mL/min/1.73 m²	2 mg once daily	4 mg once daily
eGFR 30–59 mL/min/1.73 m²	1 mg once daily	2 mg once daily
eGFR <30 mL/min/1.73 m² (not on dialysis)	Avoid	Avoid
Hemodialysis	1 mg once daily	2 mg once daily

Alternative adjustment: *Data not available*

Dosage Adjustment of Medications Eliminated by the Kidneys

Plerixafor - Selected References

Basak GW, Jaksic O, Koristek Z, et al. Identification of prognostic factors for plerixafor-based hematopoietic stem cell mobilization. Am J Hematol. 2011;86:550–3.

DiPersio JF, Stadtmauer EA, Nademanee A, et al. Plerixafor and G-CSF versus placebo and G-CSF for mobilize hematopoietic stem cells for autologous stem cell transplantation in patients with multiple myeloma. Blood. 2009;113:5720–6.

DiPersio JR, Micallef IN, Stiff PJ, et al. Phase III prospective randomized double-blind placebo-controlled trial of plerixafor plus granulocyte colony-stimulating factor compared with placebo plus granulocyte colony-stimulating factor for autologous stem-cell mobilization and transplantation for patients with non-Hodgkin's lymphoma. J Clin Oncol. 2009;27:4767–73.

Douglas KW, Parker AN, Hayden PJ, et al. Plerixafor for PBSC mobilisation in myeloma patients with advanced renal failure: safety and efficacy data in a series of 21 patients from Europe and the USA. Bone Marrow Transplant. 2012;47:18–23. doi:10.1038/bmt.2011.9.

Duarte RF, Shaw BE, Marin P, et al. Plerixafor plus granulocyte CSF can mobilize hematopoietic stem cells from multiple myeloma and lymphoma patients failing previous mobilization attempts: EU compassionate use data. Bone Marrow Transplant. 2011;46:52–8.

Giralt S, Stadtmauer EA, Harousseau JL, et al. International myeloma working group (IMWG) consensus statement and guidelines regarding the current status of stem cell collection and high-dose therapy for multiple myeloma and the role of plerixafor (AMD 3100). Leukemia. 2009;23:1904–12.

Gregory KM, Rao K, Arimistead PM. Plerixafor dosing and administration in a patient with dialysis-dependent renal failure. Ann Pharmacother. 2010;44:2028–30.

Hendrix CW, Flexner C, MacFarland RT, et al. Pharmacokinetics and safety of AMD-3100, a novel antagonist of the CXCR-4 chemokine receptor, in human volunteers. Antimicrob Agents Chemother. 2000;44:1667–73.

Hendrix CW, Collier AC, Lederman MM, et al. Safety, pharmacokinetics, and antiviral activity of AMD3100, a selective CXCR4 receptor inhibitor, in HIV-1 infection. J Acquir Immune Defic Syndr. 2004;37:1253–62.

Jacobson O, Weiss ID, Szajek L, Farber J, Kiesewetter DO. ^{64}Cu-AMD3100 – a novel imaging agent for targeting chemokine receptor CXCR4. Bioorg Med Chem. 2009;17:1486–93.

Jantuen E, Kuittinen T, Mahlamäki E, Pyörälä M, Mäntymaa P. Efficacy of pre-emptively use plerixafor in patients mobilizing poorly after chemomobilization: a single centre experience. Eur J Haematol. 2011;86:299–304.

Keating GM. Plerixafor: a review of its use in stem cell mobilization in patients with lymphoma or multiple myeloma. Drugs. 2011;71:1623–47.

Lack NA, Green B, Dale DC, et al. A pharmacokinetic-pharmacodynamic model for mobilization of CD34$^+$ hematopoietic progenitor cells by AMD3100. Clin Pharmacol Ther. 2005;77:427–36.

Lemery SJ, Hsieh MM, Smith A, et al. A pilot study evaluating the safety and CD34+ cell mobilizing activity of escalating doses of plerixafor in healthy volunteers. Br J Haematol. 2011;153:66–75.

MacFarland R, Hard ML, Scarborough R, Badel K, Calandra G. A pharmacokinetic study of plerixafor in subjects with varying degrees of renal function. Biol Blood Marrow Transplant. 2010;16:95–101.

Micallef INM, Ho AD, Klein LM, Murulkar S, Gandhi PJ, McSweeney PA. Plerixafor (Mozobil) for stem cell mobilization in patients with multiple myeloma previously treated with lenalidomide. Bone Marrow Transplant. 2011;46:350–5.

Mozobil® injection [package insert]. Cambridge: Genzyme Corp; 2010.

Pinto V, Castelli A, Gaidano G, Conconi A. Safe and effective use of plerixafor plus G-CSF in dialysis-dependent renal failure [letter]. Am J Hematol. 2010;85:461–2.

Steinberg M, Silva M. Plerixafor: a chemokine receptor-4 antagonist for mobilization of hematopoietic stem cells for transplantation after high-dose chemotherapy for non-Hodgkin's lymphoma or multiple myeloma. Clin Ther. 2010;32:821–43.

Stewart DA, Smith C, MacFarland R, Calandra G. Pharmacokinetics and pharmacodynamics of plerixafor in patients with non Hodgkin lymphoma and multiple myeloma. Biol Blood Marrow Transplant. 2009;15:39–46.

Vishnu P, Roy V, Paulsen A, Zubair AC. Efficacy and cost-benefit analysis of risk-adaptive use of plerixafor for autologous hematopoietic progenitor cell mobilization. Transfusion. 2012;52:55–62. doi:10.1111/j.1537-2995.2011.03206.x.

Wagstaff AJ. Plerixafor: in patients with non-Hodgkin's lymphoma or multiple myeloma. Drugs. 2009;69:319–26.

Dosage Adjustment of Medications Eliminated by the Kidneys

Plerixafor/Mobozil®   {Hematopoietic stem cell mobilizer}

Usual initial dose: 0.24 mg/kg subcutaneously

Usual maintenance dose: 0.24 mg/kg subcutaneously once daily for 4 days (on day 5 following 4 consecutive days of granulocyte colony stimulating factor G-CSF)

Typical maximum dose: 40 mg/day

Proportion eliminated unchanged: 70 %

Adjustment for Kidney Disease

FDA-approved product labeling: *Recommended subcutaneous dosage of plerixafor in patients with renal function impairment*

eCrCL (mL/min)	Plerixafor dosage
>50	0.24 mg/kg once daily (not to exceed 40 mg/day)
≤50	0.16 mg/kg once daily (not to exceed 27 mg/day)
Hemodialysis	Insufficient information to make dosage recommendation

Alternative adjustment: *Hemodialysis:*   *0.16 mg/kg subcutaneously X1 after 4 days of G-CSF (very limited clinical data)*

Dosage Adjustment of Medications Eliminated by the Kidneys

Polymyxin B - Selected References

Abramowicz M, Zuccotti G, Pflomm J-M, et al. Handbook of antimicrobial therapy. 19th ed. New Rochelle: The Medical Letter; 2011.

Amsden GW. Tables of antimicrobial agent pharmacology. In: Mandell GL, Bennett JE, Dolin R, editors. Mandell, Douglas, and Bennett's principles and practice of infectious diseases. Vol 1. 6th ed. Philadelphia: Elsevier; 2005. p. 634–700.

Buck AC, Cohen SL. Absorption of antibiotics during peritoneal dialysis in patients with renal failure. J Clin Pathol. 1968;21:88–92.

Chan JD, Graves JA, Dellit TH. Antimicrobial treatment and clinical outcomes of carbapenem-resistant *Acinetobacter baumannii* ventilator-associated pneumonia. J Intensive Care Med. 2010;25:343–8.

Elias LS, Konzen D, Krebs JM, Zavascki AP. The impact of polymyxin B dosage on in-hospital mortality of patients treated with this antibiotic. J Antimicrob Chemother. 2010;65:2231–7.

Falagas ME, Kasiakou AK, Tsiodras S, Michalopoulos A. The use of intravenous and aerosolized polymyxin B for the treatment of infections in critically ill patients: a review of the recent literature. Clin Med Res. 2006;4:138–46.

Hermsen ED, Sullivan CJ, Rotschafer JC. Polymyxins: pharmacology, pharmacokinetics, pharmacodynamics, and clinical applications. Infect Dis Clin North Am. 2003;17:545–62.

Hopper J, Jawetz E, Hinman F Jr. Polymyxin B in chronic pyelonephritis: observations on the safety of the drug and on its influence on the renal function. Am J Med Sci. 1953;225:402–9.

Kvitko CH, Rigatto MH, Moro AL, Zavascki AP. Polymyxin B versus other antimicrobials for the treatment of *Pseudomonas aeruginosa* bacteraemia. J Antimicrob Chemother. 2011;66:175–9.

Kwa ALH, Lim T-P, Low JGH, et al. Pharmacokinetics of polymyxin B1 in patients with multidrug-resistant gram-negative bacterial infections. Diagn Microbiol Infect Dis. 2008;60:163–7.

Kwa ALH, Abdelraouf K, Low JGH, Tam VH. Pharmacokinetics of polymyxin B in a patient with renal insufficiency: a case report [letter]. Clin Infect Dis. 2011;52:1280–1.

Mendes CAC, Cordeiro JA, Burdmann EA. Prevalence and risk factors for acute kidney injury associated with parenteral polymyxin B use. Ann Pharmacother. 2009;43:1948–55.

Oliveira MS, Prado GVB, Costa SF, Grinbaum RS, Levin AS. Ampicillin/sulbactam compared with polymyxins for the treatment of infections caused by carbapenem-resistant *Acinetobacter* spp. J Antimicrob Chemother. 2008;61:1369–75.

Oliveira MS, Prado GVB, Costa SF, Grinbaum RS, Levin AS. Polymyxin B and colistimethate are comparable as to efficacy and renal toxicity. Diagn Microbiol Infect Dis. 2009;65:431–4.

Ouderkirk, JP, Nord JA, Turett GS, Kislak JW. Polymyxin B nephrotoxicity and efficacy against nosocomial infections caused by multiresistant gram-negative bacteria. Antimicrob Agents Chemother. 2003;47:2659–62.

Parchuri S, Mohan S, Cunha BA. Extended spectrum β-lactamase-producing *Klebsiella pneumoniae* chronic ambulatory peritoneal dialysis peritonitis treated successfully with polymyxin B. Heart Lung. 2005;34:360–3.

Pastewski AA, Caruso P, Parris AR, et al. Parenteral polymyxin B use in patients with multidrug-resistant gram-negative bacteremia and urinary tract infections: a retrospective case series. Ann Pharmacother. 2008;42:1177–87.

Polymyxin B sulfate injection [package insert]. Bedford: Bedford Laboratories; 2004.

Ramasubban S, Majumdar A, Das PS. Safety and efficacy of polymyxin B in multidrug resistant sepsis and septic shock. Indian J Crit Care Med. 2008;12:153–7.

Sarria JC, Angulo-Parnett F, Kimbrough RC, McVay CS, Vidal AM. Use of polymyxin B during continuous venovenous hemodialysis. Eur J Clin Microbiol Infect Dis. 2004;23:340–1.

Sobieszczyk ME, Furuya EY, Hay CM, et al. Combination therapy with polymyxin B for the treatment of multidrug-resistant gram-negative respiratory tract infections. J Antimicrob Chemother. 2004;54:566–69.

Weinstein L, Doan T-L, Smith MA. Neurotoxicity in patients treated with intravenous polymyxin B: two case reports. Am J Health Syst Pharm. 2009;66:345–7.

Yow EM, Moyer JH. Toxicity of polymyxin B. II. Human studies with particular reference to evaluation of renal function. Arch Intern Med. 1953;92:248–57.

Zavascki AP. Dose adjustment of polymyxins for renal insufficiency [letter]. Antimicrob Agents Chemother. 2011;55:4940.

Zavascki AP, Goldani LZ, Nation RL. Polymyxin B for the treatment of multidrug-resistant pathogens: a critical review. J Antimicrob Chemother. 2007;60:1206–15.

Zavascki AP, Goldani LZ, Cao G, et al. Pharmacokinetics of intravenous polymyxin B in critically ill patients. Clin Infect Dis. 2008;47:1298–304.

Dosage Adjustment of Medications Eliminated by the Kidneys

<u>Polymyxin B</u>/Poly-Rx®   {Antibacterial}

Usual initial dose: 12,500 units/kg IV

Usual maintenance dose: 15,000–25,000 units/kg/day IV; infusions may be given every 12 h; however, the total daily dose must not exceed 25,000 units/kg/day.

Typical maximum dose: 25,000 units/kg/day

Proportion eliminated unchanged: 1 %

Adjustment for Kidney Disease

FDA-approved product labeling: *Kidney impairment*   *Reduce downward from 15,000 units/kg/day IV; infusions may be given every 12 h.*

Alternative adjustment: *Dose adjustments for polymyxin B presently are controversial; recent clinical pharmacokinetic data suggest that dose adjustment for renal impairment, no matter how severe, is neither necessary nor appropriate and that larger doses are associated with better outcomes. Other clinical experience suggests that usual doses should be decreased by 25–50 % when eCrCL is 20–50 mL/min and further decreased by 50–67 % when eCrCL is <20 mL/min.*

eCrCL >80 mL/min	*7,500–12,500 units/kg IV every 12 h*
eCrCL 50–80 mL/min	*7,500–12,500 units/kg IV every 12 h*
eCrCL 20–49 mL/min	*5,625–9,375 units/kg IV every 12 h (25 % decrease)*
eCrCL 10–19 mL/min	*2,475–4,125 units/kg IV every 12 h (67 % decrease)*
eCrCL <10 mL/min	*1,125–1,875 units/kg IV every 12 h (85 % decrease)*
Hemodialysis	*Data not available*
CAPD	*150,000 units IV every 12 h (very limited data)*
CRRT	*25,000 units/kg IV once followed by 8,000 units/kg IV daily (very limited data)*

Note: 10,000 units of polymyxin B sulfate = 1 mg of polymyxin B base

Dosage Adjustment of Medications Eliminated by the Kidneys

Polythiazide - Selected References

Aronoff GA, Bennett WM, Berns JS, et al. Drug prescribing in renal failure: dosing guidelines for adults and children. 5th ed. Philadelphia: American College of Physicians; 2007.

Baldry PE. Polythiazide in the treatment of oedema. Br J Clin Pract. 1962;16:421–3.

Cakalaroski K, Ivanovski N, Grozdanovski R, Ristovska V, Polenakovic M. Long-term diuretic therapy in patients with chronic renal failure. Clin Nephrol. 1997;48:56–8.

Ford RV. Clinical pharmacological investigation of polythiazide, a potent oral diuretic agent. Curr Ther Res Clin Exp. 1961;3:320–8.

Gold H, Kwit NT, Mehta D, Bross IDJ. Diuretic effect of polythiazide and sodium meralluride: comparison in bedfast patients with edema. JAMA. 1964;190:571–4.

Hobbs DC, Twomey TM. Kinetics of polythiazide. Clin Pharmacol Ther. 1978;23:241–6.

Klapper MS, Richard L. Polythiazide in hypertension. South Med J. 1962;55:297–300.

Kountz WB, Kheim T, Ackermann PG. Polythiazide in the treatment of the elderly and aged. Geriatrics. 1965;20:1016–22.

Renese® tablet [package insert]. New York: Pfizer Labs Division of Pfizer Inc; 1997.

Salmons JA, Martin AJ. Polythiazide in the treatment of hypertension. West J Med. 1963;4:366–8.

Samson WE. Clinical evaluation of polythiazide in hypertension and congestive heart failure: a comparative double-blind study. Am J Med Sci. 1965;249:571–5.

Scriabine A, Korol B, Kondratas B, Yu M, P'An SY, Schneider JA. Pharmacological studies with polythiazide, a new diuretic and antihypertensive. Proc Soc Exp Biol Med. 1961;107:864–72.

Scriabine A, Schreiber EC, Yu M, Wiseman EH. Renal clearance of polythiazide. Proc Soc Exp Biol Med. 1962;110:872–5.

Seller RH, Swartz C, Onesti G, Fuchs M, Brest AN, Moyer JH. The clinical pharmacology of polythiazide. Curr Ther Res Clin Exp. 1963;5:198–201.

Spiekerman RE, Achor RW, Berge KG, McGuckin WF. Antihypertensive properties of polythiazide and chlorothiazide: comparative double-blind study. JAMA. 1963;184:191–6.

Stein I, Katari G, The use of a new diuretic (polythiazide) in congestive failure and hypertension. Angiology. 1962;13:212–5.

Talso PJ, Young L, Tansey WJ. Polythiazide in the management of hypertensive disease. I. Effects of water and electrolyte metabolism. Curr Ther Res Clin Exp. 1964;6:162–8.

Tapia FA. Diuretic and antihypertensive effects of polythiazide. Curr Ther Res Clin Exp. 1961;3:365–77

Dosage Adjustment of Medications Eliminated by the Kidneys

__Polythiazide__/Renese®	{Diuretic; thiazide}	
__Usual initial dose:__	2 mg orally	
__Usual maintenance dose:__	2–4 mg orally once daily	
__Typical maximum dose:__	4 mg/day	
__Proportion eliminated Unchanged:__	25 %	

Adjustment for Kidney Disease

__FDA-approved product labeling:__	*Renal disease*	*Use with caution; cumulative effects of the drug may develop in patients with impaired renal function. May precipitate azotemia. If progressive renal impairment becomes evident, as indicated by a rising nonprotein nitrogen or blood urea nitrogen, a careful reappraisal of therapy is necessary with consideration given to withholding or discontinuing diuretic therapy.*
	Anuria	*Contraindicated*
__Alternative adjustment:__	*GFR >50 mL/min*	*1–4 mg orally every 24 h*
	GFR 10–50 mL/min	*1–4 mg orally every 24 h*
	GFR <10 mL/min	*Ineffective; preferably avoid.*
	Hemodialysis	*Ineffective; preferably avoid.*
	CAPD	*Ineffective; preferably avoid.*
	CRRT	*Not applicable; avoid.*

Potassium Chloride - Selected References

Betlach CH, Arnold JD, Frost RW, Leese PT, Gonzalez MA. Bioavailability and pharmacokinetics of a new sustained-release potassium chloride tablet. Pharm Res. 1987;4:409–11.

Cohn JN, Kowey PR, Whelton PK, Prisant LM. New guidelines for potassium replacement in clinical practice: a contemporary review by the National Council on Potassium in Clinical Practice. Arch Intern Med. 2000;160:2429–36.

Cooper BE. Implementation of an intravenous potassium policy. Hosp Pharm. 1989;24:462–4.

Hamill RJ, Robinson LM, Wexler HR, Moote C. Efficacy and safety of potassium infusion therapy in hypokalemic critically ill patients. Crit Care Med. 1991;19:694–9.

Klor-Con® caplet extend release and packet [package insert]. Minneapolis: Upsher-Smith Laboratories Inc; 2008.

Kraft MD, Btaiche IF, Sacks GS, Kudsk KA. Treatment of electrolyte disorders in adult patients in the intensive care unit. Am J Health Syst Pharm. 2005;62:1663–82.

Lim ETM, Kloo ST, Tweed WA. Efficacy of lignocaine in alleviating potassium chloride infusion pain. Anaesth Intensive Care. 1992;20:196–8.

Melikian AP, Cheng LK, Wright GJ, Cohen A, Bruce RE. Bioavailability of potassium from three dosage forms: suspension, capsule, and solution. J Clin Pharmacol. 1988;28:1046–50.

Morrill BG, Katz MD. The use of lidocaine to reduce the pain induced by potassium chloride infusion. J Intraven Nurs. 1988;11(2):105–8.

Owen P, Monahan MF, MacLaren R. Implementing and assessing an evidence-based electrolyte dosing order form in the medical ICU. Intensive Crit Care Nurs. 2008;24(1):8–19.

Potassium Chloride injection solution concentrate [package insert]. Lake Forest: Hospira Inc; 2004.

Pucino F, Danielson BD, Carlson JD, et al. Patient tolerance to intravenous potassium chloride with and without lidocaine. Drug Intell Clin Pharm. 1988;22:676–9.

Sedlacek M, Schoolwerth AC, Remillard BD. Electrolyte disturbances in the intensive care unit. Semin Dial. 2006;19:496–501.

Skoutakis VA, Carter CA, Acchiardo SR. Therapeutic assessment of Slow-K and K-Tab potassium chloride formulations in hypertensive patients treated with thiazide diuretics. Drug Intell Clin Pharm. 1987;21:445–9.

University of Colorado Hospital ICU Electrolyte Replacement Guideline, 2010.

University of Colorado Hospital Med-Surg Magnesium & Potassium Replacement Guideline, 2011.

Dosage Adjustment of Medications Eliminated by the Kidneys

__Potassium Chloride__	**{Electrolyte supplement}**
Usual initial dose:	Dosage is dependent upon the age, weight, and clinical condition of the patient as well as laboratory determinations.
Usual maintenance dose:	Dosage is dependent upon the age, weight, and clinical condition of the patient as well as laboratory determinations.
Typical maximum dose:	240 mEq/day
Proportion eliminated unchanged:	90 %

Adjustment for Kidney Disease

FDA-approved product labeling: *Should be used with great care, if at all in patients with severe renal insufficiency; in patients with diminished renal function, administration of potassium chloride may result in potassium retention.*

Alternative adjustment: *Potassium dosage in (a) ICU patients and (b) non-ICU patients (potassium replacement)*

(a) ICU patients

	Glomerular filtration rate (GFR in mL/min)		
Serum/plasma potassium level	*>50*	*25–50*	*<25*
3.3–3.7 mmol/L	*Potassium chloride solution 40 mEq via enteral route every 6 h × 4 or*	*Potassium chloride solution 40 mEq via enteral route every 12 h × 2*	*Potassium chloride solution 20 mEq via enteral route every 12 h × 2*
	If enteral route NOT available, Potassium chloride 20 mEq IV × 2 Central or 10 mEq IV × 4 Peripheral	*If enteral route NOT available Potassium chloride, 20 mEq IV × 1 Central or 10 mEq IV × 2 Peripheral*	*If enteral route NOT available, potassium chloride 10 mEq IV × 1 Central or Peripheral*
2.3–3.2 mmol/L	*Potassium chloride 20 mEq IV × 3 Central or 10 mEq IV × 6 Peripheral*	*Potassium chloride 20 mEq IV × 2 Central or 10 mEq IV × 4 Peripheral*	*Potassium chloride 20 mEq IV × 1 Central or 10 mEq IV × 2 Peripheral*
Less than or equal to 2.2 mmol/L	*Notify MD*	*Notify MD*	*Notify MD*

Note: Preferred intravenous rates: equal or less than 10 mEq/h (peripheral); equal or less than 20 mEq/h (central)

> *Maximum peripheral infusion concentration: 10 mEq/100 ml*
>
> *Maximum rate: equal or less than 40 mEq/h (emergency); Maximum intravenous dose = 240 mEq in 24 h*
>
> *Magnesium repletion should be concurrent or prior to potassium replacement.*

(b) Non-ICU patients

	Glomerular filtration rate (GFR in mL/min)		
Serum/plasma potassium level	*>50*	*25–50*	*<25*
3.3–3.7 mmol/L	*Potassium chloride solution or tablet 20 mEq PO/FT every 2 h × 3*	*Potassium chloride solution or tablet 20 mEq PO/FT every 2 h × 2*	*Potassium chloride solution or tablet 20 mEq PO/FT × 1*
If enteral route NOT available	*Potassium chloride 10 mEq IV × 4 Peripheral*	*Potassium chloride 10 mEq IV × 2 Peripheral*	*Potassium chloride 10 mEq IV × 1 Peripheral*
2.5–3.2 mmol/L	*Potassium chloride solution 20 mEq PO/FT every 2 h × 4*	*Potassium chloride solution 20 mEq PO/FT every 2 h × 3*	*Potassium chloride solution 20 mEq PO/FT every 2 h × 2*
If enteral route NOT available	*Potassium chloride 10 mEq IV × 6 Peripheral*	*Potassium chloride 10 mEq IV × 4 Peripheral*	*Potassium chloride 10 mEq IV × 2 Peripheral*
Less than or equal to .5 mmol/L	*Notify MD*	*Notify MD*	*Notify MD*

Note: Preferred intravenous rates: equal or less than 10 mEq/h peripheral. Maximum dose per day = 120 mEq

> *Magnesium repletion should be completed prior to potassium replacement*

Dosage Adjustment of Medications Eliminated by the Kidneys

Pralidoxime - Selected References

Abbara C, Rouseau JM, Lelièvre B, et al. Pharmacokinetic analysis of pralidoxime after its intramuscular injection alone or in combination with atropine-avizafone in healthy volunteers. Br J Pharmacol. 2010;161:1857–97.

Agostini M, Bianchin A. Acute renal failure from organophosphate poisoning: a case of success with haemofiltration. Hum Exp Toxicol. 2003;22:165–7.

Eddleston M, Eyer P, Worek F, et al. Pralidoxime in acute organophosphate poisoning—a randomised controlled trial. PloS Med. 2009;6:e1000104. doi:10.1371/jounal.pmed.1000104.

Houzé P, Mager DE, Risède P, Baud FJ. Pharmacokinetics and toxicodynamics of pralidoxime effects on paraoxon-induced respiratory toxicity. Toxicol Sci. 2010;116:660–72.

Jovanović D. Pharmacokinetics of pralidoxime chloride: a comparative study in healthy volunteers and in organophosphorus poisoning. Arch Toxicol. 1989;63:416–8.

Kassa J. Review of oximes in the antidotal treatment of poisonings by organophosphorus nerve agents. J Toxicol Clin Toxicol. 2002;40:803–16.

Kayouka M, Houzé P, Debray M, Baud J. Acute renal failure enhances the antidotal activity of pralidoxime toward paraoxon-induced toxicity. Toxicol Lett. 2009;189:48–56.

Kayouka M, Houzé P, Risède P, Debray M, Baud J. Acute renal failure alters the kinetics of pralidoxime in rats. Toxicol Lett. 2009;184:61–6.

Lee F, Lin J-L. Intermediate syndrome after organophosphate intoxication in patient with end-stage renal disease. Ren Fail. 2006;28:197–200.

Medicis JJ, Stork CM, Howland MA, Hoffman RS, Goldfrank LR. Pharmacokinetics following a loading dose plus a continuous infusion of pralidoxime compared with the traditional short infusion regimen in human volunteers. J Toxicol Clin Toxicol. 1996;34:289–95.

Peter JV, Moran JL, Pichamuthu K, Chacko B. Adjuncts and alternatives to oxime therapy in organophosphate poisoning—is there evidence of benefit in human poisoning? A review. Anaesth Intensive Care. 2006;47:339–50.

Protopam™ chloride injection [package insert]. Deerfield: Baxter Healthcare Corp; 2010.

Roberts DM, Buckley NA. Pharmacokinetic considerations in clinical toxicology: clinical applications. Clin Pharmacokinet. 2007;46:897–939.

Sakurada K, Matsubara K, Shimizu K, et al. Pralidoxime iodide (2-PAM) penetrates across the blood–brain barrier. Neurochem Res. 2003;28:1401–7.

Schexnayder S, James LP, Kearns GL, Farrar HC. The pharmacokinetics of continuous infusion pralidoxime in children with organophosphate poisoning. J Toxicol Clin Toxicol. 1998;36:549–55.

Sidell FR, Groff WA, Kaminskis A. Pralidoxime methanesulfonate: plasma levels and pharmacokinetics after oral administration to man. J Pharm Sci. 1972;61:1136–42.

Willems JL, Langenberg JP, Verstraete AG, et al. Plasma concentrations of pralidoxime methylsulphate in organophosphorus poisoned patients. Arch Toxicol. 1992;66:260–6.

<u>Pralidoxime (2-PAM)</u>/Protopam™	{Antidote; cholinesterase reactivator; ℞ for cholinesterase inhibiting nerve agent or organophosphate insecticide exposure}

Usual initial dose: 1–2 g IV over 15–30 min

Usual maintenance dose: After about an hour, a second dose of 1–2 g IV will be indicated if muscle weakness has not been relieved; additional doses may be given cautiously if muscle weakness persists. Ingestion of organophosphates may lead to continuing absorption; in such cases additional doses may be needed every 3–8 h; alternatively, administer a loading dose of 20–50 mg/kg (not to exceed 2,000 mg/dose) over 15–30 min followed by a continuous infusion of 10–20 mg/kg/h.

Typical maximum dose: 16 mg/kg (central nervous system toxicity limit)

Proportion eliminated unchanged: 80–90 % (as metabolites and unchanged drug)

Adjustment for Kidney Disease

FDA-approved product labeling: *Renal insufficiency* *Dosage should be reduced.*

Alternative adjustment: *Healthy adults* *16 mg/kg IV over 30 min followed by continuous IV infusion of 3.2 mg/kg/h*

Renal insufficiency *Data not available*

Pramipexole - Selected References

Antonini A, Calandrella D. Pharmacokinetic evaluation of pramipexole. Expert Opin Drug Metab Toxicol. 2011;7:1307–14.

Baba Y, Higuchi M-A, Fukuyama K, et al. Effect of chronic kidney disease on excessive daytime sleepiness in Parkinson disease. Eur J Neurol. 2011;18:1299–303.

Chwieduk CM, Curran MP. Pramipexole extended release in Parkinson's disease. CNS Drugs. 2010;24:327–36.

Deleu D, Northway MG, Hanssens Y. Clinical pharmacokinetic and pharmacodynamic properties of drugs used in the treatment of Parkinson's disease. Clin Pharmacokinet. 2002;41:261–309.

Hubble JP. Pre-clinical studies of pramipexole: clinical relevance. Eur J Pharmacol. 2000;7(Suppl 1):15–20.

Ishiguro N, Saito A, Yoloyama K, Morikawa M, Igarashi T, Tamai I. Transport of the dopamine D_2 agonist pramipexole by rat organic cation transporters OCT1 and OCT2 in kidney. Drug Metab Dispos. 2005;33:495–9.

Kompoliti K, Adler CH, Raman R, et al. Gender and pramipexole on levodopa pharmacokinetics and pharmacodynamics. Neurology. 2002;58:1418–22.

McCormack PL, Siddiqui MAA. Pramipexole in restless legs syndrome. CNS Drugs. 2007;21:429–37.

Merlino G, Serafini A, Robiony F, Valente M, Gigli GL. Clinical experience with pramipexole in the treatment of restless legs syndrome. Expert Opin Drug Metab Toxicol. 2008;4:225–35.

Miranda M, Kagi M, Fabres L, et al. Pramipexole for the treatment of uremic restless legs in patients undergoing hemodialysis. Neurology. 2004;62:831–2.

Mirapex ER® tablet extended release [package insert]. Ridgefield: Boehringer Ingelheim Pharmaceuticals Inc; 2011.

Mirapex® tablet [package insert]. Ridgefield: Boehringer Ingelheim Pharmaceuticals Inc; 2011.

Molnar MZ, Novak M, Mucsi I. Management of restless legs syndrome in patients on dialysis. Drugs. 2006;66:607–24.

Okura T, Ito R, Ishiguro N, Tamai I, Deguchi Y. Blood–brain barrier transport of pramipexole, a dopamine D_2 agonist. Life Sci. 2007;80:1564–71.

Wright CE, Sisson TL, Ichhpurani AK, Peters GH. Steady-state pharmacokinetic properties of pramipexole in healthy volunteers. J Clin Pharmacol. 1997;37:520–5.

Dosage Adjustment of Medications Eliminated by the Kidneys

<u>Pramipexole</u>/Mirapex®   **{Dopamine agonist; anti-Parkinsonian}**

Usual initial dose:	125 mcg orally
Usual maintenance dose:	1.5 mg orally three times daily
Typical maximum dose:	6 mg/day
Proportion eliminated unchanged:	80 %

Adjustment for Kidney Disease

FDA-approved product labeling: *Pramipexole dosage in Parkinson's disease patients with renal impairment*

Renal status	Starting dose (mg)	Maximum dose (mg)
Normal to mild impairment (CrCL > 60 mL/min)	*0.125 orally three times daily*	*1.5 mg orally three times daily*
Moderate impairment (CrCL 35–59 mL/min)	*0.125 orally twice*	*1.5 mg orally twice daily*
Severe impairment (CrCL 15–34 mL/min)	*0.125 orally once daily*	*1.5 orally once daily*
Very severe impairment (CrCL <15 mL/min and hemodialysis patients)	*Use has not been adequately studied in this group of patients*	

Alternative adjustment:

CrCL 20–60 mL	*For restless legs, 0.125 mg orally once daily 2 h before sleep; increase by 0.125 mg/day every 14 days to a maximum of 0.5 mg daily if necessary*
Extended release	
CrCL >50 mL/min	*0.375 mg orally once daily; based on efficacy and tolerability, after 5–7 days, dosages may be increased to 0.375 mg orally once daily and then by weekly increments of 0.375 mg/day to a maximum of 4.5 mg/day*
CrCL 30–50 mL/min	*0.375 mg orally every other day; after 1 week, dosage may be increased to 0.375 mg orally once daily and then by weekly increments of 0.375 mg/day to a maximum of 2.25 mg/day*
CrCL <30 mL/min	*Not recommended*
Hemodialysis	*For restless legs, 0.125 mg orally once daily 2 h before sleep; increase by 0.125 mg every 2–3 days to a maximum dose of 0.75 mg daily if necessary.*

Dosage Adjustment of Medications Eliminated by the Kidneys

Pregabalin - Selected References

Aperis G, Paliouras C, Zervos A, Arvanitis A, Alivanis P. The use of pregabalin in the treatment of uraemic pruritus in haemodialysis patients. J Ren Care. 2010;36:180–5.

Ben-Menachem E. Pregabalin pharmacology and its relevance to clinical practice. Epilepsia. 2004;45(Suppl 6):13–8.

Bockbrader HN, Radulovic LL, Posvar EL, et al. Clinical pharmacokinetics of pregabalin in healthy volunteers. J Clin Pharmacol. 2010;50:941–50.

Guay DRP. Pregabalin in neuropathic pain a more "pharmaceutically elegant" gabapentin? Am J Geriatr Pharmacother. 2005;3:274–87.

Healy DG, Ingle GT, Brown P. Pregabalin- and gabapentin-associated myoclonus in a patient with chronic renal failure [letter]. Mov Disord. 2009;24:2028–9.

Johannessen SI, Tomson T. Pharmacokinetic variability of newer antiepileptic drugs: when is monitoring needed? Clin Pharmacokinet. 2006;45:1061–75.

Lyrica® capsule [package insert]. New York: Parke-Davis Division of Pfizer Inc; 2011.

Lyseng-Williamson KA, Siddiqui MAA. Pregabalin: a review of its use in fibromyalgia. Drugs. 2008;68:2205–23.

Poza JJ. Management of epilepsy in the elderly. Neuropsychiatr Dis Treat. 2007;3:723–8.

Randinitis EJ, Posvar EL, Alvey CW, Sedman AJ, Cook JA, Bockbrader HN. Pharmacokinetics of pregabalin in subjects with various degrees of renal function. J Clin Pharmacol. 2003;43:277–83.

Satoh J, Yagihashi S, Baba M, et al. Efficacy and safety of pregabalin for treating neuropathic pain associated with diabetic peripheral neuropathy: a 14-week, randomized, double-blind, placebo-controlled trial. Diabet Med. 2011;28:109–16.

Shoji S, Suzuki M, Tomono Y, Bockbrader HN, Matsui S. Population pharmacokinetics of pregabalin in healthy subjects and patients with post-herpetic neuralgia or diabetic peripheral neuropathy. Br J Clin Pharmacol. 2011;72:63–76.

Yoo L, Matalon D, Hoffman RS, Goldfarb DS. Treatment of pregabalin toxicity by hemodialysis in a patient with kidney failure. Am J Kidney Dis. 2009;54:1127–30.

Dosage Adjustment of Medications Eliminated by the Kidneys

Pregabalin/Lyrica®   {**Antiepileptic; adjunctive analgesic**}

Usual initial dose: 50 mg orally

Usual maintenance dose: 50–150 mg orally two to three times daily

Typical maximum dose: 450 mg/day

Proportion eliminated unchanged: 90 %

Adjustment for Kidney Disease

FDA-approved product labeling: *Pregabalin dosage adjustment based on renal function*

CrCL (mL/min)	Total pregabalin daily dose (mg/day)*				Dose regimen
60	150	300	450	600	BID or TID
30–60	75	150	225	300	BID or TID
15–30	25–50	75	100–150	150	Once daily or BID
<15	25	25–50	50–75	75	Once daily

Supplementary dosage following hemodialysis (mg)

   On the 25 mg daily regimen: take one supplemental dose of 25 or 50 mg

   On the 25–50 mg daily regimen: take one supplemental dose of 50 or 75 mg

   On the 50–75 mg daily regimen: take one supplemental dose of 75 or 100 mg

   On the 75 mg QD regimen: take one supplemental dose of 100 or 150 mg
Total daily dose (mg/day) should be divided as indicated by dose regimen to provide mg/dose

Alternative adjustment:

GFR >50 mL/min	*50–300 mg orally every 8–12 h*
GFR 10–50 mL/min	*25–150 mg orally every 8–12 h (50 % decrease)*
GFR <10 mL/min	*25–75 mg orally once daily (75 % decrease)*
Hemodialysis	*25 mg orally every 24–48 h at bedtime; administer supplemental dose after hemodialysis on dialysis days; titrate carefully.*
CAPD	*25–75 mg orally once daily*
CRRT	*Data not available*

Dosage Adjustment of Medications Eliminated by the Kidneys

<u>Primidone</u> - Selected References

Aronoff GA, Bennett WM, Berns JS, et al. Drug prescribing in renal failure: dosing guidelines for adults and children. 5th ed. Philadelphia: American College of Physicians; 2007.

Cloyd JC, Miller KW, Leppik IE. Primidone kinetics: effects of concurrent drugs and duration of therapy. Clin Pharmacol Ther. 1981;29:402–7.

Cottrell PR, Streete JM, Berry DJ, et al. Pharmacokinetics of phenylethylmalonamide (PEMA) in normal subjects and in patients treated with antiepileptic drugs. Epilepsia. 1982;23:307–13.

El-Masri HA, Portier CJ. Physiologically based pharmacokinetics model of primidone and its metabolites phenobarbital and phenylethylmalonamide in humans, rats, and mice. Drug Metab Dispos. 1998;26:585–94.

Gareri P, Gravina T, Ferreri G, de Sarro G. Treatment of epilepsy in the elderly. Prog Neurobiol. 1999;58:389–407.

Heiertz R, Guthoff A, Bernhardt W. Primidone metabolism in renal insufficiency and acute intoxication. J Neurol. 1979;221:101–4.

Martines C, Gatti G, Sasso E, Calzetti S, Perucca E. The disposition of primidone in elderly patients. Br J Clin Pharmacol. 1990;30:607–11.

Matzke GR, Cloyd JC, Sawchuk RJ. Acute phenytoin and primidone intoxication: a pharmacokinetic analysis. J Clin Pharmacol. 1981;21:92–9.

McIntyre CW, Owen PJ. Prescribing drugs in kidney disease. In: Brenner BM, editor. Brenner & Rector's the kidney. 8th ed. Philadelphia: Saunders/Elsevier; 2008. p. 1930–55.

Mysoline® tablet [package insert]. Aliso Viejo: Valeant Pharmaceuticals North America; 2010.

Pisani F, Richens A. Pharmacokinetics of phenylethylmalonamide (PEMA) after oral and intravenous administration. Clin Pharmacokinet. 1983;8:272–6.

Stern EL. Possible phenylethylmalondiamide (PEMA) intoxication [letter]. Ann Neurol. 1977;2:356–7.

Streete JM, Berry DJ, Jones JA, Groggin MJ. Clearance of phenylethylmalonamide during haemodialysis of a patient with renal failure. Ther Drug Monit. 1990;12:281–3.

van Heijst ANP, de Jong W, Seldenrijk R, van Dijk A. Coma and crystalluria: a massive primidone intoxication treated with haemoperfusion. J Toxicol Clin Toxicol. 1983;20:307–18.

Dosage Adjustment of Medications Eliminated by the Kidneys

Primidone/Mysoline®	{Antiepileptic}

Usual initial dose:	100 mg orally
Usual maintenance dose:	250 mg orally three times daily
Typical maximum dose:	2,000 mg/day
Proportion eliminated unchanged:	30 % (plus 30 % of each dose excreted in urine as pharmacologically active phenethylmalonamide)

Adjustment for Kidney Disease

FDA-approved product labeling:	*Data not available*	
Alternative adjustment:	*GFR >50 mL/min*	*250 mg orally every12 h; may titrate to maximum 1,500 mg/day[a]*
	GFR 10–50 mL/min	*250 mg orally every 12 h[a]*
	GFR <10 mL/min	*250 mg orally every 24 h[a]*
	Hemodialysis	*250 mg orally every 24 h; administer supplemental dose after hemodialysis on dialysis days.[a]*
	CAPD	*Data not available*
	CRRT	*Data not available*

[a]*Therapeutic Drug Monitoring*

Therapeutic plasma levels:	*Primidone trough:*	*5–12 mg/L*
	Phenobarbital trough:	*15–40 mg/L*

Note that primidone clearance often increases during 4–12 weeks of continuous therapy.

Dosage Adjustment of Medications Eliminated by the Kidneys

Probenecid - Selected References

Aronoff GA, Bennett WM, Berns JS, et al. Drug prescribing in renal failure: dosing guidelines for adults and children. 5th ed. Philadelphia: American College of Physicians; 2007.

Berndt WO. Probenecid binding by renal cortical slices and homogenates. Proc Soc Exp Biol Med. 1967;126:123–6.

Bernstein A, Bronsky D, Dubin A. Successful treatment of recurrent uric acid renal calculi with probenecid (Benemid). Ann Intern Med. 1958;49:203–7.

Binder HJ, Katz LA, Spencer RP, Spiro HM. The effect of inhibitors of renal transport on the small intestine. J Clin Invest. 1966;45:1854–8.

Cunningham RF, Israili ZH, Dayton PG. Clinical pharmacokinetics of probenecid. Clin Pharmacokinet. 1981;6:135–51.

Dayton PG, Yü TF, Chen W, Berger L, West LA, Gutman AB. The physiological disposition of probenecid, including renal clearance, in man, studied by an improved method for its estimation in biological material. J Pharmacol Exp Ther. 1963;140:278–86.

Deguchi Y, Nozawa K, Yamada S, Yokoyama Y, Kimura R. Quantitative evaluation of brain distribution and blood–brain barrier efflux transport of probenecid in rats by microdialysis: possible involvement of the monocarboxylic acid transport system. J Pharmacol Exp Ther. 1997;280:551–60.

El-Sheikh AAK, van den Heuvel JJMW, Koenderink JB, Russel FGM. Effect of hypouricaemic and hyperuricaemic drugs on the renal urate efflux transporter, multidrug resistance protein 4. Br J Pharmacol. 2008;155:1066–75.

Ferris TF, Morgan WS, Levitin H. Nephrotic syndrome caused by probenecid. N Engl J Med. 1961;265:381–3.

Fravel MA, Ernst ME. Management of gout in the older adult. Am J Geriatr Pharmacother. 2011;9:271–85.

Goldfinger S, Linenberg JR, Seegmiller JE. The renal excretion of oxypurines. J Clin Invest. 1965;44:623–8.

Hanlon JT, Aspinall SL, Semla TP, et al. Consensus guidelines for oral dosing of primarily renally cleared medications in older adults. J Am Geriatr Soc. 2009;57:335–40.

Kelly WN. Pharmacologic approach to the maintenance of urate homeostasis. Nephron. 1975;14:99–115.

Probenecid and renal failure. Br Med J. 1968;3:569.

Probenecid tablet film coated [package insert]. Morgantown: Mylan Pharmaceuticals Inc; 2006.

Robbins N, Koch SE, Tranter M, Rubinstein J. The history and future of probenecid. Cardiovasc Toxicol. 2012;12:1–9. doi:10.1007/s12012-011-9145-8.

Scott JT, O'Brien PK. Probenecid, nephrotic syndrome, and renal failure. Ann Rheum Dis. 1968;27:249–52.

Sheikh MI, Stahl M. Characteristics of accumulation of probenecid by rabbit kidney cortical slices. Am J Physiol. 1977;232:F513–22.

Singh JA, Hodges JS, Asch SM. Opportunities for improving medication use and monitoring in gout. Ann Rheum Dis. 2009;68:1265–70.

Sjöberg K-H. Allopurinol therapy of gout with renal complications. Ann Rheum Dis. 1966;25:688–90.

Steele TH, Boner G. Origins of the uricosuric response. J Clin Invest. 1973;52:1368–75.

Stocker SL, Graham GG, McLachlan AJ, Williams KM, Day RO. Pharmacokinetic and pharmacodynamic interaction between allopurinol and probenecid in patients with gout. J Rheumatol. 2011;38:904–10.

Weber A, de Groot R, Ramsey B, Williams-Warren J, Smith A. Probenecid pharmacokinetics in cystic fibrosis. Dev Pharmacol Ther. 1991;16:7–12.

Dosage Adjustment of Medications Eliminated by the Kidneys

Probenecid/Benemid®   {Anti-gout; uricosuric agent}

Usual initial dose:	250 mg orally
Usual maintenance dose:	500 mg orally twice daily
Typical maximum dose:	2,000 mg/day
Proportion eliminated unchanged:	5 % (undergoes near complete renal tubular reabsorption)

Adjustment for Kidney Disease

FDA-approved product labeling:	*GFR >30 mL/min*	*Gout: 250 mg orally twice daily for 1 week followed by 500 mg orally twice daily thereafter. Given with penicillin: 1,000 mg orally at the time of single-dose β-lactam antibiotic administration or 2,000 mg daily in divided doses*
	GFR ≤30 mL/min	*May be ineffective; not recommended*
Alternative adjustment:	*GFR >50 mL/min*	*500 mg orally twice daily*
	GFR 10–50 mL/min	*Preferably avoid due to risk for nephrotoxicity.*
	GFR <10 mL/min	*Preferably avoid due to risk for nephrotoxicity.*
	Hemodialysis	*Preferably avoid due to risk for nephrotoxicity.*
	CAPD	*Preferably avoid due to risk for nephrotoxicity.*
	CRRT	*Not applicable; avoid.*

Dosage Adjustment of Medications Eliminated by the Kidneys

Procainamide - Selected References

Aronoff GA, Bennett WM, Berns JS, et al. Drug prescribing in renal failure: dosing guidelines for adults and children. 5th ed. Philadelphia: American College of Physicians; 2007.

Bauer LA, Black D, Gensler A, Sprinkle J. Influence of age, renal function and heart failure on procainamide clearance and n-acetylprocainamide serum concentrations. Int J Clin Pharmacol Ther Toxicol. 1989;27:213–6.

Brautigam RT, Schuster M, Porter S, Nydegger C, Kutalek SP. Comparison of intravenous dosing regimens for maintaining steady-state procainamide levels during programmed ventricular stimulation. Am J Cardiol. 1992;70:1086–8.

Christopher TG, Blair AD, Forrey AW, Cutler RE. Hemodialyzer clearances of gentamicin, kanamycin, tobramycin, amikacin, ethambutol, procainamide, and flucytosine, with a technique for planning therapy. J Pharmacokinet Biopharm. 1976;4:427–41.

Drayer DE, Lowenthal DT, Woosley RL, Nies AS, Schwartz A, Reidenberg MM. Cumulation of N-acetylprocainamide, an active metabolite of procainamide, in patients with impaired renal function. Clin Pharmacol Ther. 1977;22:63–9.

du Souich P, Erill S. Metabolism of procainamide in patients with chronic heart failure, chronic respiratory failure and chronic renal failure. Eur J Clin Pharmacol. 1978;14:24–7.

Funck-Brentano C, Light RT, Lineberry MD, Wright GM, Roden DM, Woosley RL. Pharmacokinetic and pharmacodynamic interaction of N-acetylprocainamide and procainamide in humans. J Cardiovasc Pharmacol. 1989;14:364–73.

Giardina E-G, Heissenbuttel RH, Bigger JT Jr. Intermittent intravenous procaine amide to treat ventricular arrhythmias: correlation of plasma concentration with effect on arrhythmia, electrocardiogram, and blood pressure. Ann Intern Med. 1973;78:183–93.

Gibson TP, Atkinson AJ Jr, Matusik E, Nelson LD, Briggs WA. Kinetics of procainamide and N-acetylprocainamide in renal failure. Kidney Int. 1977;12:422–9.

Gibson TP, Matusik J, Matuskik E, Nelson HA, Wilkinson J, Briggs WA. Acetylation of procainamide in man and its relationship to isonicotinic acid hydrazide acetylation phenotype. Clin Pharmacol Ther. 1975;17:395–9.

Grasela TH, Sheiner LB, Population pharmacokinetics of procainamide from routine clinical data. Clin Pharmacokinet. 1984;9:545–54.

Kessler KM, Kayden DS, Estes DM, et al. Procainamide pharmacokinetics in patients with acute myocardial infarction or congestive heart failure. J Am Coll Cardiol. 1986;7:1131–9.

Koch-Weser J. Pharmacokinetics of procainamide in man. Proc Ann NY Acad Sci. 1971;179:370–82.

Koch-Weser J, Klein SW. Procainamide dosage schedules, plasma concentrations, and clinical effects. JAMA. 1971;215:1454–60.

Kroboth PD, Mitchum K, Puschett JB. Use of procainamide in chronic ambulatory peritoneal dialysis: report of a case. Am J Kidney Dis. 1984;4:78–9.

Liem JB, Yee YG, Severdlow CD, Kates RF. Pharmacodynamics of procainamide in patients with ventricular tachycardia. J Clin Pharmacol. 1988;28:984–9.

Lima JJ, Goldfarb AL, Conti DR, et al. Safety and efficacy of procainamide infusions. Am J Cardiol. 1979;43:98–105.

Low CL, Phelps KR, Baile GR. Relative efficacy of haemoperfusion, haemodialysis and CAPD in the removal of procainamide and NAPA in a patient with severe procainamide toxicity. Nephrol Dial Transplant. 1996;11:881–4.

Myerberg RJ, Kessler KM, Kiem I, et al. Relationship between plasma levels of procainamide, suppression of premature ventricular complexes and prevention of recurrent ventricular tachycardia. Circulation. 1981;64:280–90.

Nguyen KPV, Thomsen G, Liem B, Swerdlow CD, Franz MR. N-Acetylprocainamide, torsades de pointes, and hemodialysis [letter]. Ann Intern Med. 1986;104:283–4.

Procainamide injection [package insert]. Lake Forest: Hospira Inc; 2007.

Procanbid® controlled release tablets [package insert]. Bristol: Monarch Pharmaceuticals Inc; 2006.

Pronestyl® capsules and tablets film coated [package insert]. Princeton: Bristol-Myers Squibb Co; 2006.

Raehl CL, Moorthy AV, Bierne GJ. Procainamide pharmacokinetics in patients on continuous ambulatory peritoneal dialysis. Nephron. 1986;44:191–4.

Roden DM, Peele SB, Higgins SB, et al. Antiarrhythmic efficacy, pharmacokinetics and safety of N-acetylprocainamide in human subjects: comparison with procainamide. Am J Cardiol. 1980;48:463–8.

Sica DA, Yonce C, Small R, Cefali E, Harford A, Poynor W. Pharmacokinetics of procainamide in continuous ambulatory peritoneal dialysis. Int J Clin Pharmacol Ther Toxicol. 1988;26:59–64.

<u>**Procainamide**</u>/**Pronestyl®, Procan® SR**   {Antiarrhythmic, class IA}

Usual initial dose:	17 mg/kg (approx 1,000 mg) IV at a rate not to exceed 50 mg/min or 500 mg orally
Usual maintenance dose:	50 μg/kg/min (range 20–80 μg/kg/min) continuous IV infusion or 50 mg/kg/day orally (250–500 mg every 3–6 h or 1,000–2,500 mg extended release every 12 h)
Typical maximum dose:	5,000 mg/day
Proportion eliminated unchanged:	50 % (depending on acetylator phenotype, an additional 20–30 % of each dose is excreted in urine as active *N*-acetylprocainamide)

Adjustment for Kidney Disease

FDA-approved product labeling:	*Renal insufficiency*	*Lesser amounts or longer intervals (than the usual dosage) may produce adequate blood concentrations and decrease the probability of dose-related adverse reactions; advancing age reduces the renal excretion of procainamide and N-acetylprocainamide independently of reductions in CrCL— compared to normal young adults, there is approximately 25 % reduction at age 50 and 50 % at age 75.*
Alternative adjustment:	*GFR >50 mL/min*	*500 mg orally every 4 h or 1,000–1,500 mg extended release every 12 h*
	GFR 10–50 mL/min	*500 mg orally every 6–12 h*
	GFR <10 mL/min	*Data not available; preferably avoid.*
	Hemodialysis	*Clearance and elimination are prolonged unpredictably; preferably avoid.*
	CAPD	*250 mg every 12 h; monitor carefully (very limited data).*
	CRRT	*Data not available; preferably avoid.*

Therapeutic Drug Monitoring

Therapeutic plasma levels:	Procainamide trough:	4–10 mg/L
	N-Acetylprocainamide (NAPA) trough:	15–25 mg/L

Dosage Adjustment of Medications Eliminated by the Kidneys

Pyridostigmine - Selected References

Aquilonius S-M, Hartvig P. Clinical pharmacokinetics of cholinesterase inhibitors. Clin Pharmacokinet. 1986;11:236–49.

Aquilonius S-M, Eckernäs S-Å, Hartvig P, Lindström B, Osterman PO. Pharmacokinetics and oral bioavailability of pyridostigmine in man. Eur J Clin Pharmacol. 1980;18:423–8.

Aronoff GA, Bennett WM, Berns JS, et al. Drug prescribing in renal failure: dosing guidelines for adults and children. 5th ed. Philadelphia: American College of Physicians; 2007.

Barber HE, Bourne GR. Pyridostigmine pharmacokinetics: evidence for an apparent capacity limited urinary elimination of the metabolites of pyridostigmine [abstract]. Br J Pharmacol. 1973;48:329-30P.

Barber HE, Calvey TN, Muir KT. The relationship between the pharmacokinetics, cholinesterase inhibition and facilitation of twitch tension of the quaternary ammonium anticholinesterase drugs, neostigmine, pyridostigmine, edrophonium, and 3-hydroxyphenytrimethyammonium. Br J Pharmacol. 1979;66:525–30.

Bishop MJ, Hornbein TF. Prolonged effect of succinylcholine after neostigmine and pyridostigmine administration in patients with renal failure. Anaesthesiology. 1983;58:384–6.

Bryer-Pfaff U, Schmezer A, Maier U, Brinkmann A, Schumm F. Neuromuscular function and plasma drug levels in pyridostigmine treatment of myasthenia gravis. J Neurol Neurosurg Psychiatry. 1990;53:502–6.

Calvey TN, Chan K. Plasma pyridostigmine levels in patients with myasthenia gravis. Clin Pharmacol Ther. 1977;21:187–93.

Chan K, Calvey TN. Renal clearance of pyridostigmine in patients with myasthenia gravis. Eur Neurol. 1977;16:69–72.

Cohan SL, Dretchen KL, Neal A. Malabsorption of pyridostigmine in patients with myasthenia gravis. Neurology. 1977;27:299–301.

Cohan SL, Pohlman JLW, Mikszewski J, O'Doherty DS. The pharmacokinetics of pyridostigmine. Neurology. 1949;26:536–9.

Cronnelly R, Stanski DR, Miller RD, Sheiner LB. Pyridostigmine kinetics with and without renal function. Clin Pharmacol Ther. 1980;28:78–81.

Marino MT, Schuster BG, Brueckner RP, Lin P, Kaminski A, Lasseter KC. Population pharmacokinetics and pharmacodynamics of pyridostigmine bromide for prophylaxis against nerve agents in humans. J Clin Pharmacol. 1998;38:227–35.

Mestinon® tablet, extended release tablet, and syrup [package insert]. Costa Mesa: Valeant Pharmaceuticals International; 2006.

Miller RD, Cullen DJ. Renal failure and postoperative respiratory failure: recurarization? Br J Anaesth. 1976;48:253–6.

Miller RD, Roderick L. Ligated renal pedicles and duration of action of neostigmine and pyridostigmine. Br J Pharmacol. 1977;60:555–8.

Oh SJ, Kim DS, Head TC, Claussen GC. Low-dose guanidine and pyridostigmine: relatively safe and effective long-term symptomatic therapy in Lambert-Eaton myasthenic syndrome. Muscle Nerve. 1997;20:1146–52.

Regonol® injection [package insert]. Princeton: Sandoz Inc; 2009.

Saltis LM, Martin BR, Traeger SM, Bonfiglio MF. Continuous infusion of pyridostigmine in the management of myasthenic crisis. Crit Care Med. 1993;21:938–40.

Shen Z-X. Pyridostigmine bromide and Gulf War syndrome. Med Hypotheses. 1998;51:235–7.

Søresen PS, Flachs H, Friis ML, Hvidberg EF, Paulson OB. Steady state kinetics of pyridostigmine in myasthenia gravis. Neurology. 1984;34:1020–4.

Stone JG, Matteo RS, Ornstein E, et al. Aging alters the pharmacokinetics of pyridostigmine. Anesth Analg. 1995;81:773–6.

White MC, De Silva P, Havard DWH. Plasma pyridostigmine levels in myasthenia gravis. Neurology. 1981;31:145–50.

White NE, Calvey TN, Chan K. Plasma concentration of pyridostigmine during the antagonism of neuromuscular block. Br J Anaesth. 1983;55:27–31.

Dosage Adjustment of Medications Eliminated by the Kidneys

Pyridostigmine/Mestinon®, Regonol®   {**Acetylcholinesterase inhibitor; ℞ for myasthenia gravis; nondepolarizing neuromuscular blocker antagonist**}

Usual initial dose:	60 mg orally
Usual maintenance dose:	60–120 mg orally every 4–6 h (average dose 600 mg (10 tablets)/day spaced to provide maximum relief) or 180–540 mg extended release once or twice daily; for reversal of neuromuscular blocking effects of nondepolarizing muscle relaxants, 0.1–0.25 mg/kg IV (with anticholinergic comedication; monitoring with use of a peripheral nerve stimulator-induced twitch response is recommended)
Typical maximum Dose:	1,500 mg/day
Proportion eliminated unchanged:	75 %

Adjustment for Kidney Disease

FDA-approved product labeling:	*Renal disease*	*Lower doses may be required; treatment should be based on titration of drug dosage to effect.*
Alternative adjustment:	*GFR >50 mL/min*	*30–60 mg orally every 4–6 h or 90–360 mg extended release once or twice daily; for myasthenic crisis, 1–4 mg/h continuous IV infusion (very limited data)*
	GFR 10–50 mL/min	*15–30 mg orally every 4–6 h or 90–180 mg extended release once or twice daily (~65 % decrease)*
	GFR <10 mL/min	*10–30 mg orally every 4–6 h or 45–90 mg extended release once or twice daily (~80 % decrease)*
	Hemodialysis	*10–30 mg orally every 4–6 h or 45–90 mg extended release once or twice daily (~80 % decrease); no supplemental post-dialysis dose*
	CAPD	*10–30 mg orally every 4–6 h or 45–90 mg extended release once or twice daily (~80 % decrease)*
	CRRT	*15–30 mg orally every 4–6 h or 90–180 mg extended release once or twice daily (~65 % decrease)*

Note: Completeness of oral absorption varies widely as do plasma levels required for adequate control of myasthenic symptoms. Accordingly, required oral dosages are broadly variable.

Q

L.K. Golightly et al. (eds.), *Renal Pharmacotherapy*,
DOI 10.1007/978-1-4614-5800-5_16, © Springer Science+Business Media New York 2013

Dosage Adjustment of Medications Eliminated by the Kidneys

Quinapril - Selected References

Accupril® tablet film coated [package insert]. New York: Parke-Davis Division of Pfizer Inc; 2009.

Aronoff GA, Bennett WM, Berns JS, et al. Drug prescribing in renal failure: dosing guidelines for adults and children. 5th ed. Philadelphia: American College of Physicians; 2007.

Begg EJ, Robson RA, Bailey RR, Lynn KL, Frank GJ, Olson SC. The pharmacokinetics and pharmacodynamics of quinapril and quinaprilat in renal impairment. Br J Clin Pharmacol. 1990;30:213–20.

Begg EJ, Robson RA, Ikram H, et al. The pharmacokinetics of quinapril and quinaprilat in patients with congestive heart failure. Br J Clin Pharmacol. 1994;37:302–4.

Blum RA, Olson SC, Kohli RK, Horvath AM, Sedman AJ, Posvar EL. Pharmacokinetics of quinapril and its active metabolite, quinaprilat, in patients on chronic hemodialysis. J Clin Pharmacol. 1990;30:938–42.

Breslin E, Posvar E, Neub M, Trenk D, Jahnchen E. Pharmacodynamic and pharmacokinetic comparison of intravenous quinaprilat and oral quinapril. J Clin Pharmacol. 1996;36:414–21.

Ferry J-J, Horvath AM, Sedman AJ, Latts JR, Colburn WA. Influence of food on the pharmacokinetics of quinapril and its active metabolite CI-928. J Clin Pharmacol. 1987;27:397–9.

Halstenson CE, Opsahl JA, Rachael K, et al. The pharmacokinetics of quinapril and its active metabolite, quinaprilat, in patients with various degrees of renal function. J Clin Pharmacol. 1992;32:344–50.

Kieback AG, Felix SB, Reffelmann T. Quinaprilat: a review of its pharmacokinetics, pharmacodynamics, toxicological data and clinical application. Expert Opin Drug Metab Toxicol. 2009;5:1337–47.

Krum H, Karrasch J, Hamer A, et al. Effect of angiotensin-converting enzyme inhibitor dosing interval on functional parameters in patients with congestive heart failure. Am Heart J. 1998;135:237–41.

McIntyre CW, Owen PJ. Prescribing drugs in kidney disease. In: Brenner BM, editors. Brenner & Rector's the kidney. 8th ed. Philadelphia: Saunders Elsevier; 2008. p. 1930–55.

Olson SC, Horvath AM, Micchniewica BM, Sedman AJ, Colburn WA, Welling G. The clinical pharmacokinetics of quinapril. Angiology. 1989;40:351–9.

Sasaki M, Maeda A, Fujimora A. Pharmacokinetic alterations of quinapril during repeated treatment in elderly subjects. Eur J Clin Pharmacol. 1998;54:347–9.

Squire IB, Macfayden RJ, Lees KR, Hillis WS, John L. Haemodynamic response and pharmacokinetics after the first dose of quinapril in patients with congestive heart failure. Br J Clin Pharmacol. 1994;38:117–23.

Swartz RD, Starmann B, Horvath AM, Olson SC, Posvar EL. Pharmacokinetics of quinapril and its active metabolite quinaprilat during continuous ambulatory peritoneal dialysis. J Clin Pharmacol. 1990;30:1136–41.

Wadworth AN, Brogden RN. Quinapril: a review of its pharmacological properties, and therapeutic efficacy in cardiovascular disorders. Drugs. 1991;41:378–99.

Yamada S, Muraoka I, Katao K, et al. Elimination kinetics of quinaprilat and perindoprilat in hypertensive patients with renal failure on haemodialysis. Biol Pharm Bull. 2003;26:872–5.

Dosage Adjustment of Medications Eliminated by the Kidneys

<u>Quinapril</u>/Accupril®

{**Antihypertensive, vasodilator, angiotensin-converting enzyme (ACE)/ renin inhibitor**}

Usual initial dose:	5 mg orally
Usual maintenance dose:	10–40 mg/day orally in one or two divided doses
Typical maximum dose:	80 mg/day
Proportion eliminated unchanged:	40 % (as quinaprilat)

Adjustment for Kidney Disease

FDA-approved product labeling: *Recommended starting doses of quinapril based on clinical and pharmacokinetic data from patients with renal impairment*

CrCL (mL/min)	Maximum recommended initial daily dose
>60	10 mg
30–60	5 mg
10–30	2.5 mg
<10	Insufficient data for dosage recommendation

Alternative adjustment:

GFR >50 mL/min	20–40 mg orally every 12–24 h
GFR 10–50 mL/min	2.5–5 mg orally every 24 h, titrate
GFR <10 mL/min	2.5 mg orally every 24 h, titrate
Hemodialysis	2.5 mg orally every 24 h, titrate; no supplemental dose after dialysis required
CAPD	2.5 mg orally every 24 h, titrate
CRRT	2.5–5 mg orally every 24 h, titrate

Dosage Adjustment of Medications Eliminated by the Kidneys

<u>Quinidine</u> - Selected References

Allen NM. Relationship between serum quinidine concentration and quinidine dosage. Pharmacotherapy. 1992;12:189–94.

Aronoff GA, Bennett WM, Berns JS, et al. Drug prescribing in renal failure: dosing guidelines for adults and children. 5th ed. Philadelphia: American College of Physicians; 2007.

Bauman JL, Bauernfeind RA, Hoff JV, Strasberg B, Swiryn S, Rosen KM. Torsade de pointes due to quinidine: observations in 31 patients. Am Heart J. 1984;107:425–30.

Bellet S, Roman LR, Boza A. Relation between quinidine serum levels and renal function: studies in normal subjects and patients with congestive heart failure. Am J Cardiol. 1971;27:368–71.

Centers for Disease Control. Availability and use of parenteral quinidine gluconate for severe or complicated malaria. MMWR Morb Mortal Wkly Rep. 2000;49:1138–40.

Collste P, Nordlander R. Quinidine dosage, with special reference to an oral loading dose schedule. Br J Clin Pharmacol. 1979;7:293–7.

Conrad KA, Molk BL, Chidsey CA. Pharmacokinetic studies of quinidine in patients with arrhythmias. Circulation. 1977;55:1–7.

Coplen SE, Antmann EM, Berlin JA, Hewitt P, Chalmers TC. Efficacy and safety of quinidine therapy for maintenance of sinus rhythm after cardioversion: a meta-analysis of randomized controlled trials. Circulation. 1990;82:1106–16.

Crevasse L. Quinidine: an update on therapeutics, pharmacokinetics and serum concentration monitoring. Am J Cardiol. 1988;62(Suppl I):22–3.

Damkier P, Brøsen K. Quinidine as a probe for CYP3A4 activity: intrasubject variability and lack of correlation with probe-based assays for CYP1A2, CYP2C9, CYP2C19, and CYP2D6. Clin Pharmacol Ther. 2000;68:199–209.

Drayer DE, Lowenthal DT, Restivo K, Schwartz A, Cook CE, Reidenberg MM. Steady-state serum levels of quinidine and active metabolites in cardiac patients with varying degrees of renal function. Clin Pharmacol Ther. 1978;24:31–9.

Eisenman DP, McKegney FP. Delirium at therapeutic serum concentrations of digoxin and quinidine. Psychosomatics. 1994;35:91–3.

Fattinger K, Vozeh S, Ha HR, Borner M, Follath F. Population pharmacokinetics of quinidine. Br J Clin Pharmacol. 1991;31:279–86.

Gillis AM, Mitchell LB, Wyse G, McDonald M, Duff HJ. Quinidine pharmacodynamics in patients with arrhythmia: effects of left ventricular function. J Am Coll Cardiol. 1995;25:989–94.

Grace AA, Camm AJ. Drug therapy: quinidine. N Engl J Med. 1998;338:35–45.

Greenblatt DJ, Pfeifer HJ, Ochs HR, et al. Pharmacokinetics of quinidine in humans after intravenous, intramuscular and oral administration. J Pharmacol Exp Ther. 1977;202:365–78.

Kessler KM, Lowenthal DT, Warner H, Gibson T, Briggs W, Reidenberg MM. Quinidine elimination in patients with congestive heart failure or poor renal function. N Engl J Med. 1974;290:706–9.

LaPointe NMA, Li P. Continuous intravenous quinidine infusion for the treatment of atrial fibrillation or flutter: a case series. Am Heart J. 2000;139:114–21.

McCollum PL, Crouch MA, Watson JE. Altered protein binding of quinidine in patients with atrial fibrillation and flutter. Pharmacotherapy. 1997;17:753–9.

Morganroth J, Hunter H. Comparative efficacy and safety of short-acting and sustained release quinidine in the treatment of patients with ventricular arrhythmia. Am Heart J. 1985;110:1176–81.

Ochs HR, Greenblatt DJ, Woo E, Franke K, Pfeifer HJ, Smith TW. Single and multiple dose pharmacokinetics of oral quinidine sulfate and gluconate. Am J Cardiol. 1978;41:770–7.

Quinidine gluconate injection [package insert]. Indianapolis: Eli Lilly and Co; 2002.

Quinidine gluconate tablet extended release [package insert]. Corona: Watson Laboratories Inc; 2007.

Quinidine sulfate tablet [package insert]. Corona: Watson Pharma Inc; 2009.

Staffeld CG, Pastan SO. Cardiac disease in patients with end-stage renal disease. Cardiol Clin. 1995;13:209–23.

Ueda CT, Williamson BJ, Dzindzio BS. Absolute quinidine bioavailability. Clin Pharmacol Ther. 1976;20:260–5.

Verme CN, Ludden TM, Clementi WA, Harris SC. Pharmacokinetics of quinidine in male patients: a population analysis. Clin Pharmacokinet. 1992;22:468–80.

Yeola SW, Rich TC, Uebele VN, Tamkun MM, Snyders DJ. Molecular analysis of a binding site for quinidine in a human cardiac delayed rectifier K$^+$ channel: role of S6 in antiarrhythmic drug binding. Circ Res. 1996;78:1105–14.

Dosage Adjustment of Medications Eliminated by the Kidneys

Quinidine/Quinidex®, Quinaglute® {Antiarrhythmic, class IA; antimalarial}

Usual initial dose: For arrhythmia, 400 mg orally (sulfate) or 648 mg orally (gluconate)

For *Plasmodium falciparum* malaria, 10–24 mg/kg IV over 2–4 h (gluconate)

Usual maintenance dose: For arrhythmia, 200 mg orally every 6 h or 324 mg (gluconate) orally every 8–12 h

For *P. falciparum* malaria, 12 mg/kg IV over 4 h every 8 h or 20 µg/kg/min continuous IV infusion

Typical maximum dose: 3,000 mg/day

Proportion eliminated unchanged: 35 % (as parent drug [~20 %] and equally and partially pharmacologically active metabolites; directly pH dependent)

Adjustment for Kidney Disease

FDA-approved product labeling: *Renal dysfunction causes the elimination of quinidine to be slowed. This can lead to quinidine toxicity if dosage is not appropriately reduced*

Alternative adjustment:

GFR >50 mL/min	*200 mg orally every 6 h (sulfate) or 324 mg orally every 8–12 h (gluconate) (100 % of usual dose)[a]*
GFR 10–50 mL/min	*200 mg orally every 6 h (sulfate) or 324 mg orally every 8–12 h (gluconate) (100 % of usual dose)[a]*
GFR <10 mL/min	*100 mg orally every 4 h (sulfate) or 162 mg orally every 8 h (gluconate) (~75 % of usual dose)[a]*
Hemodialysis	*100 mg orally every 4 h (sulfate) or 162 mg orally every 8 h (gluconate) (~75 % of usual dose); dose after dialysis[a]*
CAPD	*100 mg orally every 4 h (sulfate) or 162 mg orally every 8 h (gluconate) (~75 % of usual dose)[a]*
CRRT	*200 mg orally every 6 h (sulfate) or 324 mg orally every 8–12 h (gluconate) (100 % of usual dose)[a]*

[a]Note: Careful therapeutic drug monitoring is recommended. Specific assays, using either benzene extraction or (preferably) reverse-phase high-pressure liquid chromatography, should be utilized. A typical therapeutic trough concentration range is 2–6 mg/L

Although serum quinidine levels can be conveniently assayed and monitored, the electrocardiographic QTC interval is considered a better predictor of quinidine-induced ventricular arrhythmias. The total daily dosage should be reduced if (1) the QRS complex widens to 130 % of its pretreatment duration; (2) the QTC interval widens to 130 % of its pretreatment duration and is then longer than 500 ms; (3) P waves disappear; or (4) the patient develops significant tachycardia, symptomatic bradycardia, or hypotension

Dosage Adjustment of Medications Eliminated by the Kidneys

Quinine - Selected References

Alván G, Karlsson KK, Hellgren U, Villen T. Hearing impairment related to plasma quinine concentration in healthy volunteers. Br J Clin Pharmacol. 1991;31:409–12.

Aronoff GA, Bennett WM, Berns JS, et al. Drug prescribing in renal failure: dosing guidelines for adults and children. 5th ed. Philadelphia: American College of Physicians; 2007.

Baltodano K, Gallo BV, Weidler DJ. Verapamil vs quinine in recumbent nocturnal leg cramps in the elderly. Arch Intern Med. 1988;148:1969–70.

Centers for Disease Control. Treatment with quinidine gluconate in persons with severe *Plasmodium falciparum* infection: discontinuation of parenteral quinine. MMWR Morbid Mortal Wkly Rep. 1991;40(RR-4):21–3.

Connolly PS, Shirley EA, Wasson JH, Nierenberg DW. Treatment of nocturnal leg cramps: a crossover trial of quinine vs vitamin E. Arch Intern Med. 1992;152:1877–80.

Davies JG, Greenwood EF, Kingswood JC, Sharpstone P, Street MK. Quinine clearance in continuous venovenous hemofiltration. Ann Pharmacother. 1996;30:487–90.

Donadio JV, Whelton A, Kazyak L. Quinine therapy and peritoneal dialysis in acute renal failure complicating malarial hæmoglobinuria. Lancet. 1968;1:375–9.

Dyer JR, Davis TME, Giele C, Annus T, Garcia-Webb NJ. The pharmacokinetics and pharmacodynamics of quinine in the diabetic and non-diabetic elderly. Br J Clin Pharmacol. 1994;38:205–12.

Franke U, Proksch B, Risler T, Ehninger G. Drug monitoring of quinine by HPLC in cerebral malaria with acute renal failure treated by haemofiltration. Eur J Clin Pharmacol. 1987;33:293–6.

Kaplan JE, Benson C, Holmes KK, Brooks JT, Pau A, Masur H. Guidelines for prevention and treatment of opportunistic infections in HIV-infected adults and adolescents: recommendations from CDC, the National Institutes of Health, and the HIV Medicine Association of the Infectious Diseases Society of America. MMWR Recomm Rep. 2009;58(RR-4):1–207.

Kobrin SM, Berns JS. Quinine—a tonic too bitter for hemodialysis-associated muscle cramps? Semin Dial. 2007;20:396–401.

Lalloo DG, Shingadia D, Pasvol G, et al. UK malaria treatment guidelines. J Infect. 2007;54:111–21.

Man-Son-Hing M, Wells G. Meta-analysis of efficacy of quinine for treatment of nocturnal leg cramps in elderly people. BMJ. 1995;310:13–7.

McIntyre CW, Owen PJ. Prescribing drugs in kidney disease. In: Brenner BM, editors. Brenner & Rector's the kidney. 8th ed. Philadelphia: Saunders Elsevier; 2008. p. 1930–55.

Mirghani RA, Hellgren U, Bertilsson L, Gustafsson LL, Ericksson Ö. Metabolism and elimination of quinine in healthy volunteers. Eur J Clin Pharmacol. 2003;59:423–7.

Newton P, Keeratithakul D, Teja-Isavadharm P, Pukrittayakamee S, Kyle D, White N. Pharmacokinetics of quinine and 3-hydroxyquinine in severe falciparum malaria with acute renal failure. Trans R Soc Trop Med Hyg. 1999;93:69–72.

Notterman DA, Drayer DE, Metakis L, Reidenberg MM. Stereoselective renal tubular secretion of quinidine and quinine. Clin Pharmacol Ther. 1986;40:511–7.

Qualaquin® capsules [package insert]. Philadelphia: AR Scientific Inc; 2011.

Rimchala P, Karbwang J, Sukontason K, Banmairuroi V, Molunto P, Na-Bangchang K. Pharmacokinetics of quinine in patients with chronic renal failure. Eur J Clin Pharmacol. 1996;49:497–501.

Roca AO, Jarjoura D, Blend D, et al. Dialysis leg cramps: efficacy of quinine versus vitamin E. ASAIO J. 1992;38:M481–5.

Roy L, Leblanc M, Bannon P, Villeneuve J-P. Quinine pharmacokinetics in chronic haemodialysis patients. Br J Clin Pharmacol. 2002;54:604–9.

Sharma AM, Keller F, Boeckh M, Heitz J, Borner K. Quinine dosage in severe malaria with renal failure necessitating haemodialysis. Eur J Clin Pharmacol. 1989;36:535–6.

Sitprija V, Indrapasit S, Pochanugool C, Benyajati C, Piyaratn P. Renal failure in malaria. Lancet. 1967;1:185–8.

Trenholme GM, Williams RL, Rieckmann KH, Frischer H, Carson PE. Quinine disposition during malaria and during induced fever. Clin Pharmacol Ther. 1976;19:459–67.

White NJ, Gooareesuwan S, Warrell DA, Warrell MJ, Bunnag D, Harinasuta T. Quinine pharmacokinetics and toxicity in cerebral and uncomplicated falciparum malaria. Am J Med. 1982;73:564–72.

Dosage Adjustment of Medications Eliminated by the Kidneys

<u>Quinine</u>/Qualaquin®   {Antimalarial}

Usual initial dose:	648 mg orally
Usual maintenance dose:	648 mg orally every 8 h with food for 7 days
Typical maximum dose:	1,944 mg/day
Proportion eliminated unchanged:	20 %

Adjustment for Kidney Disease

FDA-approved product labeling:	*Severe chronic renal impairment*	*648 mg orally followed 12 h later by 324 mg orally every 12 h*
Alternative adjustment:	*GFR >50 mL/min*	*Severe or complicated malaria: loading dose 20 mg/kg IV over 4 h, followed by 10 mg/kg IV every 8 h for 48 h or until patient is able to swallow, followed by 10 mg/kg IV every 12 h or until patient is able to swallow*
		Uncomplicated malaria: 10 mg/kg (≈648 mg) orally every 8 h to complete 5–7 days quinine in total
	GFR 10–50 mL/min	*648 mg (10 mg/kg) orally every 12 h (33 % decrease)*
	GFR <10 mL/min	*648 mg orally every 24 h (in cases of severe malaria, empiric doses as large as 648 mg [10 mg/kg] every 8 h have been used successfully with attainment of effective plasma quinine levels)*
	Hemodialysis	*648 mg orally every 24 h; dose after dialysis (in cases of severe malaria, 10 mg/kg every 8 h or 15 mg/kg every 12 h has been successfully used with attainment of effective plasma quinine levels)*
	CAPD	*648 mg orally every 24 h*
	CRRT	*648 mg orally every 8–12 h or 15–20 mg/kg/day in divided doses*

R

L.K. Golightly et al. (eds.), *Renal Pharmacotherapy*,
DOI 10.1007/978-1-4614-5800-5_17, © Springer Science+Business Media New York 2013

Dosage Adjustment of Medications Eliminated by the Kidneys

Ramipril - Selected References

Altace® capsule [package insert]. Bristol: Monarch Pharmaceuticals Inc; 2011.

Aronoff GA, Bennett WM, Berns JS, et al. Drug prescribing in renal failure: dosing guidelines for adults and children. 5th ed. Philadelphia: American College of Physicians; 2007.

Aurell M, Delin K, Herlitz H, Ljungman S, Witte PU, Irmisch R. Pharmacokinetics and pharmacodynamics of ramipril in renal failure. Am J Cardiol. 1987;59(Suppl D):65–9D.

Ball SG, Julian DG, Murray GD, et al. Effect of ramipril on mortality and morbidity of survivors of acute myocardial infarction with clinical evidence of heart failure. Lancet. 1993;342:821–8.

Clase CM, Gao P, Tobe SW, et al. Estimated glomerular filtration rate and albuminuria as predictors of outcomes in patients with high cardiovascular risk: a cohort study. Ann Intern Med. 2011;154:310–8.

Debusmann ER, Ocón Pujadas JO, Lahn W, et al. Influence of renal function on the pharmacokinetics of ramipril (HOE 498). Am J Cardiol. 1987;59(Suppl D):70–8D.

Eckert HG, Badian MJ, Gantz D, Kellner H-M, Volz M. Pharmacokinetics and biotransformation of 2-[N-](S)-1-ethoxycarbonyl-3-phenylpropyl]-L-alanyl-(1S,3S,5S)-2-azabicyclo [3.3.0] octane-3-carboxylic acid (HOE 498) in rat, dog, and man. Arzneimittelforschung. 1984;34:1435–47.

Gerstein HC, Yusuf S, Mann JFE, et al. Effects of ramipril on cardiovascular and microvascular outcomes in people with diabetes mellitus: results of the HOPE study and MICRO-HOPE substudy. Lancet. 2000;355:253–9.

Gilchrist WJ, Beard K, Manhem P, Thomas EM, Robertson JIS, Ball SG. Pharmacokinetics and effects on the renin-angiotensin system of ramipril in elderly patients. Am J Cardiol. 1987;59(Suppl D):28–32D.

Harada A, Inenaga T, Washio M. Pharmacokinetics of ramipril in chronic renal failure. Curr Ther Res Clin Exp. 1988;44:200–12.

Lonn EM, Gerstein HC, Sheridan P, et al. Effect of ramipril and rosiglitazone on carotid intima-media thickness in people with impaired glucose tolerance or impaired fasting glucose: STARR (STudy of Atherosclerosis with Ramipril and Rosiglitazone). J Am Coll Cardiol. 2009;53:2028–35.

Marre M, Hailab M, Biliard A, et al. Small doses of ramipril to reduce microalbuminuria in diabetic patients with incipient nephropathy independently of blood pressure changes. J Cardiovasc Pharmacol. 1989;13(Suppl 3):S165–8.

Myer BH, Müller FO, Badian M, et al. Pharmacokinetics of ramipril in the elderly. Am J Cardiol. 1987;59(Suppl D):33–7D.

Ocón-Pujadas J, Debusmann ER, Lahn JW, Irmisch R, Mora J, Grötsch H. Pharmacodynamic effects of a single 10-mg dose of the angiotensin converting enzyme inhibitor ramipril in patients with impaired renal function. J Cardiovasc Pharmacol. 1989;13(Suppl 3):S45–8.

Ruggenenti P, Perna A, Gherardi G, et al. Renal function and requirement for dialysis in chronic nephropathy patients on long-term ramipril: REIN follow-up trial. Lancet. 1998;352:1252–6.

Ruggenenti P, Perna A, Mosconi L, et al. Randomised placebo-controlled trial of effect or ramipril on decline in glomerular filtration rate and risk of terminal renal failure in proteinuric, non-diabetic nephropathy. Lancet. 1997;349:1857–63.

Schunkert H, Kindler J, Gassmann M, et al. Pharmacokinetics of ramipril in hypertensive patients with renal insufficiency. Eur J Clin Pharmacol. 1989;37:249–56.

Shionoiri H, Ikeda Y, Kimura K, Miyakawa T, Kaneko Y. Pharmacodynamics and pharmacokinetics of single-dose ramipril in hypertensive patients with various degrees of renal function. Curr Ther Res Clin Exp. 1986;40:74–85.

Tobe SW, Clase CM, Gao P, et al. Cardiovascular and renal outcomes with telmisartan, ramipril, or both in people at high renal risk: results from the ONTARGET and TRANSCEND studies. Circulation. 2011;123:1098–107.

Todd PA, Benfield P. Ramipril: a review of its pharmacological properties and therapeutic efficacy in cardiovascular disorders. Drugs. 1990;39:110–35.

Wenting GJ, Blankestijn PJ, Poldermans D, et al. Blood pressure response of nephrectomized subjects and patients with essential hypertension to ramipril: indirect evidence that inhibition of tissue angiotensin converting enzyme is important. Am J Cardiol. 1987;59(Suppl D):92–7D.

Yusuf S, Sleight P, Dagenais G, et al. Effects of an angiotensin-converting-enzyme inhibitor, ramipril, on cardiovascular events in high-risk patients. N Engl J Med. 2000;342:145–53.

Dosage Adjustment of Medications Eliminated by the Kidneys

<u>Ramipril</u>/Altace® {**Antihypertensive, vasodilator, angiotensin-converting enzyme (ACE)/ renin inhibitor**}

Usual initial dose:	2.5 mg orally twice daily
Usual maintenance dose:	5 mg orally twice daily
Typical maximum dose:	20 mg/day
Proportion eliminated unchanged:	60 % (as parent drug and metabolites, primarily active ramiprilat)

Adjustment for Kidney Disease

FDA-approved product labeling:	*Changes in renal function may be anticipated in susceptible individuals.*	
	CrCL ≥40 mL/min	*2.5–20 mg/day orally in one or two doses*
	SCr >2.5 mg/dL or CrCL <40 mL/ min	*1.25 mg orally twice daily (25 % of usual dose), titrate*
Alternative adjustment:	*GFR >50 mL/min*	*5–10 mg orally every 24 h*
	GFR 10–50 mL/min	*2.5–7.5 mg orally every 24 h (25–50 % decrease)*
	GFR <10 mL/min	*1.25–5 mg orally every 24 h (75 % decrease)*
	Hemodialysis	*1.25–5 mg orally every 24 h; dose after dialysis*
	CAPD	*1.25–5 mg orally every 24 h*
	CRRT	*2.5–7.5 mg orally every 24 h, titrate*

Dosage Adjustment of Medications Eliminated by the Kidneys

Ranitidine (Enteral) - Selected References

Aronoff GA, Bennett WM, Berns JS, et al. Drug prescribing in renal failure: dosing guidelines for adults and children. 5th ed. Philadelphia: American College of Physicians; 2007.

Bisson C, St Laurent M, Michaud J-T, LeBel M. Pharmacokinetics and pharmacodynamics of ranitidine and famotidine in healthy elderly subjects: a double-blind, placebo-controlled comparison. Pharmacotherapy. 1993;13:3–9.

Cavagna R, Tessarin C, Cerutti M, Casol D, Cielo R. Pharmacokinetics of ranitidine in patients on continuous ambulatory peritoneal dialysis (CAPD). Clin Trials J. 1987;24:284–90.

Comstock TJ, Sica DA, Harford A, Eschelman F. Ranitidine bioavailability and disposition kinetics in patients undergoing chronic hemodialysis. Nephron. 1989;52:15–9.

Comstock TJ, Sica DA, Stone S, et al. Ranitidine accumulation in patients undergoing chronic hemodialysis. J Clin Pharmacol. 1988;28:1081–5.

Ebihara A, Ohashi K, Ikeda T, et al. Dosage regimen of ranitidine in patients with renal impairment. Int J Clin Pharmacol Res. 1989;9:1–7.

Feldman M, Burton ME. Histamine$_2$-receptor antagonists: standard therapy for acid-peptic diseases. N Engl J Med. 1990;1672–80, 1749–55.

Garg DC, Baltodano N, Jallad NS, et al. Pharmacokinetics of ranitidine in patients with renal failure. J Clin Pharmacol. 1986;26:286–91.

Gaughan WJ, Sheth VR, Francos GC, Michael HJ, Burke JF. Ranitidine-induced acute interstitial nephritis with epithelial cell foot process fusion. Am J Kidney Dis. 1993;22:337–40.

Gillett GB, Watson JD, Langford RM. Ranitidine and single-dose antacid therapy as prophylaxis against acid aspiration syndrome in obstetric practice. Anaesthesia. 1984;39:638–44.

Grant SM, Langtry HD, Brogden RN. Ranitidine: an updated review of its pharmacodynamic and pharmacokinetic properties and therapeutic use in peptic ulcer disease and other allied diseases. Drugs. 1989;37:801–70.

Hanlon JT, Aspinall SL, Semla TP, et al. Consensus guidelines for oral dosing of primarily renally cleared medications in older adults. J Am Geriatr Soc. 2009;57:335–40.

Lancaster-Smith MJ, Jaderberg ME, Jackson DA. Ranitidine in the treatment of non-steroidal anti-inflammatory drug associated gastric and duodenal ulcers. Gut. 1991;32:252–5.

Lebert PA, MacLeod SM, Mahon WA, Soldin SJ, Vandenberghe HM. Ranitidine kinetics and dynamics. I. Oral dose studies. Clin Pharmacol Ther. 1981;30:539–44.

Mcfadyen ML, Folb PI, Miller R, Keeton GR, Marks IN. Pharmacokinetics of ranitidine in patients with chronic renal failure. Eur J Clin Pharmacol. 1983;25:347–51.

McNeil JJ, Mihaly GW, Anderson A, Marshall AW, Smallwood RA, Louis WJ. Pharmacokinetics of the H$_2$-receptor antagonist ranitidine in man. Br J Clin Pharmacol. 1981;12:411–5.

Neelakantappa K, Gallo GR, Lowenstein J. Ranitidine-associated interstitial nephritis and Fanconi syndrome. Am J Kidney Dis. 1993;22:333–6.

Peden NR, Saunders JHB, Wormsley KG. Inhibition of pentagastrin-stimulated and nocturnal gastric acid secretion by ranitidine: a new H2-receptor antagonist. Lancet. 1979;1:690–2.

Pemberton LB, Schaefer N, Goehring L, Gaddis M, Arrighi DA. Oral ranitidine as prophylaxis for gastric stress ulcers in intensive care unit patients: serum concentrations and cost comparisons. Crit Care Med. 1992;21:339–42.

Price W, Coli L, Brandstetter RD, Gotz VP. Ranitidine-associated hallucinations. Eur J Clin Pharmacol. 1985;29:375–6.

Roberts CJC. Clinical pharmacokinetics of ranitidine. Clin Pharmacokinet. 1984;9:211–21.

Sica DA, Comstock T, Harford A, Eschelman F. Ranitidine pharmacokinetics in continuous ambulatory peritoneal dialysis. Eur J Clin Pharmacol. 1987;12:587–91.

Slugg PH, Haug MT, Pippenger CE. Ranitidine pharmacokinetics and adverse central nervous system reactions. Arch Intern Med. 1992;152:2325–9.

van Hecken AM, Tjandramaga TB, Mullie A, Verbesselt R, de Schepper PJ. Ranitidine: single dose pharmacokinetics and absolute bioavailability in man. Br J Clin Pharmacol. 1982;14:195–200.

Zantac® tablet film coated, effervescent, syrup [package insert]. Research Triangle Park: GlaxoSmithKline; 2011.

Dosage Adjustment of Medications Eliminated by the Kidneys

<u>**Ranitidine (Enteral)**</u>/Zantac® {Antacid; histamine H$_2$ receptor antagonist}

Usual initial dose: 150 mg orally

Usual maintenance dose: 150 mg orally twice daily or 300 mg orally after the evening meal or at bedtime

Typical maximum dose: 600 mg/day

Proportion eliminated unchanged: 80 % (30 % of an oral dose appears unchanged in urine)

Adjustment for Kidney Disease

FDA-approved product labeling:	*CrCL <50 mL/min*	*150 mg orally every 24 h. Should the patient's condition require, the frequency of dosing may be increased to every 12 h or even further with caution.*
Alternative adjustment:	*GFR >50 mL/min*	*150–300 mg orally at bedtime*
	GFR 10–50 mL/min	*75 mg orally twice daily or 150 mg orally every 24 h*
	GFR <10 mL/min	*75 orally twice daily or 150 mg orally every 24 h*
	Hemodialysis	*75 mg orally twice daily or 150 mg orally every 24 h; give after hemodialysis on dialysis days.*
	CAPD	*75 mg orally twice daily or 150 mg orally every 24 h*
	CRRT	*150 mg orally every 12–24 h*

Dosage Adjustment of Medications Eliminated by the Kidneys

Ranitidine (IV) - Selected References

Albin M, Friedlos J, Hillman K. Continuous intragastric pH measurement in the critically ill and treatment with parenteral ranitidine. Intensive Care Med. 1985;11:295–9.

Aronoff GA, Bennett WM, Berns JS, et al. Drug prescribing in renal failure: dosing guidelines for adults and children. 5th ed. Philadelphia: American College of Physicians; 2007.

Ballesteros MA, Hogan DL, Koss MA, Isenberg JI. Bolus and intravenous infusion of ranitidine: effects on gastric pH and acid secretion. A comparison of relative efficacy and cost. Ann Intern Med. 1990;112:334–9.

Ben-Joseph R, Segal R, Russell WL. Risk for adverse events among patients receiving intravenous histamine$_2$-receptor antagonists. Ann Pharmacother. 1993;27:1532–7.

Chau NP, Zech PY, Pozet N, Hadj-Aissa A. Ranitidine kinetics in normal subjects. Clin Pharmacol Ther. 1982;31:770–4.

Dixon JS, Borg-Costanzi JM, Langley SJ, Lacey LF, Toon S. The effect of renal function on the pharmacokinetics of ranitidine. Eur J Clin Pharmacol. 1994;46:167–71.

Garg DC, Baltodano N, Perez GO, Oster JR, Jallad NS, Weidler DJ. Pharmacokinetics of ranitidine after intravenous administration in hemodialysis patients. Pharmacology. 1985.32:189–93.

Garg DC, Wiedler DJ, Jallad NS, Eshelman FN. The effect of ranitidine and cimetidine on hepatic blood flow [abstract]. Clin Pharmacol Ther. 1982;31:228–9.

Gladziwa U, Krishna DR, Klotz U, et al. Pharmacokinetics of ranitidine in patients undergoing haemofiltration. Eur J Clin Pharmacol. 1988;35:427–30.

Holt RT, Graves LJ, Scheil E. Reducing costs by adjusting dosage intervals for intravenous ranitidine. Am J Hosp Pharm. 1990;47:2068–9.

Koch KM, Liu M, Davis LM, Shaw S, Yin Y. Pharmacokinetics and pharmacodynamics of ranitidine in renal impairment. Eur J Clin Pharmacol. 1997;52:229–34.

Lebert PA, Mahon WA, MacLeod SM, Soldin SJ, Fenje P, Vandenberghe HM. Ranitidine kinetics and dynamics. II. Intravenous dose studies and comparison with cimetidine. Clin Pharmacol Ther. 1981;30:545–50.

McNeil JJ, Mihaly GW, Anderson A, Marshall AW, Smallwood RA, Louis WJ. Pharmacokinetics of the H2-receptor antagonist ranitidine in man. Br J Clin Pharmacol. 1981;12:411–5.

Meffin PJ, Grgurinovich N, Brooks PM, Miners JO, Cochran M, Stranks G. Ranitidine disposition in patients with renal impairment. Br J Clin Pharmacol. 1983;16:731–4.

Morris DL, Markham SJ, Beechey A, et al. Ranitidine for stress ulceration: effect of bolus or infusion administration [abstract]. Gut. 1985;26:A106–7.

Morris DL, Markham SJ, Beechey A, et al. Ranitidine—bolus or infusion prophylaxis for stress ulcer. Crit Care Med. 1988;16:229–32.

Pachon J, Lorber MI, Bia MJ. Effects of H$_2$-receptor antagonists on renal function in cyclosporine-treated renal transplant patients. Transplantation. 1989;47:254–9.

Pickworth KK, Falcone RE, Hoogeboom JE, Santanello SA. Occurrence of nosocomial pneumonia in mechanically ventilated trauma patients: a comparison of sucralfate and ranitidine. Crit Care Med. 1993;21:1856–62.

Roberts AP, Harrison C, Dixon GT, Curtis JR. Plasma ranitidine concentrations after intravenous administration in normal volunteers and haemodialysis patients. Postgrad Med J. 1983;59:25–7.

Sanders SW, Buchi KN, Moore JG, Bishop AL. Pharmacodynamics of intravenous ranitidine after bolus and continuous infusion in patients with healed duodenal ulcers. Clin Pharmacol Ther. 1989;46:545–51.

Tsuruoka S, Sugimoto K-I, Hayasaka T, Saito T, Fujimura A. Ranitidine clearance during hemodialysis with high-flux membrane: comparison of polysulfone and cellulose acetate hemodialyzers. Eur J Clin Pharmacol. 2000;56:581–3.

Young CJ, Daneshmend TK, Roberts CJC. Pharmacokinetics of ranitidine in hepatic cirrhosis and in the elderly [abstract]. Br J Clin Pharmacol. 1982;14:152P.

Zantac® injection [package insert]. Research Triangle Park: GlaxoSmithKline; 2009.

Dosage Adjustment of Medications Eliminated by the Kidneys

<u>Ranitidine (IV)</u>/Zantac® IV	{Antacid; histamine H_2 receptor antagonist}
Usual initial dose:	50 mg IV
Usual maintenance dose:	50 mg IV every 6–8 h or 6.25 mg/h continuous IV infusion
Typical maximum dose:	400 mg/day
Proportion eliminated unchanged:	80 %

Adjustment for Kidney Disease

FDA-approved product labeling:	*CrCL <50 mL/min*	*50 mg IV every 18–24 h. Should the patient's condition require, the frequency of dosing may be increased to every 12 h or even further with caution.*
	Hemodialysis	*50 mg IV every 18–24 h; dose after dialysis*
Alternative adjustment:	*GFR >50 mL/min*	*50 mg IV every 8 h*
	GFR 10–50 mL/min	*50 mg IV every 12 h*
	GFR <10 mL/min	*50 mg IV every 24 h*
	Hemodialysis	*50 mg IV every 24 h; administer after hemodialysis on dialysis days.*
	CAPD	*50 mg IV every 24 h*
	CRRT	*50 mg IV every 12 h*

Dosage Adjustment of Medications Eliminated by the Kidneys

Ranolazine - Selected References

Abdallah H, Jerling M. Effect of hepatic impairment on the multiple-dose pharmacokinetics of ranolazine sustained-release tablets. J Clin Pharmacol. 2005;45:802–9.

Antzelevitch C, Burashnikov A, Sicouri S, Belardinelli L. Electrophysiological basis for the antiarrhythmic actions of ranolazine. Heart Rhythm. 2011;8:1281–90.

Bashore TM, Granger CB, Hranitzky P, Patel MR. Heart disease. In: McPhee SJ, Papadakis MA, Rabow MW, editors. 2011 Current medical diagnosis and treatment. 15th ed. New York: McGraw-Hill; 2011:317–415.

Chisholm JW, Morrow DA, Goldfine AB, et al. Effect of ranolazine on A1C and glucose levels in hyperglycemic patients with non-ST elevation acute coronary syndrome. Diabetes Care. 2010;33:1163–8.

Deedwania PC, Carbajal EV. Medical therapy versus myocardial revascularization in chronic coronary syndrome and stable angina. Am J Med. 2011;124:681–8.

Dobesh PP, Trujillo TC. Ranolazine: a new option in the management of chronic stable angina. Pharmacotherapy. 2007;27:1659–76.

Greene RS, Rangel RM, Edwards KL, et al. Ranolazine for the treatment of refractory angina in a veterans population. Cardiovasc Revasc Med. 2011. Epub ahead of print. doi:10.1016/j.carrev.2011.06.001.

Jerling M. Clinical pharmacokinetics of ranolazine. Clin Pharmacokinet. 2006;45:469–91.

Jerling M, Abdallah H. Effect of renal impairment on multiple-dose pharmacokinetics of extended-release ranolazine. Clin Pharmacol Ther. 2005;78:288–97.

Keating GM. Ranolazine: a review of its use in chronic stable angina pectoris. Drugs. 2008;68:2483–503.

Kumar K, Nearing BD, Carvas M, et al. Ranolazine exerts potent effects on atrial electrical properties and abbreviates atrial fibrillation duration in the intact porcine heart. J Cardiovasc Electrophysiol. 2009;20:796–802.

Morrow DA, Scirica BM, Chaitman BR, et al. Evaluation of the glycometabolic effects of ranolazine in patients with and without diabetes mellitus in the MERLIN-TIMI 36 randomized controlled trial. Circulation. 2009;119:3032–9.

Morrow DA, Scirica BM, Karwatowska-Prokopczuk E, et al. Effects of ranolazine on recurrent cardiovascular events in patients with non-ST-elevation acute coronary syndromes: the MERLIN-TIMI 36 randomized trial. JAMA. 2007;297:1775–83.

Morrow DA, Scirica BM, Sabatine MS, et al. B-type natriuretic peptide and the effect of ranolazine in patients with non-ST-segment elevation acute coronary syndromes: observations from the MERLIN-TIMI 36 (Metabolic Efficiency with Ranolazine for Less Ischemia in Non-ST-Elevation Acute Coronary Syndrome-Thrombolysis in Myocardial Infarction 36) trial. J Am Coll Cardiol. 2010;55:1189–96.

Rajamani S, Shryock JC, Belardinelli L. Rapid kinetic interactions of ranolazine with HERG K+ current. J Cardiovasc Pharmacol. 2008;51:581–9.

Ranexa® tablet film coated extended release [package insert]. Foster City: Gilead Sciences Inc; 2010.

Scirica BM, Braunwald E, Belardinelli L, et al. Relationship between nonsustained ventricular tachycardia after non-ST-elevation acute coronary syndrome and sudden cardiac death: observations from the Metabolic Efficiency with Ranolazine for Less Ischemia in Non-ST-Elevation Acute Coronary Syndrome-Thrombolysis in Myocardial Infarction 36 (MERLIN-TIMI 36) trial. Circulation. 2010;55:1189–96.

Scirica BM, Morrow DA, Hod H, et al. Effect of ranolazine, an antianginal agent with novel electrophysiological properties, on the incidence of arrhythmias in patients with non-ST-segment elevation acute coronary syndrome: results from the Metabolic Efficiency with Ranolazine for Less Ischemia in Non-ST-Elevation Acute Coronary Syndrome-Thrombolysis in Myocardial Infarction 36 (MERLIN-TIMI 36) randomized controlled trial. Circulation. 2007;116:1647–52.

Siddiqui MAA, Keam SJ. Ranolazine: a review of its use in chronic stable angina pectoris. Drugs. 2006;66:693–710.

Sossalla S, Kallmeyer B, Wagner S, et al. Altered Na+ currents in atrial fibrillation: effects of ranolazine on arrhythmias and contractility in human atrial fibrillation. J Am Coll Cardiol. 2010;55:2330–42.

Truffa AAM, Newby LK, Melloni C. Extended-release ranolazine: critical evaluation of its use in stable angina. Vasc Health Risk Manag. 2011;7:535–9.

Wang GK, Calderon J, Wang S-Y. State- and use-dependent block of muscle Nav1.4 and neuronal Nav1.7 voltage-gated Na+ channel isoforms by ranolazine. Mol Pharmacol. 2008;73:940–8.

Wasserstrom JA, Sharma R, O'Toole MJ, et al. Ranolazine antagonizes the effects of increased sodium current on intracellular calcium cycling in rat isolated intact heart. J Pharmacol Exp Ther. 2009;331:382–91.

Dosage Adjustment of Medications Eliminated by the Kidneys

<u>Ranolazine</u>/Ranexa®	**{Antianginal}**

Usual initial dose:	500 mg orally twice daily
Usual maintenance dose:	1,000 mg orally twice daily
Typical maximum dose:	2,000 mg/day
Proportion eliminated unchanged:	7 % (70 % as metabolites of uncertain activity)

Adjustment for Kidney Disease

FDA-approved product labeling: *In patients with varying degrees of renal impairment, ranolazine plasma levels increased up to 50 %. Blood pressure increases by about 15 mmHg in patients with severe renal impairment. The pharmacokinetics of ranolazine has not been assessed in patients on dialysis.*

Alternative adjustment: *In patients with kidney disease, factors other than reduced GFR contribute to the increase in plasma ranolazine concentrations.*

eCrCL 30–80 mL/min	*500 mg orally twice daily; use with cautious electrocardiographic monitoring; titrate carefully.*
eCrCL <30 mL/min	*Minimal data available; preferably avoid*

Dosage Adjustment of Medications Eliminated by the Kidneys

Repaglinide - Selected References

Bidstrup TB, Bjørnsdottir I, Sidelmann UG, Søndergård Thomsen M, Hansen KT. CYP2C8 and CYP3A4 are the principal enzymes involved in the human in vitro biotransformation of the insulin secretogogue repaglinide. Br J Clin Pharmacol. 2003;56:305–14.

Culy CR, Jarvis B. Repaglinide: a review of its therapeutic use in type 2 diabetes mellitus. Drugs. 2001;61:1625–60.

Hasslacher C, Alawi H, Böckmann G-U, et al. Safety and efficacy of repaglinide in type 2 diabetic patients with and without impaired renal function. Diabetes Care. 2003;26:886–91.

Hatorp V. Clinical pharmacokinetics and pharmacodynamics of repaglinide. Clin Pharmacokinet. 2002;41:471–83.

He J, Qiu, Z, Li N, et al. Effects of *SLCO1B1* polymorphisms on the pharmacokinetics and pharmacodynamics of repaglinide in healthy Chinese volunteers. Eur J Clin Pharmacol. 2011;67:701–7.

Kalliokoski A, Backman JT, Kurkinen KJ, Neuvonen PJ, Niemi M. Effects of gemfibrozil and atorvastatin on the pharmacokinetics of repaglinide in relation to *SLCO1B1* polymorphism. Clin Pharmacol Ther. 2008;84:488–96.

Kalliokoski A, Backman JT, Neuvonen PJ, Niemi M. Effects of the *SLCO1B1*1B* haplotype on the pharmacokinetics and pharmacodynamics of repaglinide and nateglinide. Pharmacogenet Genomics. 2008;18:937–42.

Kalliokoski A, Neuvonen M, Neuvonen PJ, Niemi M. The effect of *SLCO1B1* polymorphism on repaglinide pharmacokinetics persists over a wide dose range. Br J Clin Pharmacol. 2008;66:818–25.

Kalliokoski A, Neuvonen M, Neuvonen PJ, Niemi M. Different effects of *SLCO1B1* polymorphism on the pharmacokinetics and pharmacodynamics of repaglinide and nateglinide. J Clin Pharmacol. 2008;48:311–21.

Kalliokoski A, Neuvonen PJ, Niemi M. *SLCO1B1* polymorphism and oral antidiabetic drugs. Basic Clin Pharmacol Toxicol. 2010;107:775–81.

Kircheiner J, Roots I, Goldammer M, Rosenkranz B, Brockmöller J. Effect of genetic polymorphisms in cytochrome P450 (CYP) 2C9 and CYP2C8 on the pharmacokinetics of oral antidiabetic drugs: clinical relevance. Clin Pharmacokinet. 2005;44:1209–25.

Li J, Tian H, Li Q, et al. Improvement of insulin sensitivity and β-cell function by nateglinide and repaglinide in type 2 diabetic patients—a randomized controlled double-blind and double-dummy multicentre clinical trial. Diabetes Obes Metab. 2007;9:558–65.

Lund SS, Tarnow L, Frandsen M, et al. Impact of metformin versus the prandial insulin secretogogue, repaglinide, on fasting and postprandial glucose and lipid responses in non-obese patients with type 2 diabetes. Eur J Endocrinol. 2008;158:35–46.

Marbury TC, Ruckle JL, Hatorp V, et al. Pharmacokinetics of repaglinide in subjects with renal impairment. Clin Pharmacol Ther. 2000;67:7–15.

Massi-Benedetti M, Damsbo P. Pharmacology and clinical experience with repaglinide. Expert Opin Investig Drugs. 2000;9:885–98.

Prandin® tablet [package insert]. Princeton: Novo Nordisk Inc; 2011.

Razilawati AB, Gan SH. *CYP3A4* genetic polymorphism influences repaglinide's pharmacokinetics. Pharmacology. 2010;85:357–64.

Razilawati AB, Wahab MSA, Imran A, Ismail Z, Gan SH. Method development and validation of repaglinide in human plasma by HPLC and its application in pharmacokinetic studies. J Pharm Biomed Anal. 2007;43:1831–5.

Schumacher S, Abbasi I, Weise D, et al. Single- and multiple-dose pharmacokinetics of repaglinide in patients with type 2 diabetes and renal impairment. Eur J Clin Pharmacol. 2001;57:147–52.

Tomalik-Scharte D, Fuhr U, Hellmich M, et al. Effect of the *CYP2C8* genotype on the pharmacokinetics and pharmacodynamics of repaglinide. Drug Metab Dispos. 2011;39:927–32.

Türk T, Pietruck F, Dolff S, et al. Repaglinide in the management of new-onset diabetes mellitus after renal transplantation. Am J Transplant. 2006;6:842–6.

van Heiningen PNM, Hatorp V, Nielsen KK, et al. Absorption, metabolism and excretion of a single oral dose of 14C-repaglinide during repaglinide multiple dosing. Eur J Clin Pharmacol. 1999;55:521–5.

Yale J-F. Oral antihyperglycemic agents and renal disease: new agents, new concepts. J Am Soc Nephrol. 2005;16 (Suppl 1):S7–10.

Dosage Adjustment of Medications Eliminated by the Kidneys

Repaglinide/Prandin®	{Antidiabetic; meglitinide derivative; insulin secretogogue}	
Usual initial dose:	0.5 mg with each meal	
Usual maintenance dose:	0.5–4 mg orally with meals two, three, or four times a day	
Typical maximum dose:	16 mg/day	
Proportion eliminated unchanged:	8 %	

Adjustment for Kidney Disease

FDA-approved product labeling:	*Mild to moderate renal dysfunction*	*Initial dose adjustment does not appear to be necessary.*
	Severe renal function impairment	*Initiate therapy with 0.5 mg orally with meals; subsequently patient's dose should be carefully titrated.*
	CrCL <20 mL/min	*No data*
	Hemodialysis	*No data*
Alternative adjustment:	*eCrCL >80 mL/min*	*1–4 mg orally three times daily with meals*
	eCrCL 30–80 mL/min	*0.5–2 mg orally three times daily with meals; initiate with low doses, titrate carefully, and monitor for hypoglycemia.*
	eCrCL 5–30 mL/min	*0.5–2 mg orally three times daily with meals; initiate with low doses, titrate carefully, and monitor for hypoglycemia.*
	Hemodialysis	*0.5–2 mg orally three times daily with meals; administer after hemodialysis on dialysis days; initiate with low doses, titrate carefully, and monitor for hypoglycemia.*
	CRRT	*Not applicable; avoid*

Dosage Adjustment of Medications Eliminated by the Kidneys

Reserpine - Selected References

Abrahams DG, Wilson C. Effect of hypotensive drugs on renal function in chronic renal disease. Lancet. 1957;1:68–74.

Andreae E, Smith FE Jr. The effect of reserpine on renal plasma flow in hypertension: clinical study of fifteen patients. Am J Med Sci. 1955;230:45–8.

Aronoff GA, Bennett WM, Berns JS, et al. Drug prescribing in renal failure: dosing guidelines for adults and children. 5th ed. Philadelphia: American College of Physicians; 2007.

Bello CT, Turner LW. Reserpine as an antihypertensive in the outpatient clinic: a double-blind clinical study. Am J Med Sci. 1956;232:194–7.

Curb JD, Pressel SL, Cutler JA, et al. Effect of diuretic-based antihypertensive treatment on cardiovascular disease risk in older diabetic patients with isolated systolic hypertension. JAMA. 1996;276:1886–92.

Dustan HP, Page IH. Some factors in renal and renoprival hypertension. J Lab Clin Med. 1964;64:948–59.

Freis ED, Ari R. Clinical and experimental effects of reserpine in patients with essential hypertension. Ann N Y Acad Sci. 1954;59:45–53.

Giachetti A, Shore PA. The reserpine receptor. Life Sci. 1978;23:89–92.

Goldberg B. Renal hemodynamic effects of hypotensive drugs. I. Acute effects of hexamethonium bromide before and after reserpine. Lancet. 1957;1:74–7.

Harris R. Reserpine therapy in hypertension. J Am Geriatr Soc. 1956;4:269–75.

Hughes W, Dennis E, McConn R, Ford R, Moyer JH. Reserpine (Serpasil) in the treatment of hypertension. Am J Med Sci. 1954;228:21–35.

Hughes WM, Dennis E, Moyer JH. Treatment of hypertension with oral reserpine alone and in combination with hydralazine or hexamethonium. Am J Med Sci. 1955;229:121–34.

Kert MJ, Carleton HG, Nordyke RA, Roth SI, Westergart JP. Clinical experiences with reserpine (Serpasil) in hypertension: a preliminary report. Angiology. 1955;6:138–43.

Krogsgaard AR. The effect of intravenously injected reserpine on blood pressure, renal function and sodium excretion. Acta Med Scand. 1956;154:41–51.

Materson BJ, Cushman WC, Goldstein G, et al. Treatment of hypertension in the elderly: I. Blood pressure and clinical changes: results of a Department of Veterans Affairs Cooperative Study. Hypertension. 1990;15:348–60.

McDonald L, Goldberg B. Renal hemodynamic effects of hypotensive drugs. II. Effects of oral maintenance therapy with pentapyrrolidinium bitartrate and reserpine. Lancet. 1957;1:77–8.

McQueen EG, Doyle AE, Smirk FH. The circulatory effects of reserpine. Circulation. 1955;11:161–9.

Moyer JH, Hughes W, Huggins R. The cardiovascular and renal hemodynamic response to the administration of reserpine (Serpasil). Am J Med Sci. 1954;227:640–8.

Platt R, Sears HTN. Reserpine in severe hypertension. Lancet. 1956;1:401–3.

Redleaf PD, Tobian L. Sodium restriction and reserpine administration in experimental renal hypertension: a correlation of arterial blood pressure responses with the ionic composition of the arterial wall. Circ Res. 1958; 6:343–51.

Reserpine tablet [package insert]. Princeton: Sandoz Inc; 2011.

Savage PJ, Pressel SL, Curb JD, et al. Influence of long-term, low-dose, diuretic-based, antihypertensive therapy on glucose, lipid, uric acid, and potassium levels in older men and women with isolated systolic hypertension: the Systolic Hypertension in the Elderly Program. Arch Intern Med. 1998;158:741–51.

Wilkins RW. Clinical usage of *Rauwolfia* alkaloids, including reserpine (Serpasil). Ann N Y Acad Sci. 1954;59:36–44.

Wilson RW, Judson WE, Stone RW, Hollander W, Huckabee WE, Friedman IH. Reserpine in the treatment of hypertension: a note on the relative dosage and effects. N Engl J Med. 1954;250:477–8.

Zsotér TT, Johnson GE, DeVeber GA, Paul H. Excretion and metabolism of reserpine in renal failure. Clin Pharmacol Ther. 1973;14:325–30.

Reserpine/Serpasil®   {Antihypertensive; central monoamine-depleting agent; Rauwolfia alkaloid}

Usual initial dose: 0.5 mg orally once daily

Usual maintenance dose: 0.1–0.25 mg orally once daily

Typical maximum dose: 1 mg/day

Proportion eliminated unchanged: 1 %

Adjustment for Kidney Disease

   FDA-approved product labeling: *Caution should be exercised when treating hypertensive patients with renal insufficiency since they adjust poorly to lowered blood pressure levels.*

   Alternative adjustment:

GFR >50 mL/min	*0.1–0.25 mg orally once daily*
GFR 10–50 mL/min	*0.1–0.25 mg orally once daily*
GFR <10 mL/min	*Preferably avoid due to often delayed and unreliable responses*
Hemodialysis	*Preferably avoid due to often delayed and unreliable responses*
CAPD	*Preferably avoid due to often delayed and unreliable responses*
CRRT	*Not applicable; preferably avoid*

Dosage Adjustment of Medications Eliminated by the Kidneys

<u>Ribavirin (Oral)</u> - Selected References

Aronoff GA, Bennett WM, Berns JS, et al. Drug prescribing in renal failure: dosing guidelines for adults and children. 5th ed. Philadelphia: American College of Physicians; 2007.

Berenguer M. Treatment of chronic hepatitis C in hemodialysis patients. Hepatology. 2008;48:1690–9.

Bruchfeld A, Lindahl K, Reichard O, Carlsson T, Schvarcz R. Pegylated interferon and ribavirin for hepatitis C in haemodialysis patients. J Viral Hepat. 2006.13:316–21.

Bruchfeld A, Lindahl K, Schvarez R, Ståhle L. Dosage of ribavirin in patients with hepatitis C should be based on renal function: a population pharmacokinetic analysis. Ther Drug Monit. 2002;24:701–8.

Connor J. Ribavirin pharmacokinetics. Pediatr Infect Dis J. 1990;9(Suppl):S91–2.

Feld JJ, Lutchman G, Heller T, et al. Ribavirin improves early responses to peginterferon through enhanced interferon signaling. Gastroenterology. 2010;139:154–62.

Furusyo N, Murata M, Ogawa E, et al. Ribavirin concentration in the later stages of 48 week pegylated interferon α2b plus ribavirin therapy for chronic hepatitis C is useful for predicting virological response. J Antimicrob Chemother. 2011;66:1127–39.

Ghany MG, Strader DB, Thomas DL, Seeff LB. American Association for the Study of Liver Diseases Practice Guidelines. Diagnosis, management, and treatment of hepatitis C: an update. Hepatology. 2009;49:1335–74.

Glue P, Rouzier-Panis R, Raffanel C, et al. A dose-ranging study of pegylated interferon alfa-2b and ribavirin in chronic hepatitis C. Hepatology. 2000;32:647–53.

Jen JF, Glue P, Gupta S, Zambas D, Hajian G. Population pharmacokinetic and pharmacodynamic analysis of ribavirin in patients with chronic hepatitis C. Ther Drug Monit. 2000;22:555–65.

Jen J, Laughlin M, Chung C, et al. Ribavirin dosing in chronic hepatitis C: application of population pharmacokinetic-pharmacodynamic models. Clin Pharmacol Ther. 2002;72:349–61.

Kramer TH, Gaar GG, Ray CG, Minnich L, Copeland JG, Connor JD. Hemodialysis clearance of intravenously administered ribavirin. Antimicrob Agents Chemother. 1990;34:489–90.

Lertora JJL, Rege AB, Lacour JT, et al. Pharmacokinetics and long-term tolerance to ribavirin in asymptomatic patients infected with human immunodeficiency virus. Clin Pharmacol Ther. 1991;50:442–9.

Noureddin M, Ghany MG. Pharmacokinetics and pharmacodynamics of peginterferon and ribavirin: implications for clinical efficacy in the treatment of chronic hepatitis C. Gastroenterol Clin North Am. 2010;39:649–58.

Paroni R, Del Puppo M, Borghi C, Sirtori CR, Kienle MG. Pharmacokinetics of ribavirin and urinary excretion of the major metabolite 1,2,4-triazole-3-carboxamide in normal volunteers. Int J Clin Pharmacol Ther Toxicol. 1989;27:302–7.

Preston SL, Drusano GL, Glue P, Nash J, Gupta SK, McNamara P. Pharmacokinetics and absolute bioavailability of ribavirin in healthy volunteers as determined by stable-isotope methodology. Antimicrob Agents Chemother. 1999;43:2451–6.

Rabih SA, Agudo RG. Management of HCV infection in chronic kidney disease. Nefrologia. 2011;31:260–7.

Rebetol® capsule and oral solution [package insert]. Kenilworth: Schering Corp; 2010.

Rebetron™ injection kit [with interferon alfa-2b [package insert]. Kenilworth: Schering Corp; 2001.

Scott LJ, Perry CM. Interferon-α-2b plus ribavirin: a review of its use in the management of chronic hepatitis C. Drugs. 2002;62:507–56.

Tsubota A, Akuta N, Suzuki F, et al. Viral dynamics and pharmacokinetics in combined interferon alfa-2b and ribavirin therapy for patients infected with hepatitis C virus of genotype 1b and high pretreatment viral load. Intervirology. 2002.45:33–42.

Tsubota A, Hirose Y, Izumi N, Kumada H. Pharmacokinetics of ribavirin in combined interferon-alpha 2b and ribavirin therapy of chronic hepatitis C infection. Br J Clin Pharmacol. 2003;55:360–7.

van Vlerken LG, van Oijen MGH, van Erpecum KJ. Ribavirin concentration is a more important predictor of sustained viral response than anemia in hepatitis C patients [letter]. Gastroenterology. 2011;140:1693–4.

Wade JR, Snoeck E, Duff F, Lamb M, Jorga K. Pharmacokinetics of ribavirin in patients with hepatitis C virus. Br J Clin Pharmacol. 2006;62:710–4.

Younossi ZM, Limongi D, Stepanova M, et al. Protein pathway activation associated with sustained virologic response in patients with chronic hepatitis C treated with pegylated interferon (PEG-IFN) and ribavirin (RBV). J Proteome Res. 2011;10:774–9.

<u>Ribavirin (Oral)</u>/Rebetol®, RibaPak®, Ribasphere®, Copegus® {Antiviral; ℞ for hepatitis C}

Usual initial dose:	400 mg orally
Usual maintenance dose:	800–1,200 mg/day orally in two divided doses with food
Typical maximum dose:	1,200 mg/day
Proportion eliminated unchanged:	5–15 %

Adjustment for Kidney Disease

FDA-approved product labeling: Recommended dosing for (**a**) Rebetol, RibaPak, Ribasphere: CrCL <50 mL/min and (**b**) Copegus: CrCL ≤50 mL/min

(a) Rebetol, RibaPak, Ribasphere

Body weight	Ribavirin dose
≤75 kg	400 mg (2 capsules) orally every AM and 600 mg (3 capsules) orally every PM
>75 kg	600 mg (3 capsules) orally every AM and 600 mg (3 capsules) orally every PM
CrCL <50 mL/min	Contraindicated

(b) Copegus

	Interferon alfa-2a (Pegasys) dose	Ribavirin (Copegus) dose[a]	Duration
Hepatitis C Genotypes 1, 4	180 μg	<75 kg = 1,000 mg ≥75 kg = 1,200 mg	48 week 48 week
Hepatitis C Genotypes 2, 3	180 μg	800 mg	24 week

CrCL ≤50 mL/min: Do not use ribavirin

[a]Administer orally in two divided doses

Alternative adjustment: eCrCL ≤60 mL/min Patient safety note: See contraindication above as listed in US product labeling; potentially conflicting dose recommendations tabulated below are taken from a pilot study of 19 patients with hepatitis C infection and chronic kidney disease treated with ribavirin (Rebetol) and interferon alfa-2b (Bruchfeld et al. 2002) as well as recently published clinical practice guidelines. Plasma level monitoring is recommended.

Target ribavirin concentration at steady state

	6 μmol/L	10 μmol/L	14 μmol/L
eCrCL 60 mL/min	400 mg/day	600 mg/day	800 mg/day
eCrCL 40 mL/min	200 mg/day	400 mg/day	600 mg/day
eCrCL 20 mL/min	200 mg/day	400 mg/200 mg	400 mg/day alternate days

Hemodialysis	200 mg orally once daily
Kidney transplant	Avoid unless fibrosing cholestatic hepatitis develops
CAPD	Avoid
CRRT	400–600 mg orally twice daily

Dosage Adjustment of Medications Eliminated by the Kidneys

Rifabutin - Selected References

Aronoff GA, Bennett WM, Berns JS, et al. Drug prescribing in renal failure: dosing guidelines for adults and children. 5th ed. Philadelphia: American College of Physicians; 2007.

Bassilios N, Launay-Vacher V, Hamani A-A, et al. Pharmacokinetics and dose adjustment of rifabutin in a haemodialysis patient [letter]. Nephrol Dial Transplant. 2002;17:531–2.

Blashke TF, Skinner MH. The clinical pharmacokinetics of rifabutin. Clin Infect Dis. 1996;22(Suppl 1):S15–22.

Breda M, Pinezzola E, Strolin Benedetti M, et al. A study of the effects of rifabutin on isoniazid pharmacokinetics and metabolism in healthy volunteers. Drug Metabol Drug Interact. 1992;10:323–40.

Brogden RN, Fitton A. Rifabutin: a review of its antimicrobial activity, pharmacokinetic properties and therapeutic efficacy. Drugs. 1994;47:983–1009.

Burman WJ, Gallicano K, Peloquin C. Comparative pharmacokinetics and pharmacodynamics of the rifamycin antibacterials. Clin Pharmacokinet. 2001;40:327–41.

EBPG Expert Group on Renal Transplantation. European best practice guidelines for renal transplantation. Section IV: long-term management of the transplant recipient. IV.7.2. Late infections. Tuberculosis. Nephrol Dial Transplant. 2002;17(Suppl 4):39–43.

Gatti G, Di Biagio A, De Pascalis CR, Guerra M, Bassetti M, Bassetti D. Pharmacokinetics of rifabutin in HIV-infected patients with or without wasting syndrome. Br J Clin Pharmacol. 1999;48:704–11.

Gatti G, Papa P, Torre D, et al. Population pharmacokinetics of rifabutin in human immunodeficiency virus-infected patients. Antimicrob Agents Chemother. 1998;42:2017–23.

Hafner R, Bethel J, Standiford HC, et al. Tolerance and pharmacokinetic interactions of rifabutin and azithromycin. Antimicrob Agents Chemother. 2001;45:1572–7.

Jamis-Dow CA, Katki AG, Collins JM, Klecker RW. Rifampin and rifabutin and their metabolism by human liver esterases. Xenobiotica. 1997;27:1015–24.

Keenan N, Jeyaratnam D, Sheerin NS. Mycobacterium simiae: a previously undescribed pathogen in peritoneal dialysis peritonitis. Am J Kidney Dis. 2005;45:E75–8. doi:10.1053/j.ajkd.2005.01.040.

López-Montes A, Gallego E, López E, et al. Treatment of tuberculosis with rifabutin in a renal transplant patient. Am J Kidney Dis. 2004;44:E59–63. doi:10.1053/j.ajkd.2004.06.015

Mycobutin® capsule [package insert]. New York: Pharmacia & Upjohn Co Division of Pfizer Inc; 2010.

Narang PK, Lewis RC, Bianchine JR. Rifabutin absorption in humans: relative bioavailability and food effect. Clin Pharmacol Ther. 1992;52:335–41.

Narita M, Stambaugh JJ, Hollender ES, Jones D, Pitchenik AE, Ashkin D. Use of rifabutin with protease inhibitors for human immunodeficiency virus-infected patients with tuberculosis. Clin Infect Dis. 2000;30:779–83.

Olyaei AJ, Bennett WM. Drug dosing in elderly patients with chronic kidney disease. Clin Geriatr Med. 2009;25:459–527.

Olyaei AJ, DeMattos AM, Bennett WM. Use of drugs in patients with renal failure. In: Schrier RW, editors. Diseases of the kidney and urinary Tract. 8th ed. Philadelphia: Lippincott Williams & Wilkins; 2007. p. 2765–807.

Perucca E, Grimaldi R, Frigo GM, Sardi A, Mönig H, Ohnhaus EE. Comparative effects of rifabutin and rifampicin on hepatic microsomal enzyme activity in normal subjects. Eur J Clin Pharmacol. 1988;34:595–9.

Skinner MH, Blashke TF. Clinical pharmacokinetics of rifabutin. Clin Pharmacokinet. 1995;28:115–25.

Skinner MH, Hsieh M, Torseth J, et al. Pharmacokinetics of rifabutin. Antimicrob Agents Chemother. 1989;33:1237–41.

Sousa M, Pozniak A, Boffito M. Pharmacokinetics and pharmacodynamics of drug interactions involving rifampicin, rifabutin, and antimalarial drugs. J Antimicrob Chemother. 2008;62:872–8.

Strolin Benedetti M, Efthymiopoulos C, Sassella D, Moro E, Repetto M. Autoinduction of rifabutin metabolism in man. Xenobiotica. 1990;20:1113–9.

Weiner M, Benator D, Burman W, et al. Association between acquired rifamycin resistance and the pharmacokinetics of rifabutin and isoniazid among patients with HIV and tuberculosis. Clin Infect Dis. 2005;40:1481–91.

Zhang J, Zhu L, Stonier M, et al. Determination of rifabutin dosing regimen when administered in combination with ritonavir-boosted atazanavir. J Antimicrob Chemother. 2011;66:2075–82.

Dosage Adjustment of Medications Eliminated by the Kidneys

<u>**Rifabutin**</u>/**Mycobutin**®   {**Antitubercular**}

Usual initial dose:	300 mg orally
Usual maintenance dose:	300 mg orally once daily
Typical maximum dose:	300 mg/day
Proportion eliminated unchanged:	11 %

Adjustment for Kidney Disease

FDA-approved product labeling:	*CrCL <30 mL/min*	*150 mg orally once daily (50 % decrease)*
Alternative adjustment:	*GFR >50 mL/min*	*300 mg orally once daily*
	GFR 10–50 mL/min	*300 mg orally once daily*
	GFR <10 mL/min	*300 mg orally once daily*
	Hemodialysis	*300 mg orally once daily*
	CAPD	*150–300 mg orally once daily*
	CRRT	*300 mg orally once daily*

Dosage Adjustment of Medications Eliminated by the Kidneys

Rifampin - Selected References

Acocella G. Clinical pharmacokinetics of rifampicin. Clin Pharmacokinet. 1978;3:108–27.

Andrew OT, Schoenfeld PY, Hopewell PC, Humphreys MH. Tuberculosis in patients with end-stage renal disease. Am J Med. 1980;68:59–65.

Aronoff GA, Bennett WM, Berns JS, et al. Drug prescribing in renal failure: dosing guidelines for adults and children. 5th ed. Philadelphia: American College of Physicians; 2007.

Covic A, Goldsmith DJA, Segall L, et al. Rifampicin-induced acute renal failure: a series of 60 patients. Nephrol Dial Transplant. 1998;13:924–9.

Falagas ME, Fragoulis KN, Bliziotis IA. Oral rifampin for prevention of *S. aureus* carriage-related infections in patients with renal failure—a meta-analysis of randomized controlled trials. Nephrol Dial Transplant. 2006;21:2536–42.

Feinfeld DA, Ansari N, Nuovo M, Hussain A, Mir R. Tubulointerstitial nephritis associated with minimal self reexposure to rifampin. Am J Kidney Dis. 1999;33:e3.

Flynn CT, Rainford DJ, Hope E. Acute renal failure and rifampicin: danger of unsuspected intermittent dosage. Br Med J. 1974;2:482.

Girling DJ, Hitze KL. Adverse reactions to rifampicin. Bull World Health Organ. 1979;57:45–9.

Hall CM, Willcox PA, Swanepoel CR, Kahn D, Van Zyl Smit R. Mycobacterial infection in renal transplant recipients. Chest. 1994;106:435–9.

Heintz BH, Matzke GR, Dager WF. Antimicrobial dosing concepts and recommendations for critically ill adult patients receiving continuous renal replacement therapy or intermittent hemodialysis. Pharmacotherapy. 2009;29:562–77.

Kenny MT, Strates B. Metabolism and pharmacokinetics of the antibiotic rifampin. Drug Metab Rev. 1981;12:159–218.

Kuypers DRJ, Verleden G, Naesens M, Vanrenterghem Y. Drug interaction between mycophenolate and rifampin: possible induction of uridine diphosphate-glucuronosyltransferase. Clin Pharmacol Ther. 2005;78:81–8.

Lattes R, Radisic M, Rial M, Argento J, Casadel D. Tuberculosis in renal transplant recipients. Transpl Infect Dis. 1999;1:98–104.

Malone RS, Fish DN, Spiegel DM, Childs JM, Peloquin CA. The effect of hemodialysis on isoniazid, rifampin, pyrazinamide, and ethambutol. Am J Respir Crit Care Med. 1999;159:1580–4.

Muthukumar T, Jayakumar M, Fernando EM, Muthusethupathi MA. Acute renal failure due to rifampicin: a study of 25 patients. Am J Kidney Dis. 2002;40:690–6.

Naesens M, Kuypers DRJ, Streit F, et al. Rifampin induces alterations in mycophenolic acid glucuronidation and elimination: implications for drug exposure in renal allograft recipients. Clin Pharmacol Ther. 2006;80:509–21.

Olyaei AJ, Bennett WM. Drug dosing in elderly patients with chronic kidney disease. Clin Geriatr Med. 2009;25:459–527.

Olyaei AJ, Bennett WM. Pharmacologic approach to renal insufficiency. In: Dale DC, Federman DD, Antman K, editors. ACP Medicine, WebMD June 2007 update. Hamilton: BC Decker; 2007; NEPHROLOGY IX: Appendix A1–25.

Olyaei AJ, DeMattos AM, Bennett WM. Use of drugs in patients with renal failure. In: Schrier RW, editor. Diseases of the kidney and urinary tract. 8th ed. Philadelphia: Lippincott Williams & Wilkins; 2007. p. 2765–807.

Poole G, Stradling P, Worlledge S. Potentially serious side effects of high-dose twice-weekly rifampicin. Br Med J. 1971;3:343–7.

Rifadin® capsule and Rifadin IV® injection [package insert]. Bridgewater: Sanofi-Aventis US LLC; 2007.

Vachharajani TJ, Oza UG, Phadke AG, Kirpalani AL. Tuberculosis in renal transplant recipients: rifampicin sparing treatment protocol. Int Urol Nephrol. 2002;34:551–3.

Dosage Adjustment of Medications Eliminated by the Kidneys

Rifampin/Rifadin®	{Antitubercular; antibacterial}	
Usual initial dose:	600 mg orally or IV	
Usual maintenance dose:	10 mg/kg not to exceed 600 mg orally or IV once daily	
Typical maximum dose:	600 mg/day	
Proportion eliminated unchanged:	8–33 %	

Adjustment for Kidney Disease

FDA-approved product labeling:	*CrCL <50 mL/min*	*10 mg/kg not to exceed 600 mg orally or IV once daily (100 % of usual dose)*
	Hemodialysis	*10 mg/kg not to exceed 600 mg orally or IV once daily (100 % of usual dose)*
Alternative adjustment:	*GFR >50 mL/min*	*10 mg/kg not to exceed 600 mg orally or IV every 24 h (50–100 % of usual dose)*
	GFR 10–50 mL/min	*5–10 mg/kg not to exceed 600 mg orally or IV every 24 h (50–100 % of usual dose)*
	GFR <10 mL/min	*5–10 mg/kg not to exceed 600 mg orally or IV every 24 h (50–100 % of usual dose)*
	Hemodialysis	*5–10 mg/kg not to exceed 600 mg orally or IV every 24 h (50–100 % of usual dose); no supplemental dose after dialysis required*
	CAPD	*5–10 mg/kg not to exceed 600 mg orally or IV every 24 h (50–100 % of usual dose)*
	CVVH	*300–600 mg IV every 12–24 h*
	CVVHD	*300–600 mg IV every 12–24 h*
	CVVHDF	*300–600 mg IV every 12–24 h*

Rimantadine - Selected References

Al-jedai AH, Honaker MR, Trofe J, et al. Renal allograft loss as the result of polyomavirus interstitial nephritis after simultaneous kidney-pancreas transplantation: results with kidney retransplantation. Transplantation. 2003;75:490–4.

Aronoff GA, Bennett WM, Berns JS, et al. Drug prescribing in renal failure: dosing guidelines for adults and children. 5th ed. Philadelphia: American College of Physicians; 2007.

Atiee G, Lasseter K, Baughman S, et al. Absence of pharmacokinetic interaction between intravenous peramivir and oral oseltamivir or rimantadine in humans. J Clin Pharmacol. 2011. Epub ahead of print. doi:10.1177/0091270011414574.

Bridges CB, Fukuda K, Uyeki TM, Cox NJ, Singleton JA. Prevention and control of influenza: recommendations of the Advisory Committee on Immunization Practices (ACIP). MMWR Recomm Rep. 2002;51(RR-3):1–31.

Capparelli EV, Stevens RC, Chow MSS, Izard M, Wills RJ. Rimantadine pharmacokinetics in healthy subjects and patients with end-stage renal failure. Clin Pharmacol Ther. 1988;43:536–41.

Cirrincione-Dall G, Brennan BJ, Ballester-Sanchis RM, Navarro MT, Davies BE. Pharmacokinetics and safety of coadministered oseltamivir and rimantadine in healthy volunteers: an open-label, multiple-dose, randomized, crossover study. J Clin Pharmacol. 2011. Epub ahead of print. doi:10.1177/0091270011412960.

Flumadine® tablet and syrup [package insert]. St Louis: Forest Pharmaceuticals Inc; 2007.

Hanlon JT, Aspinall SL, Semla TP, et al. Consensus guidelines for oral dosing of primarily renally cleared medications in older adults. J Am Geriatr Soc. 2009;57:335–40.

Hayden FG, Minocha A, Spyker DA, Hoffman HE. Comparative single-dose pharmacokinetics of amantadine hydrochloride and rimantadine hydrochloride in young and elderly adults. Antimicrob Agents Chemother. 1985:28:216–21.

Hayden FG, Hoffman HE, Spyker DA. Differences in side effects of amantadine hydrochloride and rimantadine hydrochloride relate to differences in pharmacokinetics. Antimicrob Agents Chemother. 1983:23:458–64.

Olyaei AJ, Bennett WM. Drug dosing in elderly patients with chronic kidney disease. Clin Geriatr Med. 2009;25:459–527.

Olyaei AJ, DeMattos AM, Bennett WM. Use of drugs in patients with renal failure. In: Schrier RW, editor. Diseases of the kidney and urinary tract. 8th ed. Philadelphia: Lippincott Williams & Wilkins; 2007. p. 2765–807.

Schmidt AC. Antiviral therapy for influenza: a clinical and economic comparative review. Drugs. 2004;64:2031–46.

Tominack RK, Wills RJ, Gustavson LE, Hayden FG. Multiple-dose pharmacokinetics of rimantadine in elderly adults. Antimicrob Agents Chemother. 1988;32:1813–9.

Wintermeyer SM, Nahata MC. Rimantadine: a clinical perspective. Ann Pharmacother. 1995;29:299–310.

Dosage Adjustment of Medications Eliminated by the Kidneys

<u>Rimantadine</u>/Flumadine®   **{Antiviral}**

Usual initial dose: 100 mg orally

Usual maintenance dose: 100 mg orally twice daily for 7 days or, for influenza prophylaxis, for the duration of the period of peak influenza activity in the community

Typical maximum dose: 200 mg/day

Proportion eliminated unchanged: 19 %

Adjustment for Kidney Disease

FDA-approved product labeling:	*Renal insufficiency*	*Monitor for adverse effects and adjust dose as necessary.*
	Elderly nursing home patients	*100 mg orally once daily*
	CrCL ≤10 mL/min	*100 mg orally once daily*
Alternative adjustment:	*GFR >50 mL/min*	*100 mg orally twice daily*
	GFR 10–50 mL/min	*100 mg orally once daily*
	GFR <10 mL/min	*100 mg orally once daily*
	Hemodialysis	*100 mg orally once daily (supplemental dose after dialysis not required or recommended)*
	CAPD	*Data not available*
	CRRT	*100 mg orally twice daily*

Dosage Adjustment of Medications Eliminated by the Kidneys

Risedronate - Selected References

Actonel® tablet film coated [package insert]. Rockaway: Warner Chilcott (US) LLC; 2011.

Atelvia™ tablet delayed release [package insert]. Rockaway: Warner Chilcott (US) LLC; 2011.

Bobba RS, Beattie K, Parkinson B, Kumbhare D, Adachi JD. Tolerability of different dosing regimens of bisphosphonates for the treatment of osteoporosis and malignant bone disease. Drug Saf. 2006;29:1133–52.

Bock O, Felsenberg D. Bisphosphonates in the management of postmenopausal osteoporosis—optimizing efficacy in clinical practice. Clin Interv Aging. 2008;3:279–97.

Cremers SCLM, Pillai GC, Papapoulos SE. Pharmacokinetics/pharmacodynamics of bisphosphonates: use for optimasation of intermittent therapy for osteoporosis. Clin Pharmacokinet. 2005;44:551–70.

Dunn CJ, Goa KL. Risedronate: a review of its pharmacological properties and clinical use in resorptive bone disease. Drugs. 2001;61:685–712.

Fujii N, Hamano T, Mikami S, et al. Risedronate, an effective treatment for glucocorticoid-induced bone loss in CKD patients with or without concomitant active vitamin D (PRIUS-CKD). Nephrol Dial Transplant. 2007;22:1601–7.

Geusens P. Bisphosphonates for postmenopausal osteoporosis: determining duration of treatment. Curr Osteoporos Rep. 2009;7:12–7.

Miller PD, Roux C, Boonen S, Barton IP, Dunlap LE, Burgio DE. Safety and efficacy of risedronate in patients with age-related reduced renal function as estimated by the Cockroft and Gault method: a pooled analysis of nine clinical trials. J Bone Miner Res. 2005;20:2105–15.

Mitchell DY, Barr WH, Eusebio RA, et al. Risedronate pharmacokinetics and intra- and inter-subject variability upon single-dose intravenous and oral administration. Pharm Res. 2001;18:166–70.

Mitchell DY, Eusebio RA, Sacco-Gibson NA, et al. Dose-proportional pharmacokinetics of risedronate on single-dose oral administration to healthy volunteers. J Clin Pharmacol. 2000;40:258–65.

Mitchell DY, Heise MA, Pallone KA, et al. The effect of dosing regimen on the pharmacokinetics of risedronate. Br J Clin Pharmacol. 1999;48:536–42.

Mitchell DY, St Peter JV, Eusebio RA, et al. Effect of renal function on risedronate pharmacokinetics after a single oral dose. Br J Clin Pharmacol. 2000;49:215–22.

Nowacka-Cieciura E, Cieciura T, B czkowska T, et al. Bisphosphonates are effective prophylactic of early bone loss after renal transplantation. Transplant Proc. 2006;38:165–7.

Papapetrou PD. Bisphosphonate-associated adverse events. Hormones (Athens). 2009;8:96–110.

Peris P, Torra M, Olivares V, et al. Prolonged bisphosphonate release after treatment in women with osteoporosis: relation with bone turnover. Bone. 2011;49:706–9.

Russell RGG, Watts NB, Ebetino FH, Rogers MJ. Mechanisms of action of bisphosphonates: similarities and differences and their potential influence on clinical efficacy. Osteoporosis Int. 2008;19:733–59.

Strampel W, Emkey R, Civitelli R. Safety considerations with bisphosphonates for the treatment of osteoporosis. Drug Saf. 2007;30:755–63.

Torregrosa JV, Fuster D, Gentil M-Á, et al. Open-label trial: effect of weekly risedronate Immediately after transplantation in kidney recipients. Transplantation. 2010;89:1476–81.

Torregrosa JV, Fuster D, Pedroso S, et al. Weekly risedronate in kidney transplant patients with osteopenia. Transplant Int. 2007;20:708–11.

Watts NB, Diab DL. Long-term use of bisphosphonates in osteoporosis. J Clin Endocrinol Metab. 2010;95:1555–65.

Yank B, Bavbek N, Yanik T, et al. The effect of alendronate, risedronate, and raloxifene on renal functions, based on the Cockroft and Gault method, in postmenopausal women. Ren Fail. 2007;29:471–6.

Dosage Adjustment of Medications Eliminated by the Kidneys

<u>Risedronate</u>/Actonel®, Atelvia™	{Anti-osteoporotic, bisphosphonate}	
Usual initial dose:	5–150 mg orally taken at least 30 min before the first food or drink of the day; do not lie down for 30 min.	
Usual maintenance dose:	One 5-mg tablet orally taken daily or	
	One 35-mg tablet or one 35-mg delayed-release tablet orally taken once a week or	
	One 75-mg tablet orally taken on two consecutive days for a total of two tablets each month or	
	One 150-mg tablet orally taken once a month	
Typical maximum dose:	150 mg/month; usual maximal initial treatment duration = 5 years	
Proportion eliminated unchanged:	87 %	
Adjustment for Kidney Disease		
FDA-approved product labeling:	*CrCL <30 mL/min*	*Not recommended because of lack of clinical experience*
Alternative adjustment:	*eCrCL 15–30 mL/min*	*5 mg orally once daily*
	Hemodialysis	*Data not available; preferably avoid*

Dosage Adjustment of Medications Eliminated by the Kidneys

Risperidone (Oral) - Selected References

Batalla A, Vera M, Torra M, Parellada E. Antipsychotic treatment in a patient with schizophrenia undergoing hemodialysis [letter]. J Clin Psychopharmacol. 2010;30:92–4.

Borison RL, Diamond B, Pathiraja A, Meibach RC. Pharmacokinetics of risperidone in chronic schizophrenic patients. Psychopharmacol Bull. 1994;30:193–7.

de Leon J, Wynn G, Sandson NB. The pharmacokinetics of paliperidone versus risperidone. Psychosomatics. 2010;51:80–8.

Grant S, Fitton A. Risperidone: a review of its pharmacology and therapeutic potential in the treatment of schizophrenia. Drugs. 1994;48:253–73.

Gupta M, Annadatha S. Treating bipolar disorder in patients with renal failure having haemodialysis: two case reports. Clin Pract Epidemiol Ment Health. 2008;4:21. doi:10.1186/1745-0179-4-21.

Huang M-L, Van Peer A, Woestenborghs R, et al. Pharmacokinetics of the novel antipsychotic agent risperidone and the prolactin response in healthy subjects. Clin Pharmacol Ther. 1993;54:257–68.

Lin C-H, Kuo C-C, Chou L-S, et al. A randomized, double-blind comparison of risperidone versus low-dose risperidone plus low-dose haloperidol in treating schizophrenia. J Clin Psychopharmacol. 2010;30:518–25.

Llerena A, Dorado P, Peñas-Lledó EM. Relevance of CYP2D6 for risperidone pharmacokinetics, pharmacodynamics and adverse reactions. Pharmacogenomics. 2011;12:311–3.

Mannens G, Huang M-L, Meuldermans W, Hendrickx J, Woestenborghs R, Heykants J. Absorption, metabolism, and excretion of risperidone in man. Drug Metab Dispos. 1993;21:1134–41.

Mannens G, Meuldermans W, Snoeck E, Heykants J. Plasma protein binding of risperidone and its distribution in blood. Psychopharmacology (Berl). 1994;114:566–72.

Markowitz JS, DeVane CL, Liston HL, Boulton DW, Risch SC. The effects of probenecid on the disposition of risperidone and olanzapine in healthy volunteers. Clin Pharmacol Ther. 2002;71:30–8.

Maxwell RA, Sweet RA, Mulsant BH, et al. Risperidone and 9-hydroxyrisperidone concentrations are not dependent on age or creatinine clearance among elderly patients. J Geriatr Psychiatry Neurol. 2002;15:77–81.

Meltzer HY, Cola PA, Parsa M. Marked elevations of serum creatine kinase activity associated with antipsychotic drug treatment. Neuropsychopharmacology. 1996;15:395–405.

Railton CJ, Kapur B, Koren G. Subtherapeutic risperidone serum concentrations in an adolescent during hemodialysis: a pharmacological puzzle. Ther Drug Monit. 2005;27:558–61.

Risperdal® tablet, disintegrating tablet (M-Tab), and solution [package insert]. Titusville: Janssen Division of Ortho-McNeill-Janssen Pharmaceuticals Inc; 2011.

Risperdal® Consta injection extended release [package insert]. Titusville: Janssen Division of Ortho-McNeill-Janssen Pharmaceuticals Inc; 2011.

Snoeck E, Van Peer A, Sack M, et al. Influence of age, renal and liver impairment on the pharmacokinetics of risperidone in man. Psychopharmacology (Berl). 1995;122:223–9.

Vermier M, Naessens I, Remmerie B, et al. Absorption, metabolism, and excretion of paliperidone, a new monoaminergic antagonist, in humans. Drug Metab Dispos. 2008;36:769–79.

Yoo H-D, Lee S-N, Kang H-A, Cho H-Y, Lee I-K, Lee Y-B. Influence of ABCB1 genetic polymorphisms on the pharmacokinetics of risperidone in healthy subjects with CYP2D6*10/*10. Br J Pharmacol. 2011;164:433–43.

Dosage Adjustment of Medications Eliminated by the Kidneys

<u>Risperidone</u>/Risperdal®,
Risperdal® Consta

{Atypical antipsychotic; benzisoxazole derivative}

Usual initial dose:	1 mg orally twice daily
Usual maintenance dose:	2–8 mg/day orally in one or two divided doses or 25 mg IM every 2 weeks
Typical maximum dose:	16 mg/day
Proportion eliminated unchanged:	4–30 % (plus approx 40 % of each dose as metabolites including 8–30 % of the dose as active 9-hydroxyrisperidone [paliperidone])

Adjustment for Kidney Disease

FDA-approved product labeling:	*Severe renal impairment*	*The recommended initial dose is 0.5 mg twice daily. Dosage increases in these patients should be in increments of no more than 0.5 mg twice daily. Increases to dosages above 1.5 mg twice daily should generally occur at intervals of at least 1 week. In some patients, slower titration may be medically appropriate.*
Alternative adjustment:	*GFR >50 mL/min*	*1–3 mg orally twice daily*
	GFR 10–50 mL/min	*0.5–2 mg orally twice daily or 12.5 mg IM every 2 weeks*
	GFR <10 mL/min	*0.5–2 mg orally once daily; begin with modest doses and titrate carefully.*
	Hemodialysis	*0.5–4 mg orally once daily; supplemental dose after dialysis is not necessary; begin with modest doses and titrate carefully.*
	CAPD	*Data not available*
	CRRT	*Data not available*

Dosage Adjustment of Medications Eliminated by the Kidneys

Rivaroxaban - Selected References

Bauersachs R, Berkowitz SD, Brenner B, et al. Oral rivaroxaban for symptomatic venous thromboembolism. N Engl J Med. 2010;363:2499–510.

Eerenberg ES, Kamphuisen PW, Sijpkens MK, Meijers JC, Buller HR, Levi M. Reversal of rivaroxaban and dabigatran by protein complex concentrate: a randomized, placebo-controlled, crossover study in healthy subjects. Circulation. 2011;124:1573–9.

Eriksson BI, Borris LC, Friedman RJ, et al. Rivaroxaban versus enoxaparin for thromboprophylaxis after hip arthroplasty. N Engl J Med. 2008;358:2765–75.

Eriksson BI, Kakkar AK, Turpie AGG, et al. Oral rivaroxaban for the prevention of symptomatic venous thromboembolism after elective hip and knee replacement. J Bone Joint Surg Br. 2009;91:636–44.

Fox KAA, Piccini JP, Wojdyla D, et al. Prevention of stroke and systemic embolism with rivaroxaban compared with warfarin in patients with non-valvular atrial fibrillation and moderate renal impairment. Eur Heart J. 2011;32:2387–94.

Harder S. Renal profiles of anticoagulants. J Clin Pharmacol. 2011. Epub ahead of print. doi:10.1177/009127001409231.

Jiang J, Hu Y, Zhang J, et al. Safety, pharmacokinetics and pharmacodynamics of single doses of rivaroxaban – an oral, direct factor Xa inhibitor – in elderly Chinese subjects. Thromb Haemost. 2010;103:234–41.

Kakkar AK, Brenner B, Dahl WE, et al. Extended duration rivaroxaban versus short-term enoxaparin for the prevention of venous thromboembolism after total hip arthroplasty: a double-blind, randomised controlled trial. Lancet. 2008;372:31–9.

Kubitza D, Becka M, Mueck W, et al. Effect of renal impairment on the pharmacokinetics, pharmacodynamics and safety of rivaroxaban, an oral, direct factor Xa inhibitor. Br J Clin Pharmacol. 2010;70:703–12.

Kubitza D, Becka M, Roth A, Mueck W. Dose-escalation study of the pharmacokinetics and pharmacodynamics of rivaroxaban in healthy elderly subjects. Curr Med Res Opin. 2008;24:2757–65.

Kubitza D, Becka M, Wensing G, Voith B, Zuehlsdorf M. Safety, pharmacodynamics, and pharmacokinetics of BAY 59-739—an oral, direct factor Xa inhibitor—after multiple dosing in healthy male subjects. Eur J Clin Pharmacol. 2005;61:873–80.

Kubitza D, Becka M, Wensing G, Zuehlsdorf M, Mueck W. Body weight has limited influence on the safety, tolerability, pharmacokinetics, or pharmacodynamics rivaroxaban (BAY 59-739) in healthy subjects. J Clin Pharmacol. 2007;47:218–26.

Lassen MR, Ageno W, Borris LC, et al. Rivaroxaban versus enoxaparin for thromboprophylaxis after total knee arthroplasty. N Engl J Med. 2008;358:2776–86.

Mega JL, Braunwald E, Mohanavelu S, et al. Rivaroxaban versus placebo in patients with acute coronary syndromes (ATLAS ACS-TIMI 46): a randomised, double-blind, phase II trial. Lancet. 2009;374:29–38.

Mega JL, Braunwald E, Wiviott SD, et al. Rivaroxaban in patients with a recent acute coronary syndrome. N Engl J Med. 2011. Epub ahead of print. doi:10.1056/NEJMoa1112277.

Mueck W, Borris LC, Dahl OE, et al. Population pharmacokinetics and pharmacodynamics of once- and twice-daily rivaroxaban for the prevention of venous thromboembolism in patients undergoing total hip replacement. Thromb Haemost. 2008;100:453–61.

Mueck W, Eriksson BI, Bauer KA, et al. Population pharmacokinetics and pharmacodynamics of rivaroxaban – an oral, direct factor Xa inhibitor – in patients undergoing major orthopaedic surgery. Clin Pharmacokinet. 2008;47:203–16.

Patel MR, Mahafey KW, Garg J, et al. Rivaroxaban versus warfarin in nonvalvular atrial fibrillation. N Engl J Med. 2011;65:881–91.

Turpie AGG, Lassen MR, Davidson BI, et al. Rivaroxaban versus enoxaparin for thromboprophylaxis after total knee arthroplasty (RECORD4): a randomised trial. Lancet. 2009;373:1673–80.

Turpie AGG, Lassen MR, Eriksson BE, et al. Rivaroxaban for the prevention of venous thromboembolism after hip or knee arthroplasty: pooled analysis of four studies. Thromb Haemost. 2011;105:444–53.

Weitz JI, Eikelboom JW, Samama MM. New antithrombotic drugs: antithrombotic therapy and prevention of thrombosis, 9th ed: American College of Chest Physicians Evidence-Based Clinical Practice Guidelines. Chest 2012;141(2 Suppl):e120–51S. doi:10.1378/chest.11-2294.

Xarelto® tablet [package insert]. Titusville: Janssen Pharmaceuticals Inc; 2011.

Zhao X, Sun P, Zhou Y, et al. Safety, pharmacokinetics and pharmacodynamics of single/multiple doses of the oral, direct factor Xa inhibitor rivaroxaban in healthy Chinese subjects. Br J Clin Pharmacol. 2009;68:77–88.

Dosage Adjustment of Medications Eliminated by the Kidneys

Rivaroxaban/Xarelto® {Direct thrombin inhibitor; antithrombotic}

Usual initial dose:	20 mg orally
Usual maintenance dose:	10–20 mg orally once daily with the evening meal
Typical maximum dose:	20 mg/day
Proportion eliminated unchanged:	36 %

Adjustment for Kidney Disease

FDA-approved product labeling: *Nonvalvular atrial fibrillation*

CrCL >50 mL/min	*20 mg orally once daily with the evening meal*
CrCL 15–50 mL/min	*15 mg orally once daily with the evening meal; observe closely and promptly evaluate any signs or symptoms of blood loss; patients who develop acute renal failure while on rivaroxaban should discontinue treatment.*
CrCL <15 mL/min	*Avoid due to an expected increase in rivaroxaban exposure and pharmacodynamic effects in this population*

Prophylaxis of deep vein thrombosis

CrCL ≥30 mL/min	*10 mg orally once daily with the evening meal (at least 6 h after surgery for 35 days in patients undergoing hip replacement surgery or 12 days for patients undergoing knee replacement surgery)*
CrCL <30 mL/min	*Avoid due to an expected increase in rivaroxaban exposure and pharmacodynamic effects in this population, i.e., bleeding*

Alternative adjustment:

GFR >50 mL/min	*20 mg orally once daily with the evening meal (atrial fibrillation); 2.5–5 mg orally once daily (prevention of recurrent cardiovascular events in patients with acute coronary syndrome)*
GFR 30–50 mL/min	*15 mg orally once daily with the evening meal (atrial fibrillation)*
GFR <30 mL/min	*Data not available, preferably avoid*
Hemodialysis	*Data not available; preferably avoid*
CAPD	*Data not available; preferably avoid*
CRRT	*Data not available; preferably avoid*

Note: Due to exclusion of patients with GFR <30 mL/min in clinical trials and lack of experience, rivaroxaban use usually should be discouraged in these individuals in favor of unfractionated heparin, parenteral direct thrombin inhibitors, or warfarin. Patients with moderate renal impairment (CrCL 30–49 mL/min) and atrial fibrillation treated with rivaroxaban have been found to have an incidence of ischemic stroke similar to that in patients treated with warfarin, whereas this incidence was significantly reduced with rivaroxaban in patients with normal renal function.

Dosage Adjustment of Medications Eliminated by the Kidneys

Rosuvastatin - Selected References

Athyros VG, Tziomalos K, Karagiannis A, Mikhailidis DP. Statins and cardiovascular events in patients with end-stage renal disease on hemodialysis: the AURORA results suggest the need for earlier intervention [editorial]. Curr Vasc Pharmacol. 2009;7:264–6.

Ballantyne CM, Bertolami M, Hernandez Garcia HR, et al. Achieving LDL cholesterol, non-HDL cholesterol, and apolipoprotein B target levels in high-risk patients: Measuring Effective Reductions in Cholesterol Using Rosuvastatin therapY (MERCURY) II. Am Heart J. 2006;151:975.e1–9.

Burmeister JE, Miltersteiner DR, Campos BM. Rosuvastatin in hemodialysis: short-term effects on lipids and C-reactive protein. J Nephrol. 2009;22:83–9.

Crestor® tablet film coated [package insert]. Wilmington: AstraZeneca Pharmaceuticals LP; 2010.

Fellström B, Holdaas H, Jardine AG, et al. Effect of rosuvastatin on outcomes in chronic haemodialysis patients: baseline data from the AURORA study. Kidney Blood Press Res. 2007;30:314–22.

Fellström B, Jardine AG, Schmieder RE, et al. Rosuvastatin and cardiovascular events in patients undergoing hemodialysis. N Engl J Med. 2009;360:1395–407.

García-Rodríguez LA, Massó-González EL, Wallander M-A, Johansson S. The safety of rosuvastatin in comparison with other statins in over 100000 statin users in UK primary care. Pharmacoepidemiol Drug Saf. 2008;17:943–52.

Holdaas H, Holme I, Schmieder RE, et al. Rosuvastatin in diabetic hemodialysis patients. J Am Soc Nephrol. 2011;22:1335–41.

Kostapanos MS, Milionis HJ, Saougos VG, et al. Dose-dependent effect of rosuvastatin treatment on urinary protein excretion. J Cardiovasc Pharmacol Ther. 2007;12:292–7.

Marrs JC, Saseen JJ. Effects of lipid-lowering therapy on reduction of cardiovascular events in patients with end-stage renal disease requiring hemodialysis. Pharmacotherapy. 2010;30:823–9.

Martin PD, Mitchell PD, Schneck DW. Pharmacodynamic effects and pharmacokinetics of a new HMG-CoA reductase inhibitor, rosuvastatin, after morning or evening administration in healthy volunteers. Br J Clin Pharmacol. 2002;54:471–7.

Olyaei AJ, Bennett WM. Pharmacologic approach to renal insufficiency. In: Dale DC, Federman DD, Antman K, editors. ACP Medicine, WebMD June 2007 update. Hamilton: BC Decker; 2007; NEPHROLOGY IX: Appendix A1–25.

Park J-K, Meraala EMA, Muller DN, et al. Rosuvastatin protects against angiotensin II-induced renal injury in a dose-dependent fashion. J Hypertens. 2009;27:599–605.

Ridker PM, MacFayden J, Cressman M, Glynn RJ. Efficacy of rosuvastatin among men and women with moderate chronic kidney disease and elevated high-sensitivity C-reactive protein: a secondary analysis from the JUPITER (Justification for the Use of Statins in Prevention: an Intervention Trial Evaluating Rosuvastatin) trial. J Am Coll Cardiol. 2010;55:1266–73.

Sawara Y, Takei T, Uchida K, et al. Effects of lipid-lowering therapy with rosuvastatin on atherosclerotic burden in patients with chronic kidney disease. Intern Med. 2008;47:1505–10.

Sharif A, Ravindran V, Moore R, et al. The effect of rosuvastatin on insulin sensitivity and pancreatic beta-cell function in nondiabetic renal transplant recipients Am J Transplant. 2009;9:1439–45.

Stein EA, Marais AD, Ducobu J, et al. Comparison of short-term renal effects and efficacy of rosuvastatin 40 mg and simvastatin 80 mg, followed by assessment of long-term renal effects of rosuvastatin 40 mg, in patients with dyslipidemia. J Clin Lipidol. 2007;1:287–99.

Tzeng T-B, Schneck DW, Birmingham BK, et al. Population pharmacokinetics of rosuvastatin: implications of renal impairment, race, and dyslipidaemia. Curr Med Res Opin. 2008;24:2575–85.

Verma A, Ranganna KM, Reddy RS, Verma M, Gordon NF. Effect of rosuvastatin on C-reactive protein and renal function in patients with chronic kidney disease. Am J Cardiol. 2005;96:1290–2.

Vidt DG, Harris S, McTaggart F, Ditmarsch M, Sager PT, Sorof JM. Effect of short-term rosuvastatin treatment on estimated glomerular filtration rate. Am J Cardiol. 2006;97:1602–6.

Vidt DG, Ridker PM, Monyak JT, Schreiber MJ, Cressman DO. Longitudinal assessment of estimated glomerular filtration rate in apparently healthy adults: a post hoc analysis from the Jupiter study (Justification for the Use of Statins in Prevention: an Intervention Trial Evaluating Rosuvastatin). Clin Ther. 2011;33:717–25.

Whaley-Connell A, Habibi J, Nistala R, et al. Attenuation of NADPH oxidase activation and glomerular filtration barrier remodeling with statin treatment. Hypertension. 2008;51:474–80.

Dosage Adjustment of Medications Eliminated by the Kidneys

Rosuvastatin/Crestor® {**Antihypercholesterolemic agent; hydroxymethylglutaryl-coenzyme A (HMG-CoA) reductase inhibitor**}

Usual initial dose:	5 mg orally
Usual maintenance dose:	5–20 mg orally once daily
Typical maximum dose:	40 mg/day
Proportion eliminated unchanged:	10 %

Adjustment for Kidney Disease

FDA-approved product labeling: *Severe renal impairment (CrCL <30 mL/min) not on hemodialysis—dosing should be started at 5 mg once daily and not exceed 10 mg once daily.*

Alternative adjustment:

eGFR 50–80 mL/min	*5–20 mg orally once daily*
eGFR 30–49 mL/min	*5–20 mg orally once daily*
eGFR <30 mL/min	*5 mg orally once daily; titrate as necessary up to 10 mg orally once daily.*
Hemodialysis	*2.5–10 mg orally once daily*
CAPD	*Data not available*
CRRT	*Data not available*

Dosage Adjustment of Medications Eliminated by the Kidneys

Ruxolitinib - Selected References

Harrison C, Kiladjian J-J, Al-Ali HK, et al. JAK inhibition with ruxolitinib versus best available therapy for myelofibrosis. N Engl J Med. 2012;366:787–98.

Jakafi™ tablet [package insert]. Wilmington: Incyte Corp; 2011.

Mesa RA, Kanarjian H, Tefferi A, et al. Evaluating the serial use of the myelofibrosis symptom assessment form for measuring symptomatic improvement. Cancer. 2011;117:4869–77.

Ruxolitinib (*Jakafi*) for myelofibrosis. Med Lett Drugs Ther. 2012;54:27–8.

Shi JG, Chen X, Emm T, et al. The effect of CPY3A4 inhibition or induction on the pharmacokinetics and pharmacodynamics of orally administered ruxolitinib (INCB018424 phosphate) in healthy volunteers. J Clin Pharmacol. 2011. Epub ahead of print. doi:10.1177/00912700111405663.

Shi JG, Chen X, McGee RF, et al. The pharmacokinetics, pharmacodynamics, and safety of orally dosed INCB018424 phosphate in healthy volunteers. J Clin Pharmacol. 2011;51:1644–54.

Shilling AD, Nedza FM, Emm T, et al. Metabolism, excretion, and pharmacokinetics of [14C]INCB018424, a selective Janus tyrosine kinase 1/2 inhibitor, in humans. Drug Metab Dispos. 2010;38:2323–31.

Tefferi A, Litzow MR, Pardanani A. Long-term outcome of treatment with ruxolitinib in myelofibrosis [letter]. N Engl J Med. 2011;365:1455–7.

Tefferi A, Pardanani A. Serious adverse events during ruxolitinib treatment in patients with myelofibrosis. Mayo Clin Proc. 2011;86:1188–91.

Verstovsek S, Kantarjian H, Mesa RA, et al. Safety and efficacy of INCB018424, a JAK1 and JAK2 inhibitor, in myelofibrosis. N Engl J Med. 2010;363:1117–27.

Verstovsek S, Mesa RA, Gotlib J, et al. A double-blind, placebo-controlled trial of ruxolitinib for myelofibrosis. N Eng J Med. 2012;366:799–807.

Dosage Adjustment of Medications Eliminated by the Kidneys

<u>Ruxolitinib</u>/Jakafi™	{Janus tyrosine kinase 1–2 inhibitor; ℞ for myelofibrosis}

Usual initial dose: 15–20 mg orally

Usual maintenance dose: 15 mg orally twice daily for patients with a platelet count between 100 and 200×10^9/L or 20 mg orally twice daily for patients with a platelet count $>200 \times 10^9$/L; increase dose based on response to maximum.

Typical maximum dose: 25 mg orally twice daily

Proportion eliminated unchanged: 0.11 % (plus 74 % of the absorbed dose as active metabolites which confer 18 % of the pharmacodynamic actions of ruxolitinib)

Adjustment for Kidney Disease

FDA-approved product labeling:

CrCL 30–50 mL/min	*Reduce starting dose 10 mg orally twice daily in patients with a platelet count between 100 and 150×10^9/L; dose modifications should be made with careful monitoring of safety and efficacy; avoid if platelet count is $<100 \times 10^9$/L.*
CrCL 15–29 mL/min	*Reduce starting dose 10 mg orally twice daily in patients with a platelet count between 100 and 150×10^9/L; dose modifications should be made with careful monitoring of safety and efficacy; avoid if platelet count is $<100 \times 10^9$/L.*
Hemodialysis	*15 mg orally twice daily for patients with a platelet count between 100 and 200×10^9/L or 20 mg orally twice daily for patients with a platelet count $>200 \times 10^9$/L; dose modifications should be made with careful monitoring of safety and efficacy; administer after hemodialysis on dialysis days.*
CrCL <15 mL/min (not requiring hemodialysis)	*Avoid*

Alternative adjustment: *Data not available*

S

L.K. Golightly et al. (eds.), *Renal Pharmacotherapy*,
DOI 10.1007/978-1-4614-5800-5_18, © Springer Science+Business Media New York 2013

Dosage Adjustment of Medications Eliminated by the Kidneys

Salsalate - Selected References

Abraham PA, Stillman T. Salsalate exacerbation of chronic renal insufficiency: relation to inhibition of prostaglandin synthesis. Arch Intern Med. 1987;147:1674–6.

April PA, Abeles M, Baraf HSB, et al. Does the acetyl group of aspirin contribute to the antiinflammatory efficacy of salicylic acid in the treatment of rheumatoid arthritis? J Rheumatol. 1989;16:321–7.

Atkinson MH, Ménard H-A, Kalish GH. Assessment of salsalate, a nonacetylated salicylate, in the treatment of patients with arthritis. Clin Ther. 1995;17:827–37.

Chai W, Fowler DE, Liu J, Barrett EJ, Jain LA, Liu Z. Salsalate attenuates free fatty acid-induced microvascular and metabolic insulin resistance. Diabetes Care. 2011;34:1634–8.

Cowan RA, Hartnell GG, Lowdell CP, Baird IM, Leak AM. Metabolic acidosis induced by carbonic anhydrase inhibitors and salicylates in patients with normal renal function. Br Med J (Clin Res Ed). 1984;289:347–8.

Deodhar SD, Dick MM, Buchanan WW. A short-term comparative trial of salsalate and indomethacin in rheumatoid arthritis. Curr Med Res Opin. 1977;5:185–8.

Dromgoole SH, Cassell S, Furst DE, Paulus HE. Availability of salicylate from salsalate and aspirin. Clin Pharmacol Ther. 1983;34:539–45.

Dromgoole SH, Cassell S, Furst DE, Paulus HE. Metabolism of salsalate in normal subjects. J Pharm Sci. 1984;73:1657–9.

Faghihimani E, Aminorroaya A, Rezvanian H, Adibi P, Ismail-Beigi F, Amini M. Salsalate improves glycemic control in patients with newly diagnosed type 2 diabetes. Acta Diabetol. 2011. Epub ahead of print. doi:10.1007/s00592-011-039-2.

Fleischman A, Bernier R, Shoelson SE, Goldfine AB. Salsalate improves glycemia and inflammatory parameters in obese adults. Diabetes Care. 2008;31:289–94.

Goldfine AB, Fonseca V, Jablonski KA, et al. The effects of salsalate on glycemic control in patients with type 2 diabetes: a randomized trial. Ann Intern Med. 2010;152:346–57.

Harrison LI, Funk ML, Ré ON, Ober RE. Absorption, biotransformation, and pharmacokinetics of salicylsalicylic acid in humans. J Clin Pharmacol. 1981;21:401–4.

Harrison LI, Riedel DJ, Karon E, Goldlust MB, Ekholm BP. Effect of food on salsalate absorption. Ther Drug Monit. 1992;14:89–91.

Hicklin JA. Relationship of plasma salicylate levels to pain relief with two different salicylates. Curr Med Res Opin. 1978;5:572–9.

Kleinman KS, Schweitzer S, Nissenson AR. Accidental salicylate intoxication in a hemodialysis patient. Arch Intern Med. 1988;148:2277–8.

Koska J, Ortega E, Bunt JC, et al. The effect of salsalate on insulin action and glucose tolerance in obese non-diabetic patients: results of a randomised double-blind placebo-controlled study. Diabetologia. 2009;52:385–93.

Lafrance J-P, Miller DR. Selective and non-selective non-steroidal anti-inflammatory drugs and the risk of acute kidney injury. Pharmacoepidemiol Drug Saf. 2009;18:923–31.

Marchu ZA, Hanlon JT. Recognizing the risks of chronic nonsteroidal anti-inflammatory drug use in older adults. Ann Longterm Care. 2010;18:24–7.

McCarty MF. Salsalate may have broad utility in the prevention and treatment of vascular disorders and the metabolic syndrome. Med Hypotheses. 2010;75:276–81.

Rubin HS. Serum salicylate levels in osteoarthritis following oral administration of a preparation containing salicylsalicylic acid and acetylsalicylic acid. Am J Med Sci. 1964;248:31–6.

Salsalate tablet [package insert]. Livonia: Major Pharmaceuticals; 2008.

Singleton PT Jr. Salsalate: its role in the management of rheumatic disease. Clin Ther. 1980;3:80–102.

Smith PK, Gleason HL, Stoll CG, Ogorzalek S. Studies on the pharmacology of salicylates. J Pharmacol Exp Ther. 1946;87:237–55.

Williams ME, Weinblatt M, Rosa RM, et al. Salsalate kinetics in patients with chronic renal failure undergoing hemodialysis. Clin Pharmacol Ther. 1986;39:420–4.

Dosage Adjustment of Medications Eliminated by the Kidneys

<u>Salsalate</u>/Disalicylic Acid, Disalcid®, Amigesic®   {Anti-inflammatory}

Usual initial dose: 1,500 mg orally

Usual maintenance dose: 1,500 mg orally twice daily

Typical maximum dose: 4,000 mg/day

Proportion eliminated unchanged: 1 % (on a molar basis, 84 % of each dose is hydrolyzed to salicylic acid, the active anti-inflammatory compound; approximately 10 % of formed salicylic acid is eliminated unchanged in urine)

Adjustment for Kidney Disease

FDA-approved product labeling:	*Impaired renal function*	*Renal patients are at greatest risk for toxicity including renal papillary necrosis, acute renal decompensation, and other renal injury; close monitoring of renal function is advisable.*
	Advanced renal disease	*Use not recommended due to lack of information available from controlled clinical studies*
Alternative adjustment:	*Hemodialysis:*	*1,500 mg orally once followed by 750 mg orally twice daily; administer supplemental 500 mg following hemodialysis on dialysis days.*

Therapeutic drug monitoring

Therapeutic plasma levels: *Usual therapeutic (anti-inflammatory) serum salicylate trough concentration = 150–300 mg/L*

Dosage Adjustment of Medications Eliminated by the Kidneys

Saxagliptin - Selected References

Abe M, Okada K, Soma M. Antidiabetic agents in patients with chronic kidney disease and end-stage renal disease on dialysis: metabolism and clinical practice. Curr Drug Metab. 2011;12:57–69.

Aschner PJ. The role of saxagliptin with the management of type 2 diabetes mellitus: an update from the 2010 European Association for the Study of Diabetes (EASD) 46th annual meeting and the American Diabetes Association (ADA) 70th scientific session. Diabetol Metab Syndr. 2010;2:69. doi:10.1186/1758-5996-2-69.

Baetta R, Corsini A. Pharmacology of dipeptidyl peptidase-4 inhibitors: similarities and differences. Drugs. 2011;71:1441–67.

Boulton DW, Li L, Frevert EU, et al. Influence of renal or hepatic impairment on the pharmacokinetics of saxagliptin. Clin Pharmacokinet. 2011;50:253–65.

Deacon CF. Dipeptidyl peptidase-4 inhibitors in the treatment of type 2 diabetes: a comparative review. Diabetes Obes Metab. 2011;13:7–18.

Deacon CF, Holst JJ. Saxagliptin: a new dipeptidyl peptidase-4 inhibitor for the treatment of type 2 diabetes. Adv Ther. 2009;26:488–99.

Dhillon S, Weber J. Saxagliptin. Drugs. 2009;69:2103–14.

Esposito K, Cozzolino D, Bellastella G, et al. Dipeptidyl peptidase-4 inhibitors and HbA1c target of <7 % in type 2 diabetes: meta-analysis of randomized controlled trials. Diabetes Obes Metab. 2011;13:594–603.

European Medicines Agency. Onglyza: summary of product characteristics. Available at: http://www.ema.europa.eu/docs/en_GB/document_library/EPAR_-_Product_Information/human/001039/WC500044316.pdf. Accessed 13 Oct 2011.

Faknoury WK, Lereun C, Wright D. A meta-analysis of placebo-controlled clinical trials assessing the efficacy and safety of incretin-based medications in patients with type 2 diabetes. Pharmacology. 2010;86:44–57.

Göke B, Gallwitz B, Eriksson J, Hellqvist Å, Gause-Nilsson I. Saxagliptin is non-inferior to glipizide in patients with type 2 diabetes mellitus inadequately controlled on metformin alone: a 52-week randomised controlled trial. Int J Clin Pract. 2010;64:1619–31.

Golightly LK, Drayna CC, McDermott MT. Comparative clinical pharmacokinetics of dipeptidyl peptidase-4 inhibitors. Clin Pharmacokinet. 2012. Epub ahead of print. doi:10.2165/11632930-000000000-00000.

Hare KJ, Vilsbøll T, Asmar M, Deacon CF, Knop FK, Holst JJ. The glucagonostatic and insulinotropic effects of glucagon-like peptide 1 contribute equally to its glucose-lowering action. Diabetes. 2010;59:1765–70.

Holst JJ, Krarup T, Knop FK, Madsbad S, Vilsbøll T. Loss of incretin effect is a specific, important, and early characteristic of type 2 diabetes. Diabetes Care. 2011;34(Suppl 2):S251–7.

Jadzinsky M, Pfützner A, Paz-Pacheco E, Xu Z, Allen E, Chen R. Saxagliptin given in combination with metformin as initial therapy improves glycaemic control in patients with type 2 diabetes compared with either monotherapy: a randomized controlled trial. Diabetes Obes Metab. 2009;11:611–22.

Mason RP, Jacob RF, Kubant R, et al. Effect of enhanced glycemic control with saxagliptin on endothelial nitric oxide release and CD40 levels in obese rats. J Atheroscler Thromb. 2011;18:774–83.

Monami M, Cremasco F, Lamanna C, et al. Glucagon-like peptide-1 receptor agonists and cardiovascular events: a meta-analysis of randomized and clinical trials. Exp Diabetes Res. 2011;2011:215674. doi:10.1155/2011/215764.

Monami M, Marchionni N, Mannuchi E. Glucagon-like peptide-1 receptor agonists in type 2 diabetes: a meta-analysis of randomized clinical trials. Eur J Endocrinol. 2009;160:909–17.

Onglyza™ tablet [package insert]. Princeton: Bristol-Myers Squibb Co; 2009.

Patel CG, Zhang J, Li L, et al. Effect of a high-fat meal on the pharmacokinetics of saxagliptin in healthy subjects. J Clin Pharmacol. 2010;50:1211–6.

Richter B, Bandeira-Echtler E, Bergerhoff K, Lerch C. Dipeptidyl peptidase-4 (DPP-4) inhibitors for type 2 diabetes mellitus. Cochrane Database Syst Rev. 2008;(2):CD006739. doi:10.1002/14651858.CD006739.pub2.

Rosenstock J, Aguilar-Salinas C, Klein E, Nepal S, List J, Chen R. Effect of saxagliptin monotherapy in treatment-naive patients with type 2 diabetes. Curr Med Res Opin. 2009;25:2401–11.

Rosenstock J, Sankoh S, List JF. Glucose-lowering activity of the dipeptidyl peptidase-4 inhibitor saxagliptin in drug-naïve patients with type 2 diabetes. Diabetes Obes Metab. 2008;10:376–86.

Dosage Adjustment of Medications Eliminated by the Kidneys

Saxagliptin/Onglyza™   **{Antidiabetic; dipeptidyl peptidase-4 inhibitor}**

Usual initial dose:	2.5 mg orally
Usual maintenance dose:	2.5–5 mg orally once daily
Typical maximum dose:	10 mg/day
Proportion eliminated unchanged:	24 % plus 36 % as active metabolite (5-hydroxy saxagliptin)

Adjustment for Kidney Disease

FDA-approved product labeling:	*CrCL >50 mL/min*	*2.5–5 mg orally once daily*
	CrCL ≤50 mL/min	*2.5 mg orally once daily*
	Hemodialysis	*2.5 mg orally once daily; administer after hemodialysis on dialysis days.*
	CAPD	*No data*
Alternative adjustment:	*GFR >55 mL/min*	*2.5–5 mg orally once daily*
	GFR ≤55 mL/min	*2.5 mg orally once daily*

Dosage Adjustment of Medications Eliminated by the Kidneys

Silodosin - Selected References

Chapple CR, Montorsi F, Tammela TLJ, Wirth M, Koldewijn E, Fernández EF. Silodosin therapy for lower urinary tract symptoms in men with suspected benign prostatic hyperplasia: results of an international, randomized, double-blind, placebo-controlled clinical trial performed in Europe. Eur Urol. 2011;59:342–52.

Curran MP. Silodosin: treatment of the signs and symptoms of benign prostatic hyperplasia. Drugs. 2011;71:897–907.

Ishiguro M, Futabayashi Y, Ohnuki T, Ahmed M, Muramatsu I, Nagatomo T. Identification of sites of prazosin, tamsulosin and KMD-3213 with α_1-adrenergic receptor subtypes by molecular modeling. Life Sci. 2002;71:2531–41.

Ito Y, Okada A, Yasui T, et al. Efficacy of selective $\alpha 1A$ adrenoceptor antagonist silodosin in the medical expulsive therapy for ureteral stones. Int J Urol. 2011;18:672–4.

Kawabe K, Yoshida M, Homma Y. Silodosin, and new α_{1A}-adrenoceptor-selective antagonist for treating benign prostatic hyperplasia: results of a phase III randomized, placebo-controlled, double-blind study in Japanese men. BJU Int. 2006;98:1019–24.

Kobayashi K, Masumori N, Kato R, Hisasue S, Furuya R, Tsukamoto T. Orgasm is preserved regardless of ejaculatory dysfunction with selective $\alpha 1A$-blocker administration. Int J Impot Res. 2009;21:306–10.

Marks LS, Gittelman MC, Hill LA, Volinn W, Hoel G. Silodosin in the treatment of the signs and symptoms of benign prostatic hyperplasia: a 9-month, open-label extension study. Urology. 2009;74:1318–24.

Matsubara Y, Kanazawa T, Kojima Y, et al. Pharmacokinetics and disposition of silodosin (KMD-3213). Yakugaku Zasshi. 2006;126:237–45.

Moriyama N, Akiyama K, Murata S, et al. KMD-3213, a novel α_{1A}-adrenoceptor antagonist, potentially inhibits the functional α_1-adrenoceptor in human prostate. Eur J Pharmacol. 1997;331:39–42.

Nagai A, Hara R, Yokoyama T, Jo Y, Fujii T, Miyaji Y. Ejaculatory dysfunction caused by the new $\alpha 1$-blocker silodosin: a preliminary study to analyze human ejaculation using color Doppler ultrasonography. Int J Urol. 2008;15:915–8.

Nickel JC, O'Leary MP, Lepor H, et al. Silodosin for men with chronic prostates/chronic pelvic pain syndrome: results of a phase II multicenter, double-blind, placebo controlled study. J Urol. 2011;186:125–31.

Rapaflo® capsule [package insert]. Morristown: Watson Pharma Inc; 2009.

Shibata K, Foglar R, Horie K, et al. KMD-3213, a novel, potent, α_{1a}-adrenoceptor-selective antagonist: characterization using recombinant human α_1-adrenoceptors and native tissues. Mol Pharmacol. 1995;48:250–8.

Tanaka T, Zhang Li, Suzuki F, Muramatsu I. Alpha-1 adrenoceptors: evaluation of receptor subtype-binding kinetics in intact arterial tissues and comparison of membrane binding. Br J Pharmacol. 2004;141:468–76.

Tsumura H, Satoh T, Ishiyama H, et al. Comparison of prophylactic naftopidil, tamsulosin, and silodosin for ^{125}I brachytherapy-induced lower urinary tract symptoms in patients with prostate cancer: randomized controlled trial. Int J Radiat Oncol Biol Phys. 2011;81:385–92.

Watanabe T, Ozono S, Kageyama S. A randomized crossover study comparing patient preference for tamsulosin and silodosin in patients with lower urinary tract symptoms associated with benign prostatic hypertrophy. J Int Med Res. 2011;39:129–42.

Yamada S, Ito Y, Tsukada H. α_1-Adrenoceptors and muscarinic receptors in voiding function—binding characteristics of therapeutic agents in relation to the pharmacokinetics. Br J Clin Pharmacol. 2011;72:205–17.

Yamada S, Okura T, Kimura R. In vivo demonstration of the α_{1A}-adrenoceptor subtype selectivity of KMD-3213 in rat tissues. J Pharmacol Exp Ther. 2001;296:160–7.

Yoshida M, Kudoh J, Homma Y, Kawabe K. Safety and efficacy of silodosin for the treatment of benign prostatic hyperplasia. Clin Interv Aging. 2011;6:161–72.

Yu H-J, Lin AT-L, Yang SS-D, et al. Non-inferiority of silodosin to tamsulosin in treating patients with lower urinary tract symptoms (LUTS) associated with benign prostatic hyperplasia (BPH). BJU Int. 2011;108:1843–8.

Zhou Y, Sun P-H, Liu Y-W, Zhao X, Meng L, Cui Y-M. Safety and pharmacokinetic studies of silodosin, a new α_{1A}-adrenoceptor selective antagonist, in healthy Chinese male subjects. Biol Pharm Bull. 2011;34:1240–5.

Dosage Adjustment of Medications Eliminated by the Kidneys

<u>Silodosin</u>/Rapaflo™   {Adrenergic α₁ blocker; ℞ for benign prostatic hypertrophy}

Usual initial dose: 8 mg orally

Usual maintenance dose: 8 mg orally once daily with a meal

Typical maximum dose: 8 mg/day

Proportion eliminated unchanged: 33 % (primarily as active glucuronide conjugate metabolites)

Adjustment for Kidney Disease

    FDA-approved product labeling: *CrCL 51–80 mL/min*   *8 mg orally once daily with food*

                                                 CrCL 30–50 mL/min   *4 mg orally once daily with food*

                                                 CrCL <30 mL/min   *Contraindicated*

    Alternative adjustment: *Data not available*

Dosage Adjustment of Medications Eliminated by the Kidneys

Sitagliptin - Selected References

Barzilai N, Guo H, Mahoney EM, et al. Efficacy and tolerability of sitagliptin monotherapy in elderly patients with type 2 diabetes: a randomized, double-blind, placebo-controlled trial. Curr Med Res Opin. 2011;27:1049–58.

Bergman A, Ebel D, Liu F, et al. Absolute bioavailability of sitagliptin, an oral dipeptidyl peptidase-4 inhibitor, in healthy volunteers. Biopharm Drug Dispos. 2007;28:315–22.

Bergman A, Mistry GC, Luo W-L, et al. Dose-proportionality of a final market image sitagliptin formulation, an oral dipeptidyl peptidase-4 inhibitor, in healthy volunteers. Biopharm Drug Dispos. 2007;28:307–13.

Bergman AJ, Smith W, Cote J, et al. Effect of renal insufficiency on the pharmacokinetics of sitagliptin, a dipeptidyl peptidase-4 inhibitor. Diabetes Care. 2007;30:1862–4.

Bergman AJ, Stevens C, Zhao YY, et al. Pharmacokinetic and pharmacodynamic properties of multiple oral doses of sitagliptin, a dipeptidyl peptidase-IV inhibitor: a double-blind, randomized, placebo-controlled study in healthy male volunteers. Clin Ther. 2006;28:55–72.

Chan JCN, Scott R, Ferreira JCA, et al. Safety and efficacy of sitagliptin in patients with type 2 diabetes and chronic renal insufficiency. Diabetes Obes Metab. 2008;10:545–55.

Deacon CF. Dipeptidyl peptidase-4 inhibitors in the treatment of type 2 diabetes: a comparative review. Diabetes Obes Metab. 2011;13:7–18.

Esposito K, Cozzolino D, Bellastella G, et al. Dipeptidyl peptidase-4 inhibitors and HbA1c target of <7 % in type 2 diabetes: meta-analysis of randomized controlled trials. Diabetes Obes Metab. 2011;13:594–603.

Golightly LK, Drayna CC, McDermott MT. Comparative clinical pharmacokinetics of dipeptidyl peptidase-4 inhibitors. Clin Pharmacokinet. 2012. Epub ahead of print. doi:10.2165/11632930-000000000-00000.

Hare KJ, Vilsbøll T, Asmar M, Deacon CF, Knop FK, Holst JJ. The glucagonostatic and insulinotropic effects of glucagon-like peptide 1 contribute equally to its glucose-lowering action. Diabetes. 2010;59:1765–70.

Herman GA, Bergman A, Liu F, et al. Pharmacokinetics and pharmacodynamic effects of the oral DPP-4 inhibitor sitagliptin in middle-aged obese subjects. Clin Pharmacol Ther. 2006;46:876–86.

Herman GA, Stevens C, Van Dyck K, et al. Pharmacokinetics and pharmacodynamics of sitagliptin, an inhibitor of dipeptidyl peptidase IV, in healthy subjects: results from two randomized, double-blind, placebo-controlled studies with single oral doses. Clin Pharmacol Ther. 2005;78:75–88.

Herman GA, Stevens C, Yi B, Kipnes M. Tolerability and pharmacokinetics of metformin and the dipeptidyl peptidase-4 inhibitor sitagliptin when co-administered in patients with type 2 diabetes. Curr Med Res Opin. 2006;22:1939–47.

Holst JJ, Krarup T, Knop FK, Madsbad S, Vilsbøll T. Loss of incretin effect is a specific, important, and early characteristic of type 2 diabetes. Diabetes Care. 2011;34(Suppl 2):S251–7.

Januvia® tablet [package insert]. Whitehouse Station: Merck & Co Inc; 2010.

Lerner JM, Babura R, Edwards CMB. Renal impairment with sitagliptin: is there a need for active monitoring of potential renal toxicity? Br J Hosp Med. 2011;72:412–3.

Migoya EM, Bergeron R, Miller JL, et al. Dipeptidyl peptidase-4 inhibitors administered in combination with metformin result in an additive increase in the plasma concentration of active GLP-1. Clin Pharmacol Ther. 2010;88:801–8.

Migoya EM, Stevens CH, Bergman AJ, et al. Effect of moderate hepatic insufficiency on the pharmacokinetics of sitagliptin. Can J Clin Pharmacol. 2009;16:e165–70.

Nauck MA, Meininger G, Sheng D, Terranella L, Stein PP. Efficacy and safety of the dipeptidyl peptidase-4 inhibitor, sitagliptin, compared with the sulfonylurea, glipizide, in patients with type 2 diabetes inadequately controlled on metformin alone: a randomized, double-blind, non-inferiority trial. Diabetes Obes Metab. 2007;9:194–205.

Richter B, Bandeira-Echtler E, Bergerhoff K, Lerch C. Dipeptidyl peptidase-4 (DPP-4) inhibitors for type 2 diabetes mellitus. Cochrane Database Syst Rev. 2008;(2):CD006739. doi:10.1002/14651858.CD006739.pub2.

Scheen AJ. Pharmacokinetic and pharmacodynamic evaluation of sitagliptin plus metformin. Expert Opin Drug Metab Toxicol. 2010;6:1265–76.

Seck T, Nauck M, Sheng D, et al. Safety and efficacy of treatment with sitagliptin or glipizide in patients with type 2 diabetes inadequately controlled on metformin: a 2-year study. Int J Clin Pract. 2010;64:562–76.

Vincent SH, Reed JR, Bergman AJ, et al. Metabolism and excretion of the dipeptidyl peptidase 4 inhibitor [¹⁴C]sitagliptin in humans. Drug Metab Dispos. 2007;35:533–8.

Dosage Adjustment of Medications Eliminated by the Kidneys

<u>**Sitagliptin**</u>/Januvia®   **{Antidiabetic; dipeptidyl peptidase-4 inhibitor}**

Usual initial dose: 100 mg orally

Usual maintenance dose: 100 mg orally once daily

Typical maximum dose: 100 mg/day

Proportion eliminated unchanged: 79 %

Adjustment for Kidney Disease

    FDA-approved product labeling: *CrCL ≥50 mL/min or*

                                      SCr ≤1.7 mg/dL in men or

                                        SCr ≤1.5 mg/dL in women   *100 mg orally once daily*

                                        CrCL 30–50 mL/min or

                                        SCr 1.7–3 mg/dL in men or

                                        SCr 1.5–2.5 mg/dL in women   *50 mg orally once daily*

                                        CrCL <30 mL/min or

                                        SCr >3 mg/dL in men or

                                        SCr >2.5 mg/dL in women or

                                        ESRD requiring hemodialysis   *25 mg orally once daily; may be given*
                                        or peritoneal dialysis   *without regard to time of dialysis*

        Alternative adjustment: *Data not available*

Dosage Adjustment of Medications Eliminated by the Kidneys

Sodium Citrate and Citric Acid - Selected References

Bauer E, Derfler K, Juokhadar C, Drumi W. Citrate kinetics in patients receiving long-term hemodialysis therapy. Am J Kidney Dis. 2005;46:903–7.

Cytra-2 oral solution [package insert]. Madison: Cypress Pharmaceutical Inc; 2011.

Hermite L, Quenot J-P, Nadji A, et al. Sodium citrate versus saline catheter locks for non-tunneled hemodialysis central venous catheters in critically ill adults: a randomized controlled trial. Intensive Care Med. 2011. Epub ahead of print. doi:10.1007/s00134-011-2422-y.

Kozik-Jaromin J, Nier V, Heemann U, et al. Citrate pharmacokinetics and calcium levels during high-flux dialysis with regional citrate anticoagulation. Nephrol Dial Transplant. 2009;24:2244–51.

Kramer L, Bauer E, Joukhadar C, et al. Citrate pharmacokinetics and metabolism in cirrhotic and noncirrhotic critically ill patients. Crit Care Med. 2003;31:2450–5.

Maki DG, Ash SR, Winger RK, Lavin P. A novel antimicrobial and antithrombotic lock solution for hemodialysis catheters: a multicenter, controlled, randomized trial. Crit Care Med. 2011;39:613–20.

Moran JE, Ash SR, Beathard GA, et al. Locking solutions for hemodialysis catheters: heparin and citrate—a position paper by ASDIN. Semin Dial. 2008;21:490–2.

Morgera S, Scholle C, Melzer C, et al. A simple, safe and effective citrate anticoagulation protocol for the Genius® dialysis system in acute renal failure. Nephron Clin Pract. 2004;98:c35–40. doi:10.1159/000079925.

Phisitkul S, Khanna A, Simoni J, et al. Amelioration of metabolic acidosis in patients with low GFR reduced kidney endothelin production and kidney injury, and better preserved GFR. Kidney Int. 2010;77:617–23.

Pierce DA, Rocco MV. Trisodium citrate: an alternative to unfractionated heparin for hemodialysis catheters. Pharmacotherapy. 2010;30:1150–8.

<u>**Sodium Citrate and Citric Acid**</u>/Bicitra®, Cytra-2   {Systemic alkalizer}

Usual initial dose:	10–30 mL diluted in 30–90 mL of water orally
Usual maintenance dose:	10–30 mL diluted in 30–90 mL of water orally after meals and at bedtime daily
Typical maximum dose:	120 mL/day
Proportion eliminated unchanged:	5 %

Adjustment for Kidney Disease

FDA-approved product labeling:	*Low urinary output*	*Use with caution; periodic examinations and determinations of serum electrolytes, particularly sodium bicarbonate level, should be carried out.*
	Severe renal impairment	*Contraindicated*
Alternative adjustment:	*GFR 20–59 mL/min*	*1 mL (1 mEq)/kg/day orally in three divided doses (limited data)*

Dosage Adjustment of Medications Eliminated by the Kidneys

Solifenacin - Selected References

Callegari E, Malhotra B, Bungay PJ, et al. A comprehensive non-clinical evaluation of the CNS penetration potential of antimuscarinic agents for the treatment of overactive bladder. Br J Clin Pharmacol. 2011;72:235–46.

Chapple CR, Martinez-García R, Selvaggi L, et al. A comparison of the efficacy and tolerability of solifenacin succinate and extended release tolterodine at treating overactive bladder: results of the STAR trial. Eur Urol. 2005;48:464–70.

Doroshyenko O, Fuhr U. Clinical pharmacokinetics and pharmacodynamics of solifenacin. Clin Pharmacokinet. 2009;48:281–302.

Herschorn S, Pommerville P, Stothers L, et al. Tolerability of solifenacin and oxybutynin immediate release in older (>65 years) and younger (<65 years) patients with overactive bladder: sub-analysis from a Canadian, randomized, double-blind study. Curr Med Res Opin. 2011;27:375–82.

Herschorn S, Stothers L, Carlson K, et al. Tolerability of 5 mg solifenacin once daily versus 5 mg oxybutynin immediate release 3 times daily: results of the VECTOR trial. J Urol. 2010;183:1892–8.

Herschorn S, Vicente C, Piwko C. Canadian cost-effectiveness analysis of solifenacin compared to oxybutynin immediate release in patients with overactive bladder. J Med Econ. 2010;13:588–15.

Hsaio S-M, Chang T-C, Wu W-Y, Chen C-H, Yu H-J, Lin H-H. Comparisons of urodynamic effects, therapeutic efficacy and safety of solifenacin versus tolterodine for female overactive bladder syndrome. J Obstet Gynaecol Res. 2011;37:1084–91.

Jakobsen SM, Kersten H, Molden E. Evaluation of brain anticholinergic activities of spasmolytic drugs using a high-throughput radio receptor bioassay. J Am Geriatr Soc. 2011;59:501–5.

Kaplan SA, McCammon K, Fincher R, Fakhoury A, He W. Safety and tolerability of solifenacin add-on therapy to α-blocker treated men with residual urgency and frequency. J Urol. 2009;182:2825–30.

Kessler TM, Bachmann LM, Minder C, et al. Adverse event assessment of antimuscarinics for treating overactive bladder: a network meta-analytic approach. PLoS One. 2011;6:e16718. doi:10.1371/journal.pone.0016718.

Kim DS, Kyung YS, Woo SH, Chang YS, Kim H-J. Efficacy of anticholinergics for chronic prostatitis/chronic pelvic pain syndrome in young and middle-aged patients: a single-blinded, prospective, multi-center study. Int Neurourol J. 2011;15:172–5.

Krauwinkel WJJ, Smulders RA, Mulder H, Swart PJ, Taekema-Roelvink MEJ. Effect of age on the pharmacokinetics of solifenacin in men and women. Int J Clin Pharmacol Ther. 2005;43:227–38.

Lowenstein L, Kenton K, Mueller ER, et al. Solifenacin objectively decreases urinary sensation in women with overactive bladder syndrome. Int Urol Nephrol. 2011. Epub ahead of print. doi:10.1007/s11255-011-0059-y.

Meek PD, Evang SD, Tadrous M, Roux-Lirange D, Triller DM, Gumustop B. Overactive bladder drugs and constipation: a meta-analysis of randomized, placebo-controlled trials. Dig Dis Sci. 2011;56:7–18.

Paquette A, Gou P, Tannenbaum C. Systematic review and meta-analysis: do clinical trials testing antimuscarinic agents for overactive bladder adequately measure central nervous system adverse events? J Am Geriatr Soc. 2011;59:1332–9.

Smulders RA, Smith NN, Krauwinkel WJ, Hoon TJ. Pharmacokinetics, safety, and tolerability of solifenacin in patients with renal insufficiency. J Pharmacol Sci. 2007;103:67–74.

Takao T, Tsujimura A, Yamamoto K, et al. Solifenacin may improve sleep quality in patients with overactive bladder and sleep disturbance. Urology. 2011;78:648–52.

Uchida T, Krauwinkel WJ, Mulder H, Smulders RA. Food does not affect the pharmacokinetics of solifenacin, a new muscarinic receptor antagonist: results of a randomized crossover trial. Br J Clin Pharmacol. 2004;58:4–7.

van Rey F, Heesakkrs J. Solifenacin in multiple sclerosis patients with overactive bladder: a prospective study. Adv Urol. 2011;2011:834753. doi:10.1155/2011/834753.

Vesicare® tablet [package insert]. Research Triangle Park: Astellas Pharma US Inc and GlaxoSmithKline; 2011.

Yamaguchi O, Kakizaki H, Homma Y, et al. Solifenacin as add-on therapy for overactive bladder symptoms in men treated for lower urinary tract symptoms—ASSIST, randomized controlled study. Urology. 2011;78:126–33.

Yokoyama O, Yamaguchi O, Kakizaki H, et al. Efficacy of solifenacin on nocturia in Japanese patients with overactive bladder: impact on sleep evaluated by bladder diary. J Urol. 2011;186:170–4.

Zaitsu M, Mikami K, Ishida N, Takeuchi T. Comparative evaluation of the safety and efficacy of long-term use of imidafenacin and solifenacin in patients with overactive bladder: a prospective, open, randomized parallel-group trial (the LIST study). Adv Urol. 2011;2011:854697. doi:10.1155/2011/854697.

Dosage Adjustment of Medications Eliminated by the Kidneys

<u>Solifenacin</u>/Vesicare® {**Anticholinergic agent; ℞ for overactive bladder or urge incontinence**}

Usual initial dose:	5 mg orally
Usual maintenance dose:	5–10 mg orally once daily
Typical maximum dose:	10 mg/day
Proportion eliminated unchanged:	15 %

Adjustment for Kidney Disease

FDA-approved product labeling:	*CrCL ≥30 mL/min*	*5–10 mg orally once daily*
	CrCL <30 mL/min	*5 mg orally once daily*
Alternative adjustment:	*Data not available*	

Dosage Adjustment of Medications Eliminated by the Kidneys

Sorafenib - Selected References

Akaza H, Tsukamoto T, Murai M, Nakajima K, Naito S. Phase II study to investigate the efficacy, safety, and pharmacokinetics of sorafenib in Japanese patients with advanced renal cell carcinoma. Jpn J Clin Oncol. 2007;37:755–62.

Awada A, Gil T, Whenham N, et al. Safety and pharmacokinetics of sorafenib combined with capecitabine in patients with advanced solid tumors: results of a phase I trial. J Clin Pharmacol. 2011. Epub ahead of print. doi:10.1177/0091270010386226.

Awada A, Hendlisz A, Gil T, et al. Phase I safety and pharmacokinetics of BAY 43–9006 administered for 21 days on/7 days off in patients with advanced, refractory solid tumors. Br J Cancer. 2005;92:1855–61.

Clark JW, Eder JP, Ryan D, Lathia C, Lenz H-J. Safety and pharmacokinetics of the dual action Raf kinase and vascular endothelial growth factor receptor inhibitor, BAY 43–9006, in patients with advanced, refractory solid tumors. Clin Cancer Res. 2005;11:5472–80.

Crump M, Hedley D, Kamel-Reid S, et al. A randomized phase I clinical and biologic study of two schedules of sorafenib in patients with myelodysplastic syndrome or acute myeloid leukemia: a NCIC (National Cancer Institute of Canada) clinical trials group study. Leuk Lymphoma. 2010;51:252–60.

Dahut WL, Scripture C, Posadas E, et al. A phase II clinical trial of sorafenib in androgen-independent prostate cancer. Clin Cancer Res. 2008;14:209–14.

Hilger RA, Richly H, Grubert M, et al. Pharmacokinetics of sorafenib in patients with renal impairment undergoing hemodialysis. Int J Clin Pharmacol Ther. 2009;47:61–4.

Hornecker M, Blanchet B, Billemont B, et al. Saturable absorption of sorafenib in patients with solid tumors: a population model. Invest New Drugs. 2011. Epub ahead of print. doi:10.1007/s10637-011-9760-z.

Hoshino-Yoshino A, Kato M, Nakano K, Ishigai M, Kudo T, Ito K. Bridging from preclinical to clinical studies for tyrosine kinase inhibitors based on pharmacokinetics/pharmacodynamics and toxicokinetics/toxicodynamics. Drug Metab Pharmacokinet. 2011. Epub ahead of print. doi:10.2133/dmpk.DMPK-11-RG-043.

Jain L, Woo S, Gardner ER, et al. Population pharmacokinetic analysis of sorafenib in patients with solid tumors. Br J Clin Pharmacol. 2011;72:294–305.

Kennoki T, Kondo T, Kimata N, et al. Clinical results and pharmacokinetics of sorafenib in chronic hemodialysis patients with metastatic renal cell carcinoma. Jpn J Clin Oncol. 2011;41:647–55.

Khan G, Golshayan A, Elson P, et al. Sunitinib and sorafenib in metastatic renal cell carcinoma patients with renal insufficiency. Ann Oncol. 2010;21:1618–22.

Miller AA, Murry DJ, Owzar K, et al. Phase I and pharmacokinetic study of sorafenib in patients with hepatic or renal dysfunction: CALGB 60301. J Clin Oncol. 2009;27:1800–5.

Minami H, Kawad K, Ebi H, et al. Phase I and pharmacokinetic study of sorafenib, an oral multikinase inhibitor, in Japanese patients with advanced refractory solid tumors. Cancer Sci. 2008;99:1492–8.

Moore M, Hirte HW, Siu L, et al. Phase I study to determine the safety and pharmacokinetics of the novel Raf kinase and VEGFR inhibitor BAY 43–9006, administered for 28 days on/7 days off in patients with advanced, refractory solid tumors. Ann Oncol. 2005;16:1688–94.

Nexavar® tablet film coated [package insert]. Wayne: Bayer HealthCare Pharmaceuticals Inc; 2011.

Okamoto I, Miyazaki M, Morinaga R, et al. Phase I clinical and pharmacokinetic study of sorafenib in combination with carboplatin and paclitaxel in patients with advanced non-small cell lung cancer. Invest New Drugs. 2010;28:844–53.

Poller B, Wagenaar E, Tang SC, Schinkel AH. Double-transduced MDCKII cells to study human P-glycoprotein (ABCB1) and breast cancer resistance protein (ABCG2) interplay in drug transport across the blood–brain barrier. Mol Pharmacol. 2011;8:571–82.

Pratz KW, Cho E, Levis MJ, et al. A pharmacodynamic study of sorafenib in patients with relapsed and refractory acute leukemias. Leukemia. 2010;24:1437–44.

Shinsako K, Mizuno T, Terada T, et al. Tolerable sorafenib therapy for a renal cell carcinoma patient with hemodialysis: a case study. Int J Clin Oncol. 2010;15:512–4.

Strumberg D, Clark JW, Awada A, et al. Safety, pharmacokinetics, and preliminary antitumor activity of sorafenib: a review of four phase I trials in patients with advanced refractory solid tumors. Oncologist. 2007;12:426–37.

van Erp NP, Gelderblom H, Guchelaar H-J. Clinical pharmacokinetics of tyrosine kinase inhibitors. Cancer Treat Rev. 2009;35:692–706.

Dosage Adjustment of Medications Eliminated by the Kidneys

<u>**Sorafenib**</u>/Nexavar®   {Antineoplastic; tyrosine kinase and vascular endothelial growth factor (VEGF) inhibitor}

Usual initial dose:	400 mg orally
Usual maintenance dose:	400 mg orally twice daily without food
Typical maximum dose:	800 mg/day
Proportion eliminated unchanged:	19 % (as active and inactive metabolites)

Adjustment for Kidney Disease

FDA-approved product labeling: *No dosage adjustment is necessary in patients with mild, moderate, or severe renal impairment not undergoing dialysis.*

Alternative adjustment:

eCrCL ≥60 mL/min	*400 mg orally twice daily without food*
eCrCL 40–59 mL/min	*400 mg orally twice daily without food*
eCrCL 20–39 mL/min	*200 mg orally twice daily without food*
eCrCL <20 mL/min	*Insufficient data; dose not defined*
Hemodialysis	*200 orally once or twice daily (Note: At least one patient has been reported to tolerate extended treatment with 400 mg orally twice daily with no clinical, biochemical, or hematological evidence of toxicity.)*

Note: Neurological, hematological, cardiovascular, or other considerations may suggest further dosage adjustments.

Dosage Adjustment of Medications Eliminated by the Kidneys

Sotalol - Selected References

Advani SV, Singh BN. Pharmacodynamic, pharmacokinetic and antiarrhythmic properties of *d*-sotalol, the dextro-isomer of sotalol. Drugs. 1995;49:664–79.

Anttila M, Arstila M, Pfeffer M, Tikkanen R, Fallinkoski V, Sundquist H. Human pharmacokinetics of sotalol. Acta Pharmacol Toxicol. 1976;39:118–28.

Aronoff GA, Bennett WM, Berns JS, et al. Drug prescribing in renal failure: dosing guidelines for adults and children. 5th ed. Philadelphia: American College of Physicians; 2007.

Barbey JT, Sale ME, Woosley RL, Shi J, Melikian AP, Hinderling PH. Pharmacokinetic, pharmacodynamic, and safety evaluation of an accelerated dose titration regimen of sotalol in healthy middle-aged subjects. Clin Pharmacol Ther. 1999;66:91–9.

Berglund G, Descamps R, Thomis JA. Pharmacokinetics of sotalol after chronic administration to patients with renal insufficiency. Eur J Clin Pharmacol. 1980;18:321–6.

Betapace AF® [package insert]. Wayne: Bayer HealthCare Pharmaceuticals Inc; 2010.

Blair AD, Burgess ED, Maxwell BM, Cutler RE. Sotalol kinetics in renal insufficiency. Clin Pharmacol Ther. 1981;29:457–63.

Brown HC, Carruthers SG, Kelly JG, McDevitt DG, Shanks RG. Observations on the efficacy and pharmacokinetics of sotalol after oral administration. Eur J Clin Pharmacol. 1976;9:367–72.

Dumas M, d'Athis P, Besancenot JF, et al. Variations of sotalol kinetics in renal insufficiency. Int J Clin Pharmacol Ther Toxicol. 1989;27:486–9.

Fiset C, Philippon F, Gilbert M, Turgeon J. Stereoselective disposition of (±)-sotalol at steady-state conditions. Br J Clin Pharmacol. 1993;36:75–7.

Funck-Brentano C. Pharmacokinetic and pharmacodynamic profiles of d-sotalol and d,l-sotalol. Eur Heart J. 1993;14(Suppl H):30–5.

Huynh-Do U, Wahl C, Sulzer M, Bühler H, Keusch G. Torsade de pointes during low-dosage sotalol therapy in haemodialysis patients. Nephrol Dial Transplant. 1996;11:1153–4.

Ishizaki T, Hirayama H, Tawara K, Nakaya H, Sato M, Sato K. Pharmacokinetics and pharmacodynamics in young normal and elderly hypertensive subjects: a study using sotalol as a model drug. J Pharmacol Exp Ther. 1990;212:173–81.

Mulder VX, Oudemans-van Stratten MH, Zandstra DF, Franssen EJF. Massive ingestion of cardiac drugs: toxicokinetic aspects of digoxin and sotalol during hemofiltration. Clin Toxicol (Phila). 2010;48:218–21.

Patrick GM, Pollock CA, Ibels LS, Caterson RJ. Sotalol and end-stage renal failure [letter]. Aust NZ J Med. 1994;24:31–2.

Pratt CM, Camm AJ, Cooper W, et al. Mortality in the Survival with ORal D-Sotalol (SWORD) trial: why did patients die? Am J Cardiol. 1998;81:869–76.

Rizza C, Valderrabano M, Singh BN. Recurrent torsades de pointes after sotalol therapy for symptomatic paroxysmal atrial fibrillation in a patient with end-stage renal disease. J Cardiovasc Pharmacol Ther. 1999;4:129–34.

Schnelle K, Klein G, Schinz A. Studies on the pharmacokinetics and pharmacodynamics of the beta-adrenergic blocking agent sotalol in normal man. J Clin Pharmacol. 1979;19:516–22.

Singh BN, Deedwania P, Nademanee K, Ward A, Sorkin EM. Sotalol: a review of its pharmacodynamic and pharmacokinetic properties, and therapeutic use. Drugs. 1987;34:311–49.

Singh SN, Lazin A, Cohen A, Johnson M, Fletcher RD. Sotalol-induced torsades de pointes successfully treated with hemodialysis after failure of conventional therapy. Am Heart J. 1991;121:601–2.

Somberg JC, Preston RA, Ranade V, Molnar J. Developing a safe intravenous sotalol dosing regimen. Am J Ther. 2010.17:365–72.

Sotalol hydrochloride injection for intravenous use [package insert]. Lake Bluff: Academic Pharmaceutical Inc; 2009.

Sundquist HK, Anttila M, Forsström J, Kasanen A. Serum levels and half-life of sotalol in chronic renal failure. Ann Clin Res. 1975;7:442–6.

Tjandramaga TB, Verbeeck JTR, Verbesselt R, Verberckmoes R, de Schepper PJ. The effect of end-stage renal failure and haemodialysis on the elimination kinetics of sotalol. Br J Clin Pharmacol. 1976;3:259–65.

van den Uum SHM, van den Merkhof LFM, Lucassen AMJ, Wuis EW, Diemont W. Successful haemodialysis in sotalol-induced torsade de pointes in a patient with progressive renal failure. Nephrol Dial Transplant. 1997;12:331–3.

Dosage Adjustment of Medications Eliminated by the Kidneys

Sotalol/Betapace®, Betapace AF®, Sorine®   {Antiarrhythmic, class II/III}

Usual initial dose:	80 mg orally twice daily or 75 mg IV over 5 h
Usual maintenance dose:	120–160 mg orally twice daily or 75 mg IV over 5 h every 12 h
Typical maximum dose:	640 mg/day orally or 150 mg/day IV
Proportion eliminated unchanged:	90 %

Adjustment for Kidney Disease

FDA-approved product labeling:

Sotalol dosing for (a) ventricular arrhythmias in renal function impairment and (b) atrial fibrillation in renal function impairment

CrCL (mL/min)	Dosage
(a)	
>60	*80 mg orally or 75 mg IV over 5 h every 12 h*
30–59	*80 mg orally or 75 mg IV over 5 h every 24 h*
10–29	*80 mg orally every 36–48 h (IV use not recommended)*
<10	*Oral dose should be individualized (IV use not recommended)*
(b)	
>60	*80 mg orally or 75 mg IV over 5 h every 12 h*
40–60	*80 mg orally or 75 mg IV over 5 h every 24 h*
<40	*Contraindicated*

Alternative adjustment:

GFR >50 mL/min	*80–160 mg orally every 12 h*
GFR 10–50 mL/min	*80–160 mg orally every 24–48 h*
GFR <10 mL/min	*80–160 mg orally every 48–72 h*
Hemodialysis	*80–160 mg orally every 48–72 h; administer after hemodialysis on dialysis days.*
CAPD	*80–160 mg orally every 48–72 h*
CRRT	*80–160 mg orally every 24–48 h; titrate.*

Note: Electrocardiographic considerations such as QT interval prolongation may suggest further dosage adjustments.

Dosage Adjustment of Medications Eliminated by the Kidneys

Spironolactone - Selected References

Aldactone® tablet film coated [package insert]. New York: GD Searle LLC Division of Pfizer Inc; 2008.

Aronoff GA, Bennett WM, Berns JS, et al. Drug prescribing in renal failure: dosing guidelines for adults and children. 5th ed. Philadelphia: American College of Physicians; 2007.

Butler JV, McAvoy H, McEnroy D, Mulkerrin EC. Spironolactone therapy for older patients—the impact of renal dysfunction. Arch Gerontol Geriatr. 2002;35:45–9.

Chua D, Lo A, Lo C. Spironolactone use in heart failure patients with end-stage renal disease on hemodialysis: is it safe? Clin Cardiol. 2010;33:604–8.

Edwards NC, Ferro C, Kirkwood H, et al. Effect of spironolactone on left ventricular systolic and diastolic function in patients with early stage chronic kidney disease. Am J Cardiol. 2010;106:1505–11.

Edwards NC, Steeds RP, Chue CD, Stewart P, Ferro C, Townend J. The safety and efficacy of spironolactone in patients with mild-moderate kidney disease. Br J Clin Pharmacol. 2012;73:447–54.

Feinfeld DA, Carvounis CP. Fatal hyperkalemia and hyperchloremic acidosis: association with spironolactone in the absence of renal impairment. JAMA. 1978;240:1516.

Goland S, Naugolny V, Korbut Z, Rozen I, Caspi A, Malnick S. Appropriateness and complications of the use of spironolactone in patients at a heart failure clinic. Eur J Intern Med. 2011;22:424–7.

Guney I, Selcuk NY, Altintepe L, Atalay H, Başarali MK, Büyükbaş S. Antifibrotic effects of aldosterone receptor blocker (spironolactone) in patients with chronic kidney disease. Ren Fail. 2009;31:779–84.

Hammer F, Edwards NC, Hughes BA, et al. The effect of spironolactone upon corticosteroid hormone metabolism in patients with early stage chronic kidney disease. Clin Endocrinol (Oxf). 2010;73:566–72.

Hanlon JT, Aspinall SL, Semla TP, et al. Consensus guidelines for oral dosing of primarily renally cleared medications in older adults. J Am Geriatr Soc. 2009;57:335–40.

Herman E, Rado J. Fatal hyperkalemic paralysis associated with spironolactone: observation on a patient with severe renal disease and refractory edema. Arch Neurol. 1966;15:74–7.

Manning RT, Behrle FC. Use of spironolactone in renal edema: effectiveness and association with hyperkalemia. JAMA. 1961;176:769–71.

McInnes GT, Perkins RM, Shelton JR, Harrison IR. Dose–response relationships for spironolactone at steady state. Clin Pharmacol Ther. 1981;29:679–86.

McInnes GT, Shelton JR, Harrison IR. Steady-state relative potency of aldosterone antagonists: spironolactone and prorenoate. Clin Pharmacol Ther. 1982;31:317–23.

Mehdi UF, Adams-Huet B, Raskin P, Vega GL, Toto RD. Addition of angiotensin receptor blockade or mineralocorticoid antagonism to maximal angiotensin-converting enzyme inhibition in diabetic nephropathy. J Am Soc Nephrol. 2009;20:2641–50.

Monte EG, Polanco AAN, Toribio MJ, et al. Addition of spironolactone to dual blockade of renin angiotensin system dramatically reduces severe proteinuria in renal transplant patients: an uncontrolled pilot study at 6 months. Transplant Proc. 2010;42:2899–901.

Neale TJ, Lynn KL, Bailey RR. Spironolactone-associated aggravation of renal function impairment. N Z Med J. 1976;83:147–9.

Raebel MA, Ross C, Xu S, et al. Diabetes and drug-associated hyperkalemia: effect of potassium monitoring. J Gen Intern Med. 2010;25:326–33.

Schrier RW, Masoumi A, Elhassan E. Aldosterone: role in edematous disorders, hypertension, chronic renal failure, and metabolic syndrome. Clin J Am Soc Nephrol. 2010;5:1132–40.

Sengul E, Sahin T, Sevin E, Yilmaz A. Effect of spironolactone on urinary protein excretion in patients with chronic kidney disease. Ren Fail. 2009;31:928–32.

Tamirisa KP, Aaronson KD, Koelling TM. Spironolactone-induced renal insufficiency and hyperkalemia in patients with heart failure. Am Heart J. 2004;148:971–8.

Vukusich A, Kunstmann S, Varela C, et al. A randomized, double-blind, placebo-controlled trial of spironolactone on carotid intima-media thickness in nondiabetic hemodialysis patients. Clin J Am Soc Nephrol. 2010;5:1380–7.

Wei L, Struthers AD, Fahey T, Watson AD, MacDonald TM. Spironolactone use and renal toxicity: population based longitudinal analysis. BMJ. 2010;340:c1768. doi:10.1136/bmj.c1768.

Dosage Adjustment of Medications Eliminated by the Kidneys

Spironolactone/Aldactone®	{Diuretic; aldosterone antagonist}
Usual initial dose:	25 mg orally
Usual maintenance dose:	12.5–200 mg orally once daily
Typical maximum dose:	400 mg/day
Proportion eliminated unchanged:	30 %

Adjustment for Kidney Disease

FDA-approved product labeling:	*Anuria, acute renal insufficiency, significant impairment of renal excretory function*	*Contraindicated*
Alternative adjustment:	*GFR >50 mL/min*	*25–100 mg orally every 12–24 h*
	GFR 30–50 mL/min	*12.5–25 mg orally every 12–24 h*
	GFR <30 mL/min	*Preferably avoid due to risk for hyperkalemia.*
	Hemodialysis	*Preferably avoid due to risk for hyperkalemia.*
	CAPD	*Preferably avoid due to risk for hyperkalemia.*
	CRRT	*Preferably avoid due to risk for hyperkalemia.*

Note: Preliminary studies in patients with chronic kidney disease and other comorbidities suggest that spironolactone may be associated with certain cardio- and reno-protective effects; additional clinical trial experience is necessary before spironolactone may be considered generally safe for use in these patients.

Note also: In patients with heart failure, dosage usually should be limited to 25 mg orally once daily due to risks for serious electrolyte disorders with higher dosages.

Dosage Adjustment of Medications Eliminated by the Kidneys

Stavudine - Selected References

Aronoff GA, Bennett WM, Berns JS, et al. Drug prescribing in renal failure: dosing guidelines for adults and children. 5th ed. Philadelphia: American College of Physicians; 2007.

Brady KA, Boston RC, Aldrich JL, MacGregor RR. Stavudine entry into cerebrospinal fluid after single and multiple doses in patients infected with human immunodeficiency virus. Pharmacotherapy. 2005;25:10–7.

Cretton EM, Zhou Z, Kidd LB, et al. In vitro and in vivo disposition and metabolism of 3'-deoxy-2',3'-didehydrothymidine. Antimicrob Agents Chemother. 1993;37:1816–25.

Dudley MN, Graham KK, Kaul S, et al. Pharmacokinetics of stavudine in patients with AIDS or AIDS-related complex. J Infect Dis. 1992;166:480–5.

Gallant JE, Staszewski S, Pozniak AL, et al. Efficacy and safety of tenofovir DF vs stavudine in combination therapy in antiretroviral-naive patients: a 3-year randomized trial. JAMA. 2004;292:191–201.

Grasela DM, Stoltz RR, Barry M, et al. Pharmacokinetics of single-dose oral stavudine in subjects with renal impairment and in subjects requiring hemodialysis. Antimicrob Agents Chemother. 2000;44:2149–53.

Gupta SK, Eustace JA, Winston JA, et al. Guidelines for the management of chronic kidney disease in HIV-infected patients: recommendations of the HIV Medicine Section of the Infectious Diseases Society of America. Clin Infect Dis. 2005;40:1559–85.

Horton CM, Dudley MN, Kaul S, et al. Population pharmacokinetics of stavudine (d4T) in patients with AIDS or advanced AIDS-related complex. Antimicrob Agents Chemother. 1995;39:23049–15.

Hurst M, Noble S. Stavudine: an update of its use in the treatment of HIV infection. Drugs. 1999;58:919–49.

Kaul S, Christofalo B, Raymond RH, Steward MB, Macleod CM. Effect of food on the bioavailability of stavudine n subjects with human immunodeficiency virus infection. Antimicrob Agents Chemother. 1998;42:2295–8.

Lea AP, Faulds D. Stavudine: a review of its pharmacodynamic and pharmacokinetic properties and clinical potential in HIV infection. Drugs. 1996;51:846–64.

Mokrzycki MH, Harris C, May H, Lau J, Palmisano J. Lactic acidosis associated with stavudine administration: a report of five cases. Clin Infect Dis. 2000;30:198–200.

Moyle G. Toxicity of antiretroviral nucleoside and nucleotide analogues: is mitochondrial toxicity the only mechanism? Drug Saf. 2000;23:467–81.

Nelson M, Azwa A, Sokwala A, Harania RS, Stebbing J. Fanconi syndrome and lactic acidosis associated with stavudine and lamivudine therapy. AIDS. 2008;22:1374–6.

Panhard X, Legrand M, Taburet A-M, Diquet B, Goujard C, Mentré F, COPHAR 1 ANRS 102 Study Group. Population pharmacokinetic analysis of lamivudine, stavudine and zidovudine in controlled HIV-infected patients on HAART. Eur J Clin Pharmacol. 2007;63:1019–29.

Rana KZ, Dudley MN. Clinical pharmacokinetics of stavudine. Clin Pharmacokinet. 1997;33:276–84.

Schaad HJ, Petty BG, Grasela DM, Christofalo B, Raymond R, Stewart M. Pharmacokinetics and safety of stavudine (d4T) in patients with severe hepatic impairment. Antimicrob Agents Chemother. 1997;41:2793–6.

Seifert RD, Steward MB, Sramek JJ, Conrad J, Kaul S, Cutler NR. Pharmacokinetics of co-administered didanosine and stavudine in HIV-seropositive male patients. Br J Clin Pharmacol. 1994;38:405–10.

Taburet A-M, Gerard L, Legrand M, Guy A, Verthelot J-M. Antiretroviral drug removal by haemodialysis [letter]. AIDS. 2000;14:902–3.

Tortolani DR, Russell JW, Whiterock VJ, et al. Prodrugs of 2',3'-didehydro-3'-deoxythymidine (d4T): synthesis, antiviral activity, and rapid pharmacokinetic evaluation. J Pharm Sci. 1994;83:339–43.

Tourret J, Tostivint I, Tézenas Du Montcel S, et al. Antiretroviral drug dosing errors in HIV-infected patients undergoing hemodialysis. Clin Infect Dis. 2007;4:775–84.

Zerit® capsule and powder for solution [package insert]. Princeton: Bristol-Myers Squibb Company; 2010.

Dosage Adjustment of Medications Eliminated by the Kidneys

Stavudine (d4T)/Zerit®   {Nucleoside reverse transcriptase inhibitor antiretroviral}

Usual initial dose: 15 mg orally (body weight <60 kg); 20 mg (weight ≥60 kg)

Usual maintenance dose: 30 mg orally twice daily (weight <60 kg); 40 mg orally twice daily (weight ≥60 kg)

Typical maximum dose: 80 mg/day

Proportion eliminated unchanged: 70 %

Adjustment for Kidney Disease

FDA-approved product labeling: *Stavudine dosage adjustment for renal impairment*

CrCL (mL/min)	Recommended dose	
	Patient weight ≥60 kg	*Patient weight <60 kg*
>50	*40 mg every 12 h*	*30 mg every 12 h*
26–50	*20 mg every 12 h*	*15 mg every 12 h*
10–25	*20 mg every 24 h*	*15 mg every 24 h*

Hemodialysis: 15 mg orally every 24 h (weight <60 kg); 20 mg orally every 24 h (weight ≥60 kg); dose after hemodialysis on dialysis days

Alternative adjustment:

GFR >50 mL/min	*30 mg orally every 12 h (if <60 kg); 40 mg every 12 h (if ≥60 kg)*
GFR 21–50 mL/min	*15 mg orally every 12–24 h (if <60 kg); 20 mg every 12–24 h (if ≥60 kg)*
GFR 10–20 mL/min	*15 mg orally every 24 h (if <60 kg); 20 mg every 24 h (if ≥60 kg)*
Hemodialysis	*15 mg orally every 24 h (if <60 kg); 20 mg every 24 h (if ≥60 kg); administer after hemodialysis on dialysis days.*
CAPD	*Data not available*
CRRT	*30 mg orally every 12 h (if <60 kg); 40 mg every 12 h (if ≥60 kg)*

Dosage Adjustment of Medications Eliminated by the Kidneys

Streptomycin - Selected References

Akaho E, Maekawa T, Uchinashi M, Kanamori R. A study of streptomycin blood level information of patients undergoing hemodialysis. Biopharm Drug Dispos. 2002;23:47–52.

Aronoff GA, Bennett WM, Berns JS, et al. Drug prescribing in renal failure: dosing guidelines for adults and children. 5th ed. Philadelphia: American College of Physicians; 2007.

Beaney GPE. Otolaryngeal problems arising during the management of severe renal failure. J Laryngol Otol. 1964;78:507–15.

Beck PR, Thomson RB, Chaudhuri AKR. Aminoglycoside antibiotics and renal function: changes in urinary γ-glutamyl-transferase excretion. J Clin Pathol. 1977;30:432–7.

Dick JC, Stevenson JS. Streptomycin serum levels in the treatment of renal tuberculosis. Br J Urol. 1952;24:179–87.

Edwards KDG, Whyte HM. Streptomycin poisoning in renal failure: an indication for treatment with an artificial kidney. Br Med J. 1959;1:752–4.

Ellard GA. Chemotherapy of tuberculosis for patients with renal impairment [editorial]. Nephron. 1993;64:169–81.

Erlanson P, Lundgren A. Ototoxic side effects following treatment with streptomycin, dihydrostreptomycin, and kanamycin: connection with dosage and renal function; preventive measures. Acta Med Scand. 1964;176:147–63.

Forgit EJ, Menzies D. Adverse reactions to first-line antituberculosis drugs. Expert Opin Drug Saf. 2006;5:231–49.

Fujita K, Fujita HM. Comparative study on renal accumulation of aminoglycoside antibiotics. Int J Clin Pharmacol Ther Toxicol. 1985;23:47–51.

Hettig RA, Adcock JD. Studies on the toxicity of streptomycin for man: a preliminary report. Science. 1946;103:355–7.

Holdiness MR. Clinical pharmacokinetics of the antituberculosis drugs. Clin Pharmacokinet. 1984;9:511–44.

Kucers A, Bennett NMcK, Kemp RJ. The use of antibiotics: a comprehensive review with clinical emphasis. 4th ed. Philadelphia: JB Lippincott Co; 1987. p. 585–600.

Kunin CM, Finland M. Persistence of antibiotics in blood of patients with acute renal failure. III. Penicillin, streptomycin, erythromycin and kanamycin. J Clin Invest. 1959;38:1509–19.

Lattimer JK, Wechsler H, Spirito AL. Treatment of renal tuberculosis with triple-drug therapy: use of a combination of streptomycin, isoniazid, and sodium aminosalicylic acid. JAMA. 1956;160:544–6.

Lindholm DD. Antibiotic persistence during renal failure and hemodialysis. Am Heart J. 1967;73:841–2.

Luft FC, Bloch R, Sloan RS, Yum MN, Costello R, Maxwell DR. Comparative nephrotoxicity of aminoglycoside antibiotics in rats. J Infect Dis. 1978;138:541–5.

Letona JM-L, Barbolla L, Frieyro E, Bouza E, Gilsanz F, Fernández MN. Immune haemolytic anaemia and renal failure induced by streptomycin. Br J Haematol. 1977;35:561–71.

Ockerblad NF, Weltmer RP. Renal tuberculosis with special reference to cases of long standing and those treated with streptomycin. J Urol. 1948;59:674–81.

Papadimitriou M, Memmos D, Metaxas P. Tuberculosis in patients on regular haemodialysis. Nephron. 1979;24:53–7.

Peloquin CA. Mycobacterium avium complex infection: pharmacokinetic and pharmacodynamic considerations that may improve clinical outcomes. Clin Pharmacokinet. 1997;32:132–44.

Peloquin CA, Benning SE. Intravenous streptomycin [letter]. Ann Pharmacother. 1993;27:1546–7.

Prasad JS, Krishnaswamy K. Streptomycin pharmacokinetics in malnutrition. Chemotherapy. 1978;24:333–7.

Sirotta HH, Jones DH. The effect of streptomycin on the cochlear and vestibular mechanism in patients treated primarily for renal tuberculosis. Laryngoscope. 1948;58:1287–93.

Streptomycin sulfate injection [package insert]. New York: Roerig Division of Pfizer Inc; 2006.

Sturdy A, Goodman A, José RJ, et al. Multidrug-resistant tuberculosis (MDR-TB) treatment in the UK: a study of injectable use and toxicity in practice. J Antimicrob Chemother. 2011;66:1815–20.

Thomson AH, Coote J, MacPherson L, Gordon J. Bayesian estimation of streptomycin pharmacokinetics. Ther Drug Monit. 1992;14:522–4.

Walker RJ, Lazaro VA, Duggin GG, Horvath JS, Tiller DJ. Synergistic toxicity of cyclosporin A and streptomycin in renal epithelial cell cultures. Res Commun Chem Pathol Pharmacol. 1988;62:447–60.

Zhu M, Burman WJ, Jaresko GS, Berning SE, Jelliffe RW, Peloquin CA. Population pharmacokinetics of intravenous and intramuscular streptomycin in patients with tuberculosis. Pharmacotherapy. 2001;21:1037–45.

Dosage Adjustment of Medications Eliminated by the Kidneys

<u>Streptomycin</u>	{Antibacterial; aminoglycoside}
Usual initial dose:	15 mg/kg (max 1,000 mg) IM
Usual maintenance dose:	15 mg/kg (max 1,000 mg) IM once daily or 25–30 mg/kg (max 1,500 mg) IM twice weekly
Typical maximum dose:	1,500 mg/day
Proportion eliminated unchanged:	90 %

Adjustment for Kidney Disease

<table>
<tr><td>FDA-approved product labeling:</td><td colspan="2">Extreme caution must be exercised in selecting a dosage regimen in the presence of preexisting renal insufficiency. In patients >60 years of age, the drug should be used at a reduced dosage due to increased risk of toxicity.</td></tr>
<tr><td>Alternative adjustment:</td><td>GFR >50 mL/min</td><td>15 mg/kg (max 1,000 mg) IM or IV over 30 min every 24 h; after definite clinical improvement is noted—often within 2 weeks—dosage should be reduced to 750–1,000 mg IM given 2–3 times weekly, and if mycobacterial sputum smears are negative, streptomycin usually may be dropped from combination antimycobacterial treatment regimens.</td></tr>
<tr><td></td><td>GFR 10–50 mL/min</td><td>15 mg/kg (max 1,000 mg) IM or IV over 30 min every 24–72 h</td></tr>
<tr><td></td><td>GFR <10 mL/min</td><td>15 mg/kg (max 1,000 mg) IM or IV over 30 min every 72–96 h</td></tr>
<tr><td></td><td>Hemodialysis</td><td>1,000 mg IM or IV over 30 min every 72–96 h; administer 500–1,000 mg IM after hemodialysis on dialysis days.</td></tr>
<tr><td></td><td>CAPD</td><td>Add to dialysate qs 20–40 mg/L</td></tr>
<tr><td></td><td>CRRT</td><td>15 mg/kg (max 1,000 mg) IM or IV over 30 min every 24–72 h; monitor levels.</td></tr>
</table>

Note: Renal function should be monitored carefully; patients with renal impairment and/or nitrogen retention should receive reduced dosages.

The peak serum concentration in individuals with kidney disease should not exceed 20–25 mg/L, and trough concentrations generally should be ≤4 mg/L. Usual maximum total dose over a course of therapy is 120 g, unless no other therapeutic options exist.

Dosage Adjustment of Medications Eliminated by the Kidneys

Sulfadoxine and Pyrimethamine - Selected References

Barnes KI, Little F, Mabuza A, et al. Increased gametocytemia after treatment: an early parasitological indicator of emerging sulfadoxine-pyrimethamine resistance in falciparum malaria. J Infect Dis. 2008;197:1605–13.

Barnes KI, Little F, Smith PJ, Evans A, Watkins WM, White NJ. Sulfadoxine-pyrimethamine pharmacokinetics in malaria: pediatric dosing implications. Clin Pharmacol Ther. 2006;80:582–96.

Bustos DG, Lazaro JE, Gay F, et al. Pharmacokinetics of sequential and simultaneous treatment with the combination chloroquine and sulfadoxine-pyrimethamine in acute uncomplicated *Plasmodium falciparum* malaria in the Philippines. Trop Med Int Health. 2002;7:584–91.

Dzinjalamala FK, Macheso A, Kublin JG, et al. Association between the pharmacokinetics and in vivo therapeutic efficacy of sulfadoxine-pyrimethamine in Malawian children. Antimicrob Agents Chemother. 2005;49:3601–6.

Edstein MD. Pharmacokinetics of sulfadoxine and pyrimethamine after Fansidar® administration in man. Chemotherapy. 1987;33:229–33.

Edwards G, Winstanley PA, Ward SA. Clinical pharmacokinetics in the treatment of tropical diseases: some applications and limitations. Clin Pharmacokinet. 1994;27:150–65.

Fansidar® tablet [package insert]. Nutley: Roche Laboratories Inc; 2004.

Gatton ML, Martin LB, Cheng Q. Evolution of resistance to sulfadoxine-pyrimethamine in *Plasmodium falciparum*. Antimicrob Agents Chemother. 2004;48:2116–23.

Green MD, van Eijk AM, van ter Kuile FO, et al. Pharmacokinetics of sulfadoxine-pyrimethamine in HIV-infected and uninfected pregnant women in western Kenya. J Infect Dis. 2007;196:1403–8.

Hellgren U, Kihamia CM, Bergqvist Y, Lebbad M, Premji Z, Rombo L. Standard and reduced doses of sulfadoxine-pyrimethamine for treatment of Plasmodium falciparum malaria in Tanzania, with determination of drug concentrations and susceptibility in vitro. Trans R Soc Trop Med Hyg. 1990;84:469–73.

Kaplan JE, Benson C, Holmes KK, Brooks JT, Pau A, Masur H. Guidelines for prevention and treatment of opportunistic infections in HIV-infected adults and adolescents: recommendations from CDC, the National Institutes of Health, and the HIV Medicine Association of the Infectious Diseases Society of America. MMWR Recomm Rep. 2009;58(RR-4):1–207.

Karbwang J, Back DJ, Bunnag D, Breckenridge AM. Pharmacokinetics of mefloquine in combination with sulfadoxine-pyrimethamine and primaquine in male Thai patients with falciparum malaria. Bull World Health Organ. 1990;68:633–8.

Karbwang J, Bunnag D, Breckenridge AM, Back DJ. The pharmacokinetics of mefloquine when given alone or in combination with sulfadoxine and pyrimethamine in Thai male and female subjects. Eur J Clin Pharmacol. 1987;32:173–7.

Karunajeewa HA, Salman S, Mueller I, et al. Pharmacokinetic properties of sulfadoxine-pyrimethamine in pregnant women. Antimicrob Agents Chemother. 2009;53:4368–76.

Lalloo DG, Shingadia D, Pasvol G, et al. UK malaria treatment guidelines. J Infect. 2007;54:111–21.

Mansor SM, Navaratnam V, Mohamad M, et al. Single dose kinetic study of the triple combination of mefloquine/sulphadoxine/pyrimethamine (Fansimef®) in healthy male volunteers. Br J Clin Pharmacol. 1989;27:381–6.

Newton CRJC, Winstanley PA, Watkins WM, et al. A single dose of intramuscular sulfadoxine-pyrimethamine as an adjunct to quinine in the treatment of severe malaria: pharmacokinetics and efficacy. Trans R Soc Trop Med Hyg. 1993;87:207–10.

Obua C, Hellgren U, Ntale M, et al. Population pharmacokinetics of chloroquine and sulfadoxine and treatment response in children with malaria: suggestions for an improved dose regimen. Br J Clin Pharmacol. 2007;65:493–501.

Olliaro P, Pinoges L, Checchi F, Vaillant M, Guthmann J-P. Risk associated with asymptomatic parasitaemia occurring post-antimalarial treatment. Trop Med Int Health. 2008;13:83–90.

Plourde PJ, McCarthy A, Houston S, et al. Committee to Advise on Tropical Medicine and Travel of the Public Health Agency of Canada. Canadian recommendations for the prevention of malaria and treatment of malaria among international travelers – 2009. Can Commun Dis Rep. 2009;35(Suppl 1):1–82.

Schwartz DE, Weidekamm E, Mimica I, Heizmann P, Portmann R. Multiple-dose pharmacokinetics of the antimalarial drug Fansimef® (pyrimethamine + sulfadoxine + mefloquine) in healthy subjects. Chemotherapy. 1987;33:1–8.

Wang NS, Guo XB, Liu QD, Fu LC, Li GQ, Arnold K. Pharmacokinetics of the combination pyrimethamine with sulfadoxine and Mefloquine (Fansimef) in Chinese volunteers and the relative bioavailability of a lacquered tablet. Chemotherapy. 1990;36:177–84.

Watkins WM, Mosobo M. Treatment of *Plasmodium falciparum* malaria with pyrimethamine-sulfadoxine: selective pressure for resistance is a function of elimination half-life. Trans R Soc Trop Med Hyg. 1993;87:75–8.

Sulfadoxine and Pyrimethamine/
Fansidar®   {Antimalarial}

Usual initial dose:

Treatment of acute malaria (caution, drug resistance is common in some areas), two to three tablets (1,000–1,500 mg sulfadoxine/50–75 mg pyrimethamine) swallowed whole, not chewed, with plenty of fluids after a meal as a single dose; *prevention* of malaria (caution, not recommended due to risks of severe exfoliative dermatological reactions), one tablet (500 mg sulfadoxine/25 mg pyrimethamine) swallowed whole, not chewed, with plenty of fluids after a meal beginning 1 or 2 days before arrival in an endemic area

Usual maintenance dose:

Prevention of malarial—one tablet (500 mg sulfadoxine/25 mg pyrimethamine) orally once weekly or two tablets (1,000 mg sulfadoxine/50 mg pyrimethamine) orally every 2 weeks swallowed whole, not chewed, with plenty of fluids after a meal during the stay in an endemic area and continuing for 4–6 weeks after return

Typical maximum dose:

Three tablets (1,500 mg sulfadoxine/75 mg pyrimethamine)

Proportion eliminated unchanged:

Specific data not available; both sulfadoxine and pyrimethamine are eliminated mainly via the kidneys.

Adjustment for Kidney Disease

FDA-approved product labeling:

Impaired renal function	*The risk of toxic reactions may be greater in these patients.*
Renal failure	*Repeated prophylactic (prolonged) use is contraindicated.*

Alternative adjustment: *Data not available*

Dosage Adjustment of Medications Eliminated by the Kidneys

Sulfamethoxazole and Trimethoprim (Enteral) - Selected References

Adam WR, Henning M, Dawborn JK. Excretion of trimethoprim and sulphamethoxazole in patients with renal failure. Aust N Z J Med. 1973;3:383–7.

Bergan T, Brodwall EK, Vik-Mo, Årnstad U. Pharmacokinetics of sulfadiazine, sulphamethoxazole and trimethoprim in patients with varying renal function. Infection. 1979;7(Suppl 4):S382–7.

de Jongh CA, Wade JC, Finley RS, et al. Trimethoprim/sulfamethoxazole versus placebo: a double-blind comparison of infection prophylaxis in patients with small cell carcinoma of the lung. J Clin Oncol. 1983;1:302–7.

Denneberg T, Ekberg M, Ericson C, Hanson A. Co-trimoxazole in the long-term treatment of pyelonephritis with normal and impaired renal function. Scand J Infect Dis Suppl. 1976;8(8):61–6.

Dijkmans BAC, van Hooff JP, de Wolff FA, Mattie H. The effect of co-trimoxazole on serum creatinine. Br J Clin Pharmacol. 1981;12:701–3.

Fox BC, Sollinger HW, Belzer FO, Maki DG. A prospective, randomized, double-blind study of trimethoprim-sulfamethoxazole for prophylaxis of infection in renal transplantation: clinical efficacy, absorption of trimethoprim-sulfamethoxazole, effects on the microflora, and the cost-benefit of prophylaxis. Am J Med. 1990;89:255–74.

Gilbert DN. Urinary tract infections in patients with chronic renal insufficiency. Clin J Am Soc Nephrol. 2006;1:327–31.

Glasson P, Favre H. Treatment of peritonitis in continuous ambulatory peritoneal dialysis patients with co-trimoxazole. Nephron. 1984;36:65–7.

Goff JB, Schlegel JU, O'Dell RM. Urinary excretion of nalidixic acid, sulfamethoxazole and nitrofurantoin in patients with reduced renal function. J Urol. 1968;99:371–5.

Heintz BH, Matzke GR, Dager WF. Antimicrobial dosing concepts and recommendations for critically ill adult patients receiving continuous renal replacement therapy or intermittent hemodialysis. Pharmacotherapy. 2009;29:562–77.

Leoung GS, Stanford JF, Giordano MF, et al. Trimethoprim-sulfamethoxazole (TMP-SMZ) dose escalation versus direct rechallenge for *Pneumocystis carinii* pneumonia prophylaxis in human immunodeficiency virus-infected patients with previous adverse reaction to TMP-SMZ. J Infect Dis. 2001;184:992–7.

Maki DG, Fox BC, Kuntz Sollinger HW, Belzer. A prospective, randomized, double-blind study of trimethoprim-sulfamethoxazole for prophylaxis of infection in renal transplantation: side effect of trimethoprim-sulfamethoxazole, interaction with cyclosporine. J Lab Clin Med. 1992;119:11–24.

Olyaei AJ, DeMattos AM, Bennett WM. Use of drugs in patients with renal failure. In: Schrier RW, editor. Diseases of the kidney and urinary tract. 8th ed. Philadelphia: Lippincott Williams & Wilkins; 2007. p. 2765–807.

Ortengren B, Magni L, Bergan T. Development of sulphonamide-trimethoprim combinations for urinary tract infections. Part 3: pharmacokinetic characterization of sulphadiazine and sulphamethoxazole given with trimethoprim. Infection. 1979;7(Suppl 4):S371–81.

Perazella MA. Trimethoprim-induced hyperkalemia: clinical data, mechanism, prevention and management. Drug Saf. 2000;22:227–36.

Septra® and Septra® DS tablet [package insert]. Bristol: Monarch Pharmaceuticals Inc; 2007.

Stevens RC, Laizure SC, Sanders PL, Stein DS. Multiple-dose pharmacokinetics of 12 milligrams of trimethoprim and 60 milligrams of sulfamethoxazole per kilogram of body weight per day in healthy volunteers. Antimicrob Agents Chemother. 1993;37:448–52.

Stevens RC, Laizure SC, Williams CL, Stein DS. Pharmacokinetics and adverse effects of 20-mg/kg/day trimethoprim and 100 mg/kg/day sulfamethoxazole in healthy adult subjects. Antimicrob Agents Chemother. 1991;35:1884–90.

Tasker PRW, MacGregor GA, de Wardener HE, Thomas RD, Jones NF. Use of co-trimoxazole in chronic renal failure. Lancet. 1973;1:1216–8.

Van Scoy RE, Wilson WR. Antimicrobial agents in adult patients with renal insufficiency: initial dosage and general recommendations. Mayo Clin Proc. 1987;62:1142–5.

Varoquaux O, Lajoie D, Gobert C, et al. Pharmacokinetics of the trimethoprim-sulphamethoxazole combination in the elderly. Br J Clin Pharmacol. 1985;20:575–81.

Wade JC, Schimpff SC, Hargadon MT, Fortner CL, Young VM, Wiernik PH. A comparison of trimethoprim-sulfamethoxazole plus nystatin with gentamicin plus nystatin in the prevention of infections in acute leukemia. N Engl J Med. 1981;304:1057–6.

Welling PG, Craig WA, Amidon GL, Kunin CM. Pharmacokinetics of trimethoprim and sulfamethoxazole in normal subjects and in patients with renal failure. J Infect Dis. 1973;128(Suppl):S556–66.

Dosage Adjustment of Medications Eliminated by the Kidneys

Sulfamethoxazole and Trimethoprim (Enteral)/
Co-trimoxazole,TMP-SMX, Bactrim™, Septra®, Sulfatrim®   {Antibacterial; sulfonamide}

Usual initial dose:	800/160 mg orally
Usual maintenance dose:	800/160 mg (1 DS tablet, 2 SS tablets, or 20-mL suspension) enterally every 12 h for 10–14 days
Typical maximum dose:	20 mg (trimethoprim)/kg/day
Proportion eliminated unchanged:	85 %/67 %

Adjustment for Kidney Disease

FDA-approved product labeling: *Sulfamethoxazole and trimethoprim dosage for patients wit impaired renal function*

CrCL (mL/min)	Recommended dosage regimen
>30	*Usual standard regimen*
15–30	*One-half the usual regimen*
<15	*Use not recommended*

Alternative adjustment:

GFR >50 mL/min	*800/160 mg enterally every 12 h for 10–14 days*
	Serious/life-threatening infections, 12–20 mg (trimethoprim)/kg/day in two to three divided doses
	Prophylaxis of Pneumocystis carinii infection, 150 mg (trimethoprim)/m²/day in two divided doses on 3 consecutive days each week
GFR 10–50 mL/min	*800/160 mg enterally once followed by 400/80 mg enterally every 12 h*
GFR <10 mL/min	*Avoid unless no suitable alternative exists; if necessary, 800/160 mg enterally once followed by 400/80 mg enterally every 24 h*
Hemodialysis	*800/160 mg enterally once followed by 400/80 mg enterally every 24 h; administer after hemodialysis on dialysis days.*
CAPD	*800/160 mg enterally every 24 h or add parenteral sulfamethoxazole-trimethoprim to each bag of intraperitoneal dialysate to attain concentrations of sulfamethoxazole 80 mg/L and trimethoprim 16 mg/L three to four times daily for up to 2 weeks*
CRRT	*2.5–7.5 mg (trimethoprim)/kg enterally every 12 h*

Note: Some authorities suggest that due to attainment of low, potentially subtherapeutic drug concentrations in urine, sulfamethoxazole-trimethoprim should be avoided for the treatment of urinary tract infections in patients with GFR <50 mL/min/1.73 m².

Dosage Adjustment of Medications Eliminated by the Kidneys

Sulfamethoxazole and Trimethoprim (IV) - Selected References

Abramowicz M, Zuccotti G, Pflomm J-M, et al., editors. Handbook of antimicrobial therapy. 19th ed. New Rochelle: The Medical Letter; 2011.

Bennett WM, Craven R. Urinary tract infections in patients with severe renal disease: treatment with ampicillin and trimethoprim-sulfamethoxazole. JAMA. 1976;236:946–8.

Caterson RJ, Collett PV, Hood VL, et al. Trimethoprim/sulfamethoxazole and renal function in transplant patients. Clin Pharmacol Ther. 1978;23:553–7.

Craig WA, Kunin CM. Trimethoprim-sulfamethoxazole: pharmacodynamic effects of urinary pH and impaired renal function: studies in humans. Ann Intern Med. 1973;78:491–7.

Curkovic I, Lüthi B, Franzen D, Ceschi A, Rudiger A, Corti N. Trimethoprim/sulfamethoxazole pharmacokinetics in two patients undergoing continuous venovenous hemodiafiltration. Ann Pharmacother. 2010;44:1669–72.

Gilbert DN. Urinary tract infections in patients with chronic renal insufficiency. Clin J Am Soc Nephrol. 2006;1:327–31.

Gleckman R, Gantz NM, Joubert DW. Intravenous sulfamethoxazole-trimethoprim: pharmacokinetics, therapeutic indications, and adverse reactions. Pharmacotherapy. 1981;1:206–11.

Heintz BH, Matzke GR, Dager WF. Antimicrobial dosing concepts and recommendations for critically ill adult patients receiving continuous renal replacement therapy or intermittent hemodialysis. Pharmacotherapy. 2009;29:562–77.

Hughes WT, Rivera GK, Schell MJ, Thornton D, Lott L. Successful intermittent chemoprophylaxis for Pneumocystis carinii pneumonitis. N Engl J Med. 1987;316:1627–32.

Jelliffe RW, Gomis P, Tahani B, Ruskin J, Sattler FR. A population pharmacokinetic model of trimethoprim in patients with Pneumocystis pneumonia, made with parametric and nonparametric methods. Ther Drug Monit. 1997;19:450–9.

Joos B, Schmidli M, Keusch G. Pharmacokinetics of antimicrobial agents in anuric patients during continuous venovenous haemofiltration. Nephrol Dial Transplant. 1996;11:1582–5.

Kagaya H, Miura M, Niioka T, et al. Influence of NAT2 polymorphisms on sulfamethoxazole pharmacokinetics in renal transplant recipients. Antimicrob Agents Chemother. 2011. Epub ahead of print. doi:10.1128/AAC.05037-11.

Markowitz N, Quinn EL, Saravolatz LD. Trimethoprim-sulfamethoxazole compared with vancomycin for the treatment of Staphylococcus aureus infection. Ann Intern Med. 1992;117:390–8.

Medina I, Mills J, Leoung G, et al. Oral therapy for Pneumocystis carinii pneumonia in the acquired immunodeficiency syndrome: a controlled trial of trimethoprim-sulfamethoxazole versus trimethoprim-dapsone. N Engl J Med. 1990;323:776–82.

Noto H, Kaneko Y, Takano T, Kurokawa K. Severe hyponatremia and hyperkalemia induced by trimethoprim-sulfamethoxazole in patients with Pneumocystis carinii pneumonia. Intern Med. 1995;34:96–9.

Olyaei AJ, DeMattos AM, Bennett WM. Use of drugs in patients with renal failure. In: Schrier RW, editor. Diseases of the kidney and urinary tract. 8th ed. Philadelphia: Lippincott Williams & Wilkins; 2007. p. 2765–807.

Quintilani R, Levitz RE, Nightingale CH. Potential role of trimethoprim-sulfamethoxazole in the treatment of serious hospital-acquired bacterial infections. Rev Infect Dis. 1987;9(Suppl 2):S160–7.

Sharpstone Pl. The renal handling of trimethoprim and sulphamethoxazole in man. Postgrad Med J. 1969;45(Nov Suppl):38–42.

Sulfamethoxazole and trimethoprim injection [package insert]. Irvine: Teva Parenteral Medicines Inc; 2011.

Van Scoy RE, Wilson WR. Antimicrobial agents in adult patients with renal insufficiency: initial dosage and general recommendations. Mayo Clin Proc. 1987;62:1142–5.

Vree TB, Hekster YA, Baars AM, Damsma JE, van der Kleijn E. Pharmacokinetics of sulphamethoxazole in man: effects of urinary pH and urine flow on metabolism and renal excretion of sulphamethoxazole and its metabolite N_4-aceytylsulphamethoxazole. Clin Pharmacokinet. 1978;3:319–29.

Vree TB, Hekster YA, Damsma JE, van der Kleijn E, O'Reilly WJ. Pharmacokinetics of N_1-acetyl- and N_4-aceytylsulphamethoxazole in man. Clin Pharmacokinet. 1979;4:310–9.

Winston DJ, Lau WK, Gale P, Young LS. Trimethoprim-sulfamethoxazole for the treatment of Pneumocystis carinii pneumonia. Ann Intern Med. 1980;92:762–9.

Wofsy CB. Use of trimethoprim-sulfamethoxazole in the treatment of Pneumocystis carinii pneumonitis in patients with the acquired immunodeficiency syndrome. Rev Infect Dis. 1987;9(Suppl 2):S184–94.

Dosage Adjustment of Medications Eliminated by the Kidneys

Sulfamethoxazole and Trimethoprim (IV)/
Co-trimoxazole, TMP-SMX, Bactrim™, Septra®   {Antibacterial}

Usual initial dose:	10 mg (trimethoprim)/kg IV
Usual maintenance dose:	*Pneumocystis carinii pneumonia*: 5 mg (trimethoprim)/kg IV every 6–8 h (15–20 mg [trimethoprim]/kg/day) for 14–21 days
	Severe urinary tract infections and shigellosis: 8–10 mg (trimethoprim)/kg/day IV in two to four equally divided doses for up to 14 days
Typical maximum dose:	20 mg (trimethoprim)/kg/day
Proportion eliminated unchanged:	85 %/67 %

Adjustment for Kidney Disease

FDA-approved product labeling: *Sulfamethoxazole and trimethoprim dosage for patients wit impaired renal function*

CrCL (mL/min)	Recommended dosage regimen
>30	Usual standard regimen
15–30	One-half the usual regimen
<15	Use not recommended

Alternative adjustment:

GFR >50 mL/min	4–5 mg (trimethoprim)/kg IV every 6 h (16–20 mg [trimethoprim]/kg/day)
GFR 10–50 mL/min	4–5 mg (trimethoprim)/kg IV every 12 h (8–10 mg [trimethoprim]/kg/day)
GFR <10 mL/min	Avoid unless no suitable alternative exists; if necessary, 2.5–5 mg (trimethoprim)/kg IV every 24 h
Hemodialysis	2.5–5 mg (trimethoprim)/kg IV every 24 h; administer after hemodialysis on dialysis days.
CVVH	2.5–7.5 mg (trimethoprim)/kg IV every 12 h
CVVHD	4–5 mg (trimethoprim)/kg IV every 6–8 h
CVVHDF	4–5 mg (trimethoprim)/kg IV every 6–8 h

Note: Authorities suggest that due to attainment of low, potentially subtherapeutic drug concentrations in urine, sulfamethoxazole-trimethoprim should be avoided for the treatment of urinary tract infections in patients with GFR <50 mL/min/1.73 m².

Dosage Adjustment of Medications Eliminated by the Kidneys

<u>Sunitinib</u> - Selected References

Adams VR, Leggas M. Sunitinib malate for treatment of metastatic renal cell carcinoma and gastrointestinal tumors. Clin Ther. 2007;29:1338–53.

Bello CL, Sherman L, Zhou J, et al. Effect of food on the pharmacokinetics of sunitinib malate (SU11248), a multi-targeted receptor tyrosine kinase inhibitor: results from a phase I study in healthy subjects. Anticancer Drugs. 2006;17:353–8.

Britten CD, Kabbinavar F, Hecht JR, et al. A phase I and pharmacokinetic study of sunitinib administered daily for 2 weeks, followed by a 1-week off period. Cancer Chemother Pharmacol. 2008;61:515–24.

Desar IME, Burger DM, Van Hoesel QGCM, Beijnen JH, Van Herpen CML, Van der Graaf WTA. Pharmacokinetics of sunitinib in an obese patient with a GIST [letter]. Ann Oncol. 2009;20:599–600.

Di Gion P, Kanefendt F, Lindauer A, et al. Clinical pharmacokinetics of tyrosine kinase inhibitors: focus on pyrimidines, pyridines and pyrroles. Clin Pharmacokinet. 2011;50:551–603.

Escudier B, Roigas J, Gillessen S, et al. Phase II study of sunitinib administered in a continuous once-daily dosing regimen in patients with cytokine-refractory metastatic renal cell carcinoma. J Clin Oncol. 2009;27:4068–75.

Faivre S, Delbaldo C, Vera K, et al. Safety, pharmacokinetic, and antitumor activity of SU11248, a novel oral multitarget tyrosine kinase inhibitor, in patients with cancer. J Clin Oncol. 2006;24:25–35.

Fiedler W, Serve H, Döhner H, et al. A phase I study of SU11248 in the treatment of patients with refractory or resistant acute myeloid leukemia (AML) or not amenable to conventional therapy for the disease. Blood. 2005;105:986–93.

Gallagher DJ, Al-Ahmadie H, Ostrovnaya I, et al. Sunitinib in urothelial cancer: clinical, pharmacokinetic, and immunohistochemical study of predictors of response. Eur Urol. 2011;60:344–9.

Gurevich F, Perazella MA. Renal effects of anti-angiogenesis therapy: update for the internist. Am J Med. 2009;122:322–8.

Hartmann JT, Haap M, Kopp H-G, Lipp H-P. Tyrosine kinase inhibitors—a review on pharmacology, metabolism and side effects. Curr Drug Metab. 2009;10:470–81.

Hoshino-Yoshino A, Kato M, Nakano K, Ishigai M, Kudo T. Bridging from preclinical to clinical studies for tyrosine kinase inhibitors based on pharmacokinetics/pharmacodynamics and toxicokinetics/toxicodynamics. Drug Metab Pharmacokinet. 2011. Epub ahead of print. doi:10.2133/dmpk.DMPK-11-RG-043.

Houk BE, Bello CL, Kang D, Amantea M. A population pharmacokinetic meta-analysis of sunitinib malate (SU11248) and its primary metabolite (SU12662) in healthy volunteers and oncology patients. Clin Cancer Res. 2009;15:2497–506.

Izzedine H, Etienne-Grimaldi MC, Renée N, Vignot S, Milano G. Pharmacokinetics of sunitinib in hemodialysis [letter]. Ann Oncol. 2009;20:392–3.

Kawahara H, Noguchi K, Katayama K, Mitsubishi J, Sugimoto Y. Pharmacological interaction with sunitinib is abolished by a germ-line mutation (1291T>C) of *BCRP/ABCG2* gene. Cancer Sci. 2010;101:1493–500.

Khosravan R, Toh M, Garrett M, et al. Pharmacokinetics and safety of sunitinib malate in subjects with impaired renal function. J Clin Pharmacol. 2010;50:472–81.

Lindauer A, Di Gion P, Kanefendt F, et al. Pharmacokinetic/pharmacodynamic modeling of biomarker response to sunitinib in healthy volunteers. Clin Pharmacol Ther. 2010;87:601–8.

Mannavola D, Coco P, Vannuchi G, et al. A novel tyrosine-kinase selective inhibitor, sunitinib, induces transient hypothyroidism by blocking iodine uptake. J Clin Endocrinol Metab. 2007;92:3531–4.

Sablin M-P, Dreyer C, Colichi C, et al. Benefits from pharmacological and pharmacokinetic properties of sunitinib for clinical development. Expert Opin Drug Metab Toxicol. 2010;6:1005–15.

Sutent® capsule [package insert]. New York: Pfizer Labs Division Pfizer Inc; 2011.

van der Veidt AAM, Eechoute K, Geiderblom H, et al. Genetic polymorphisms associated with a prolonged progression-free survival in patients with metastatic renal cell cancer treated with sunitinib. Clin Cancer Res. 2011;17:620–9.

van Erp NP, Baker SD, Zandvliet AS, et al. Marginal increase of sunitinib exposure by grapefruit juice. Cancer Chemother Pharmacol. 2011;67:695–703.

van Erp NP, Gelderblom H, Guchelar H-J. Clinical pharmacokinetics of tyrosine kinase inhibitors. Cancer Treat Rev. 2009;35:692–706.

van Erp NP, van der Veidt AA, Haanen JB, et al. Pharmacogenetic pathway analysis for determination of sunitinib-induced toxicity. J Clin Oncol. 2009;26:4406–12.

Dosage Adjustment of Medications Eliminated by the Kidneys

Sunitinib/Sutent®	{Antineoplastic; tyrosine kinase and vascular endothelial growth factor (VEGF) inhibitor}
Usual initial dose:	50 mg orally
Usual maintenance dose:	*Gastrointestinal stromal tumor* (GIST) or *renal cell carcinoma* (RCC)—50 mg orally once daily for 4 weeks on treatment followed by 2 weeks off
	Progressive, well-differentiated pancreatic neuroendocrine tumor (pNET)—37.5 mg orally once daily continuously without a scheduled off-treatment period
Typical maximum dose:	50 mg/day
Proportion eliminated unchanged:	<12 %

Adjustment for Kidney Disease

FDA-approved product labeling:	*Renal impairment*	*No dose modification is necessary in patients with diminished excretory kidney function, except as noted below.*
Alternative adjustment:	*CrCL ≥30 mL/min*	*GIST and RCC, 50 mg orally once daily for 4 weeks on treatment followed by 2 weeks off; pNET, 37.5 mg orally once daily continuously*
	CrCL <30 mL/min	*GIST and RCC, 50 mg orally once daily for 4 weeks on treatment followed by 2 weeks off; pNET, 37.5 mg orally once daily continuously (no change)*
	Hemodialysis	*GIST and RCC, 50 mg orally once daily for 4 weeks on treatment followed by 2 weeks off; pNET, 37.5 mg orally once daily continuously; doses may be administered without regard to time of dialysis.*

Note: Due to decreased systemic assimilation, total exposure to both sunitinib and its active metabolite may be diminished by approximately 50 % in patients receiving chronic hemodialysis as compared to those with normal renal function; in these patients, initial dosages should be the same as in those with normal kidneys, but subsequent doses may be gradually increased up to twofold (to 75–100 mg/day) based on overall patient tolerability.

T

L.K. Golightly et al. (eds.), *Renal Pharmacotherapy*,
DOI 10.1007/978-1-4614-5800-5_19, © Springer Science+Business Media New York 2013

Dosage Adjustment of Medications Eliminated by the Kidneys

Tadalafil - Selected References

Adcirca® tablet [package insert]. Indianapolis: Lung Rx Subsidiary of United Therapeutics and Eli Lilly and Co; 2011.

Arif SA, Poon H. Tadalafil: a long-acting phosphodiesterase-5 inhibitor for the treatment of pulmonary arterial hypertension. Clin Ther. 2011;33:993–1004.

Basu A, Ryder REJ. New treatment options for erectile dysfunction in patients with diabetes mellitus. Drugs. 2004;64:2667–88.

Berez PB. The successful use of phosphodiesterase type 5 inhibitors to treat the syndrome of cor pulmonale and prerenal azotemia with diuresis of anasarca (CorPRADA). South Med J. 2010;103:116–20.

Forgue ST, Patterson BE, Bedding AW, et al. Tadalafil pharmacokinetics in healthy subjects. Br J Clin Pharmacol. 2005;61:280–8.

Forgue ST, Phillips DL, Bedding AW, et al. Effects of gender, age, diabetes mellitus and renal and hepatic impairment on tadalafil pharmacokinetics. Br J Clin Pharmacol. 2006;63:24–35.

Francis SH, Corbin JD. Molecular mechanisms and pharmacokinetics of phosphodiesterase-5 antagonists. Curr Urol Rep. 2003;4:457–67.

Gupta M, Kovar A, Meibohm B. The clinical pharmacokinetics of phosphodiesterase-5 inhibitors for erectile dysfunction. J Clin Pharmacol. 2005;45:987–1003.

Kalambokis GN, Kosta P, Pappas K, Tsianos EV. Haemodynamic and renal effects of tadalafil in patients with cirrhosis [letter]. World J Gastroenterol. 2010;16:5009–10.

Koka S, Das A, Zhu S-G, Durrant D, Xi L, Kukreja RC. Long-acting phosphodiesterase-5 inhibitor tadalafil attenuates doxorubicin-induced cardiomyopathy without interfering with chemotherapeutic effect. J Pharmacol Exp Ther. 2010;334:1023–30.

Luks AM, Swenson ER. Medication and dosage considerations in the prophylaxis and treatment of high-altitude illness. Chest. 2008;133:744–55.

Mehrotra N, Gupta M, Kovar A, Meibohm B. The role of pharmacokinetics and pharmacodynamics in phosphodiesterase-5 inhibitor therapy. Int J Impot Res. 2006;19:253–64.

Montorsi F, Verheyden B, Meuleman E, et al. Long-term safety and tolerability of tadalafil in the treatment of erectile dysfunction. Eur Urol. 2004;45:339–45.

Porst H, Padma-Nathan H, Giuliano F, Anglin G, Varanese L, Rosen R. Efficacy of tadalafil for the treatment of erectile dysfunction at 24 and 36 hours after dosing: a randomized controlled trial. Urology. 2003;62:121–6.

Raheem AA, Kell P. Patient preference and satisfaction in erectile dysfunction therapy: a comparison of the three phosphodiesterase-5 inhibitors sildenafil, vardenafil and tadalafil. Patient Prefer Adherence. 2009;3:99–104.

Ring BJ, Patterson BE, Mitchell MI, et al. Effect of tadalafil on cytochrome P450 3A4-mediated clearance: studies in vitro and in vivo. Clin Pharmacol Ther. 2005;77:63–75.

Staab A, Tillmann C, Forgue ST, et al. Population dose–response model for tadalafil in the treatment of male erectile dysfunction. Pharm Res. 2004;21:1463–70.

Supuran CT, Mastrolorenzo A, Barbaro G, Scozzafava A. Phosphodiesterase 5 inhibitors—drug design and differentiation based on selectivity, pharmacokinetic and efficacy profiles. Curr Pharm Des. 2006;12:3459–65.

Tay EL-W, Geok-Mui MK, Poh-Hoon MC, Yip J. Sustained benefit of tadalafil in patients with pulmonary arterial hypertension with prior response to sildenafil: a case series of 12 patients [letter]. Int J Cardiol. 2008;125:416–7.

Trocóniz IF, Tillmann C, Staab A, Rapado J, Forgue ST. Tadalafil population pharmacokinetics in patients with erectile dysfunction. Eur J Clin Pharmacol. 2007;63:583–90.

Wrishko RE, Dingemanse J, Yu A, Darstein C, Phillips DL, Mitchell MI. Pharmacokinetic interaction between tadalafil and bosentan in healthy male subjects. J Clin Pharmacol. 2008;48:610–18.

Wrishko R, Sorsaburu S, Wong D, Strawbridge A, McGill J. Safety, efficacy, and pharmacokinetic overview of low-dose daily administration of tadalafil. J Sex Med. 2009;6:2039–48.

Dosage Adjustment of Medications Eliminated by the Kidneys

<u>Tadalafil</u>/Adcirca™   {Phosphodiesterase-5 enzyme inhibitor; ℞ for pulmonary arterial hypertension}

Usual initial dose:	40 mg orally
Usual maintenance dose:	40 mg orally once daily
Typical maximum dose:	40 mg/day
Proportion eliminated unchanged:	36 % (primarily as metabolites)

Adjustment for Kidney Disease

FDA-approved product labeling:	*CrCL >80 mL/min*	*40 mg orally once daily*
	CrCL 51–80 mL/min	*20 mg orally once daily; may increase to 40 mg once daily based on individual tolerability*
	CrCL 31–50 mL/min	*20 mg orally once daily; may increase to 40 mg once daily based on individual tolerability*
	CrCL <30 mL/min	*Avoid*
	Hemodialysis	*Avoid*
	CRRT	*Data not available*
Alternative adjustment:	*Data not available*	

Dosage Adjustment of Medications Eliminated by the Kidneys

Tamsulosin - Selected References

Flomax® capsule [package insert]. Ridgefield: Boehringer Ingelheim Pharmaceuticals Inc; 2011.

Franco-Salinas G, de al Rosette JJMCH, Michel MC. Pharmacokinetics and pharmacodynamics of tamsulosin in its modified-release and oral controlled absorption system formulations. Clin Pharmacokinet. 2010;49:177–88.

Hussein MM. Does tamsulosin increase stone clearance after shockwave lithotripsy of renal stones? A prospective, randomized controlled study. Scand J Urol Nephrol. 2010;44:27–31.

Kamimura H, Oishi S, Matsushima H, et al. Identification of cytochrome P450 isoenzymes involved in metabolism of the α_1-adrenoceptor blocker tamsulosin in human liver microsomes. Xenobiotica. 1998;28:909–22.

Koiso K, Akaza H, Kikuchi K, et al. Pharmacokinetics of tamsulosin hydrochloride in patients with renal impairment: effects of α_1-acid glycoprotein. J Clin Pharmacol. 1996;36:1029–38.

Korstanje C, Drauwinkel W, van Doesum-Wolters FLC. Tamsulosin shows a higher unbound drug fraction in human prostate than in plasma: a basis for uroselectivity? Br J Clin Pharmacol. 2011;72:218–25.

Lyseng-Williamson KA, Jarvis B, Wagstaff AJ. Tamsulosin: an update of its role in the management of lower urinary tract symptoms. Drugs. 2002;62:135–67.

Matsushima H, Kamimura H, Soeishi Y, Watanabe T, Higuchi S, Miyazaki M. Plasma protein binding of tamsulosin hydrochloride in renal disease: role of α_1-acid glycoprotein and possibility of binding interactions. Eur J Clin Pharmacol. 1999;55:437–43.

Matsushima H, Kamimura H, Soeishi Y, Watanabe T, Higuchi S, Tsunoo M. Pharmacokinetics and plasma protein binding of tamsulosin hydrochloride in rats, dogs, and humans. Drug Metab Dispos. 1998;26:240–5.

Miller J, Tarter TH. Combination therapy with dutasteride and tamsulosin for the treatment of symptomatic enlarged prostate. Clin Interv Aging. 2009;4:251–8.

Miyazawa Y, Blum RA, Schentag JJ, et al. Pharmacokinetics and safety of tamsulosin in subjects with normal and impaired renal or hepatic function. Curr Ther Res Clin Exp. 2001;62:603–21.

Ohkura T, Yamada S, Deguchi Y, et al. Ex vivo occupancy by tamsulosin of α_1-adrenoceptors in rat tissues in relation to the plasma concentration. Life Sci. 1998;24:2147–59.

Rolan P, Terpstra IJ, Clarke C, Mullins F, Visser JN. A placebo-controlled pharmacodynamic and pharmacokinetic interaction study between tamsulosin and acenocoumarol. Br J Clin Pharmacol. 2003;55:314–16.

Soeishi Y, Matsushima H, Watanabe T, Higuchi S, Cornelissen K, Ward J. Absorption, metabolism and excretion of tamsulosin hydrochloride in man. Xenobiotica. 1996;26:637–45.

Stevens HNE, Speakman M. Behaviour and transit of tamsulosin oral controlled absorption system in the gastrointestinal tract. Curr Med Res Opin. 2006;22:2323–8.

Taguchi K, Schäfers RF, Michel MC. Radioreceptor assay analysis of tamsulosin and terazosin pharmacokinetics. Br J Clin Pharmacol. 1998;45:49–55.

Troost J, Tatami S, Tsuda Y, et al. Effects of strong CYP2D6 and 3A4 inhibitors, paroxetine and ketoconazole, on the pharmacokinetics and cardiovascular safety of tamsulosin. Br J Clin Pharmacol. 2011;72:247–56.

Witte DG, Brune ME, Katwala SP, et al. Modeling of relationships between pharmacokinetics and blockade of agonist-induced elevation of intraurethral pressure and mean arterial pressure in conscious dogs treated with α_1-adrenoceptor antagonists. J Pharmacol Exp Ther. 2002;300:495–504.

Wolzt M, Fabrizii V, Dorner GT, et al. Pharmacokinetics of tamsulosin in subjects with normal and varying degrees of impaired renal function: an open-label single-dose and multiple-dose study. Eur J Clin Pharmacol. 1998;54:367–73.

Zatoun OM, Yakoubi R, Zahran AR, et al. Tamsulosin and doxazosin as adjunctive therapy following shock-wave lithotripsy of renal calculi: randomized controlled trial. Urol Res. 2011; E-pub ahead of print. doi: 10.1007/s00240-011-0410-x.

Zheng S, Liu LR, Yuan HC, Wei Q. Tamsulosin as adjunctive treatment after shockwave lithotripsy in patients with upper urinary tract stones: a systematic review and meta-analysis. Scand J Urol Nephrol. 2010;44:425–32.

Dosage Adjustment of Medications Eliminated by the Kidneys

<u>Tamsulosin</u>/Flomax®   {Adrenergic α1 blocker; ℞ for benign prostatic hypertrophy}

Usual initial dose: 0.4 mg orally

Usual maintenance dose: 0.4–0.8 mg orally once daily

Typical maximum dose: 0.8 mg/day

Proportion eliminated unchanged: 9 %

Adjustment for Kidney Disease

    FDA-approved product labeling: *CrCL ≥10 mL/min*   *0.4–0.8 mg/day*

                                                 CrCL <10 mL/min   *Has not been studied in patients with end-stage renal disease*

    Alternative adjustment: *eCrCL ≥10 mL/min*   *0.4–0.8 mg/day*

                                                 eCrCL <10 mL/min   *0.4 mg/day*

                                                 Hemodialysis   *0.4 mg/day (very limited data)*

                                                 CRRT   *Not applicable; preferably avoid*

Dosage Adjustment of Medications Eliminated by the Kidneys

Tapentadol - Selected References

Buynak R, Shapiro DY, Okamoto A, et al. Efficacy and safety of tapentadol extended release for the management of low back pain: results of a prospective, randomized, double-blind, placebo- and active-controlled phase III study. Expert Opin Pharmacother. 2010;11:1787–804.

Daniels S, Casson E, Stegmann J-U, et al. A randomized, double-blind, placebo-controlled phase 3 study of the relative efficacy and tolerability of tapentadol IR and oxycodone IR for acute pain. Curr Med Res Opin. 2009;25:1551–61.

Drug Enforcement Administration, Department of Justice. Schedules of controlled substances: placement of tapentadol into schedule II. Final rule. Fed Regist. 2009;74:23790–3.

Etropolski M, Kelly K, Okamoto A, Rauschkolb C. Comparable efficacy and superior gastrointestinal tolerability (nausea, vomiting, constipation) of tapentadol compared with oxycodone hydrochloride. Adv Ther. 2011;28:401–17.

Hale M, Upmalis D, Okamoto A, Lange C, Rauschkolb C. Tolerability of tapentadol immediate release in patients with lower back pain or osteoarthritis of the hip or knee over 90 days: a randomized, double-blind study. Curr Med Res Opin. 2009;25:1095–104.

Hartrick C, Van Hove I, Stegmann J-U, Oh C, Upmalis D. Efficacy and tolerability of tapentadol immediate release and oxycodone HCl immediate release in patients awaiting primary joint replacement surgery for end-stage joint disease: a 10-day, phase III, randomized, double-blind, active- and placebo-controlled study. Clin Ther. 2009;31:260–71.

Kleinert R, Lange C, Steup A, et al. Single dose analgesic efficacy of tapentadol in postsurgical dental pain: the results of a randomized, double-blind, placebo-controlled study. Anesth Analg. 2008;107:2048–55.

Kneip C, Terlinden R, Beier H, Chen G. Investigations into the drug-drug interaction potential of tapentadol in human liver microsomes and fresh human hepatocytes. Drug Metab Lett. 2008;2:67–75.

Kwong WJ, Özer-Stillman I, Miller JD, Haber NA, Russell MW, Kavanagh S. Cost-effective analysis of tapentadol immediate release for the treatment of acute pain. Clin Ther. 2010;32:1768–81.

Nucynta® ER extended release oral tablet [package insert]. Titusville: Janssen Pharmaceuticals Inc; 2011.

Nucynta® immediate release oral tablet [package insert]. Titusville: Janssen Pharmaceuticals Inc; 2011.

Riemsma R, Forbes C, Harker J, et al. Systematic review of tapentadol in chronic severe pain. Curr Med Res Opin. 2011;27:1907–30.

Schröder W, Tzschentke TM, Terlinden R, et al. Synergistic interaction between the two mechanisms of action of tapentadol in analgesia. J Pharmacol Exp Ther. 2011;337:312–20.

Schwartz S, Etropolski M, Shapiro DY, et al. Safety and efficacy of tapentadol ER in patients with painful diabetic neuropathy: results of a randomized-withdrawal, placebo-controlled trial. Curr Med Res Opin. 2011;27:151–62.

Smit JW, Oh C, Rengelshausen R, et al. Effects of acetaminophen, naproxen, and acetylsalicylic acid on tapentadol pharmacokinetics: results of two randomized, open-label, crossover, drug-drug interaction studies. Pharmacotherapy. 2010;30:25–34.

Stegmann J-U, Weber H, Steup A, Okamoto A, Upmalis D, Daniels S. The efficacy and tolerability of multiple-dose tapentadol immediate release for the relief of acute pain following orthopedic (bunionectomy) surgery. Curr Med Res Opin. 2008;24:3185–96.

Terlinden R, Kögel BY, Englberger W, Tzschentke TM. In vitro and in vivo characterization of tapentadol metabolites. Methods Find Exp Clin Pharmacol. 2010;32:31–8.

Terlinden R, Ossig J, Fliegert F, Lange C, Göhler K. Absorption, metabolism, and excretion of ^{14}C-labeled tapentadol HCl in healthy male subjects. Eur J Drug Metab Pharmacokinet. 2007;32:163–9.

Tzschentke TM, Christoph T, Kögel B, et al. (−)-(1R,2R)-3-(3-dimethylamino-1-ethyl-2-methyl-propyl)-phenol hydrochloride (tapentadol HCl): a novel μ-opioid receptor agonist/norepinephrine reuptake inhibitor with broad-spectrum analgesic properties. J Pharmacol Exp Ther. 2007;323:265–76.

Wade WE, Spruill WJ. Tapentadol hydrochloride: a centrally acting oral analgesic. Clin Ther. 2009;31:2804–18.

Xu XS, Smit JW, Lin R, Stuyckens K, Terlinden R, Nandy P. Population pharmacokinetics of tapentadol immediate release (IR) in healthy subjects and patients with moderate or severe pain. Clin Pharmacokinet. 2010;49:671–82.

Dosage Adjustment of Medications Eliminated by the Kidneys

Tapentadol/Nucynta®, Nucynta ER®   {Analgesic; opioid μ-receptor agonist}

Usual initial dose:	50 mg orally
Usual maintenance dose:	50–100 mg orally every 4–6 h as necessary depending on pain intensity or 50 mg extended-release [ER] tablet orally every 12 h (opioid-naïve patients) or 100–250 mg orally every 12 h (patients currently receiving chronic opioid therapy)
Typical maximum dose:	600 mg/day
Proportion eliminated unchanged:	3 % (~80 % of the absorbed dose is eliminated in urine as pharmacologically inactive glucuronide metabolites)

Adjustment for Kidney Disease

FDA-approved product labeling:	*Mild to moderate renal impairment*	*Tapentadol exposure increases in renal impairment; use with caution: (immediate-release/film-coated tablets) 50–100 mg orally every 4–6 h as necessary depending on pain intensity or (extended-release [ER] tablet) 50 mg orally every 12 h (for opioid-naïve patients) or 100–250 mg orally every 12 h (for patients currently receiving chronic opioid therapy)*
	Severe renal impairment	*Use not recommended due to lack of data in this population*
Alternative adjustment:	*Data not available*	

Dosage Adjustment of Medications Eliminated by the Kidneys

Telavancin - Selected References

Clouse FL, Hovde LB, Rotschafer JC. In vitro evaluation of the activities of telavancin, cefazolin, and vancomycin against methicillin-susceptible and methicillin-resistant *Staphylococcus aureus* in peritoneal dialysate. Antimicrob Agents Chemother. 2007;51:4521–4.

Goldberg MR, Wong SL, Shaw J-P, Kitt MM, Barriere SL. Lack of effect of moderate hepatic impairment on the pharmacokinetics of telavancin. Pharmacotherapy. 2010;30:35–42.

Goldberg MR, Wong SL, Shaw J-P, Kitt MM, Barriere SL. Single-dose pharmacokinetics and tolerability of telavancin in elderly men and women. Pharmacotherapy. 2010;30:806–11.

Gotfried MH, Shaw P-J, Benton BM, et al. Intrapulmonary distribution of intravenous telavancin in healthy subjects and effect of pulmonary surfactant on in vitro activities of telavancin and other antibiotics. Antimicrob Agents Chemother. 2008;52:92–7.

Hegde SS, Reyes N, Wiens T, et al. Pharmacodynamics of telavancin (TD-6424), a novel bactericidal agent, against gram-positive bacteria. Antimicrob Agents Chemother. 2004;48:3043–50.

Leonard SN, Vidaillac C, Rybak MJ. Activity of telavancin against *Staphylococcus aureus* strains with various vancomycin susceptibilities in an in vitro pharmacokinetic/pharmacodynamic model with simulated endocardial vegetations. Antimicrob Agents Chemother. 2009;53:2928–33.

Lodise TP Jr, Gotfried M, Barriere S, Drusano GL. Telavancin penetration into human epithelial lining fluid determined by population pharmacokinetic modeling and Monte Carlo simulation. Antimicrob Agents Chemother. 2008;52:2300–4.

Lunde CS, Rexer CH, Hartouni SR, Axt S, Benton BM. Fluorescence microscopy demonstrates enhanced targeting of telavancin to the division septum of Staphylococcus aureus. Antimicrob Agents Chemother. 2010;54:2198–200.

MacGowan AP, Noel AR, Tamaselli S, Elliott HC, Bowker KE. Pharmacodynamics of telavancin studied in an in vitro pharmacokinetic model of infection. Antimicrob Agents Chemother. 2011;55:867–73.

Miró JM, García-de-la-Mária C, Armero Y, et al. Efficacy of telavancin in the treatment of experimental endocarditis due to glycopeptide-intermediate *Staphylococcus aureus*. Antimicrob Agents Chemother. 2007;51:2373–7.

Odenholt I, Löwdin E, Cars O. Pharmacodynamic effects of telavancin against methicillin-resistant and methicillin-susceptible Staphylococcus aureus strains in the presence of albumin or serum and in an in vitro kinetic model. Antimicrob Agents Chemother. 2007;51:3311–6.

Patel JH, Churchwell MD, Seroogy JD, Barriere SL, Grio M, Mueller B. Telavancin and hydroxypropyl-β-cyclodextrin clearance during continuous renal replacement therapy: an in vitro study. Int J Artif Organs. 2009;32:745–51.

Reyes N, Skinner R, Kaniga K, et al. Efficacy of telavancin (TD-6424), a rapidly bactericidal lipoglycopeptide with multiple mechanisms of action, in a murine model of pneumonia induced by methicillin-resistant *Staphylococcus aureus*. Antimicrob Agents Chemother. 2005;49:4344–6.

Rubinstein E, Lalani T, Corey GR, et al. Telavancin versus vancomycin for hospital-acquired pneumonia due to gram-positive pathogens. Clin Infect Dis. 2011;52:31–40.

Saravolatz DD, Stein GE, Johnson LB. Telavancin: a novel lipoglycopeptide. Clin Infect Dis. 2009;49:1908–14.

Shaw J-P, Cheong J, Goldberg MR, Kitt MM. Mass balance and pharmacokinetics of [^{14}C]telavancin following intravenous administration to healthy male volunteers. Antimicrob Agents Chemother. 2010;54:3365–71.

Shaw JP, Seroogy J, Kaniga K, Higgins DL, Kitt M, Barriere S. Pharmacokinetics, serum inhibitory and bactericidal activity, and safety of telavancin in healthy subjects. Antimicrob Agents Chemother. 2005;49:195–201.

Sun HK, Duchin K, Nightingale CH, Shaw J-P, Seroogy J, Nicolau DP. Tissue penetration of telavancin after intravenous administration in healthy subjects. Antimicrob Agents Chemother. 2006;50:788–90.

Vibativ™ injection [package insert]. Deerfield: Astellas Pharma US Inc; 2009.

Wong SL, Barriere SL, Kitt MM, Goldberg MR. Multiple-dose pharmacokinetics of intravenous telavancin in healthy male and female subjects. J Antimicrob Chemother. 2008;62:780–3.

Wong SL, Goldberg MR, Ballow CH, Kitt MM, Barriere SL. Effect of telavancin on the pharmacokinetics of the cytochrome P450 3A probe substrate midazolam: a randomized, double-blind, crossover study in healthy subjects. Pharmacotherapy. 2010;30:136–43.

Wong SL, Sörgel F, Kinzig M, Goldberg MR, Kitt MM, Barriere SL. Lack of pharmacokinetic drug interactions following concomitant administration of telavancin with aztreonam or piperacillin/tazobactam in healthy participants. J Clin Pharmacol. 2009;49:816–23.

Dosage Adjustment of Medications Eliminated by the Kidneys

Telavancin/Vibativ™   {Antibacterial; glycopeptide}

Usual initial dose:	10 mg/kg IV
Usual maintenance dose:	10 mg/kg IV every 24 h
Typical maximum dose:	15 mg/kg/day
Proportion eliminated unchanged:	76 %

Adjustment for Kidney Disease

FDA-approved product labeling: *Telavancin dosage adjustment in adult patients with renal impairment*

CrCL (mL/min)	Telavancin dosage
>50	10 mg/kg every 24 h
30–50	7.5 mg/kg every 24 h
10–29	10 mg/kg every 48 h
<10	Insufficient data to make specific dosage adjustment recommendations
Hemodialysis	Insufficient data to make specific dosage adjustment recommendations

Alternative adjustment:

GFR <10 mL/min	Presently (January 2012), too few data are available to enable determination of appropriate dose levels. To increase its solubility, telavancin injection contains hydroxypropyl-β-cyclodextrin (HPCD)—as compared with patients without renal impairment, systemic clearance of this solvent has been shown to be significantly diminished, leading to accumulation. Until such time as clinical trial data are available to confirm safety, telavancin probably should be avoided in these patients
Hemodialysis	Presently (February 2012), too few data are available to enable determination of appropriate dose levels. Following administration of 7.5 mg/kg IV, 6 % of the administered dose was recovered in dialysate following 4 h of hemodialysis. In vitro experiments have shown that continuous hemodialysis may be sufficient to prevent HPCD accumulation
CRRT	Presently (February 2012), too few data are available to enable determination of appropriate dose levels. A bovine blood model using a polysulfone hemodiafilter reported a mean telavancin sieving coefficient ranging from 0.25 to 0.31. In vitro experiments have shown that CRRT may be sufficient to prevent HPCD accumulation

Dosage Adjustment of Medications Eliminated by the Kidneys

Telithromycin - Selected References

Alferova IV, Vostrov SN, Portnoy YA, Lubenko IT, Zinner SH, Firsov AA. Comparative pharmacodynamics of telithromycin and clarithromycin with *Streptococcus pneumoniae* and *Staphylococcus aureus* in an in vitro dynamic model: focus on clinically achievable antibiotic concentrations. Int J Antimicrob Agents. 2005;26:197–204.

Aronoff GA, Bennett WM, Berns JS, et al. Drug prescribing in renal failure: dosing guidelines for adults and children. 5th ed. Philadelphia: American College of Physicians; 2007.

Bhargava V, Lenfant B, Perrett, Pascual M-H, Sultan E, Montay G. Lack of effect of food on the bioavailability of a new ketolide antibacterial, telithromycin. Scand J Infect Dis. 2002;34:823–6.

Brinker AD, Wassel RT, Lyndly J, et al. Telithromycin-associated hepatotoxicity: clinical spectrum and causality assessment of 42 cases. Hepatology. 2009;49:250–7.

Cantalloube C, Bhargava V, Sultan E, Vacheron F, Batista I, Montay G. Pharmacokinetics of the ketolide telithromycin after single and repeated doses in patients with hepatic impairment. Int J Antimicrob Agents. 2003;22:112–21.

Ciervo CA, Shi J. Pharmacokinetics of telithromycin: application to dosing in the treatment of community-acquired respiratory tract infections. Curr Med Res Opin. 2005;21:1641–50.

Edlund C, Alván G, Barkholt L, Vacheron F, Nord CE. Pharmacokinetics and comparative effects of telithromycin (HMR 3647) and clarithromycin on the oropharyngeal and intestinal microflora. J Antimicrob Chemother. 2000;46:741–9.

Gattinger R, Urbauer E, Traunmüller F, et al. Pharmacokinetics of telithromycin in plasma and soft tissues after single-dose administration to healthy volunteers. Antimicrob Agents Chemother. 2004;48:4650–3.

Kadota J-I, Ishimatsu Y, Iwashita T, et al. Intrapulmonary pharmacokinetics of telithromycin, a new ketolide, in healthy Japanese volunteers. Antimicrob Agents Chemother. 2002;46:917–21.

Ketek® tablet film coated [package insert]. Bridgewater: Sanofi-Aventis US LLC; 2010.

Khair OA, Andrews JM, Honeybourne D, Jevons G, Vacheron F, Wise R. Lung concentrations of telithromycin after oral dosing. J Antimicrob Chemother. 2001;47:837–40.

Lee JH, Lee MG. Effects of acute renal failure on the pharmacokinetics of telithromycin in rats: negligible effects of increase in CYP3A1 on the metabolism of telithromycin. Biopharm Drug Dispos. 2007;28:157–66.

Mandel GL, Coleman E. Uptake, transport, and delivery of antimicrobial agents by human polymorphonuclear neutrophils. Antimicrob Agents Chemother. 2001;45:1794–8.

Muller-Serieys C, Soler P, Cantalloube C, et al. Brochopulmonary disposition of the ketolide telithromycin (HMR 3647). Antimicrob Agents Chemother. 2001;45:3104–8.

Namour F, Wessels DH, Pascual MH, Reynolds D, Sultan E, Lenfant B. Pharmacokinetics of the new ketolide telithromycin (HMR 3647) administered in ascending single and multiple doses. Antimicrob Agents Chemother. 2001;45:170–5.

Perret C, Lenfant B, Weinling E, Wessels DH, Schoultz HE, Montay G, Sultan E. Pharmacokinetics and absolute oral bioavailability of an 800-mg oral dose of telithromycin in healthy young and elderly volunteers. Chemotherapy. 2002;48:217–23.

Shi J, Chapel S, Montay G, et al. Effect of ketoconazole on the pharmacokinetics and safety of telithromycin and clarithromycin in older subjects with renal impairment. Int J Clin Pharmacol Ther. 2005;43:123–33.

Shi J, Montay G, Bhargava VO. Clinical pharmacokinetics of telithromycin, the first ketolide antibacterial. Clin Pharmacokinet. 2005;44:915–34.

Shi J, Montay G, Chapel S, et al. Pharmacokinetics and safety of the ketolide telithromycin in patients with renal impairment. J Clin Pharmacol. 2004;44:234–44.

Tintillier M, Kirch L, Almpanis C, Cosyns J-P, Pochet J-M, Cuvelier C. Telithromycin-induced acute interstitial nephritis: a first case report. Am J Kidney Dis. 2004;44: 25–7.

Yamaguchi S, Zhao YL, Nadai M, et al. Involvement of the drug transporters P glycoprotein and multidrug resistance-associated protein Mrp2 in telithromycin transport. Antimicrob Agents Chemother. 2006;50:80–7.

Zhanel GG, Johanson C, Laing N, Hisanaga T, Wierzbowski A, Hoban DJ. Pharmacodynamic activity of telithromycin at simulated clinically achievable free-drug concentrations in serum and epithelial lining fluid efflux (*mefE*)-producing macrolide-resistant *Streptococcus pneumoniae* for which telithromycin MICs vary. Antimicrob Agents Chemother. 2005;49:1943–9.

Dosage Adjustment of Medications Eliminated by the Kidneys

<u>Telithromycin</u>/Ketek® {Antibacterial; ketolide}

Usual initial dose: 800 mg orally

Usual maintenance dose: 800 mg orally once every 24 h for 7–10 days

Typical maximum dose: 800 mg/day

Proportion eliminated unchanged: 18 % in healthy subjects, 6 % in patients with severe renal impairment

Adjustment for Kidney Disease

FDA-approved product labeling:	*CrCL ≥30 mL/min*	*800 mg orally once every 24 h for 7–10 days*
	CrCL <30 mL/min	*600 mg orally once daily*
	CrCL <30 mL/min with coexisting hepatic impairment	*400 mg orally once daily*
	Hemodialysis	*600 mg orally once daily; administer after hemodialysis on dialysis days*
Alternative adjustment:	*GFR >50 mL/min*	*800 mg orally once daily*
	GFR 10–50 mL/min	*800 mg orally once daily (no adjustment needed)*
	GFR <10 mL/min	*600 mg orally once daily (no adjustment needed)*
	Hemodialysis	*600 mg orally once daily; administer after hemodialysis on dialysis days*
	CAPD	*Data not available*
	CRRT	*800 mg orally once daily (no adjustment needed unless clearance <30 mL/min, then 600 mg orally once daily)*

Dosage Adjustment of Medications Eliminated by the Kidneys

Tenofovir - Selected References

Abramowicz M, Zuccotti G, Pflomm J-M, et al., editors. Handbook of antimicrobial therapy. 19th ed. New Rochelle: The Medical Letter; 2011.

Aronoff GA, Bennett WM, Berns JS, et al. Drug prescribing in eenal failure: dosing guidelines for adults and children. 5th ed. Philadelphia: American College of Physicians; 2007.

Barditch-Crovo P, Deeks SG, Collier A, et al. Phase I/II trial of the pharmacokinetics, safety, and antiretroviral activity of tenofovir disoproxil fumarate in human immunodeficiency virus-infected adults. Antimicrob Agents Chemother. 2001;45:2733–9.

Birkus G, Hitchkock JMJ, Cihlar T. Assessment of mitochondrial toxicity in human cells treated with tenofovir comparison with other nucleoside reverse transcriptase inhibitors. Antimicrob Agents Chemother. 2002;46716–23.

Cihlar T, Birkus G, Greenwlt DE, Hitchcock MJM. Tenofovir exhibits low cytotoxicity in various human cell types: comparison with other nucleoside reverse transcriptase inhibitors. Antiviral Res. 2002;54:37–45.

de la Prada FJ, Prados AM, Tugores A, Uriol M, Saus C, Morey A. Insuficiencia renal agua y disfunción tubular proximal en paciente diagnosticado de infección VIH tratado con tenofovir. Nefrología. 2006;26:626–30.

Deeks SG, Barditch-Crovo P, Leitman PS, et al. Safety, pharmacokinetics, and antiretroviral activity of intravenous 9-[2-(R)-(phosponomethoxy)propyl]adenine, a novel anti-human immunodeficiency virus (HIV) therapy, in HIV-infected adults. Antimicrob Agents Chemother. 1998;42:2380–4.

Gallant JE, Parish MA, Keruly JC, Moore RD. Changes in renal function associated with tenofovir disoproxil fumarate treatment, compared with nucleoside reverse-transcriptase inhibitor treatment. Clin Infect Dis. 2005;40:1194–8.

Gupta SK, Eustace JA, Winston JA, et al. Guidelines for the management of chronic kidney disease in HIV-infected patients: recommendations of the HIV Medicine Section of the Infectious Diseases Society of America. Clin Infect Dis. 2005;40:1559–85.

Irizarry-Alvarado JM, Dwyer JP, Brumble LM, Alvarez S, Mendez JC. Proximal tubular dysfunction associated with tenofovir and didanosine causing Fanconi syndrome and diabetes insipidus: a report of 3 cases. AIDS Read. 2009;19:114–21.

Kearney BP, Flaherty JF, Shah J. Tenofovir disoproxil fumarate: clinical pharmacology and pharmacokinetics. Clin Pharmacokinet. 2004;43:595–612.

Kohler JJ, Hosseini SH, Green E, et al. Tenofovir renal proximal tubular toxicity is regulated by OAT1 and MRP4 transporters. Lab Invest. 2011;91:852–8.

Lebrecht D, Venhoff AC, Kirschner J, Wiech T, Venhoff N, Walder UA. Mitochondrial tubulopathy in tenofovir disoproxil fumarate-treated rats. J Acquir Immune Defic Syndr. 2009;51:258–63.

Manosuthi W, Mankatitham W, Lueangniyomkul A, et al. Renal impairment after switching from stavudine/lamivudine to tenofovir/lamivudine in NNRTI-based antiretroviral regimens. AIDS Res Ther. 2010;7:37. doi: 10.1186/1742-6405-7-37.

Marcellin P, Heathcote EJ, Buti M, et al. Tenofovir disoproxil fumarate versus adefovir dipivoxil for chronic hepatitis B. N Engl J Med. 2008;359:2442–55.

Murphy MD, O'Hearn M, Chou S. Fatal lactic acidosis and acute renal failure after addition of tenofovir to an antiretroviral regimen containing didanosine. Clin Infect Dis. 2003;36:1082–5.

Peyrière H, Reynes J, Rouanet I, et al. Renal tubular dysfunction associated with tenofovir therapy: report of 7 cases. J Acquir Immune Defic Syndr. 2004;35:269–73.

Rollot F, Nazel E-M, Chauvelot-Moachon L, et al. Tenofovir-related Fanconi syndrome with nephrogenic diabetes insipidus in a patient with acquired immunodeficiency syndrome: the role of lopinavir-ritonavir-didanosine. Clin Infect Dis. 2003;37:e174–6.

Thompson MA, Aberg JA, Cahn P, et al. Antiretroviral treatment of adult HIV infection: 2010 recommendations of the International AIDS Society—USA Panel. JAMA. 2010;304:321–33.

Tordato F, Lepri AC, Ciccooni P, et al. Evaluation of glomerular filtration rate in HIV-1-infected patients before and after combined antiretroviral therapy exposure. HIV Med. 2011;12:4–13.

Vidal F, Domingo JC, Guallar J, et al. In vitro cytotoxicity and mitochondrial toxicity of tenofovir alone and in combination with other antiretrovirals in human renal proximal tubule cells. Antimicrob Agents Chemother. 2006;50:3824–32.

Viread® [package insert]. Foster City: Gilead Sciences Inc; 2011.

Willig JH, Westgfall AO, Allison J, et al. Nucleoside reverse-transcriptase inhibitor dosing errors in an outpatient HIV clinic in the electronic medical record era. Clin Infect Dis. 2007;45:658–61.

Zimmermann AE, Pizzoferrato T, Bedford J, Morris A, Hoffman R, Braden G. Tenofovir-associated acute and chronic kidney disease: a case of multiple drug interactions. Clin Infect Dis. 2006;42:283–90.

Dosage Adjustment of Medications Eliminated by the Kidneys

Tenofovir/Viread®   **{Antiretroviral; nucleoside reverse transcriptase inhibitor}**

Usual initial dose:	300 mg orally
Usual maintenance dose:	300 mg orally once daily
Typical maximum dose:	300 mg/day
Proportion eliminated unchanged:	75 %

Adjustment for Kidney Disease

FDA-approved product labeling: *Tenofovir dosage adjustment for patients with altered creatinine clearance*

CrCL (mL/min)	Tenofovir dosage
≥50	300 mg every 24 h
30–49	300 mg every 48 h
10–29	300 mg every 72–96 h
<10	No data
Hemodialysis	300 mg every 7 days or after ~12 h of hemodialysis
CRRT	No data

Alternative adjustment:

GFR >50 mL/min	300 mg orally every 24 h
GFR 30–50 mL/min	Preferably avoid unless no suitable alternative exists; if indeed necessary, 300 mg orally every 48 h
GFR 10–29 mL/min	Preferably avoid unless no suitable alternative exists; if indeed necessary, 300 mg orally every 72–96 h
GFR <10 mL/min	Data not available
Hemodialysis	Preferably avoid unless no suitable alternative exists; if indeed necessary, 300 mg orally every 7 days or after ~12 h of emodialysis
CAPD	Data not available
CRRT	Data not available

Dosage Adjustment of Medications Eliminated by the Kidneys

Terbinafine - Selected References

Back DJ, Tjia JF. Comparative effects of the antimycotic drugs ketoconazole, fluconazole, Itraconazole and terbinafine on the metabolism of cyclosporin by human liver microsomes. Br J Clin Pharmacol. 1991;32:624–6.

Debruyne D, Coquerel A. Pharmacokinetics of antifungal agents in onychomycoses. Clin Pharmacokinet. 2001;40:441–72.

Faegemann J, Zehender H, Millerioux L. Levels of terbinafine in plasma, stratum corneum, dermis-epidermis (without stratum corneum), sebum, hair and nails during and after 250 mg terbinafine orally once daily for 7 and 14 days. Clin Exp Dermatol. 1994;19:121–6.

Finielz P. Tinea capitis in adult renal transplant recipient [letter]. Nephron. 1999;82:86.

Finlay AY. Pharmacokinetics of terbinafine in the nail. Br J Dermatol. 1992;126(Suppl 39):28–32.

Gupta AK, Ryder JE, Lynch LE, Tavakkol A. The use of terbinafine in the treatment of onychomycosis in adults and special populations: a review of the evidence. J Drugs Dermatol. 2005;4:302–8.

Harari S. Current strategies in the treatment of invasive Aspergillus infections in immunocompromised patients. Drugs. 1999;58:621–31.

Iverson SL, Uetrecht JP. Identification of a reactive metabolite of terbinafine: insights into terbinafine-induced hepatotoxicity. Chem Res Toxicol. 2001;14:175–81.

Jensen P, Lehne G, Fauchald P, Simonsen S. Effect of oral terbinafine treatment on cyclosporin pharmacokinetics in organ transplant recipients with dermatophyte nail infection. Acta Derm Venereol. 1996;76:280–1.

Kovarik JM, Kirkesseli S, Humbert H, Grass P, Kutz K. Dose-proportional pharmacokinetics of terbinafine and its N-demethylated metabolite in healthy volunteers. Br J Dermatol. 1992;126(Suppl 39):8–13.

Kovarik JM, Mueller EA, Zehender H, Denquël J, Caplain H, Millerioux L. Multiple-dose pharmacokinetics and distribution in tissue of terbinafine and metabolites. Antimicrob Agents Chemother. 1995;39:2738–41.

Lamisil® tablet [package insert]. East Hanover: Novartis Pharmaceuticals Corp; 2011.

Lee KH, Kim YS, Chung HS, Park K. Study of the efficacy and tolerability of oral terbinafine in the treatment of onychomycosis in renal transplant patients. Transplant Proc. 1996;28:1488–9.

Li JYZ, Young TY, Grove DI, Coates PTH. Successful control of Scedosporium prolificans septic arthritis and probable osteomyelitis without radical surgery in a long-term renal transplant recipient. Transpl Infect Dis. 2008;10:63–5.

Long CC, Hill SA, Thomas RC, et al. Effect of terbinafine on the pharmacokinetics of cyclosporin in humans. J Invest Dermatol. 1994;102:740–3.

Madani S, Barilla D, Cramer J, Wang Y, Paul C. Effect of terbinafine on the pharmacokinetics and pharmacodynamics of desipramine in healthy volunteers identified as cytochrome P450 2D6 (CYP2D6) extensive metabolizers. J Clin Pharmacol. 2002;42:1211–8.

Magagnin CM, Stopiglia CDO, Vieira FJ, et al. Antifungal susceptibility of dermatophytes isolated from patients with chronic renal failure. An Bras Dermatol. 2011;86:694–701.

McClellan KJ, Wiseman LR, Markham A. Terbinafine: an update of its use in superficial mycoses. Drugs. 1999;58:179–202.

Muñoz P, Singh N, Bouza E. Treatment of solid organ transplant patients with invasive fungal infections: should a combination of antifungal drugs be used? Curr Opin Infect Dis. 2006;19:365–70.

Nedelman J, Cramer JA, Robbins B, et al. The effect of food on the pharmacokinetics of multiple-dose terbinafine in young and elderly healthy subjects. Biopharm Drug Dispos. 1997;18:127–38.

Nedelman JR, Gibiansky E, Robins RA, et al. Pharmacokinetics and pharmacodynamics of multiple-dose terbinafine. J Clin Pharmacol. 1996;36:452–61.

Shah IA, Whiting PH, Omar G, Ormerod AD, Burke MD. The effects of retinoids and terbinafine on the human hepatic microsomal metabolism of cyclosporin. Br J Dermatol. 1993;129:395–8.

Vickers AEM, Sinclair JR, Zollinger M, et al. Multiple cytochrome P-450s involved in the metabolism of terbinafine suggest a limited potential for drug-drug interactions. Drug Metab Dispos. 1999;27:1029–38.

Villars V, Jones TC. Clinical efficacy and tolerability of terbinafine (Lamisil)—a new topical and systemic fungicidal drug for treatment of dermatomycoses. Clin Exp Dermatol. 1989;14:124–7.

Zhang Y-Q, Xu X-G, Li F-Q, Wei H, Chen H-D, Li-YH. Co-existence of cutaneous alternariosis and tinea corporis in a renal transplant recipient. Med Mycol. 2011;49:435–8.

Dosage Adjustment of Medications Eliminated by the Kidneys

<u>Terbinafine</u>/Lamisil® {Antifungal}

Usual initial dose: 250 mg orally

Usual maintenance dose: 250 mg orally once daily for 6 weeks (fingernail onychomycosis) or 12 weeks (toenail onychomycosis)

Typical maximum dose: 500 mg/day

Proportion eliminated unchanged: Nil (80 % of an absorbed dose is eliminated in urine as metabolites with minimal antifungal activity)

Adjustment for Kidney Disease

FDA-approved product labeling:	*CrCL <50 mL/min*	*The clearance of terbinafine is decreased by approximately 50 % compared to normal volunteers*
Alternative adjustment:	*SCr >300 μmol/L (>3.6 mg/dL)*	*125 mg orally once daily for 6–12 weeks*
		Note: Limited data suggest that terbinafine may be successfully used in renal transplant recipients with stable renal function and superficial or certain invasive fungal infections in doses of 250 mg orally once daily (monitor for liver function and possible drug-drug interactions with immunosuppressants, antidepressants, and other medicines)

Terbutaline - Selected References

Andersson K-E, Nyberg L. Pharmacokinetics of terbutaline therapy. Eur J Respir Dis. 1984;65(Suppl 134):165–70.

Aronoff GA, Bennett WM, Berns JS, et al. Drug prescribing in renal failure: dosing guidelines for adults and children. 5th ed. Philadelphia: American College of Physicians; 2007.

Blake PG, Ryan F. Rhabdomyolysis and acute renal failure after terbutaline overdose. Nephron. 1989;53:76–7.

Borgström L, Nyberg L, Jönsson S, Lindberg C, Paulson J. Pharmacokinetic evaluation in man of terbutaline given as separate enantiomers and as the racemate. Br J Clin Pharmacol. 1989;27:49–56.

Davies DS. Pharmacokinetics of terbutaline after oral administration. Eur J Respir Dis. 1984;65(Suppl 134):111–7.

Fagerström P-O. Pharmacokinetics of terbutaline after parenteral administration. Eur J Respir Dis. 1984;65(Suppl 134):101–10.

Hochhaus G, Möllmann H. Pharmacokinetic/pharmacodynamic characteristics of the β-2 agonists terbutaline, salbutamol and fenoterol. Int J Clin Pharmacol Ther Toxicol. 1992;30:342–62.

Lyrenäs S, Grahnén A, Lindberg B, Lönnerholm G. Pharmacokinetics of terbutaline in pregnancy. Br J Clin Pharmacol. 29:619–23.

Nyberg L. Pharmacokinetic parameters of terbutaline in healthy man: an overview. Eur J Respir Dis. 1984;65(Suppl 134):149–60.

Petersen AH, Korsatko S, Köhler G, et al. The effect of terbutaline on the absorption of pulmonary administered insulin in subjects with asthma. Br J Clin Pharmacol. 2010;69:271–8.

Sowinski KM, Cronin D, Mueller BA, Kraus MA. Subcutaneous terbutaline use in CKD to reduce potassium concentrations. Am J Kidney Dis. 2005;45:1040–5.

Terbutaline sulfate injection [package insert]. Bedford: Bedford Laboratories; 2004.

Terbutaline sulfate tablet [package insert]. Philadelphia: Lannett Company Inc; 2011.

Walle T, Walle UK. Stereoselective sulphate conjugation of racemic terbutaline by human liver cytosol. Br J Clin Pharmacol. 1990;30:127–33.

Dosage Adjustment of Medications Eliminated by the Kidneys

<u>Terbutaline</u>/Bricanyl®   {Bronchodilator; β_2-adrenergic agonist}

Usual initial dose: 0.25 mg subcutaneously or 5 mg orally

Usual maintenance dose: 0.25 mg subcutaneously; may repeat in 15–30 min or 5 mg orally every 6 h
                                   during three times daily during the hours that the patient is usually awake
                                   (reduce to 2.5 mg orally three times daily if side effects are particularly
                                   disturbing)

Typical maximum dose: 0.5 mg subcutaneously/4-h period or 15 mg/day orally

Proportion eliminated unchanged: 55 %

Adjustment for Kidney Disease

FDA-approved product labeling: *There are no reports of any clinical pharmacokinetic studies investigating dose
proportionality, effect of food, or special population studies with terbutaline*

Alternative adjustment: *GFR >50 mL/min*   *0.25 mg subcutaneously; may repeat in 15–30 min or
17.5–30 µg/min continuous IV infusion or 5 mg orally
every 6 h three times daily during the hours that the
patient is usually awake (reduce to 2.5 mg orally three
times daily if side effects are particularly disturbing)*

GFR 10–50 mL/min   *0.125 mg subcutaneously; may repeat in 15–30 min or
8.75–15 µg/min continuous IV infusion (50 % decrease);
avoid oral administration*

GFR <10 mL/min   *Data not available; preferably avoid*

Hemodialysis   *7 µg/kg subcutaneously*

CAPD   *Data not available; preferably avoid*

CRRT   *0.25 mg subcutaneously; may repeat in 15–30 min or
17.5–30 µg/min IV; avoid oral administration*

Dosage Adjustment of Medications Eliminated by the Kidneys

Tetracycline - Selected References

Abramowicz M, Zuccotti G, Pflomm J-M, et al., editors. Handbook of antimicrobial therapy. 19th ed. New Rochelle: The Medical Letter; 2011.

Aronoff GA, Bennett WM, Berns JS, et al. Drug prescribing in renal failure: dosing guidelines for adults and children. 5th ed. Philadelphia: American College of Physicians; 2007.

Babu E, Takeda M, Narikawa S, et al. Human organic anion transporters mediate the transport of tetracycline. Jpn J Pharmacol. 2002;88:69–76.

Bihorac A, Özener Ç, Ako lu, E, Kullu S. Tetracycline-induced acute interstitial nephritis as a cause of acute renal failure. Nephron. 1999;81:72–5.

Brugh R III, Rous SN, Rosenblum RP. Severe metabolic acidosis as a complication of intravenous tetracycline therapy. J Urol. 1977;117:395–6.

Clausen G, Nagy Z, Szalay L, Aukland K. Mechanisms of oliguric renal failure induced by tetracycline infusions. Scand J Clin Lab Invest. 1975;35:625–33.

Eastwood JB, Bailey RR, Curtis JR, Gower PE, de Wardener HE. Tetracycline and renal failure [letter]. Lancet. 1970;2:262–3.

Edwards OM, Huskisson EC, Taylor RT. Azotaemia aggravated by tetracycline. Br Med J. 1970;1:26–7.

Greenberg PA, Sanford JP. Removal and absorption of antibiotics in patients with renal failure undergoing peritoneal dialysis: tetracycline, chloramphenicol, kanamycin, and colistimethate. Ann Intern Med. 1967;66:465–79.

Heaton PC, Fenwick SR, Brewer DE. Association between tetracycline or doxycycline and hepatotoxicity: a population based case–control study. J Clin Pharm Ther. 2007;32:483–7.

Kucers A, Bennett NMcK, Kemp RJ. The use of antibiotics: a comprehensive review with clinical emphasis. 4th ed. Philadelphia: JB Lippincott Co; 1987. p. 979–1044.

Kunin CM. Council on drugs: nephrotoxicity of antibiotics. JAMA. 1967;202:204–8.

Levister E, Becker KL. Tetracycline and renal tubular function. Curr Ther Res Clin Exp. 1969;11:638–40.

Lew HT, French SW. Tetracycline nephrotoxicity and nonoliguric acute renal failure. Arch Intern Med. 1966;118:123–8.

Little PJ, Bailey RR. Tetracyclines and renal failure. N Z Med J. 1970;72:183–4.

Mavromatis F. Tetracycline nephropathy: case report with renal biopsy. JAMA. 1965;193:191–4.

Miller CS, McGarity GJ. Tetracycline-induced renal failure after dental treatment. J Am Dent Assoc. 2009;140:56–60.

Phillips ME, Eastwood JB, Curtis JR, Gower PE, de Wardener HE. Tetracycline poisoning in renal failure. Br Med J. 1974;2:149–51.

Reudy J. The effects of peritoneal dialysis on the physiological disposition of oxacillin, ampicillin and tetracycline in patients with renal disease. Can Med Assoc J. 1966;94:257–61.

Romas NA, Clark I. The distribution of tetracycline in renal tissue during pyelonephritis. J Urol. 1969;102:541–6.

Shils ME. Renal disease and the metabolic effects of tetracycline. Ann Intern Med. 1963;58:389–408.

Sirota JH, Saltzman A. The renal clearance and plasma protein binding of aureomycin in man. J Pharmacol Exp Ther. 1950;100:210–18.

Stott RB, Cameron JS, Ogg CS, Toseland P. Tetracyclines and impaired renal function [letter]. Lancet. 1971;2:1378–9.

Taneja OP, Grover NK, Thakur LC, Bhatia VN. Effects of blood levels of tetracycline and oxytetracycline on hepatic and renal functions in normal subjects. Chemotherapy. 1974;20:201–11.

Tetracycline hydrochloride capsule [package insert]. Corona: Watson Pharma Inc; 2010.

Wegienka Weller JM. Renal tubular acidosis caused by degraded tetracycline. Arch Intern Med. 1964;114:232–5.

Whelton A. Tetracyclines in renal insufficiency: resolution of a therapeutic dilemma. Bull N Y Acad Med. 1978;54:223–56.

Dosage Adjustment of Medications Eliminated by the Kidneys

<u>Tetracycline</u>/Sumycin®, Aureomycin™   {Antibacterial}

Usual initial dose:	250 mg
Usual maintenance dose:	250–500 mg orally two to four times daily
Typical maximum dose:	2,000 mg/day
Proportion eliminated unchanged:	60 %

Adjustment for Kidney Disease

FDA-approved product labeling: *If renal impairment exists, even usual oral or parenteral doses may lead to excessive systemic accumulation of the drug and possible liver toxicity. Under such conditions, lower than usual total doses are indicated, and, if therapy is prolonged, serum level determinations of the drug may be advisable*

Alternative adjustment:

GFR >50 mL/min	*250–500 mg orally every 8–12 h*
GFR 10–50 mL/min	*Preferably avoid unless no suitable alternative exists; if indeed necessary, 250–500 mg orally every 12–24 h*
GFR <10 mL/min	*Preferably avoid unless no suitable alternative exists; if indeed necessary, 250–500 mg orally every 24 h*
Hemodialysis	*Preferably avoid unless no suitable alternative exists; if indeed necessary, 250–500 mg orally every 24 h*
CAPD	*Preferably avoid unless no suitable alternative exists; if indeed necessary, 250–500 mg orally every 24 h*
CRRT	*Not applicable; avoid*

Dosage Adjustment of Medications Eliminated by the Kidneys

Thiopental - Selected References

Aronoff GA, Bennett WM, Berns JS, et al. Drug prescribing in renal failure: dosing guidelines for adults and children. 5th ed. Philadelphia: American College of Physicians; 2007.

Barratt RL, Graham GG, Torda TA. Kinetics of thiopentone in relation to site of sampling. Br J Anaesth. 1984;56:1385–90.

Bishoff KB, Dedrick RL. Thiopental pharmacokinetics. J Pharm Sci. 1968;57:1346–51.

Bluth M, Berenyi KJ, Urban BJ. Anesthesia for patients on renal dialysis. Anesth Analg. 1969;48:420–6.

Burch PG, Stanski DR. Decreased protein binding and thiopental kinetics. Clin Pharmacol Ther. 1982;32:212–7.

Burch PG, Stanski DR. The role of metabolism and protein binding in thiopental anesthesia. Anesthesiology. 1983;58:146–52.

Christensen JH, Andreasen F, Jansen J. Influence of age and sex on the pharmacokinetics of thiopentone. Br J Anaesth. 1981;53:1189–95.

Christensen JH, Andreasen F, Jansen J. Pharmacokinetics and pharmacodynamics of thiopentone: a comparison between young and elderly patients. Anaesthesia. 1982;37:398–404.

Christensen JH, Andreasen F, Jansen J. Pharmacokinetics and pharmacodynamics of thiopental in patients undergoing renal transplantation. Acta Anaesthesiol Scand. 1983;27:513–6.

Dogan Z, Yuzbasioglu F, Kurutas EB, et al. Thiopental improves renal ischemia-reperfusion injury. Ren Fail. 2010;32:391–5.

Gaspari F, Marraro G, Penna GF, Valsecchi R, Bonati M. Elimination kinetics of thiopentone in mothers and their newborn infants. Eur J Clin Pharmacol. 1985;28:321–5.

Gronheim MM, Van Hamme MJ. Pharmacokinetics of thiopentone: effects of enflurane and nitrous oxide anaesthesia and surgery. Br J Anaesth. 1978;50:1237–42.

Habibi B, Basty R, Chodez S, Prunat A. Thiopental-related immune hemolytic anemia and renal failure: specific involvement of red-cell antigen-1. N Engl J Med. 1985;312:353–5.

Habif DV, Papper EM, Fitzpatrick HF, Lowrance P, Smythe McC, Bradley SE. The renal and hepatic blood flow, glomerular filtration rate, and urinary output of electrolytes during cyclopropane, ether, and thiopental anesthesia, operation, and the immediate postoperative period. Surgery. 1950;30:241–55.

Homer TD, Stanski DR. The effect of increasing age on thiopental disposition and anesthetic requirement. Anesthesiology. 1985;62:714–24.

Huynh F, Mabasa VH, Ensom MHH. A critical review: does thiopental continuous infusion warrant therapeutic drug monitoring in the critical care population? Ther Drug Monit. 2009;31:153–69.

Kessler P, Lischke V, Hecker M. Etomidate and thiopental inhibit the release of endothelium-derived hyperpolarizing factor in the human renal artery. Anesthesiology. 1996;84:1485–8.

Lebowitz PW, Cote ME, Daniels AL, Bonventre JV. Comparative renal effects of midazolam and thiopental in humans. Anesthesiology. 1983;59:381–4.

Morgan DJ, Blackman GL, Paull JD, Wolf LJ. Pharmacokinetics and plasma binding of thiopental. I: studies in surgical patients. Anesthesiology. 1981;54:468–73.

Papper EM, Habif DV, Bradley SE. Studies of renal and hepatic function in normal man during thiopental, cyclopropane and high spinal anesthesia [abstract]. J Clin Invest. 1950;29:838.

Pentothal® injection [package insert]. Lake Forest: Hospira Inc; 2004.

Samuel JR, Powell D. Renal transplantation: anaesthetic experience in 100 cases. Anaesthesia. 1970;25:165–76.

Srivastava K, Hatanaka T, Katayama K, Koizumi T. Pharmacokinetic and pharmacodynamic consequences of thiopental in renal dysfunction in rats: evaluation with electroencephalography. Chem Pharm Bull. 1998;21:1327–33.

Stanski DR, Maitre PO. Population pharmacokinetics and pharmacodynamics of thiopental: the effect of age revisited. Anesthesiology. 1990;72:412–22.

Stanski DR, Mihm FG, Rosenthal MH, Kalman SN. Pharmacokinetics of high-dose thiopental used in cerebral resuscitation. Anesthesiology. 1980;53:169–71.

Yuzer H, Yuzbasioglu F, Cialik H, et al. Effects of intravenous anesthetics on renal ischemia/reperfusion injury. Ren Fail. 2009;31:290–6.

Dosage Adjustment of Medications Eliminated by the Kidneys

<u>Thiopental</u>/Pentothal®	**{General anesthetic; antiepileptic; short-acting barbiturate}**
Usual initial dose:	Rapid induction of anesthesia: 3–4 mg/kg IV in two to four fractional doses
	Seizures/refractory status epilepticus: 3–5 mg/kg IV followed by 1–2 mg/kg every 2–3 min until seizures are controlled (maximum 10 mg/kg)
	Increased intracranial pressure in neurosurgical patients: 1.5–3.5 mg/kg IV
Usual maintenance dose:	Anesthesia: 25–50 mg IV as needed or whenever the patient moves
	Seizures: 3–5 mg/kg/h as a continuous IV infusion
Typical maximum dose:	10 mg/kg
Proportion eliminated unchanged:	Minimal; pharmacologically inactive biotransformation products are eliminated in urine

Adjustment for Kidney Disease

FDA-approved product labeling:	*Renal dysfunction, increased blood urea nitrogen*	*Relatively contraindicated*
Alternative adjustment:	*GFR >50 mL/min*	*3–4 mg/kg IV*
	GFR 10–50 mL/min	*3–4 mg/kg IV (100 % of usual dose)*
	GFR <10 mL/min	*2–3 mg/kg IV (~75 % of usual dose)*
	Hemodialysis	*Data not available*
	CAPD	*Data not available*
	CRRT	*3–4 mg/kg IV (100 % of usual dose)*

Dosage Adjustment of Medications Eliminated by the Kidneys

Ticarcillin and Clavulanate - Selected References

Abramowicz M, Zuccotti G, Pflomm J-M, et al., editors. Handbook of antimicrobial therapy. 19th ed. New Rochelle: The Medical Letter; 2011.

Aronoff GA, Bennett WM, Berns JS, et al. Drug prescribing in renal failure: dosing guidelines for adults and children. 5th ed. Philadelphia: American College of Physicians; 2007.

Brittain DC, Scully BE, Neu HC. Ticarcillin plus clavulanic acid in the treatment of pneumonia and other serious infections. Am J Med. 1985;79(Suppl 5B):81–3.

Dalet F, del Rio G, Torrelias A. Ticarcillin/clavulanate in severe infection in patients with varying renal function. J Antimicrob Chemother. 1989;24(Suppl B):131–9.

Davies M, Morgan JR, Anand C. Administration of ticarcillin to patients with severe renal failure. Chemotherapy. 1974;20:339–41.

Ervin FR, Bullock WE. Clinical and pharmacological studies of ticarcillin in gram-negative infections. Antimicrob Agents Chemother. 1976;9:94–101.

Fuchs PC, Jones RN, Barry AL, et al. Effect of clavulanic acid on the susceptibility of clinical anaerobic bacteria to ticarcillin: a multicenter study. Diagn Microbiol Infect Dis. 1988;9:47–50.

Heintz BH, Matzke GR, Dager WF. Antimicrobial dosing concepts and recommendations for critically ill adult patients receiving continuous renal replacement therapy or intermittent hemodialysis. Pharmacotherapy. 2009;29:562–77.

Höffken G, Tetzel H, Koeppe P, Lode H. The pharmacokinetics of ticarcillin, clavulanic acid and their combination. J Antimicrob Chemother. 1986;17(Suppl C):47–55.

Imada A, Itagaki N, Hasegawa H, Horiuchi A. Comparative study of the pharmacokinetics of various β-lactams after intravenous and intraperitoneal administration in patients undergoing continuous ambulatory peritoneal dialysis. Drugs. 1988;35(Suppl 2):82–7.

Jungbluth GL, Cooper DL, Doyle GD, Chudzik GM, Jusko WJ. Pharmacokinetics of ticarcillin and clavulanic acid (Timentin) in relation to renal function. Antimicrob Agents Chemother. 1986;30:896–900.

Koeppe P, Höffler D, Hulla FW. Pharmacokinetic studies on clavulanate potentiated ticarcillin in normal subjects and patients with renal insufficiency. Arzneimittelforschung. 1987;37:203–8.

Moriyama B, Henning SA, Neuhauser WM, Danner RL, Walsh TJ. Continuous-infusion β-lactam antibiotics during continuous venovenous hemofiltration for the treatment of resistant gram-negative bacteria. Ann Pharmacother. 2009;43:1324–7.

Munckhof WJ, Carney J, Neilson G, et al. Continuous infusion of ticarcillin-clavulanate for home treatment of serious infections: clinical efficacy, safety, pharmacokinetics and pharmacodynamics. Int J Antimicrob Agents. 2005;25:514–22.

Parry MF, Neu HC. Pharmacokinetics of ticarcillin in patients with abnormal renal function. J Infect Dis. 1978;133:46–9.

Pasadakis P, Thodis E, Euthimiadou A, et al. Treatment of CAPD peritonitis with clavulanate potentiated ticarcillin. Adv Perit Dial. 1992;8:238–41.

Pastorek JG Jr, Aldridge KE, Cunningham GL, et al. Comparison of ticarcillin plus clavulanic acid with cefoxitin in the treatment of female pelvic infection. Am J Med. 1985;79(Suppl 5B):161–3.

Rodriguez V, Inagaki J, Bodey GP. Clinical pharmacology of ticarcillin (α-carboxyl-3-thienylmethyl penicillin, BRL 2288). Antimicrob Agents Chemother. 1973;4:31–6.

Scully BE, Chin N-X, Neu HC. Pharmacology of ticarcillin combined with clavulanic acid in humans. Am J Med. 1985;79(Suppl 5B):39–43.

Timentin® injection [package insert]. Research Triangle Park: GlaxoSmithKline; 2011.

Trotman RL, Williamson JC, Shoemaker M, Salzer WL. Antibiotic dosing in critically ill adult patients receiving continuous renal replacement therapy. Clin Infect Dis. 2005;41:1159–66.

Watson ID, Boulton-Jones M, Stewart MJ, Henderson I, Payton CD. Pharmacokinetics of clavulanic acid-potentiated ticarcillin in renal failure. Ther Drug Monit. 1987;9:139–47.

Watson ID, Stewart MJ, Platt DJ. Clinical pharmacokinetics of enzyme inhibitors in antimicrobial chemotherapy. Clin Pharmacokinet. 1988;15:133–64.

Wise R, Reeves DS, Parker AS. Administration of ticarcillin, a new antipseudomonal antibiotic, in patients undergoing dialysis. Antimicrob Agents Chemother. 1974;5:119–20.

Dosage Adjustment of Medications Eliminated by the Kidneys

<u>**Ticarcillin and Clavulanate**</u>/Timentin®　　{**Antibacterial; extended-spectrum penicillin/β-lactamase inhibitor**}

Usual initial dose:	3.1 g IV
Usual maintenance dose:	3.1 g IV every 4–6 h
Typical maximum dose:	18.6 g/day
Proportion eliminated unchanged:	70 %/45 %

Adjustment for Kidney Disease

FDA-approved product labeling:　*Ticarcillin/clavulanate administration in renal function impairment*

CrCL (mL/min)	Dosage
>60	3.1 g every 4 h
30–60	2 g every 4 h
10–30	2 g every 8 h
<10	2 g every 12 h
<10 with hepatic function impairment	2 g every 24 h
Peritoneal dialysis	3.1 g every 12 h
Hemodialysis	2 g every 12 h supplemented with 3.1 g after each dialysis

Alternative adjustment:

GFR >50 mL/min	3.1 g IV every 4 h or 9.3–12.4 g/24 h continuous IV infusion
GFR 10–50 mL/min	3.1 g IV every 8–12 h
GFR <10 mL/min	2 g IV every 12 h
Hemodialysis	2 g IV every 12 h; administer supplemental 3.1 g IV after hemodialysis on dialysis days
CAPD	3.1 g IV every 12 h or add to peritoneal dialysate qs 320 mg/L in each exchange for 10 days
CVVH	2 g IV every 6–8 h
CVVHD	3.1 g IV every 6–8 h
CVVHDF	3.1 g IV every 6 h

Dosage Adjustment of Medications Eliminated by the Kidneys

Tiludronate - Selected References

Bonjour P-P, Ammann P, Barbier A, Caverzasio J, Rizzoli R. Tiludronate: bone pharmacology and safety. Bone. 1995;17(5 Suppl): 473S–7S.

de la Piedra C, Rapado A, Díaz Diego EM, et al. Variable efficacy of bone remodeling biochemical markers in the management of patients with Paget's disease of bone treated with tiludronate. Calcif Tissue Int. 1996;59:95–9.

Deal C. Osteoporosis therapies: bisphosphonates, SERMs, PTH, and new therapies. Clin Rev Bone Miner Metab. 2005;3:125–41.

Devogelaer JP, Malghem J, Stasse P, de Deuxchaisnes CN. Biological and radiological responses to oral etidronate and tiludronate in Paget's disease of bone. Bone. 1997;20:259–61.

Dumon JC, Magritte A, Body JJ. Efficacy and safety of the bisphosphonate tiludronate for the treatment of tumor-associated hypercalcemia. Bone Miner. 1991;15:257–66.

Fraser WD, Stamp TC, Creek RA, Sawyer JP, Picot C. A double-blind, multicentre, placebo-controlled study of tiludronate in Paget's disease of the bone. Postgrad Med J. 1997;73:496–502.

Maier GA, Lockwood GF, Oppermann JA, et al. Characterization of the highly variable bioavailability of tiludronate in normal volunteers using population pharmacokinetic methodologies. Eur J Drug Metab Pharmacokinet. 1999;24:249–54.

McClung MR, Tou CKP, Goldstein NH, Picot C. Tiludronate therapy for Paget's disease of bone. Bone. 1995;17 (5 Suppl):493S–6S.

Morales-Piga A. Tiludronate. A new treatment for an old ailment: Paget's disease of bone. Expert Opin Pharmacother. 1999;1:157–70.

Morales-Piga A, Del Pino J, Rapado A, Diaz-Curiel M, Pallares M, Gonzalez-Macias J. Comparison of the efficacy and bioequivalence of two oral formulations of tiludronate in the treatment of Paget's disease of bone. Clin Ther. 1997;19:963–74.

Neer RM. Skeletal safety of tiludronate. Bone. 1995;17(5 Suppl):501S–3S.

Reginster JYL. Oral tiludronate: pharmacological properties and potential usefulness in Paget's disease of bone and osteoporosis. Bone. 1992;13:351–4.

Reginster JY, Christiansen C, Roux C, Fechtenbaum J, Rouillon A, Tou KP. Intermittent cyclic tiludronate in the treatment of osteoporosis. Osteoporos Int. 2001;12:169–77.

Reginster JY, Colson F, Morlock G, Combe B, Ethgen D, Geusens P. Evaluation of the efficacy and safety of oral tiludronate in Paget's disease of bone: a double-blind, multiple-dosage, placebo-controlled study. Arthritis Rheum. 1992;35:967–74.

Reginster JY, Lecart MP, Deroisy R, Ethgen D, Zegels B, Franchimont P. Paget's disease of bone treated with a five day course of oral tiludronate. Ann Rheum Dis. 1993;52:54–7.

Roux C, Gennari C, Farrerons J, et al. Comparative prospective, double-blind, multicenter study of the efficacy of tiludronate and etidronate in the treatment of Paget's disease of bone. Arthritis Rheum. 1995;38:851–8.

Sansom LN, Necciari J, Thiercelin JF. Human pharmacokinetics of tiludronate. Bone. 1995;17(5 Suppl):479S–83S.

Schwietert HR, Peeters PAM, Dingemanse J, et al. Multiple dose pharmacokinetics of tiludronate in healthy volunteers. Eur J Clin Pharmacol. 1996;51:175–81.

Siris ES, Lyles KW, Singer F, Meunier PJ. Medical management of Paget's disease of bone: indications for treatment and review of current therapies. J Bone Miner Res. 2006;21(Suppl 2):P94–8.

Skelid® tablet [package insert]. Bridgewater: Sanofi-Aventis US LLC; 2006.

Yoshida M, Tokuda H, Ishisaki A, et al. Tiludronate inhibits prostaglandin F2α-induced vascular endothelial growth factor synthesis in osteoblasts. Mol Cell Endocrinol. 2005;236:59–66.

Dosage Adjustment of Medications Eliminated by the Kidneys

<u>Tiludronate</u>/Skelid®   {**Hypocalcemic agent; bisphosphonate; ℞ for Paget's disease**}

Usual initial dose:	400 mg orally
Usual maintenance dose:	400 mg orally once daily 2 h before breakfast for 3 months
Typical maximum dose:	800 mg/day
Proportion eliminated unchanged:	60 %

Adjustment for Kidney Disease

FDA-approved product labeling:	*CrCL ≥30 mL/min*	*400 mg orally once daily before breakfast for 3 months*
	CrCL <30 mL/min	*Not recommended due to lack of clinical experience*
Alternative adjustment:	*eCrCL ≥30 mL/min*	*400–600 mg orally once daily before breakfast for 3 months*
	eCrCL <30 mL/min	*Data not available; preferably avoid*

Dosage Adjustment of Medications Eliminated by the Kidneys

Tinzaparin - Selected References

Barrett JS, Gibiansky E, Hull RD, et al. Population pharmacodynamics in patients receiving tinzaparin for the prevention and treatment of deep vein thrombosis. Int J Clin Pharmacol Ther. 2001;39:431–45.

Barrett JS, Hainer JW, Kornhauser DM, et al. Anticoagulant pharmacodynamics of tinzaparin following 175 IU/kg subcutaneous administration to healthy volunteers. Thromb Res. 2001;101:243–54.

Branham K, Varrier M, Asgari E, Makanjuola D. Comparison of Tinzaparin™ and unfractionated heparin as anticoagulation on haemodialysis: equal safety, efficacy and economical parity. Nephron Clin Pract. 2008;110:c107–13. doi: 10.1159/000158561.

Davenport A. Low-molecular-weight heparin as an alternative anticoagulant to unfractionated heparin for routine outpatient haemodialysis treatments. Nephrology (Carlton). 2009;14:455–61.

Egfjord M, Rosenlund L, Hedegaard B, et al. Dose titration study of tinzaparin, a low molecular weight heparin, in patients on hemodialysis. Artif Organs. 1998;22:633–7.

Farooq V, Hegarty J, Chandrasekar T, et al. Serious adverse incidents with usage of low molecular weight heparins in patients with kidney disease. Am J Kidney Dis. 2004;43:531–7.

George-Phillips KL, Bungard TJ. Use of low-molecular weight heparin to bridge therapy in obese patients and in patients with renal dysfunction. Pharmacotherapy. 2006;26:1479–90.

Hainer JW, Sherrard DJ, Swan SK, et al. Intravenous and subcutaneous weight-based dosing of the low molecular weight heparin tinzaparin (Innohep) in end-stage renal disease patients undergoing chronic hemodialysis. Am J Kidney Dis. 2002;40:531–8.

Hoy SM, Scott LJ, Plosker GL. Tinzaparin sodium: a review of its use in the prevention and treatment of deep vein thrombosis and pulmonary embolism, and in the prevention of clotting in the extracorporeal circuit during haemodialysis. Drugs. 2010;70:1319–47.

Hull RD, Pineo GF, Brant R, et al. Home therapy of venous thrombosis with long-term LMWH versus usual care: patient satisfaction and post-thrombotic syndrome. Am J Med. 2009;122:762–9.

Innohep® injection. Boulder: Celgene Corp; 2008.

Leiorovicz A, Siguret V, Mottier D. Safety profile of tinzaparin versus subcutaneous unfractionated heparin in elderly patients with impaired renal function treated for deep vein thrombosis: the Innohep® in Renal Insufficiency Study (IRIS). Thromb Res. 2011;128:27–34.

Lim W, Dentali F, Eikelboom JW, Crowther MA. Meta-analysis: low-molecular-weight heparin and bleeding in patients with severe renal insufficiency. Ann Intern Med. 2006;144:673–84.

Mahé I, Aghassarian M, Drouet L, et al. Tinzaparin and enoxparin given at prophylactic dose for eight days in medical elderly patients with impaired renal function: a comparative pharmacokinetic study. Thromb Haemost. 2007;97:581–6.

Malo J, Jodcoeur C, Theriault F, Lachaine J, Senecal L. Comparison between standard heparin and tinzaparin for haemodialysis catheter lock. ASAIO J. 2010;56:42–7.

Nagge J, Crowther M, Hirsch J. Is impaired renal function a contraindication to the use of low-molecular-weight heparin? Arch Intern Med. 2002;162:2605–9.

Natescu EA, Spinler SA, Wittowsky A, Dager WE. Low-molecular-weight heparins in renal impairment and obesity: available evidence and clinical practice recommendations across medical and surgical settings. Ann Pharmacother. 2009;43:1064–83.

Pettigrew M, Soltys GIM, Bell RZ, et al. Tinzaparin reduces health care resource use for anticoagulation in hemodialysis. Hemodial Int. 2011;15:273–9.

Romera A, Cairols MA, Vila-Coll R, et al. A randomized open-label trial comparing long-term sub-cutaneous low-molecular-weight heparin compared with oral-anticoagulant therapy in the treatment of deep venous thrombosis. Eur J Vasc Endovasc Surg. 2009;37:349–56.

Sabry A, Taha M, Nada M, Al Fawzan F, Alsaran K. Anticoagulation therapy during haemodialysis: a comparative study between two heparin regimens. Blood Coagul Fibrinolysis. 2009;20:57–62.

Siguret V, Gouin-Thibault I, Pautas E, Leizorovicz A. No accumulation of the peak anti-factor Xa activity of tinzaparin in elderly patients with moderate-to-severe renal impairment. J Thromb Haemost. 2011;9:1966–72.

Simpson HKI, Baird J, Allison M, et al. Long-term use of the low molecular weight heparin tinzaparin in haemodialysis. Haemostasis. 1996;26:90–7.

Dosage Adjustment of Medications Eliminated by the Kidneys

<u>Tinzaparin</u>/Innohep®	{Antithrombotic; low-molecular-weight heparin}
Usual initial dose:	175 units/kg subcutaneously
Usual maintenance dose:	175 units/kg subcutaneously every 24 h for at least 6 days and until the patient is adequately anticoagulated with warfarin and INR is at least 2.0 on two consecutive days
Typical maximum dose:	175 units/kg/day
Proportion eliminated unchanged:	90 %

Adjustment for Kidney Disease

FDA-approved product labeling:	*Renal insufficiency (CrCL >60 mL/min)*	*Elderly patients and patients with renal insufficiency may show reduced elimination of tinzaparin. It should be used with care in these patients*
	CrCL ≤60 mL/min	*Contraindicated*
Alternative adjustment:	*CrCL ≤60 mL/min*	*175 units/kg subcutaneously every 24 h*
	Hemodialysis	*To prevent thrombosis of the extracorporeal/access circuit, 75 units/kg IV just before each hemodialysis and, to provide continuous thromboprophylaxis, 75 units/kg subcutaneously once daily on off-dialysis days*
		For hemodialysis catheter lock, 2,000 units per catheter line
		Note: The above dose and/or route recommendations for use in patients with renal impairment are contrary to FDA-approved labeling. Although low-molecular-weight heparins generally are contraindicated in severe kidney disease, tinzaparin, with its higher-than-average molecular weight distribution and correspondingly reduced potential for bioaccumulation in patients with renal impairment, is a possible exception. In Europe, it is the number one most prescribed agent for prevention of access thrombosis. Discouraging, however, is the fact that a large-scale randomized trial (IRIS) that compared treatment of deep vein thrombosis in elderly patients with renal insufficiency with either tinzaparin or heparin was terminated prematurely due to a higher rate of mortality in the tinzaparin group (11.5 %) as compared to heparin (6.3 %, p = 0.035). The preponderance of death in tinzaparin-treated patients was not attributable to recurrent thrombosis or bleeding. Rather, the mortality difference appeared to be due to overrepresentation of cardiovascular disease, malignancy, serious infections, and leg paralysis in the tinzaparin group
	CRRT	*Data not available*

Dosage Adjustment of Medications Eliminated by the Kidneys

Tirofiban - Selected References

Aggrastat® injection [package insert]. Somerset: Medicure International Inc; 2007.

Armstrong P, DeCaní J, Hirsch J, et al. Inhibition of the platelet glycoprotein IIb/IIIa receptor tirofiban in unstable angina and non-Q-wave myocardial infarction: the Platelet Receptor Inhibition in Ischemic Syndrome Management in Patients Limited by Unstable Signs and Symptoms (PRISM-PLUS) study. N Engl J Med. 1998;338:1488–97.

Barrett JS, Murphy G, Peerlinck K, et al. Pharmacokinetics and pharmacodynamics of MK-383, a selective non-peptide platelet glycoprotein IIb/IIIa receptor antagonist, in healthy men. Clin Pharmacol Ther. 1994;56:377–88.

Berger PB, Best PJM, Topol EJ, et al. The relation of renal function to ischemic and bleeding outcomes with 2 different glycoprotein IIb/IIIa inhibitors: the Do Tirofiban and ReoPro Give Similar Efficacy Outcome (TARGET) trial. Am Heart J. 2005;149:869–75.

Eikelboom JW, Hirsch J, Spencer FA, Baglin TP, Weitz JI. Antiplatelet drugs: antithrombotic therapy and prevention of thrombosis, 9th ed: American College of Chest Physicians Evidence-Based Practice Guidelines. Chest. 2012;141(2 Suppl): e89–119S. doi: 10.1378/chest.11.2293.

Friedland S, Eisenberg MJ, Shimony A. Meta-analysis of randomized controlled trials of intracoronary versus intravenous administration of glycoprotein IIb/IIIa inhibitors during percutaneous coronary intervention for acute coronary syndrome. Am J Cardiol. 2011;108:1244–51.

Hermanides RS, van Werkum JW, Ottervanger JP, et al. The effect of pre-hospital glycoprotein IIb-IIIa inhibitors on angiographic outcome in STEMI patients who are candidates for primary PCI. Catheter Cardiovasc Interv. 2011; Epub ahead of print. doi: 10.1002/ccd.23165.

Huynh T, Piazza N, DiBattiste PM, et al. Analysis of bleeding complications associated with glycoprotein IIb/IIIa receptors blockade in patients with high-risk acute coronary syndromes: insights from the PRISM-PLUS study. Int J Cardiol. 2005;100:73–8.

Januzzi JL, Cannon CP, DiBattiste PM, Murphy S, Weintraub W, Braunwald E. Effects of renal insufficiency on early invasive management in patients with acute coronary syndromes (the TACTICS-TIMI 18 trial). Am J Cardiol. 2002;90:1246–9.

Januzzi JL Jr, Snapin SM, DiBattiste PM, Jang I-K, Theroux P. Benefits and safety of tirofiban among acute coronary syndrome patients with mild to moderate renal insufficiency: results from the Platelet Receptor Inhibition in Ischemic Syndrome Management in Patients Limited by Unstable Signs and Symptoms (PRISM-PLUS) trial. Circulation. 2002;105:2361–6.

Kimmelstiel C, Badar J, Covic L, et al. Pharmacodynamics and pharmacokinetics of the platelet GPIIb/IIIa inhibitor tirofiban in patients undergoing percutaneous coronary intervention: implications for adjustment of tirofiban and clopidogrel dosage. Thromb Res. 2005;116:55–66.

Kondo K, Umemura K. Clinical pharmacokinetics of tirofiban, a nonpeptide glycoprotein IIb/IIIa receptor antagonist: comparison with the monoclonal antibody abciximab. Clin Pharmacokinet. 2002;41:187–95.

Koster A, Chew D, Merkle F, et al. Extracorporeal elimination of large concentrations of tirofiban by zero-balanced ultrafiltration during cardiopulmonary bypass: an in vitro investigation. Anesth Analg. 2004;99:989–92.

Koster A, Kukucka M, Bach F, et al. Anticoagulation during cardiopulmonary bypass in patients with heparin-induced thrombocytopenia type II and renal impairment using heparin and the platelet glycoprotein IIb-IIIa antagonist tirofiban. Anesthesiology. 2001;94:245–51.

Koster A, Loebe M, Mertzlufft F, Kuppe H, Hetzer R. Cardiopulmonary bypass in a patient with heparin-induced thrombocytopenia II and impaired renal function using heparin and the platelet GP IIb/IIIa inhibitor tirofiban as anticoagulant. Ann Thorac Surg. 2000;70:2160–1.

Link A, Girndt M, Selejan S, Rbah R, Böhm M. Tirofiban preserves platelet loss during continuous renal replacement therapy in a randomised prospective open-blinded pilot study. Crit Care. 2008;12:R111. doi: 10.1186/cc6998.

McClellan KJ, Goa KL. Tirofiban: a review of its use in acute coronary syndromes. Drugs. 1998;56:1067–80.

Sethi A, Bahekar A, Doshi H, et al. Tirofiban use with clopidogrel and aspirin decreases adverse cardiovascular events after percutaneous coronary intervention for ST-elevation myocardial infarction: a meta-analysis of randomized trials. Can J Cardiol. 2011;27:548–54.

Vickers S, Theoharides AD, Arison B, et al. In vitro and in vivo studies on the metabolism of tirofiban. Drug Metab Dispos. 1999;27:1360–6.

Dosage Adjustment of Medications Eliminated by the Kidneys

<u>Tirofiban</u>/Aggrastat®	**{Glycoprotein IIb/IIIa antagonist; platelet aggregation inhibitor}**
Usual initial dose:	0.4 mcg/kg/min IV for 30 min
Usual maintenance dose:	0.1 mcg/kg/min IV
Typical maximum dose:	0.1 mcg/kg/min
Proportion eliminated unchanged:	65 %

Adjustment for Kidney Disease

FDA-approved product labeling:	*CrCL ≥30 mL/min*	*0.4 mcg/kg/min IV for 30 min and then 0.1 mcg/kg/min*
	CrCL <30 mL/min	*Patients with severe renal insufficiency should receive half the usual rate of infusion*

Alternative adjustment:

<u>*Acute coronary syndrome*</u>

eCrCL <30 mL/min   *0.2 mcg/kg/min IV for 30 min followed by 0.05 mcg/kg/ min continuous IV infusion (50 % decrease); infusion should be continued through angiography and for 12–24 h after angioplasty, with IV heparin, according to the manufacturers' weight-based rate table for 50 mcg/mL infusion solutions*

Tirofiban dosage adjustment by weight

Patient weight (kg)	*Most patients (CrCL ≥30 mL/min)*		*Severe renal impairment (CrCL <30 mL/min)*	
	30-min loading infusion rate (mL/h)	*Maintenance infusion rate (mL/h)*	*30-min loading infusion rate (mL/h)*	*Maintenance infusion rate (mL/h)*
30–37	*16*	*4*	*8*	*2*
38–45	*20*	*5*	*10*	*3*
46–54	*24*	*6*	*12*	*3*
55–62	*28*	*7*	*14*	*4*
63–70	*32*	*8*	*16*	*4*
71–79	*36*	*9*	*18*	*5*
80–87	*40*	*10*	*20*	*5*
88–95	*44*	*11*	*22*	*6*
96–104	*48*	*12*	*24*	*6*
105–112	*52*	*13*	*26*	*7*
113–120	*56*	*14*	*28*	*7*
121–128	*60*	*15*	*30*	*8*
129–137	*64*	*16*	*32*	*8*
138–145	*68*	*17*	*34*	*9*
146–153	*72*	*18*	*36*	*9*

<u>*Platelet preservation in cardiogenic shock/CRRT*</u>

CVVHD   *0.2 mcg/kg/min IV for 30 min followed by 0.05 mcg/kg/min continuous IV infusion (limited data)*

<u>*Anticoagulation during cardiopulmonary bypass (CPB)*</u>

eCrCL <50 mL/min   *10 mcg/kg IV bolus followed by 0.15 mcg/kg/min continuous IV infusion until 1 h before conclusion of CPB (limited data)*

Tizanidine - Selected References

Backman JT, Schröder MT, Neuvonen PJ. Effects of gender and moderate smoking on the pharmacokinetics and effects of the CYP1A2 substrate tizanidine. Eur J Clin Pharmacol. 2008;64:17–24.

Emre M, Leslie GC, Muir C, Part NJ, Pokorny R, Roberts RC. Correlations between dose, plasma concentrations, and antispastic action of tizanidine (Sirdalud®). J Neurol Neurosurg Psychiatry. 1994;57:1355–9.

Henney HR III, Runyan JD. A clinically relevant review of tizanidine hydrochloride dose relationships to pharmacokinetics, drug safety and effectiveness in healthy subjects and patients. Int J Clin Pract. 2008;62:314–24.

Kabita Y, Orita H, Kamimura M, et al. Symptomatic bradycardia probably due to tizanidine hydrochloride in a chronic hemodialysis patient. Ther Apher Dial. 2005;9:74–7.

Kaddar N, Vigneault P, Pilote S, Patoine D, Simard C, Drolet B. Tizanidine (Zanaflex): a muscle relaxant that may prolong the QT interval by blocking I_{Kr}. J Cardiovasc Pharmacol Ther. 2011; E-pub ahead of print. doi: 10.1177/1074248410395020.

Olvey EL, Armstrong EP, Grizzle AJ. Contemporary pharmacologic treatments for spasticity of the upper limb after stroke: a systematic review. Clin Ther. 2010;32:2282–303.

Roberts RC, Part NJ, Pokorny R, Muir C, Leslie GC, Emre M. Pharmacokinetics and pharmacodynamics of tizanidine. Neurology. 1994;44(Suppl 9):S29–31.

Shah J, Wesnes KA, Kovelesky RA, Henney HR III. Effects of food on the single-dose pharmacokinetics/pharmacodynamics of tizanidine capsules and tablets in healthy volunteers. Clin Ther. 2006;28:1308–17.

Shellenberger MK, Groves L, Shah J, Novack GD. A controlled pharmacokinetic evaluation of tizanidine and baclofen at steady state. Drug Metab Dispos. 1999;27:201–4.

Tse FLS, Jaffe JM, Bhuta S. Pharmacokinetics of orally administered tizanidine in healthy volunteers. Fundam Clin Pharmacol. 1987;1:479–88.

Zanaflex® capsule and tablet [package insert]. Hawthorne: Accorda Therapeutics Inc; 2010.

Dosage Adjustment of Medications Eliminated by the Kidneys

<u>Tizanidine</u>/Zanaflex®   {Antispasmodic; α_2-adrenergic agonist}

Usual initial dose:	4 mg orally
Usual maintenance dose:	8 mg orally every 6–8 h as necessary
Typical maximum dose:	36 mg/day
Proportion eliminated unchanged:	60 %

Adjustment for Kidney Disease

FDA-approved product labeling:	*CrCL ≥25 mL/min*	*8 mg orally every 6–8 h as necessary*
	CrCL <25 mL/min	*Use with caution as clearance is reduced by more than 50 %. In these patients, during titration, the individual doses should be reduced. If higher doses are required, individual doses rather than dosing frequency should be increased. These patients should be monitored closely for the onset or increase in severity of the common adverse events (dry mouth, somnolence, asthenia, and dizziness) as indicators of potential overdose*
Alternative adjustment:	*Hemodialysis*	*2 mg orally once daily; titrate according to response and tolerance*

Dosage Adjustment of Medications Eliminated by the Kidneys

Tobramycin - Selected References

Abramowicz M, Zuccotti G, Pflomm J-M, et al., editors. Handbook of antimicrobial therapy. 19th ed. New Rochelle: The Medical Letter; 2011.

Bauer LA, Blouin RA. Influence of age on tobramycin pharmacokinetics in patients with normal renal function. Antimicrob Agents Chemother. 1981;20:587–9.

Bunke CM, Aronoff GR, Luft FC. Pharmacokinetics of common antibiotics used in continuous ambulatory peritoneal dialysis. Am J Kidney Dis. 1983;3:114–7.

Chelluri L, Warren J, Jastremski MS. Pharmacokinetics of a 3 mg/kg body weight loading dose of gentamicin or tobramycin in critically ill patients. Chest. 1989;95:1295–7.

Contrepois A, Brion N, Garaud J-J, et al. Renal disposition of gentamicin, dibekacin, tobramycin, netilmicin, and amikacin in humans. Antimicrob Agents Chemother. 1985;27:520–4.

Gatell JM, Ferran F, Araujo V, et al. Univariate and multivariate analyses of risk factors predisposing to auditory toxicity in patients receiving aminoglycosides. Antimicrob Agents Chemother. 1987;31:1383–7.

Heintz BH, Matzke GR, Dager WF. Antimicrobial dosing concepts and recommendations for critically ill adult patients receiving continuous renal replacement therapy or intermittent hemodialysis. Pharmacotherapy. 2009;29:562–77.

Heintz BH, Thompson GR III, Dager WE. Clinical experience with aminoglycosides in dialysis-dependent patients: risk factors for mortality and reassessment of current dosing practices. Ann Pharmacother. 2011;45:1338–45.

Jaffe G, Meyers BR, Hirschman SZ. Pharmacokinetics of tobramycin in patients with stable renal impairment, patients undergoing peritoneal dialysis, and patients on chronic hemodialysis. Antimicrob Agents Chemother. 1974;5:611–6.

Joos B, Schmidli M, Keusch G. Pharmacokinetics of antimicrobial agents in anuric patients during continuous venovenous haemofiltration. Nephrol Dial Transplant. 1996;11:1582–5.

Koo J, Tight R, Rajkumr V, Hawa Z. Comparison of once-daily versus pharmacokinetic dosing of aminoglycosides in elderly patients. Am J Med. 1996;101:177–83.

Kuang D, Verbine A, Ronco C. Pharmacokinetics and antimicrobial dosing adjustment in critically ill patients during continuous renal replacement therapy. Clin Nephrol. 2007;67:267–84.

Lockwood WR, Bower JD. Tobramycin and gentamicin concentrations in the serum of normal and anephric patients. Antimicrob Agents Chemother. 1973;3:125–9.

Mars RL, Moles K, Pope K, Hargrove, P. Use of intraperitoneal aminoglycosides for treating peritonitis in end-stage renal disease patients receiving continuous ambulatory peritoneal dialysis and continuous cycling peritoneal dialysis. Adv Perit Dial. 2000;16:280–4.

Matzke GR, Halstenson CE, Keane WF. Hemodialysis elimination rates and clearance of gentamicin and tobramycin. Antimicrob Agents Chemother. 1984;25:128–30.

Mohamed OHK, Wahba I, Watnick S, et al. Administration of tobramycin in the beginning of the dialysis session: a novel intradialytic dosing regimen. Clin J Am Soc Nephrol. 2007;2:694–99.

Nikolaidis P, Vas S, Lawson V, et al. Is intraperitoneal tobramycin ototoxic in CAPD patients? Perit Dial Int. 1991;11:156–61.

Nimmo CR, Mamdani F, Baker A, Jewesson P. Development and implementation of simplified aminoglycoside empiric dosing guidelines. Pharmacotherapy. 1993;13:407–14.

Pai MP, Nafziger AN, Bertino JS Jr. Simplified estimation of aminoglycoside pharmacokinetics in underweight and obese adult patients. Antimicrob Agents Chemother. 2011;55:4006–11.

Prins JM, Weverling GJ, de Blok K, van Ketel RJ, Speelman P. Validation and nephrotoxicity of a simplified once-daily aminoglycoside dosing schedule and guidelines for monitoring therapy. Antimicrob Agents Chemother. 1996;40:2494–9.

Sarrubbi FA Jr, Hull JH. Amikacin serum concentrations: prediction of levels and dosage guidelines. Ann Intern Med. 1978;89:612–8.

Schentag JJ, Lasezkay G, Cumgo TJ, Plaut ME, Jusko WJ. Accumulation pharmacokinetics of tobramycin. Antimicrob Agents Chemother. 1978;13:649–56.

Tobramycin in sodium chloride injection [package insert]. Lake Forest: Hospira Inc; 2011.

Weinstein AJ, Karchmer AW, Moellering RC Jr. Tobramycin concentrations during peritoneal dialysis. Antimicrob Agents Chemother. 1973;4:432–4.

Xuan D, Lu, Nicolau DP, Nightingale CH. Population pharmacokinetics of tobramycin in hospitalized patients receiving once-daily dosing regimen. Int J Antimicrob Agents. 2000;15:185–91.

Dosage Adjustment of Medications Eliminated by the Kidneys

<u>**Tobramycin**</u>/Nebcin®   {Antibacterial; aminoglycoside}

Usual initial dose: 2–7 mg/kg IV (actual body weight [ABW] or ideal [IBW]+0.4(ABW – IBW) if ABW>IBW)

Usual maintenance dose: 3–5 mg/kg/day IV in two to three divided doses*

Typical maximum dose: 10 mg/kg/day

Proportion eliminated unchanged: 95 %

Adjustment for Kidney Disease

FDA-approved product labeling: *CrCL ≤70 mL/min*   *Following a loading dose (1 mg/kg), the amount of an adjusted dose can be determined by multiplying the normal dose (above) by the percent of normal dose (to be given in the usual two to three divided daily dose regimen) from the nomogram (Fig. 19.1)*

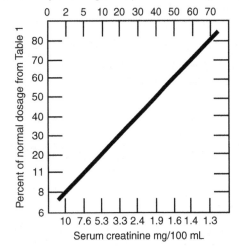

Fig. 19.1 Reduced dosage nomogram. Scales have been adjusted to facilitate dosage calculations

Alternative adjustment: *GFR >50 mL/min*   *2–2.5 mg/kg IV once followed by 1.7 mg/kg every 8–12 h or 4–7 mg/kg (9 mg/kg lean body mass in obese patients) IV every 24 h**

GFR 10–50 mL/min   *2–2.5 mg/kg IV once followed by 1.7 mg/kg IV every 24–48 h* (if pre-dose plasma level is within desired range, usually ≤1 mg/L)**

GFR <10 mL/min   *1.7 mg/kg IV every 72 h (if pre-dose plasma level is within desired range, usually ≤1 mg/L)**

Hemodialysis   *1–1.7 mg/kg IV at the end of each dialysis (if pre-dose plasma level is within desired range, usually ≤1 mg/L) or 1.5 mg/kg IV given within the first 30 min of high-flux hemodialysis**

CAPD   *Add to dialysate qs 4–8 mg/L for multiple exchanges or add 5 mg/kg to a single exchange dwelled for a minimum of 6 h**

CVVHD or CVVHDF   *1.5–2.5 mg/kg IV every 24–48 h (if pre-dose plasma level is within desired range, usually ≤1 mg/L)**

*Therapeutic drug monitoring

Therapeutic plasma levels: *Peak:*   *6–10 mg/L (conventional dosing)*

Trough: *<2 mg/L; patients on extended-interval dosing generally should be re-dosed when levels fall below 1 mg/L*

Dosage Adjustment of Medications Eliminated by the Kidneys

Tolmetin - Selected References

Aronoff GA, Bennett WM, Berns JS, et al. Drug prescribing in renal failure: dosing guidelines for adults and children. 5th ed. Philadelphia: American College of Physicians; 2007.

Ayres JW, Weidler DJ, MacKichan J, et al. Pharmacokinetics of tolmetin with and without concomitant administration of antacid in man. Eur J Clin Pharmacol. 1977;12:421–8.

Bender WL, Whelton A, Beschorner WE, Darwish MO, Hall-Craggs M, Solez K. Interstitial nephritis, proteinuria, and renal failure caused by nonsteroidal anti-inflammatory drugs: immunologic characterization of the inflammatory infiltrate. Am J Med. 1984;76:1006–12.

Cressman WA, Wortham F, Plostnieks J. Absorption and excretion of tolmetin in man. Clin Pharmacol Ther. 1976;19:224–33.

Franchimont P, Hauwaert C, Mailleux E. Concentrations of tolmetin in plasma and synovial fluid after a single intake in patients with rheumatoid arthritis. Eur J Rheumatol Inflamm. 1981;4:387–91.

Furst DE, Dromgoole SH, Desiraju R, Paulus HE. Clinical pharmacology of tolmetin: comparisons in rheumatoid arthritis patients and normal volunteers. J Clin Pharmacol. 1983;23:329–35.

Furst DE, Dromgoole SH, Fow S, Landaw EM. Comparison of tolmetin kinetics in rheumatoid arthritis and matched healthy controls. J Clin Pharmacol. 1983;23:557–62.

Gasparich JP, Mayo ME. Comparative effects of four prostaglandin synthesis inhibitors on the obstructed kidney in the dog. J Urol. 1986;135:1088–90.

Grindel JM. The pharmacokinetic and metabolic profile of the antiinflammatory agent tolmetin in laboratory animals and man. Drug Metab Rev. 1981;12:363–77.

Grindel JM, Migdalof BH, Plostnieks J. Absorption and excretion of tolmetin in arthritic patients. Clin Pharmacol Ther. 1979;26:122–8.

Hyneck ML, Smith PC, Munafo A, McDonagh AF, Benet LZ. Disposition and irreversible plasma protein binding of tolmetin in humans. Clin Pharmacol Ther. 1988;44:107–14.

Katz SM, Capaldo R, Everts EA, DiGregorio JG. Tolmetin: association with reversible renal failure and acute interstitial nephritis. JAMA. 1981;17:243–5.

Liyanage SP, Steele CF. Tolmetin in osteoarthrosis of the hip and knee: double-blind crossover trials. Curr Med Res Opin. 1977–1978;5:299–305.

McIntyre CW, Owen PJ. Prescribing drugs in kidney disease. In: Brenner BM, editor. Brenner and Rector's the kidney. 8th ed. Philadelphia: Saunders Elsevier; 2008. p. 1930–55.

Munafo A, Hyneck ML, Benet LZ. Pharmacokinetics and irreversible binding of tolmetin and its glucuronide esters in the elderly. Pharmacology. 1993;47:309–17.

Noordewier B, Stygles VG, Hook JB, Gussin RZ. Effect of tolmetin on renal function and prostaglandin synthesis. J Pharmacol Exp Ther. 1978;204:461–8.

Pascoe MD, Gordon GD, Temple-camp CRE. Tolmetin-induced acute renal failure: a case report. S Afr Med J. 1986;70:232–3.

Pérez-Urizar J, Flores-Murrietta FJ, Castañeda-Hernández G. Effect of experimental hypoalbuminemia on the plasma protein binding of tolmetin. Life Sci. 2002;71:1015–22.

Pritchard JF, O'Neill PJ, Affrime MB, Lowenthal DT. Influence of uremia and hemodialysis on the plasma protein binding of tolmetin. Pharmacology. 1984;29:312–9.

Radford MG, Holley KE, Grande JP, et al. Reversible membranous nephropathy associated with the use of nonsteroidal anti-inflammatory drugs. JAMA. 1996;276:466–9.

Selley ML, Glass J, Triggs EJ, Thomas J. Pharmacokinetic studies of tolmetin in man. Clin Pharmacol Ther. 1975;17:599–605.

Shaw GR, Anderson WR. Multisystem failure and hepatic microvesicular fatty metamorphosis associated with tolmetin ingestion. Arch Pathol Lab Med. 1991;115:818–21.

Tolmetin capsule [package insert]. Morgantown: Mylan Pharmaceuticals Inc; 2008.

van Duk RA, Rico PB, Hoitsma A, Kunst VAJM. Immune hemolytic anemia associated with tolmetin and suprofen. Transfusion. 1989;29:638–41.

Dosage Adjustment of Medications Eliminated by the Kidneys

<u>Tolmetin</u>/Tolectin®	**{Anti-inflammatory; analgesic; nonsteroidal anti-inflammatory drug}**
Usual initial dose:	400 mg orally
Usual maintenance dose:	400–600 mg orally three times daily
Typical maximum dose:	1,800 mg/day
Proportion eliminated unchanged:	10 % (plus 72 % of each absorbed dose as the primary oxidative metabolite)

Adjustment for Kidney Disease

FDA-approved product labeling: *Acute interstitial nephritis, with hematuria and proteinuria, and occasionally nephritic syndrome has been reported in patients treated with tolmetin. Renal toxicity also has been seen in patients in whom renal prostaglandins have a compensatory role in the maintenance of renal perfusion. In these patients, administration of an NSAID may cause a dose-dependent reduction in prostaglandin formation and, secondarily, in renal blood flow, which may precipitate overt renal decompensation. Patients at greatest risk of this reaction are those with impaired renal function, heart failure, and liver dysfunction, those taking diuretics and ACE inhibitors, and the elderly*

	Advanced renal disease	*No information is available; use is not recommended*
Alternative adjustment:	*GFR >50 mL/min*	*400 mg orally three times daily*
	GFR 10–50 mL/min	*400 mg orally three times daily*
	GFR <10 mL/min	*400 mg orally three times daily*
	Hemodialysis	*Data not available*
	CAPD	*Data not available*
	CRRT	*Not applicable; preferably avoid*

Dosage Adjustment of Medications Eliminated by the Kidneys

Tolterodine - Selected References

Anderson RU, MacDiarmid S, Kell S, Barada JH, Serels S, Goldberg RP. Effectiveness and tolerability of extended-release oxybutynin vs extended-release tolterodine in women with or without prior anticholinergic treatment for overactive bladder. Int Urogynecol J Pelvic Floor Dysfunct. 2006;17:502–11.

Brynne N, Dalén P, Alván G, Bertilsson L, Gustafsson LL. Influence of CYP2D6 polymorphism on the pharmacokinetics and pharmacodynamics of tolterodine. Clin Pharmacol Ther. 1998;63:529–39.

Brynne N, Forslund C, Hallén B, Gustafsson LL, Bertilsson L. Ketoconazole inhibits the metabolism of tolterodine in subjects with deficient CYP2D6 activity. Br J Clin Pharmacol. 1999;48:564–72.

Detrol® LA capsule, extended release [package insert]. New York: Pharmacia & Upjohn Division of Pfizer Inc; 2011.

Detrol® tablet film coated [package insert]. New York: Pharmacia & Upjohn Division of Pfizer Inc; 2011.

Drutz HP, Appell RA, Gleason D, Klimberg I, Radomski S. Clinical efficacy and safety of tolterodine compared to oxybutinin and placebo in patients with overactive bladder. Int Urogynecol J Pelvic Floor Dysfunct. 1999;10:283–9.

Frenkl T, Railkar R, Shore N, et al. Evaluation of an experimental urodynamic platform to identify treatment effects: a randomized, placebo-controlled, crossover study in patients with overactive bladder. Neurourol Urodyn. 2011; E-pub ahead of print. doi: 10.1002/nau.21094.

Juss JK, Radhamma AKJ, Forsyth DR. Tolterodine-induced hyponatremia. Age Ageing. 2005;34:524–5.

Larsson G, Hallén B, Nilvebrant L. Tolterodine in the treatment of overactive bladder: analysis of the pooled phase II efficacy and safety data. Urology. 1999;53:990–8.

Lawrence M, Guay DRP, Benson SR, Anderson MJ. Immediate-release oxybutinin versus tolterodine in detrusor overactivity: a population analysis. Pharmacotherapy. 2000;20:470–5.

Lv JL, Tang QN, Hui JH, Lu FD. Efficacy of tolterodine for medical treatment of intramural ureteral stone with vesical irritability. Urol Res. 2011;39:213–6.

Malhotra BK, Darsey E, Crownover P, Fang J, Glue P. Comparison of pharmacokinetic variability of fesoterodine vs tolterodine extended release in cytochrome P450 2D6 extensive and poor metabolizers. Br J Clin Pharmacol. 2011;72:226–34.

Malhotra BK, Glue P, Sweeney K, Anziano R, Mancuso J, Wicker P. Thorough QT study with recommended and supratherapeutic doses of tolterodine. Clin Pharmacol Ther. 2007;81:377–85.

Millard R, Tuttle J, Moore K, et al. Clinical efficacy and safety of tolterodine compared to placebo in detrusor overactivity. J Urol. 1999;161:1551–5.

Nilvebrant L, Hallén B, Larsson G. Tolterodine – a new bladder selective muscarinic receptor antagonist: preclinical pharmacological and clinical data. Life Sci. 1997;60:1129–36.

Oishi M, Chiba K, Malhotra B, Suwa T. Effect of CYP2D6*10 genotype on tolterodine pharmacokinetics. Drug Metab Dispos. 2010;38:1456–63.

Oishi M, Chiba K, Malhotra B, Suwa T. Pharmacokinetics of tolterodine in Japanese and Koreans: physiological and stochastic assessment of ethnic differences. Drug Metab Pharmacokinet. 2011;26:236–41.

Olsson B, Brynne N, Johansson C, Arnberg H. Food increases the bioavailability of tolterodine but not effective exposure. J Clin Pharmacol. 2001;41:298–301.

Olsson B, Szamosi J. Multiple dose pharmacokinetics of a new once daily extended release tolterodine formulation versus immediate release tolterodine. Clin Pharmacokinet. 2001;40:227–36.

Paquette A, Gou P, Tannenbaum C. Systematic review and meta-analysis: do clinical trials testing antimuscarinic agents for overactive bladder adequately measure central nervous system adverse events? J Am Geriatr Soc. 2011;59:1332–9.

Postlind H, Danielson Å, Lindgren A, Andersson SHG. Tolterodine, a new muscarinic receptor antagonist, is metabolized by cytochromes P450 3D6 and 3A in human liver microsomes. Drug Metab Dispos. 1998;26:289–93.

Rentzhog L, Stanton SL, Cardozo L, Nelson E, Fall M, Abrams P. Efficacy and safety of tolterodine in patients with detrusor instability: a dose-ranging study. Br J Urol. 1998;81:42–8.

Siami P, Seidman LS, Lama D. A multicenter, prospective, open-label study of tolterodine extended-release 4 mg for overactive bladder: the Speed of Onset of Therapeutic Assessment Trial (STAT). Clin Ther. 2002;24:606–28.

Van Kerrebroeck PEVA, Amarenco G, Thüroff JW, et al. Dose-ranging study of tolterodine in patients with detrusor hyperreflexia. Neurourol Urodyn. 1998;17:499–512.

Dosage Adjustment of Medications Eliminated by the Kidneys

<u>**Tolterodine**</u>/Detrol®   {**Anticholinergic agent; ℞ for overactive bladder or urge incontinence**}

Usual initial dose: 2 mg orally

Usual maintenance dose: 1–2 mg orally twice daily or 2–4 mg LA orally once daily

Typical maximum dose: 4 mg/day

Proportion eliminated unchanged: 1–2 % (plus 3–12 % of the absorbed dose as active oxidative metabolite)

Adjustment for Kidney Disease

FDA-approved product labeling:	*CrCL ≥30 mL/min*	*1–2 mg orally twice daily or 2–4 mg LA once daily*
	CrCL 10–30 mL/min	*1 mg twice daily or 2 mg LA once daily*
	CrCL <10 mL/min	*No data; use not recommended*
Alternative adjustment:	*Data not available*	

Dosage Adjustment of Medications Eliminated by the Kidneys

Tolvaptan - Selected References

Berl T, Quittnat-Pelletier F, Verbalis JG, et al. Oral tolvaptan is safe and effective in chronic Hyponatremia. J Am Soc Nephrol. 2010;21:705–12.

Blair JEA, Pang PS, Schrier RW, et al. Changes in renal function during hospitalization and soon after discharge in patients admitted for worsening heart failure in the placebo group of the EVEREST trial. Eur Heart J. 2011;32:2563–72.

Cárdenas A, Ginès P, Marotta P, et al. Tolvaptan, an oral vasopressin antagonist, in the treatment of hyponatremia in cirrhosis. J Hepatol. 2011; E-pub ahead of print. doi: 10.1016/j.jhep.2011.08.020.

Chiong JR, Kim S, Lin J, Christian R, Dasta JF. Evaluation of costs associated with tolvaptan-mediated length-of-stay reduction among heart failure patients with Hyponatremia in the US, based on the EVEREST trial. J Med Econ. 2011; E-pub ahead of print. doi: 10.3111/13696998.2011.643329.

Gheorghiade M, Gattis WA, O'Connor CM, et al. Effects of tolvaptan, a vasopressin antagonist, in patients hospitalized with worsening heart failure: a randomized controlled trial. JAMA. 2004;291:1963–71.

Gheorghiade M, Konstam MA, Burnett JC Jr, et al. Short-term clinical effects of tolvaptan, an oral vasopressin antagonist, in patients hospitalized for heart failure: the EVEREST clinical status trials. JAMA. 2007;297:1332–43.

Hauptman PJ, Zimmer C, Udelson J, et al. Comparison of two doses and dosing regimens of tolvaptan in congestive heart failure. J Cardiovasc Pharmacol. 2005;46:609–14.

Higashihara E, Torres VE, Chapman AB, et al. Tolvaptan in autosomal dominant polycystic kidney disease: three years' experience. Clin J Am Soc Nephrol. 2011;6:2499–507.

Irazabal MV, Torres VE, Hogan MC, et al. Short-term effects of tolvaptan on renal function and volume in patients with autosomal dominant polycystic kidney disease. Kidney Int. 2011;80:295–301.

Kim SR, Hasunuma T, Sato O, Okada T, Kondo M, Azuma J. Pharmacokinetics, pharmacodynamics and safety of tolvaptan, a novel, oral, selective nonpeptide AVP V2-receptor antagonist: results of single- and multiple-dose studies in healthy male Japanese volunteers. Cardiovasc Drugs Ther. 2011;25(Suppl 1):S5–17.

Pang PS, Gheorghiade M, Dihu J, et al. Effects of tolvaptan on physician-assessed symptoms and signs in patients hospitalized with acute heart failure syndromes: analysis from the Efficacy of Vasopressin Antagonism in Heart Failure Outcome Study with Tolvaptan (EVEREST) trials. Am Heart J. 2011;161:1067–72.

Pitt B, Gheorghiade M. Vasopressin V1 receptor-mediated aldosterone production as a result of selective V2 receptor antagonism: a potential explanation for the failure of tolvaptan to reduce cardiovascular outcomes in the EVEREST trial. Eur Heart J. 2011;13:1261–3.

Samsca™ tablet [package insert]. Rockville: Otsuka Pharmaceutical Co; 2009.

Schrier RW, Gross P, Gheorghiade M, et al. Tolvaptan, a selective oral vasopressin V_2-receptor antagonist, for hyponatremia. N Engl J Med. 2006;355:2099–112.

Shoaf SE, Bramer SL, Bricmont P, Zimmer CA. Pharmacokinetic and pharmacodynamic interaction between tolvaptan, a non-peptide AVP antagonist, and furosemide or hydrochlorothiazide. J Cardiovasc Pharmacol. 2007;50:213–22.

Shoaf SE, Bricmont P, Mallikaarjun S. Effect of CYP3A4 inhibition and induction on the pharmacokinetics and pharmacodynamics of tolvaptan a non-peptide AVP antagonist in healthy subjects. Br J Clin Pharmacol. 2011; E-pub ahead of print. doi: 10.1111/j.1365-2125.2011.04114.x.

Shoaf SE, Wang Z, Bricmont P, Mallikaarjun S. Pharmacokinetics, pharmacodynamics, and safety of tolvaptan, a nonpeptide AVP antagonist, during ascending single-dose studies in healthy subjects. J Clin Pharmacol. 2007;47:1498–507.

Torres AC, Wickham EP, Biskobing DM. Tolvaptan for the management of syndrome of inappropriate antidiuretic hormone secretion: lessons learned in titration of dose. Endocr Pract. 2011;17:e97–100. doi: 10.4158/EP10386.CR.

Udelson JE, Bilsker M, Hauptman PJ, et al. A multicenter, randomized, double-blind, placebo-controlled study of tolvaptan monotherapy compared to furosemide and the combination of tolvaptan and furosemide in patients with heart failure and systolic dysfunction. J Card Fail. 2011;17:973–81.

Udelson JE, Orlandi C, Ouyang J, et al. Acute hemodynamic effects of tolvaptan, a vasopressin V_2 receptor blocker, in patients with symptomatic heart failure and systolic dysfunction. J Am Coll Cardiol. 2008;52:1540–5.

Yi S, Jeon H, Yoon SH, et al. Pharmacokinetics and pharmacodynamics of oral tolvaptan administered in 15- to 60-mg single doses to healthy Korean males. J Cardiovasc Pharmacol. 2011; E-pub ahead of print. doi: 10.1097/FJC.0b013e318241e89c.

Dosage Adjustment of Medications Eliminated by the Kidneys

<u>Tolvaptan</u>/Samsca™ {Vasopressin receptor antagonist; ℞ for hypovolemic/euvolemic hyponatremia}

Usual initial dose:	15 mg orally once daily
Usual maintenance dose:	30–60 mg orally once daily
Typical maximum dose:	60 mg/day
Proportion eliminated unchanged:	1 %

Adjustment for Kidney Disease

FDA-approved product labeling:	*CrCL ≥80 mL/min*	*15–60 mg orally once daily*
	CrCL 10–79 mL/min	*15–60 mg orally once daily*
	CrCL <10 mL/min	*No data, not recommended*
	Hemodialysis	*No data, not recommended*
	Anuria	*Contraindicated; no benefit can be expected*
Alternative adjustment:	*Data not available*	

Dosage Adjustment of Medications Eliminated by the Kidneys

Topiramate - Selected References

Bialer M, Doose DR, Murthy B, et al. Pharmacokinetic interactions of topiramate. Clin Pharmacokinet. 2004;43:763–80.

Britzi M, Perucca E, Soback S, et al. Pharmacokinetic and metabolic investigation of topiramate disposition in healthy subjects in the absence and in the presence of enzyme induction by carbamazepine. Epilepsia. 2005;46:378–84.

Browning L, Parke D Jr, Liu-DeRyke X, Shah A, Coplin WM, Rhoney DH. Possible removal of topiramate by continuous renal replacement therapy. J Neurol Sci. 2010;288:186–9.

Christensen J, Højskov CS, Dam M, Poulsen JH. Plasma concentration of topiramate correlates with cerebrospinal fluid concentrations. Epilepsia. 2001;23:529–33.

Contin M, Riva R, Albani F, Avoni P, Baruzzi A. Topiramate therapeutic monitoring in patients with epilepsy: effect of concomitant antiepileptic drugs. Ther Drug Monit. 2002;24:332–7.

Doose DR, Brodie MJ, Wilson EA, et al. Topiramate and lamotrigine pharmacokinetics during repetitive monotherapy and combination therapy in epilepsy patients. Epilepsia. 2003;44:917–22.

Garvey WT, Ryan DH, Look M, et al. Two-year sustained weight loss and metabolic benefits with controlled-release phentermine/topiramate in obese and overweight adults (SEQUEL): a randomized, placebo-controlled, phase 3 extension study. Am J Clin Nutr. 2010;95:297–308.

Izzedine H, Launay-Vacher V, Deray G. Topiramate-induced renal tubular acidosis [letter]. Am J Med. 2004;116:281–2.

Lacerda C, Krummel T, Sabourdy Ryvlin P, Hirsch E. Optimizing therapy of seizures in patients with renal or hepatic dysfunction. Neurology. 2006;67(Suppl 4):S28–33.

Lindberger M, Tomson T, Öhman I, Wallstedt L, Ståhle L. Estimation of topiramate in subdural cerebrospinal fluid, subcutaneous extracellular fluid, and plasma: a single case microdialysis study. Epilepsia. 1999;40:800–2.

Lyseng-Williamson KA, Yang LPH. Topiramate: a review of its use in the treatment of epilepsy. Drugs. 2007;67:2231–56.

McIntyre CW, Owen PJ. Prescribing drugs in kidney disease. In: Brenner BM, editor. Brenner and Rector's the kidney. 8th ed. Philadelphia: Saunders Elsevier; 2008. p. 1930–55.

Mirza NA, Alfirevic A, Jorgensen A, Marson AG, Pirmohamed M. Metabolic acidosis with topiramate and zonisamide: an assessment of its severity and predictors. Pharmacogenet Genomics. 2011;21:297–302.

Mirza N, Marson AG, Pirmohamed M. Effect of topiramate on acid–base balance: extent, mechanism and effects. Br J Clin Pharmacol. 2009;68:655–61.

Perucca E. A pharmacological and clinical review on topiramate, a new antiepileptic drug. Pharmacol Res. 1997;35:241–56.

Ramsay RE, Uthman B, Pryor FM, et al. Topiramate in older patients with partial-onset seizures: a pilot double-blind, dose-comparison study. Epilepsia. 2008;49:1180–5.

Rosenfeld WE. Topiramate: a review of preclinical, pharmacokinetic, and clinical data. Clin Ther. 1997;19:1294–308.

Rosenfeld WE, Kiao S, Kramer LD, et al. Comparison of the steady-state pharmacokinetics of topiramate and valproate in patients with epilepsy during monotherapy and concomitant therapy. Epilepsia. 1997;38:324–33.

Sacré A, Jouret F, Manicourt D, Devuyst O. Topiramate induces type 3 renal tubular acidosis by inhibiting renal carbonic anhydrase [letter]. Nephrol Dial Transplant. 2006;21:2995–6.

Shank RP, Doose DR, Streeter AJ, Bialer M. Plasma and whole blood pharmacokinetics of topiramate: the role of carbonic anhydrase. Epilepsy Res. 2005;63:103–12.

Shank RP, Maryanoff BE. Molecular pharmacodynamics, clinical therapeutics, and pharmacokinetics of topiramate. CNS Neurosci Ther. 2008;14:120–42.

Shiber JR. Severe non-anion gap metabolic acidosis induced by topiramate: a case report. J Emerg Med. 2010;38:494–6.

Suppes T. Review of the use of topiramate for treatment of bipolar disorders. J Clin Psychopharmacol. 2002;22:599–609.

Topamax® capsule, coated pellets and tablet, coated [package insert]. Titusville: Ortho-McNeil Neurologics Division of Ortho-McNeill-Janssen Pharmaceuticals Inc; 2008.

Vovk T, Jakovljević MB, Kos MK, Janković SM, Mrhar A, Grabnar I. A nonlinear mixed effects modeling analysis of topiramate: pharmacokinetics in patients with epilepsy. Biol Pharm Bull. 2010;33:1176–82.

Wilner A, Raymond, Pollard R. Topiramate and metabolic acidosis. Epilepsia. 1999;40:792–5.

Zanotta N, Raggi ME, Radice L, Degrate A, Bresolin N, Zucca C. Clinical evidence with topiramate dosing and serum levels in patients with epilepsy. Seizure. 2006;15:86–92.

Dosage Adjustment of Medications Eliminated by the Kidneys

Topiramate/Topamax®   {**Antiepileptic; adjunctive analgesic; ℞ for alcoholism or migraine**}

Usual initial dose:	25 mg orally twice daily
Usual maintenance dose:	100–200 mg orally twice daily (epilepsy) or 50 mg orally twice daily (migraine)
Typical maximum dose:	1,600 mg/day
Proportion eliminated unchanged:	70 %

Adjustment for Kidney Disease

FDA-approved product labeling:		*The major route of elimination of unchanged topiramate and its metabolites is via the kidney. Dosage adjustment may be required in patients with reduced renal function.*
	CrCL ≤70 mL/min	*50–100 mg orally twice daily (epilepsy) or 25 mg orally twice daily (migraine) (50 % decrease)*
	Hemodialysis	*A supplemental dose of topiramate may be required. The actual adjustment should take into account (1) the duration of dialysis period, (2) the clearance rate of the dialysis system being used, and (3) the effective clearance of topiramate in the patient being dialyzed*
Alternative adjustment:	*GFR >50 mL/min*	*200 mg orally every 12 h*
	GFR 10–50 mL/min	*100 mg orally every 12 h (50 % decrease)*
	GFR <10 mL/min	*25–50 mg enterally every 12 h (75 % decrease)*
	Hemodialysis	*50 mg orally every 12 h; dose after hemodialysis on dialysis days (50 % decrease)*
	CAPD	*25–50 mg orally every 12 h (75 % decrease)*
	CVVHDF	*100–200 mg enterally every 12 h*

Dosage Adjustment of Medications Eliminated by the Kidneys

Topotecan (Oral) - Selected References

Aronoff GA, Bennett WM, Berns JS, et al. Drug prescribing in renal failure: dosing guidelines for adults and children. 5th ed. Philadelphia: American College of Physicians; 2007.

Brogden RN, Wiseman LR. Topotecan: a review of its potential in advanced ovarian cancer. Drugs. 1998;56:709–23.

Creemers GJ, Gerrits CJH, Eckhardt JR, et al. Phase I and pharmacologic study of oral topotecan administered twice daily for 21 days to adult patients with solid tumors. J Clin Oncol. 1997;15:1087–93.

Dennis MJ, Beijnen JH, Grochow LB, van Warmerdam LJC. An overview of the clinical pharmacology of topotecan. Semin Oncol. 1997;24(Suppl 5):S5–12.

Herben VMM, ten Bokkel Huinink WW, Beijnen JH. Clinical pharmacokinetics of topotecan. Clin Pharmacokinet. 1996;31:85–102.

Hycamtin® capsule [package insert]. Research Triangle Park: GlaxoSmithKline; 2011.

Dosage Adjustment of Medications Eliminated by the Kidneys

__Topotecan (Oral)__/Hycamtin®   {__Antineoplastic; topoisomerase inhibitor__}

__Usual initial dose:__	2.3 mg/m^2
__Usual maintenance dose:__	2.3 mg/m^2 orally once daily for five consecutive days repeated every 21 days
__Typical maximum dose:__	2.3 mg/m^2/day
__Proportion eliminated unchanged:__	20 %

Adjustment for Kidney Disease

__FDA-approved product labeling:__	*CrCL 50–80 mL/min*	*2.3 mg/m^2 orally once daily for five consecutive days repeated every 21 days*
	CrCL 30–49 mL/min	*1.8 mg/m^2 orally once daily for five consecutive days repeated every 21 days*
	CrCL <30 mL/min	*Insufficient data are available to provide a dosage recommendation; risk of toxic reactions may be greater in patients with impaired renal function*
__Alternative adjustment:__	*Data not available*	

Note: Hematological and other considerations may suggest further dosage adjustments.

693

Dosage Adjustment of Medications Eliminated by the Kidneys

Topotecan (IV) - Selected References

Aronoff GA, Bennett WM, Berns JS, et al. Drug prescribing in renal failure: dosing guidelines for adults and children. 5th ed. Philadelphia: American College of Physicians; 2007.

Brogden RN, Wiseman LR. Topotecan: a review of its potential in advanced ovarian cancer. Drugs. 1998;56:709–23.

Dennis MJ, Beijnen JH, Grochow LB, van Warmerdam LJC. An overview of the clinical pharmacology of topotecan. Semin Oncol. 1997;24(Suppl 5):S5–12.

Gallo JM, Laub PB, Rowinsky EK, Grochow LB, Baker SD. Population pharmacokinetic model for topotecan derived from phase I clinical trials. J Clin Oncol. 2000;18:2459–67.

Grochow LB, Rowinsky EK, Johnson R, et al. Pharmacokinetics and pharmacodynamics of topotecan in patients with advanced cancer. Drug Metab Dispos. 1992;20:706–13.

Haas NB, LaCreta FP, Walczak J, et al. Phase I/pharmacokinetic study of topotecan by 24-hour continuous infusion weekly. Cancer Res. 1994;54:1220–6.

Herben VMM, ten Bokkel Huinink WW, Beijnen JH. Clinical pharmacokinetics of topotecan. Clin Pharmacokinet. 1996;31:85–102.

O'Dwyer PJ, LaCreta FP, Haas NB, et al. Clinical, pharmacokinetic and biological studies of topotecan. Cancer Chemother Pharmacol. 1994;34(Suppl):S46–52.

O'Reilly S, Rowinsky EK, Slichenmyer W, et al. Phase I and pharmacologic study of topotecan in patients with impaired renal function. J Clin Oncol. 1996;14:3062–73.

Rowinsky EK, Adjei A, Donehower RC, et al. Phase I pharmacodynamic study of the topoisomerase I-inhibitor topotecan in patients with refractory acute leukemia. J Clin Oncol. 1994;12:2193–203.

Rowinsky EK, Grochow LB, Hendricks CB, et al. Phase I pharmacologic study of topotecan: a novel topoisomerase inhibitor. J Clin Oncol. 1992;10:647–56.

Saltz L, Sirott M, Young C, et al. Phase I clinical and pharmacology study of topotecan given daily for 5 consecutive days to patients with advanced solid tumors, with attempt at dose intensification using recombinant granulocyte colony-stimulating factor. J Natl Cancer Inst. 1993;85:1499–507.

Sung C, Blaney SM, Cole DE, Balis FM, Dedrick RL. A pharmacokinetic model of topotecan clearance from plasma and cerebrospinal fluid. Cancer Res. 1994;54:5118–22.

Topotecan injection solution concentrate [package insert]. Lake Forest: Hospira Inc; 2011.

van Warmerdam LJC, Creemers G-J, Rodenhuis S, et al. Pharmacokinetics and pharmacodynamics of topotecan given on a daily-times-five schedule in phase II clinical trials using a limited-sampling procedure. Cancer Chemother Pharmacol. 1996;38:254–60.

van Warmerdam LJC, ten Bokkel Huinink WW, Rodenhuis S, et al. Phase I clinical and pharmacokinetic study of topotecan administered by a 24-hour continuous infusion. J Clin Oncol. 1995;13:1768–76.

van Warmerdam LJC, Verweij J, Schellens JHM, et al. Pharmacokinetics and pharmacodynamics of topotecan administered daily for 5 days every 3 weeks. Cancer Chemother Pharmacol. 1995;35:237–45.

Dosage Adjustment of Medications Eliminated by the Kidneys

<u>Topotecan (IV)</u>/Hycamtin® IV   {Antineoplastic; topoisomerase inhibitor}

Usual initial dose: 1.5 mg/m^2 IV

Usual maintenance dose: 1.5 mg/m^2 IV daily for five consecutive days, starting on day 1 of a 21-day course (ovarian cancer, non-small cell lung cancer); in the absence of tumor progression, a minimum of four courses is recommended

Typical maximum dose: 1.5 mg/m^2/day

Proportion eliminated unchanged: 50 %

Adjustment for Kidney Disease

FDA-approved product labeling:	*CrCL 40–60 mL/min*	*1.5 mg/m^2 IV daily for five consecutive days, starting on day 1 of a 21-day course (ovarian cancer, non-small cell lung cancer) (no change/adjustment needed)*
	CrCL 20–39 mL/min	*0.75 mg/m^2 IV daily for five consecutive days starting on day 1 of a 21-day course (cervical cancer or ovarian cancer, non-small cell lung cancer)*
	CrCL <20 mL/min	*Insufficient data are available to provide a dosage recommendation*
Alternative adjustment:	*GFR 40–59 mL/min*	*1–1.5 mg/m^2 IV daily for 5 consecutive days starting on day one of a 21-day course (extensively pretreated patients may require further dose reductions)*
	GFR 20–39 mL/min	*0.5–1 mg/m^2 IV daily for 5 consecutive days starting on day one of a 21-day course (extensively pretreated patients may require further dose reductions)*
	GFR <20 mL/min	*Data not available; preferably avoid*
	Hemodialysis	*Data not available; preferably avoid*
	CAPD	*Data not available; preferably avoid*
	CRRT	*0.75 mg/m^2 IV on days 1, 2, and 3 followed by cisplatin on day 1 repeated every 21 days*

Note: Hematological and other considerations may suggest further dosage adjustments

Dosage Adjustment of Medications Eliminated by the Kidneys

Tositumomab and ^{131}I-Tositumomab - Selected References

Bexxar® dosimetric and therapeutic kit [package insert]. Seattle: Corixa Corp, 2004.

Davies AJ. A review of tositumomab and I^{131} tositumomab radioimmunotherapy for the treatment of follicular lymphoma. Expert Opin Biol Ther. 2005;5:577–88.

Kaminski MS, Tuck M, Estes J, et al. ^{131}I-tositumomab therapy as initial treatment for follicular lymphoma. N Engl J Med. 2005;352:441–9.

Kaminski MS, Radford JA, Gregory SA, et al. Re-treatment with I-131 tositumomab in patients with non-Hodgkin's lymphoma who had previously responded to I-131 tositumomab. J Clin Oncol. 2005;23:7985–93.

Kaminski MS, Zasadny KR, Francis IR, et al. Radioimmunotherapy of B-cell lymphoma with [^{131}I]anti-B1 (anti-CD20) antibody. N Engl J Med. 1993;329:459–65.

Klemens S, Wolf I, Baumgartl H-J, et al. Biodistribution and kinetics of 131I-lablled anti-CD20 MAB IDEC-C2B8 (rituximab) in relapsed non-Hodgkin's lymphoma. Eur J Nucl Med. 2002;29:1276–82.

Mones JV, Coleman M, Kostakoglu L, et al. Dose-attenuated radioimmunotherapy with tositumomab and iodine 131 tositumomab in patients with recurrent non-Hodgkin's lymphoma (NHL) and extensive bone marrow involvement. Leuk Lymphoma. 2007;48:342–8.

Scheidhauer K, Wolf I, Baumgartl H-J, et al. Biodistribution and kinetics of ^{131}I-labelled anti-CD20 MAB IDEC-C2B8 (rituximab) in relapsed non-Hodgkin's lymphoma. Eur J Nucl Med. 2002;29:1276–82.

Wahl RL. Tositumomab and ^{131}I therapy in non-Hodgkin's lymphoma. J Nucl Med. 2005:46(Suppl):128–40.

Dosage Adjustment of Medications Eliminated by the Kidneys

<u>__Tositumomab and ^{131}I-Tositumomab__</u>/Bexxar®   **{Antineoplastic; monoclonal antibody; radiopharmaceutical}**

Usual initial dose: Dosimetric step—450 mg IV (tositumomab) and 35 mg IV (^{131}I-tositumomab)

Usual maintenance dose: Therapeutic step—450 mg IV (tositumomab) and 35 mg IV (^{131}I-tositumomab) with detailed adjustment according to gamma camera dose calibrator procedures and biodistribution studies

Typical maximum dose: 450 mg IV (tositumomab) and 35 mg IV (^{131}I-tositumomab)

Proportion eliminated unchanged: 98 %

Adjustment for Kidney Disease

    FDA-approved product labeling: *[131]I- tositumomab and iodine-131 are excreted primarily by the kidneys. Impaired renal function may decrease the rate of excretion of the radiolabeled iodine and increase patient exposure to the radioactive component of the tositumomab and ^{131}I-tositumomab therapeutic regimen. There are no data regarding the safety of administration of the tositumomab and ^{131}I-tositumomab therapeutic regimen in patients with impaired renal function*

    Alternative adjustment: *Data not available*

Dosage Adjustment of Medications Eliminated by the Kidneys

Tramadol - Selected References

Aronoff GA, Bennett WM, Berns JS, et al. Drug prescribing in renal failure: dosing guidelines for adults and children. 5th ed. Philadelphia: American College of Physicians; 2007.

Barnung SK, Treschow M, Borgbjerg FM. Respiratory depression following oral tramadol in patient with impaired renal function. Pain. 1997;71:111–2.

Bodalia B, McDonald CJ, Smith KJ, O'Brien C, Cousens L. A comparison of the pharmacokinetics, clinical efficacy, and tolerability of once-daily tramadol tablets with normal release tramadol capsules. J Pain Symptom Manage. 2003;25:142–9.

Elsing B, Blaschke G. Achiral and chiral high-performance liquid chromatographic determination of tramadol and its major metabolite in urine after oral administration of racemic tramadol. J Chromatogr. 1993;612:223–30.

Gan SH, Ismail R, Adnan WAW, Zulmi W, Jelliffe RW. Population pharmacokinetic modelling of tramadol with application of the NPEM algorithms. J Clin Pharm Ther. 2004;29:455–63.

Grond S, Sablotzki A. Clinical pharmacology of tramadol. Clin Pharmacokinet. 2004;43:879–923.

Hui-Chen L, Yang Y, Na W, Ming D, Jian-Fang L, Hong-Yuan X. Pharmacokinetics of the enantiomers of *trans*-tramadol and its active metabolite, *trans-O*-desmethytramadol, in healthy male and female Chinese volunteers. Chirality. 2004;16:112–8.

Izzedine H, Launay-Vacher V, Abbara C, Aymard G, Bassilos N, Deray G. Pharmacokinetics of tramadol in a hemodialysis patient [letter]. Nephron. 2002;92:755–6.

Klotz U. Tramadol—the impact of its pharmacokinetic and pharmacodynamic properties on the clinical management of pain. Arzneimittelforschung. 2003;53:681–7.

Levine B, Ramcharitar V, Smialek JE. Tramadol distribution in four postmortem cases. Forensic Sci Int. 1997;86:43–8.

Liu H-C, Liu T-J, Yang Y-Y, Hou Y-N. Pharmacokinetics of enantiomers of *trans*-tramadol and its active metabolite, *trans-O*-demethyltramadol, in human subjects. Acta Pharmacol Sin. 2001;22:91–6.

Marks JL, Colebatch AN, Buchbinder R, Edwards CJ. Pain management for rheumatoid arthritis and cardiovascular or renal comorbidity (review). Cochrane Database Syst Rev. 2011;(10):CD008952. doi: 10.1002/14651858.CD008952.pub2.

Moore KA Cina S, Jones R, Selby DM, Levine B, Smith ML. Tissue distribution of tramadol and metabolites in an overdose fatality. Am J Forensic Med Pathol. 1999;20:98–100.

Niscola P, Scaramucci L, Vischini G, et al. The use of major analgesics in patients with renal dysfunction. Curr Drug Targets. 2010;11:752–8.

Pedersen RS, Damkier P, Brøsen K. Enantioselective pharmacokinetics of tramadol in CYP2D6 extensive and poor metabolizers. Eur J Clin Pharmacol. 2006;62:513–21.

Quetglas EG, Azanza R, Cardenas E, Sádaba B, Campanero MA. Stereoselective pharmacokinetic analysis of tramadol and its main phase I metabolites in healthy subjects after intravenous and oral administration of racemic tramadol. Biopharm Drug Dispos. 2007;28:19–33.

Sachdeva DK, Jolly BT. Tramadol overdose requiring prolonged opioid antagonism [letter]. Am J Emerg Med. 1997;15:217–8.

Scott LJ, Perry CM. Tramadol: a review of its use in postoperative pain. Drugs. 2000;60:139–76.

Slanař O, Nobilis M, Kvétina J, Matoušková O, Idle JR, Perlík F. Pharmacokinetics of tramadol is affected by *MDR1* polymorphism *C3435T* [letter]. Eur J Clin Pharmacol. 2007;63:419–21.

Stamer UM, Stüber F, Muders T, Musshof F. Respiratory depression with tramadol in a patient with renal impairment and CYP2D6 gene duplication. Anesth Analg. 2008;107:926–9.

Stubhaug A, Grimstad J, Breivik H. Lack of analgesic effect of 50 and 100 mg oral tramadol after orthopedic surgery: a randomized, double-blind, placebo and standard active drug comparison. Pain. 1995;62:111–8.

Tzvetkov MV, Saadatmand AR, Lötsch J, Tegeder I, Stingl JC, Brockmöller J. Genetically polymorphic OCT1: another piece in the puzzle of the variable pharmacokinetics of the opioidergic drug tramadol. Clin Pharmacol Ther. 2011;90:143–50.

Ultram® tablet, coated [package insert]. Raritan: PriCara Division of Ortho-McNeil-Janssen Pharmaceuticals Inc; 2009.

Valadares de Moraes N, Luaretti GR, Napolitano MN, Santos NR, Godoy ALPC, Lanchote VL. Enantioselective analysis of unbound tramadol, *O*-desmethyltramadol and *N*-desmethyltramadol in plasma by ultrafiltration and LC-MS/MS: application to clinical pharmacokinetics. J Chromatogr B Analyt Technol Biomed Life Sci. 2012;880:140–7.

Dosage Adjustment of Medications Eliminated by the Kidneys

<u>**Tramadol**</u>/Ultram®	{**Analgesic, centrally acting**}

Usual initial dose: 25 mg orally

Usual maintenance dose: 25 mg orally every morning, increasing by 25 mg/day every 3 days to 100 mg/day (25 mg orally four times daily); thereafter, the total daily dose may be increased by 50 mg as tolerated every 3 days to reach 200 mg/day (50 mg four times daily); after titration, 50–100 mg can be administered *prn* for pain relief every 4–6 h, not to exceed 400 mg/day

Typical maximum dose: 400 mg/day

Proportion eliminated unchanged: 95 %

Adjustment for Kidney Disease

FDA-approved product labeling: *Impaired renal function results in a decreased rate and extent of excretion of tramadol and its active metabolite*

	CrCL <30 mL/min	*50–100 mg orally every 12 h as needed; maximum 200 mg/day*
	Hemodialysis	*50–100 mg orally every 12 h as needed; maximum 200 mg/day; dose after hemodialysis on dialysis days*
Alternative adjustment:	*GFR >50 mL/min*	*50–100 mg orally every 4–6 h as needed for pain relief, not to exceed 400 mg/day*
	GFR 10–50 mL/min	*50–100 mg orally every 6–12 h as needed for pain*
	GFR <10 mL/min	*50 mg orally every 12 h as needed for pain*
	Hemodialysis	*50 mg orally every 12 h as needed for pain; administer after hemodialysis on dialysis days*
	CAPD	*50 mg orally every 12 h as needed for pain*
	CRRT	*Not applicable; preferably avoid*

Dosage Adjustment of Medications Eliminated by the Kidneys

Trandolapril - Selected References

Aepfelbacher FC, Messerli FH, Nunez E, Michalewica L. Cardiovascular effects of a trandolapril/verapamil combination in patients with mild to moderate essential hypertension. Am J Cardiol. 1997;79:826–8.

Aronoff GA, Bennett WM, Berns JS, et al. Drug prescribing in renal failure: dosing guidelines for adults and children. 5th ed. Philadelphia: American College of Physicians; 2007.

Bakris GL, Gaxiola E, Messerli FH, et al. Clinical outcomes in the diabetes cohort of the International Verapamil SR-Trandolapril Study. Hypertension. 2004;44:637–42.

Bakris GL, Weir MR, DeQuattro V, McMahon FG. Effects of an ACE inhibitor/calcium antagonist combination on proteinuria in diabetic nephropathy. Kidney Int. 1998;54:1283–9.

Bevan EG, McInnes GT, Aldigier JC, et al. Effect of renal function on the pharmacokinetics and pharmacodynamics of trandolapril. Br J Clin Pharmacol. 1993;35:128–35.

Danielson B, Querin S, LaRochelle P, et al. Pharmacokinetics and pharmacodynamics of trandolapril after repeated administration of 2 mg to patients with chronic renal failure and healthy control subjects. J Cardiovasc Pharmacol. 1994;23(Suppl 4):S50–9.

Gokel Y, Paydas S, Duru M. High-dose verapamil-trandolapril induced rhabdomyolysis and acute renal failure [letter]. Am J Emerg Med. 2000;18:738–9.

Hemmelder MH, de Zeeuw D, de Jong PE. Antiproteinuric efficacy of verapamil in comparison to trandolapril in non-diabetic renal disease. Nephrol Dial Transplant. 1999;14:98–104.

Ichihara A, Hayashi M, Kaneshiro Y, et al. Low doses of losartan and trandolapril improve arterial stiffness in hemodialysis patients. Am J Kidney Dis. 2005;45:866–74.

Kümler T, Gislason GH, Kober L, Gustafsson F, Schou M, Torp-Pedersen C. Renal function at the time of a myocardial infarction maintains prognostic value for more than 10 years. BMC Cardiovasc Disord. 2011;11:37. doi: 10.1186/1471-2261-11-37.

Mavik® tablet. North Chicago: Abbott Laboratories; 2011.

McIntyre CW, Owen PJ. Prescribing drugs in kidney disease. In: Brenner BM, editors. Brenner and Rector's the kidney. 8th ed. Philadelphia: Saunders Elsevier; 2008. p. 1930–55.

Oka K, Imai E, Moriyama T, et al. A clinicopathological study of IgA nephropathy in renal transplant recipients: beneficial effect of angiotensin-converting enzyme inhibitor. Nephrol Dial Transplant. 2000;15:689–95.

Pepine CJ, Handberg EM, Cooper-DeHoff RM, et al. A calcium antagonist vs a non-calcium antagonist hypertension treatment strategy for patients with coronary heart disease. The International Verapamil-Trandolapril Study (INVEST): a randomized controlled trial. JAMA. 2003;290:2805–16.

Remuzzi G, Macia M, Ruggenenti P. Prevention and treatment of diabetic renal disease in type 2 diabetes: the BENEDICT study. J Am Soc Nephrol. 2006;17(4 Suppl 2):S90–7.

Shoda J, Kanno Y, Suzuki H. A five-year comparison of the renal protective effects of angiotensin-converting enzyme inhibitors and angiotensin receptor blockers in patients with non-diabetic nephropathy. Intern Med. 2006;45:193–8.

Solomon SD, Rice MM, Jablonski KA, et al. Renal function and effectiveness of angiotensin-converting enzyme inhibitor therapy in patients with chronic stable coronary disease in the Prevention of Events with ACE inhibition (PEACE) trial. Circulation. 2006;114:26–31.

Song JC, White CM. Clinical pharmacokinetics and selective pharmacodynamics of new angiotensin converting enzyme inhibitors: an update. Clin Pharmacokinet. 2002;41:207–24.

van der Ent M, Remme WJ, de Leeuw PW, Bartels GL. Renal hemodynamic effects in patients with moderate to severe heart failure during chronic treatment with trandolapril. Cardiovasc Drugs Ther. 1998;12:395–403.

Wiseman LR, McTavish D. Trandolapril: a review of its pharmacodynamics and pharmacokinetic properties, and therapeutic use in essential hypertension. Drugs. 1994;48:71–90.

Dosage Adjustment of Medications Eliminated by the Kidneys

<u>Trandolapril</u>/Mavik®   **{Antihypertensive, vasodilator, angiotensin converting enzyme (ACE)/renin inhibitor}**

Usual initial dose:	1 mg orally once daily in nonblack and 2 mg orally once daily in black patients
Usual maintenance dose:	2–4 mg orally once daily
Typical maximum dose:	8 mg/day
Proportion eliminated unchanged:	33 %

Adjustment for Kidney Disease

FDA-approved product labeling:	*CrCL < 30 mL/min*	*Recommended starting dose is 0.5 mg daily; subsequently titrate to the optimal response*
Alternative adjustment:	*GFR >50 mL/min*	*1–4 mg orally once daily*
	GFR 10–50 mL/min	*0.5–4 mg orally once daily*
	GFR <10 mL/min	*0.5–2 mg orally once daily (50 % decrease)*
	Hemodialysis	*0.5–2 mg orally once daily (50 % decrease)*
	CAPD	*0.5–2 mg orally once daily (50 % decrease)*
	CRRT	*1–4 mg orally once daily*

Dosage Adjustment of Medications Eliminated by the Kidneys

Tranexamic Acid - Selected References

Al Ameel T, West M. Tranexamic acid treatment of life-threatening hematuria in polycystic kidney disease. Int J Nephrol. 2011;2011:203579. doi: 10.4061/2011/203579.

Aronoff GA, Bennett WM, Berns JS, et al. Drug prescribing in renal failure: dosing guidelines for adults and children. 5th ed. Philadelphia: American College of Physicians; 2007.

Brown JR, Birkmeyer NJO, O'Connor GT. Meta-analysis comparing the effectiveness and adverse outcomes of antifibrinolytic agents in cardiac surgery. Circulation. 2007;115:2801–13.

Cesati V, Sandreli L, Speziali G, Calori G, Grasso MA, Spagnolo S. Hemostatic effects of tranexamic acid in elective thoracic aortic surgery: a prospective, randomized, double-blind, placebo-controlled study. J Thorac Cardiovasc Surg. 2002;123:1084–91.

Cyclocapron® injection [package insert]. New York: Pharmacia & Upjohn Division of Pfizer Inc; 2011.

Fernández-Lucas M, Liaño F, Navarro JF, Sastre JL, Quereda C, Ortuño J. Acute renal failure secondary to antifibrinolytic therapy [letter]. Nephron. 1995;69:478–9.

Fiechtner BK, Nuttall GA, Johnson ME, et al. Plasma tranexamic acid concentrations during cardiopulmonary bypass. Anesth Analg. 2001;92:1131–6.

Galbuser M, Remuzzi G, Boccardo P. Treatment of bleeding in dialysis patients. Semin Dial. 2009;22:279–86.

Henry DA, Carless PA, Moxey AJ, et al. Anti-fibrinolytic use for minimizing perioperative allogeneic blood transfusion (review). Cochrane Database Syst Rev. 2011;(3):CD001886. doi: 10.1002/14651858.CD001886.pub4.

Katsaros D, Petricevic M, Snow NJ, Woodhall DD, van Bergen R. Tranexamic acid reduces postbypass blood use: a double-blinded, prospective, randomized study of 210 patients. Ann Thorac Surg. 1996;61:1131–5.

Keyl C, Uhl R, Beyersdorf F, et al. High-dose tranexamic acid is related to increased risk of generalized seizures after aortic valve replacement. Eur J Cardiothorac Surg. 2011;39:e114–21. doi: 10.1016/j.ejcts.2010.12.030.

Kimura S, Odawara J, Aoki T, et al. Use of tranexamic acid for disseminated intravascular coagulation with excessive fibrinolysis associated with aortic dissection in a patient with chronic renal failure. Int J Hematol. 2009;89:549–52.

Kitimura H, Matsui I, Itoh N, et al. Tranexamic acid-induced visual impairment in a hemodialysis patient. Clin Exp Nephrol. 2003;7:311–4.

Koo J-R, Lee Y-K, Kim Y-S, Cho W-Y, Kim H-K, Won N-H. Acute renal cortical necrosis caused by an antifibrinolytic drug (tranexamic acid). Nephrol Dial Transplant. 1999;14:750–2.

Lysteda® tablet [package insert]. Parsippany: Ferring Pharmaceuticals Inc; 2011.

Martin K, Knorr J, Breuer T, et al. Seizures after open heart surgery: comparison of ε-aminocaproic acid and tranexamic acid. J Cardiothorac Vasc Anesth. 2011;25:20–5.

Mezzano D, Panes O, Muñoz B, et al. Tranexamic acid inhibits fibrinolysis, shortens the bleeding time and improves platelet function in patients with chronic renal failure. Thromb Haemost. 1999;82:1250–4.

Moore KA, Morin E, Marenco T, Lavigne JR, Morelli G. Pharmacokinetic studies in women of 2 novel oral formulations of tranexamic acid therapy for heavy menstrual bleeding. Am J Ther. 2011; E-pub ahead of print. doi: 10.1097/MJT.0b013e318205427a.

Nutall GA, Gutierrez MC, Dewey JD, et al. A preliminary study of a new tranexamic acid dosing schedule for cardiac surgery. J Cardiothorac Vasc Anesth. 2008;22:230–5.

Odabaş AR, Çetinkaya R, Selçuk Y, Kaya H, Coşkun Ū. Tranexamic acid-induced acute renal cortical necrosis in a patient with haemophilia A [letter]. Nephrol Dial Transplant. 2001;16:189–90.

Šabovič M, Laver J, Vujkovac B. Tranexamic acid is beneficial as adjunctive therapy in treating major upper gastrointestinal bleeding in dialysis patients. Nephrol Dial Transplant. 2003;18:1388–91.

Šabovič M, Zupan IP, Salobir B, et al. The effect of long term, low-dose tranexamic acid treatment on platelet dysfunction and haemoglobin levels in haemodialysis patients. Thromb Haemost. 2005;1245–50.

Sander M, Spies CD, Martiny V, Rosenthal C, Wernecke K-D, von Heymann C. Mortality associated with administration of high-dose tranexamic acid and aprotinin in primary open-heart procedures: a retrospective analysis. Crit Care. 2010;14:R148. doi: 10.1186/cc9216.

Vujkovac B, Šabovič M. Treatment of subdural and intracerebral haematomas in a haemodialysis patient with tranexamic acid. Nephrol Dial Transplant. 2000;15:107–9.

Dosage Adjustment of Medications Eliminated by the Kidneys

<u>Tranexamic Acid</u>/Lysteda®, Cyklokapron® {**Hemostatic agent; antifibrinolytic**}

Usual initial dose: 1,300 mg orally or 10 mg/kg IV

Usual maintenance dose: 1,300 mg orally three times daily (max duration 5 days) or 10 mg/kg IV three to four times daily

Typical maximum dose: 3,900 mg/day orally

Proportion eliminated unchanged: 95 %

Adjustment for Kidney Disease

FDA-approved product labeling:

Tranexamic acid dosage adjustment for patients with renal impairment

SCr (mg/dL[a])	Adjusted dose	Total daily dose (mg)	Maximum duration
>1.4 to ≤2.8	1,300 mg twice daily	2,600	5 days
>2.8 to ≤5.7	1,300 mg once daily	1,300	5 days
>5.7	650 mg once daily	650	5 days

SCr (mg/dL[a])	IV tranexamic acid dosage
1.36–2.83	10 mg/kg twice daily
2.83–5.66	10 mg/kg daily
>5.66	10 mg/kg every 48 h or
	5 mg/kg every 24 h

[a]Not calibrated or traceable to isotope dilution mass spectrometry (IDMS) standards

Alternative adjustment:

GFR >50 mL/min	10 mg/kg/dose IV three to four times daily
GFR 10–50 mL/min	6.25 mg/kg/dose IV three to four times daily (75 % decrease)
GFR <10 mL/min	2.5 mg/kg/dose IV three to four times daily (90 % decrease)
Hemodialysis	Avoid unless no suitable alternative exists; if indeed necessary, 5 mg/kg IV every 24 h
CAPD	Avoid unless no suitable alternative exists; if indeed necessary, 5 mg/kg IV every 24 h
CRRT	6.25 mg/kg/dose IV up to four times daily (75 % decrease)

Dosage Adjustment of Medications Eliminated by the Kidneys

Triamterene - Selected References

Aronoff GA, Bennett WM, Berns JS, et al. Drug prescribing in renal failure: dosing guidelines for adults and children. 5th ed. Philadelphia: American College of Physicians; 2007.

Daudon M, Jungers P. Drug-induced renal calculi: epidemiology, prevention and management. Drugs. 2004;64:245–75.

Dyckner T, Wester PO. Intracellular magnesium loss after diuretic administration. Drugs. 1984;28(Suppl 1):161–6.

Dyrenium® capsule [package insert]. Sarasota: Wellspring Pharmaceutical Corp; 2009.

Farge D, Turner MW, Roy DR, Jothy S. Dyazide-induced reversible acute renal failure associated with intracellular crystal deposition. Am J Kidney Dis. 1986;8:445–9.

Favre L, Glasson P, Vallotton MB. Reversible acute renal failure from combined triamterene and indomethacin. Ann Intern Med. 1982;96:317–20.

Gilfrich HJ, Kremer G, Möhrke W, Mutschler E, Völger K-D. Pharmacokinetics of triamterene after i.v. administration to man: determination of bioavailability. Eur J Clin Pharmacol. 1983;25:237–41.

Hanlon JT, Aspinall SL, Semla TP, et al. Consensus guidelines for oral dosing of primarily renally cleared medications in older adults. J Am Geriatr Soc. 2009;57:335–40.

Hasegawa J, Lin ET, Williams RL, Sörgel F, Benet LZ. Pharmacokinetics of triamterene and its metabolite in man. J Pharmacokinet Biopharm. 1982;10:507–23.

Hollenberg NK, Mickiewicz CW. Postmarketing surveillance in 70,898 patients treated with triamterene/hydrochlorothiazide combination (Maxzide). Am J Cardiol. 1989;63(4):37–41B.

Jick H, Dinan BJ, Hunter JR. Triamterene and renal stones. J Urol. 1982;127:224–5.

Kleeman CR, Okun R, Heller RJ. The renal regulation of sodium and potassium in patients with chronic renal failure (CRF) and the effect of diuretics on the excretion of these ions. Ann N Y Acad Sci. 1966;139:520–39.

Knauf H, Möhrke W, Mutschler E. Delayed elimination of triamterene and its active metabolite in chronic renal failure. Eur J Clin Pharmacol. 1983;24:453–6.

Lustermans FAT. A simple method for assessing patient compliance in triamterene therapy. Curr Ther Res Clin Exp. 1986;29:952–60.

Möhrke W, Knauf H, Mutschler E. Pharmacokinetics and pharmacodynamics of triamterene and hydrochlorothiazide and their combination in volunteers. Int J Clin Pharmacol Ther. 1997;35:447–52.

Mutschler E, Gilfrich HJ, Knauf H, Möhrke W, Völger K-D. Pharmacokinetics of triamterene. Clin Exp Hypertens A. 1983;5:249–69.

Pierratos A, Couture RA, Hierlihy PJ, Bell RC, Levine DZ. Bartter's syndrome, nephrocalcinosis and renal insufficiency. CMAJ. 1989;141:1055–7.

Roy LF, Villeneuve J-P, Dumont A, et al. Irreversible renal failure associated with triamterene. Am J Nephrol. 1991;11:486–8.

Sörgel F, Hasegawa J, Lin ET, Williams RL. Oral triamterene disposition. Clin Pharmacol Ther. 1985;38:306–12.

van Meyel JJM, Smits P, Gribnau FWJ. Absence of magnesium sparing effect of a single dose of triamterene in combination with frusemide in healthy male adults. Br J Clin Pharmacol. 1990;30:774–7.

Walker BR, Hoppe RC, Alexander F. Effect of triamterene on the renal clearance of calcium, magnesium, phosphate, and uric acid in man. Clin Pharmacol Ther. 1972;13:245–50.

Watson RA, Ettinger B, Deshon GE, Agee RE, Oldroyd NO. Triamterene stone: advantage of crystallographic analysis. Urology. 1981;18:238–40.

Weinberg MS, Quigg RJ, Salant DJ, Bernard DB. Anuric renal failure precipitated by indomethacin and triamterene. Nephron. 1985;40:216–8.

White DJ, Nancollas GH. Triamterene and renal stone formation. J Urol. 1982;127:593–7.

White DJ, Nancollas GH. Triamterene and renal stone formation: the influence of triamterene and triamterene stones on calcium oxalate crystallization. Calcif Tissue Int. 1987;40:79–84.

Williams RL, Thornhill D, Upton RA, et al. Absorption and disposition of two combination formulations of hydrochlorothiazide and triamterene: influence of age and renal function. Clin Pharmacol Ther. 1986;40:226–32.

Yarlagadda SG, Perazella MA. Drug-induced crystal nephropathy: an update. Expert Opin Drug Saf. 2008;7:147–58.

Dosage Adjustment of Medications Eliminated by the Kidneys

Triamterene/Dyrenium®   {**Diuretic; potassium-sparing agent**}

Usual initial dose: 50 mg orally

Usual maintenance dose: 100 mg orally twice daily after meals

Typical maximum dose: 300 mg/day

Proportion eliminated unchanged: 4 % (plus 51 % of the absorbed dose as active primary hydroxylated sulfate conjugate metabolite)

Adjustment for Kidney Disease

FDA-approved product labeling:	*Severe or progressive kidney disease or anuria/ CrCL <10 mL/min*	*Contraindicated*
Alternative adjustment:	*GFR >50 mL/min*	*50–150 mg every 12 h*
	GFR 10–50 mL/min	*Avoid due to risk for hyperkalemia and cardiac irregularities*
	GFR <10 mL/min	*Avoid due to risk for hyperkalemia and cardiac irregularities*
	Hemodialysis	*Avoid due to risk for hyperkalemia and cardiac irregularities*
	CAPD	*Avoid due to risk for hyperkalemia and cardiac irregularities*
	CRRT	*Not applicable; avoid*

Dosage Adjustment of Medications Eliminated by the Kidneys

Trimethoprim - Selected References

Ahlmén J, Brorson J-E. Pharmacokinetics of trimethoprim given in single daily doses for three days. Scand J Infect Dis. 1982;14:143–5.

Alappan R, Perazella MA, Buller GK. Hyperkalemia in hospitalized patients treated with trimethoprim-sulfamethoxazole. Ann Intern Med. 1996;124:316–20.

Aronoff GA, Bennett WM, Berns JS, et al. Drug prescribing in renal failure: dosing guidelines for adults and children. 5th ed. Philadelphia: American College of Physicians; 2007.

Bergan T, Brodwell EK, Vik-Mo H, Ånstad U. Pharmacokinetics of sulphadiazine, sulphamethoxazole and trimethoprim in patients with varying renal function. Infection. 1979;7(Suppl 4):S382–7.

Brogden RN, Carmine AA, Heel RC, Speight TM, Avery GS. Trimethoprim: a review of its antibacterial activity, pharmacokinetics and therapeutic use in urinary tract infections. Drugs. 1982;23:405–30.

Bushby SRM, Hitchings GH. Trimethoprim, a sulphonamide potentiator. Br J Pharmacol Chemother. 1968;33:72–90.

Darrell JH, Garrod LP, Waterworth PM. Trimethoprim: laboratory and clinical studies. J Clin Pathol. 1968;21:202–9.

Eiam-Ong S, Kurtzman NA, Sabatini S. Studies on the mechanism of trimethoprim-induced hyperkalemia. Kidney Int. 1996;49:1372–8.

Friesen WT, Hekster YA, Vree TB. Trimethoprim: clinical use and pharmacokinetics. Drug Intell Clin Pharm. 1981;15:325–30.

Gleckman R, Blagg N, Joubert DW. Trimethoprim: mechanisms of action, antimicrobial activity, bacterial resistance, pharmacokinetics, adverse reactions, and therapeutic indications. Pharmacotherapy. 1981;1:14–20.

Grüneberg RN, Kolbe R. Trimethoprim in the treatment of urinary infections in hospital. Br Med J. 1969;1:545–7.

Hoppu K, Koskimies O, Tuomisto J. Trimethoprim pharmacokinetics in children with renal insufficiency. Clin Pharmacol Ther. 1987;42:181–6.

Kaplan SA, Weinfeld RE, Cotler S, Abruzzo CW, Alexander K. Pharmacokinetic profile of trimethoprim in dog and man. J Pharm Sci. 1970;59:358–63.

Kastrup J, Petersen P, Bartram R, Hansen JM. The effect of trimethoprim on serum creatinine. Br J Urol. 1985;57:265–8.

Kucers A, Bennett NMcK, Kemp RJ. The use of antibiotics: a comprehensive review with clinical emphasis. 4th ed. Philadelphia: JB Lippincott Co; 1987. p.1118–202.

McIntyre CW, Owen PJ. Prescribing drugs in kidney disease. In: Brenner BM, editors. Brenner and Rector's the kidney. 8th ed. Philadelphia: Saunders Elsevier; 2008. p. 1930–55.

Myre SA, McCann J, First MR, Cluxton RH Jr. Effect of trimethoprim on serum creatinine in healthy and chronic renal failure volunteers. Ther Drug Monit. 1987;9:161–5.

Nolte H, Büttner H. Pharmacokinetics of trimethoprim and its combination with sulfamethoxazole in man after single and chronic oral administration. Chemotherapy. 1973;18:274–84.

Odlind B, Hartvig P, Fjellström KE, Lindström B, Bengtsson S. Steady state pharmacokinetics of trimethoprim 300 mg once daily in healthy volunteers assessed by two independent methods. Eur J Clin Pharmacol. 1984;26:393–7.

Perazella MA. Trimethoprim-induced hyperkalemia: clinical data, mechanism, prevention and management. Drug Saf. 2000;22:227–36.

Proloprim® tablet [package insert]. Bristol: Monarch Pharmaceuticals Inc; 2003.

Reeves DS, Wilkinson RJ. The pharmacokinetics of trimethoprim and trimethoprim/sulphonamide combinations, including penetration into body tissues. Infection. 1979;7(Suppl 4):S330–41.

Schwartz DE, Ziegler WH. Assay and pharmacokinetics of trimethoprim in man and animals. Postgrad Med J. 1969;45 (Suppl):32–7.

Smith GW, Cohen SB. Hyperkalaemia and non-oliguric renal failure associated with trimethoprim [letter]. BMJ. 1994;308:454.

Velázquez H, Perazalla MA, Wright FS, Ellison DH. Renal mechanism of trimethoprim-induced hyperkalemia. Ann Intern Med. 1993;119:296–301.

Watson ID, Stewart MJ, McIntosh SJ. Pharmacokinetics of two dosage levels of trimethoprim to 'steady-state' in normal volunteers. J Int Med Res. 1983;11:137–44.

Dosage Adjustment of Medications Eliminated by the Kidneys

<u>Trimethoprim</u>/Primsol®, Proloprim®   {Antibacterial; purine biosynthesis blocker}

Usual initial dose:	100 mg orally
Usual maintenance dose:	100 mg orally every 12 h or 200 mg orally every 24 h for 10 days
Typical maximum dose:	15–20 mg/kg/day
Proportion eliminated unchanged:	75 %

Adjustment for Kidney Disease

FDA-approved product labeling:	*CrCL 15–30 mL/min*	*50 mg orally every 12 h*
	CrCL <15 mL/min	*Not recommended*
Alternative adjustment:	*GFR >50 mL/min*	*100 mg orally every 12 h or 200 mg orally every 24 h*
	GFR 31–50 mL/min	*100 mg orally every 12 h*
	GFR 10–20 mL/min	*100 mg orally every 12–24 h*
	GFR <10 mL/min	*100 mg orally every 24 h*
	Hemodialysis	*100 mg orally every 24 h; administer after hemodialysis on dialysis days*
	CAPD	*100 mg orally every 24 h*
	CRRT	*2.5–5 mg/kg enterally every 12 h (mild infections) or 10 mg/kg enterally every 12 h (severe infections)*

Dosage Adjustment of Medications Eliminated by the Kidneys

Trimetrexate - Selected References

Allegra CJ, Jenkins J, Weiss RB, et al. A phase I and pharmacokinetic study of trimetrexate using a 24-hour continuous-infection schedule. Invest New Drugs. 1990;8:159–66.

Aronoff GA, Bennett WM, Berns JS, et al. Drug prescribing in renal failure: dosing guidelines for adults and children. 5th ed. Philadelphia: American College of Physicians; 2007.

Bishop JF, Raghaven D, Olver IN, Reece P, Morris R, Friedlander ML. A phase I study of trimetrexate (NSC 352122) administered by 5-day continuous intravenous infusion. Cancer Chemother Pharmacol. 1989;24:246–50.

Fitton B, Wagstaff AJ, McTavish D. Trimetrexate: a review of its pharmacodynamic and pharmacokinetic properties and therapeutic potential in the treatment of *Pneumocystis carinii* pneumonia. Drugs. 1995;49:563–76.

Grochow LB, Noe DA, Dole GB, et al. Phase I trial of trimetrexate glucuronate on a five-day bolus schedule: clinical pharmacology and pharmacodynamics. J Natl Cancer Inst. 1989;81:124–30.

Grochow LB, Noe DA, Ettinger DS, Donehower RC. A phase I trial of trimetrexate glucuronate (NSC 352122) given every 3 weeks: clinical pharmacology and pharmacodynamics. Cancer Chemother Pharmacol. 1989;24:314–20.

Ho DHW, Covington WP, Legha SS, Newman RA, Krakoff IH. Clinical pharmacology of trimetrexate. Clin Pharmacol Ther. 1987;42:351–6.

Huan SD, Legha SS, Raber MN, Krakoff IH. Phase I studies of trimetrexate using single and weekly dose schedules. Invest New Drugs. 1991;9:199–206.

Hudes GR, LaCreta F, DeLap RJ, Grillo-Lopez AJ, Catalano R, Comis RL. Phase I clinical and pharmacological trial of trimetrexate in combination with 5-fluorouracil. Cancer Chemother Pharmacol. 1989;24:117–22.

Hudes GR, LaCreta F, Walczak J, et al. Pharmacokinetic study of trimetrexate in combination with cisplatin. Cancer Res. 1991;51:3080–7.

Koda RT, Dubé RP, Li WY, Chatterjee DJ, Stansell JD, Sattler FR. Pharmacokinetics of trimetrexate and dapsone in AIDS patients with *Pneumocystis carinii* pneumonia. J Clin Pharmacol. 1999;39:268–74.

Lin JT, Cashmore AR, Baker M, et al. Phase I studies with trimetrexate: clinical pharmacology, analytical methodology, and pharmacokinetics. Cancer Res. 1987;47:609–16.

Marshall JL, DeLap RJ. Clinical pharmacokinetics and pharmacology of trimetrexate. Clin Pharmacokinet. 1994;26:190–200.

Neutrexin® injection powder lyophilized for solution [package insert]. Gathersberg: Medimmune Oncology Inc; 2000.

Reece PA, Morris RG, Bishop JF, Olver IN, Raghavan D. Pharmacokinetics of trimetrexate administered by five-day continuous infusion to patients with advanced cancer. Cancer Res. 1987;47:2996–9.

Stewart JA, McCormack JJ, Tong W, et al. Phase I clinical and pharmacokinetic study of trimetrexate using a daily ×5 schedule. Cancer Res. 1988;48:5029–35.

Dosage Adjustment of Medications Eliminated by the Kidneys

<u>Trimetrexate</u>/Neutrexin®	{**Antiparasitic; folate antagonist; antineoplastic; ℞ for Pneumocystis carinii pneumonia in immunocompromised patients**}

Usual initial dose: 45 mg/m^2 IV

Usual maintenance dose: 45 mg/m^2 IV once daily over 60 min (must be administered with concurrent leucovorin protection)

Typical maximum dose: 45 mg/m^2/day

Proportion eliminated unchanged: 30 %

Adjustment for Kidney Disease

FDA-approved product labeling:	*SCr >2.5 mg/dL*	*Interrupt therapy; avoid*
Alternative adjustment:	*GFR >50 mL/min*	*45 mg/m^2 IV every 24 h (with concurrent leucovorin)*
	GFR 10–50 mL/min	*Data not available*
	GFR <10 mL/min:	*Avoid due to risk for hematological toxicity*
	Hemodialysis	*Data not available*
	CAPD	*Data not available*
	CRRT	*Data not available*

Note: Hematological and other considerations may suggest further dosage adjustments

Tromethamine - Selected References

Atik M. Prevention of acute renal failure: an experimental study and a preliminary clinical report. Am J Surg. 1964;108: 384–92.

Bleich HL, Schwartz WB. Tris buffer (THAM): an appraisal of its physiologic effects and clinical usefulness. N Engl J Med. 1966;274:782–7.

Brasch H, Thies E, Iven H. Pharmacokinetics of TRIS (hydroxymethy-)aminomethane in healthy subjects and in patients with metabolic acidosis. Eur J Clin Pharmacol. 1982;22:257–64.

Chiu C-J, Shaftan GW, Limson A, Rosen PN. Renal blood flow in induced hypotension: the effects of THAM and sodium bicarbonate. J Cardiovasc Surg (Torino). 1967;8:149–54.

Goetz RH, Selmonosky CA, State D. The effect of the amine buffer tris (hydroxymethyl) amino methane (THAM) on the renal blood flow during hemorrhagic shock. Surg Gynecol Obstet. 1963;117:715–21.

Jacobs RP, Korobkin M, Lieberman RS, Seidlitz L, Carlson EL. Reversal of oliguria and renal cortical ischemia of hemorrhagic shock in the dog with tris (hydroxymethyl) amino methane (THAM): hemodynamic studies. Invest Radiol. 1975;10:273–83.

Neville WE, Scicchitano L, Maben H, Banuchi F, Peacock H. Cardiopulmonary bypass with large volume nonblood perfusate: experimental and clinical observations. Circulation. 1965;31(Suppl 1):130–6.

Nahas GG. The clinical pharmacology of THAM [tris(hydroxymethyl)aminomethane]. Clin Pharmacol Ther. 1963;4: 784–803.

Nahas GG. The use of buffers in the management of respiratory failure. Ann N Y Acad Sci. 1965;121:871–2.

Russ M, Deja M, Ott S, et al. Experimental high-volume hemofiltration with predilutional tris-hydroxymethylaminomethane for correction of low tidal volume ventilation-induced acidosis. Artif Organs. 2011;e108–17.

Saito S, Smith LL, Saito I. Prevention and treatment of acute renal failure: an experimental study. Am J Surg. 1965;110: 1982–7.

Teschan PE, Lawson NL. Studies in acute renal failure: prevention by osmotic diuresis, and observations on the effect of plasma and extracellular expansion. Nephron. 1966;3:1–16.

THAM® injection solution [package insert]. Lake Forest: Hospira Inc; 2005.

Thompson RG, Moulder RV, Harrison RW, Daicoff GR. Tromethamine (Talatrol) for acidosis therapy in surgery. Surg Clin North Am. 1963;43:179–86.

<u>**Tromethamine**</u>/THAM®   {**Alkalinizing agent; H⁺ acceptor**}

Usual initial dose:	300–700 mL IV (total mL equivalent to weight [kg] × base deficit [mEq/L] × 1.1)
Usual maintenance dose:	500–1,000 mL IV
Typical maximum dose:	15 mL/kg/h (~1,100 mL over 1 h)
Proportion eliminated unchanged:	75 %

Adjustment for Kidney Disease

FDA-approved product labeling:	*Renal disease or reduced urinary output*	*Extreme care should be exercised because of potential hyperkalemia and the possibility of decrease of excretion of tromethamine. Use cautiously with electrocardiographic monitoring and frequent serum potassium determinations*
	Uremia and anuria	*Contraindicated*
Alternative adjustment:	*Data not available*	

Dosage Adjustment of Medications Eliminated by the Kidneys

Trospium - Selected References

Bödeker R-H, Madersbacher H, Neumeister C, Zellner M. Dose escalation improves therapeutic outcome: post hoc analysis of data from a 12-week, multicentre, double-blind, parallel-group trial of trospium chloride in patients with urge incontinence. BMC Urol. 2010;10:15. doi: 10.1186/1471-2490-10-15.

Dallegari E, Malhotra B, Bungay PJ, et al. Comprehensive non-clinical evaluation of the CNS penetration potential of antimuscarinic agents for the treatment of overactive bladder. Br J Clin Pharmacol. 2011;72:235–46.

Doroshyenko O, Jetter A, Ddenthal KP, Fuhr U. Clinical pharmacokinetics of trospium chloride. Clin Pharmacokinet. 2005;44:701–20.

Halaska M, Ralph G, Wiedemann A, et al. Controlled, double-blind, multicentre clinical trial to investigate long-term tolerability and efficacy of trospium chloride in patients with detrusor instability. World J Urol. 2003;20:392–9.

Höfner K, Oelke M, Machtens S, Grünewald V. Trospium chloride – an effective drug in the treatment of overactive bladder and detrusor hyperreflexia. World J Urol. 2001;19:336–43.

Kessler TM, Bachman LM, Minder C, et al. Adverse event assessment of antimuscarinics for treating overactive bladder: a network meta-analytic approach. PLoS One. 2011;6:e16718. doi: 10.1371/journal.pone.0016718.

MacDiarmid SA, Ellsworth PI, Ginsberg DA, Oefelein Sussman DO. Safety and efficacy of once-daily trospium chloride extended-release in male patients with overactive bladder. Urology. 2011;77:24–9.

Michael MC, Hegde SS. Treatment of the overactive bladder syndrome with muscarinic receptor antagonists – a matter of metabolites? Naunyn Schmiedebergs Arch Pharmacol. 2006;374:79–85.

Nabi G, Cody JD, Hay-Smith J, Herbison GP. Anticholinergic drugs versus placebo for overactive bladder syndrome in adults (review). Cochrane Database Syst Rev. 2006;(4):CD0037181. doi: 10.1002/14651858.CD003781.pub2.

Paquette A, Gou P, Tannenbaum C. Systematic review and meta-analysis: do clinical trials testing antimuscarinic agents for overactive bladder adequately measure central nervous system adverse events? J Am Geriatr Soc. 2011;59:1332–9.

Rovner ES. Trospium chloride in the management of overactive bladder. Drugs. 2004;64:2433–46.

Sanctura® tablet [package insert]. Irvine: Allergan Inc; 2011.

Sand PK, Johnson TM II, Rovner ES, Ellsworth PI, Oefelein MG, Staskin DR. Trospium chloride once-daily extended release is efficacious and tolerated in elderly subjects (aged ≥75 years) with overactive bladder syndrome. BJU Int. 2011;107:612–20.

Schröder S. Ketter A, Zaigler M, et al. Absorption pattern of trospium chloride along the human gastrointestinal tract assessed using local enteral administration. Int J Clin Pharmacol Ther. 2004;42:543–9.

Schwantes U, Topfmeier P. Importance of pharmacological and physicochemical properties for tolerance of antimuscarinic drugs in the treatment of detrusor instability and detrusor hyperreflexia—chances for improvement of therapy. Int J Clin Pharmacol Ther. 1999;37:209–18.

Silver N, Sandage B, Sabounjian LA, Schwiderski U, Shipley J, Harnett M. Pharmacokinetics of once-daily trospium chloride 60 mg extended release and twice-daily trospium chloride 20 mg in healthy adults. J Clin Pharmacol. 2010;50:143–50.

Singh-Franco D, Machado C, Tuteja S, Zapantis A. Trospium chloride for the treatment of overactive bladder with urge incontinence. Clin Ther. 2005;27:511–30.

Staskin DR, Cardozo L. Baseline incontinence severity is predictive of the percentage of patients continent after receiving trospium chloride extended release. Int J Clin Pract. 2009;63:973–6.

Staskin DR, Harnett MD. Effect of trospium chloride on somnolence and sleepiness in patients with overactive bladder. Curr Urol Rep. 2004;5:423–6.

Staskin D, Kay G, Tannenbaum C, et al. Trospium chloride has no effect on memory testing and is assay undetectable in the central nervous system of older patients with overactive bladder. Int J Clin Pract. 2010;64:1294–300.

Wenge B, Geyer J, Bönisch H. Oxybutinin and trospium are substrates of the human organic anion cation transporters. Naunyn Schmiedebergs Arch Pharmacol. 2011;383:203–8.

Zellner M, Madersbacher H, Palmtag H, Stöhrer M, Bödeker R-H. Trospium chloride and oxybutinin hydrochloride in a German study of adults with urinary urge incontinence: results of a 12-week, multicenter, randomized, double-blind, parallel-group, flexible-dose noninferiority trial. Clin Ther. 2009;31:2519–39.

Zinner N, Gittelman M, Harris R, Susset J, Kanellos A, Auerbach S. Trospium chloride improves overactive bladder symptoms: a multicentre phase III trial. J Urol. 2004;171:2311–5.

Dosage Adjustment of Medications Eliminated by the Kidneys

Trospium/Sanctura®   {**Anticholinergic agent; ℞ for overactive bladder or urge incontinence**}

Usual initial dose:	20 mg orally
Usual maintenance dose:	20 mg orally twice daily at least 1 h before meals or given on an empty stomach
Typical maximum dose:	60 mg/day
Proportion eliminated unchanged:	70 % of an absorbed dose (bioavailability $\approx$ 10 %)

Adjustment for Kidney Disease

FDA-approved product labeling:	*CrCL <30 mL/min*	*20 mg orally once daily at bedtime*
Alternative adjustment:	*Data not available*	

V

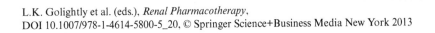

L.K. Golightly et al. (eds.), *Renal Pharmacotherapy*,
DOI 10.1007/978-1-4614-5800-5_20, © Springer Science+Business Media New York 2013

Dosage Adjustment of Medications Eliminated by the Kidneys

Valacyclovir - Selected References

Asahi T, Tsutsui M, Wakasugi M, et al. Valacyclovir neurotoxicity: clinical experience and a review of the literature. Eur J Neurol. 2009;16:457–60.

Bruxelle J, Pinchinat S. Effectiveness of antiviral treatment on acute phase of herpes zoster and development of post herpetic neuralgia: review of international publications. Med Mal Infect. 2011. Epub ahead of print. doi:10.1016/j.medmal.2011.11.001.

Corey L, Wald A, Patel R, et al. Once-daily valacyclovir to reduce the risk of transmission of genital herpes. N Engl J Med. 2004;350:11–20.

Das V, Peraldi M-N, Legendre C. Adverse neuropsychiatric effects of cytomegalovirus prophylaxis with valaciclovir in renal transplant recipients. Nephrol Dial Transplant. 2006;21:1395–401.

De Keyzer K, Van Laecke S, Peeters P, Vanholder R. Human cytomegalovirus and kidney transplantation: a clinician's update. Am J Kidney Dis. 2011;58:118–26.

Hanlon JT, Aspinall SL, Semla TP, et al. Consensus guidelines for oral dosing of primarily renally cleared medications in older adults. J Am Geriatr Soc. 2009;57:335–40.

Helldén A, Lycke J, Vander T, Svensson J-O, Odar-Cederlöf I, Ståhle L. The aciclovir metabolite CMMG is detectable in the CSF of subjects with neuropsychiatric symptoms during aciclovir and valaciclovir treatment. J Antimicrob Chemother. 2006;57:945–9.

Höglund M, Ljungman P, Weller S. Comparable acyclovir exposures produced by oral valaciclovir and intravenous aciclovir in immunocompromised cancer patients. J Antimicrob Chemother. 2001;47:855–61.

Lapolla W, DiGiorgio C, Haitz K, et al. Incidence of post-herpetic neuralgia after combination treatment with gabapentin and valacyclovir in patients with acute herpes zoster: open-label study. Arch Dermatol. 2011;147:901–7.

Leone PA, Trottier S, Miller JM. Valacyclovir for episodic treatment of genital herpes: a shorter 3-day treatment course compared with 5-day treatment. Clin Infect Dis. 2002;34:958–62.

Lowrance D, Neumayer AH-H, Legendre CM, et al. Valacyclovir for the prevention of cytomegalovirus disease after renal transplantation. N Engl J Med. 1999;340:1462–70.

Mugwanya K, Baeten JM, Mugo NR, Irungu E, Ngure K, Celum C. High-dose valacyclovir HSV-2 suppression results in greater reduction in plasma HIV-1 levels compared with standard dose acyclovir among HIV-1/HSV-2 coinfected persons: a randomized, crossover trial. J Infect Dis. 2011;204:1912–7.

Reischig T, Jindra P, Mareš J, et al. Valacyclovir for cytomegalovirus prophylaxis reduces the risk of acute renal allograft rejection. Transplantation. 2005;79:317–24.

Reischig T, Jindra P, Švecová M, Kormunda S, Opatrný K Jr, Třeška V. The impact of cytomegalovirus disease and asymptomatic infection on acute renal allograft rejection. J Clin Virol. 2006;36:146–51.

Reishig T, Němcová J, Vaněček T, et al. Intragraft cytomegalovirus infection: a randomized trial of valacyclovir prophylaxis versus pre-emptive therapy in renal transplant recipients. Antivir Ther. 2010;15:23–30.

Reischig T, Opatmy K Jr, Bouda M, Treska V, Jindra P, Svecova M. A randomized prospective controlled trial of oral ganciclovir versus oral valacyclovir for prophylaxis of cytomegalovirus disease after renal transplantation. Transpl Int. 2002;15:615–22.

Reitano M, Tyring S, Lang W, et al. Valaciclovir for the suppression of recurrent genital herpes simplex virus infection: a large-scale dose range-finding study. J Infect Dis. 1998;178:603–10.

Smith JP, Weller S, Johnson B, Nicotera J, Luther JM, Haas DW. Pharmacokinetics of acyclovir and its metabolites in cerebrospinal fluid and systemic circulation after administration of high-dose valacyclovir in subjects with normal and impaired renal function. Antimicrob Agents Chemother. 2010;54:1146–51.

Soul-Lawton J, Seaber E, On N, Wooton R, Rolan P, Posner J. Absolute bioavailability and metabolic disposition of valaciclovir, the L-valyl ester of acyclovir, following oral administration to humans. Antimicrob Agents Chemother. 1995;39:2759–64.

Stathoulopoulou F, Dhillon S, Thodis H, Stathakis C, Vargemezis V. Evaluation of valaciclovir dosage reduction in continuous ambulatory peritoneal dialysis patients. Nephron. 2002;91:164–6.

Tiyssaubt ND, Tan MBP, Nicholls K, Walker RG, Cohney SJ. Low-dose valaciclovir and cytomegalovirus immunoglobulin to prevent cytomegalovirus disease in high-risk renal transplant recipients. Nephrology (Carlton). 2011;16:113–7.

Valtrex® caplet [package insert]. Research Triangle Park: GlaxoSmithKline; 2011.

Weller S, Blum R, Doucette M, et al. Pharmacokinetics of the acyclovir prodrug valaciclovir after escalating single- and multiple-dose administration to normal volunteers. Clin Pharmacol Ther. 1993;54:595–605.

Dosage Adjustment of Medications Eliminated by the Kidneys

Valacyclovir/Valtrex®   {Antiviral}

Usual initial dose:	1,000 mg orally
Usual maintenance dose:	500–1,000 mg orally two to three times daily
Typical maximum dose:	8,000 mg/day
Proportion eliminated unchanged:	46 %

Adjustment for Kidney Disease

FDA-approved product labeling: *Valacyclovir dosage recommendations for adults with renal impairment*

Indications	Normal dosage regimen (CrCL ≥50 mL/min)	CrCL (mL/min) 30–49	10–29	<10
Cold sores (Herpes labialis): do not exceed 1 day of treatment	Two 2-g doses taken 12 h apart	Two 1-g doses taken 12 h apart	Two 500-mg doses taken 12 h apart	500 mg single dose
Genital herpes: initial episode	1 g every 12 h	No reduction	1 g every 24 h	500 mg every 24 h
Genital herpes: recurrent episode	500 mg every 12 h	No reduction	500 mg every 24 h	500 mg every 24 h
Genital herpes: suppressive therapy				
Immunocompetent patients	1 g every 24 h	No reduction	500 mg every 24 h	500 mg every 24 h
Alternate dose for immunocompetent patients with recurrences/year	500 mg every 24 h	No reduction	500 mg every 48 h	500 mg every 48 h
HIV-infected patients	500 mg every 12 h	No reduction	500 mg every 24 h	500 mg every 24 h
Herpes zoster	1 g every 8 h	1 g every 12 h	1 g every 24 h	500 mg every 24 h

Alternative adjustment:		
	GFR >75 mL/min	1,000 mg orally every 8 h; 2,000 mg orally four times daily for prophylaxis of cytomegalovirus disease following kidney transplantation
	GFR 51–75 mL/min	1,000 mg orally every 8–12 h; 1,500 mg orally four times daily for prophylaxis of cytomegalovirus disease following kidney transplantation
	GFR 25–50 mL/min	1,000 mg orally every 12 h; 1,500 mg orally three times daily for prophylaxis of cytomegalovirus disease following kidney transplantation
	GFR 10–24 mL/min	1,000 mg orally every 24 h; 1,500 mg orally two times daily for prophylaxis of cytomegalovirus disease following kidney transplantation
	GFR <10 mL/min	500 mg orally every 24 h; 1,500 mg orally every 24 h for prophylaxis of cytomegalovirus disease following kidney transplantation
	Hemodialysis	500 mg orally every 24 h; dose after hemodialysis on dialysis days
	CAPD	500 mg orally every 24 h
	CRRT	Not applicable; (consider IV acyclovir)

Dosage Adjustment of Medications Eliminated by the Kidneys

Valganciclovir - Selected References

Ayala E, Greene J, Sandin R, et al. Valganciclovir is safe and effective as pre-emptive therapy for CMV infection in allogeneic hematopoietic stem cell transplantation. Bone Marrow Transplant. 2006;37:851–6.

Caldés A, Colom H, Armendariz Y, et al. Population pharmacokinetics of ganciclovir after intravenous ganciclovir and oral valganciclovir administration in solid organ transplant patients infected with cytomegalovirus. Antimicrob Agents Chemother. 2009;53:4816–24.

Caldés A, Gil-Vernet S, Armendariz Y, et al. Sequential treatment of cytomegalovirus infection or disease with a short course of intravenous ganciclovir followed by oral valganciclovir: efficacy, safety, and pharmacokinetics. Transplant Infect Dis. 2010;12:204–12.

Chamberlain CE, Penzak SR, Alfaro RM, et al. Pharmacokinetics of low and maintenance dose valganciclovir in kidney transplant recipients. Am J Transplant. 2008;8:1297–302.

Czock D, Scholle C, Rasche FM, Schaarschmidt D, Keller F. Pharmacokinetics of valganciclovir and ganciclovir in renal impairment. Clin Pharmacol Ther. 2002;72:142–50.

Gabardi S, Magee CC, Baroletti SA, Powelson JA, Can JL, Chandraker AK. Efficacy and safety of low-dose valganciclovir for prevention of cytomegalovirus disease in renal transplant recipients: a single-center, retrospective analysis. Pharmacotherapy. 2004;24:1323–30.

Kalpoe JS, Schippers EF Eling Y, Sijpkens YW, de Fijter JW, Kroes ACM. Similar reduction of cytomegalovirus DNA load by oral valganciclovir and intravenous ganciclovir on pre-emptive therapy after renal and renal-pancreas transplantation. Antivir Ther. 2005;10:119–23.

Leone F, Akl A, Giral M, et al. Six months anti-viral prophylaxis significantly decreased cytomegalovirus disease compared with no anti-viral prophylaxis following renal transplantation. Transpl Int. 2010;23:897–906.

Manuel O, Pascual M. Perrottet N, et al. Ganciclovir exposure under a 450 mg daily dosage of valganciclovir for cytomegalovirus prevention in kidney transplantation: a prospective study. Clin Transplant. 2010;24:794–800.

Martin DF, Sierra-Madero J, Walmsley S, et al. A controlled trial of valganciclovir as induction therapy for cytomegalovirus retinitis. N Engl J Med. 2002;346:1119–26.

McIntyre CW, Owen PJ. Prescribing drugs in kidney disease. In: Brenner BM, editors. Brenner & Rector's the kidney. 8th ed. Philadelphia: Saunders Elsevier; 2008, p. 1930–55.

Perrottet N, Csajka C, Pascual M, et al. Population pharmacokinetics of ganciclovir in solid-organ transplant recipients receiving oral valganciclovir. Antimicrob Agents Chemother. 2009;53:3017–23.

Perrottet N, Decosterd LA, Meylan P, Pascual M, Biollaz J, Buclin T. Valganciclovir in adult solid organ transplant recipients: pharmacokinetic and pharmacodynamic characteristics and clinical interpretation of plasma concentration measurements. Clin Pharmacokinet. 2009;48:399–418.

Perrottet N, Manuel O, Lamoth F, et al. Variable viral clearance despite adequate ganciclovir plasma levels during valganciclovir treatment for cytomegalovirus disease in D+/R- transplant recipients. BMC Infect Dis. 2010;10:2. doi:10.1186/1471-2334-10-2.

Perrottet N, Robatel C, Meylan P, et al. Disposition of valganciclovir during continuous renal replacement therapy in two lung transplant recipients. J Antimicrob Chemother. 2008;61:1332–5.

Reishig T, Jindra P, Hes O, Švecová M, Klaboch J, Třeška V. Valacyclovir prophylaxis versus preemptive valganciclovir therapy to prevent cytomegalovirus disease after renal transplantation. Am J Transplant. 2008;18:69–77.

Reishig T, Němcová J, Vaněček T, et al. Intragraft cytomegalovirus infection: a randomized trial of valacyclovir prophylaxis versus pre-emptive therapy in renal transplant recipients. Antivir Ther. 2010;15:23–30.

Spinner ML, Saab G, Casabar E, Bowman LJ, Storch GA, Brennan DC. Impact of prophylactic versus preemptive valganciclovir on long-term renal allograft outcomes. Transplantation. 2010;90:412–8.

Sugawara M, Huang W, Fei Y-J, Leibach FH, Ganapathy V, Ganapathy ME. Transport of valganciclovir, a ganciclovir prodrug, via peptide transporters PEPT1 and PEPT2. J Pharm Sci. 2000;89:781–9.

Valcyte® tablet and powder for solution [package insert]. South San Francisco: Genentech USA Inc; 2010.

Welker H, Farhan M, Humar A, Washington C. Ganciclovir pharmacokinetics parameters do not change when extending valganciclovir prophylaxis from 100 to 200 days. Transplantation. 2010;90:1414–9.

Wiltshire H, Hirankarn S, Farrell C, et al. Pharmacokinetic profile of ganciclovir after its oral administration and from its prodrug, valganciclovir, in solid organ transplant recipients. Clin Pharmacokinet. 2005;44:495–507.

Dosage Adjustment of Medications Eliminated by the Kidneys

Valganciclovir/Valcyte®   {Antiviral; nucleoside analog; ℞ for cytomegalovirus}

Usual initial dose:	900 mg orally
Usual maintenance dose:	900 mg orally one to two times daily
Typical maximum dose:	1,800 mg/day
Proportion eliminated unchanged:	90 %

Adjustment for Kidney Disease

FDA-approved product labeling: *Valganciclovir dose modifications in patients with impaired renal function*

CrCL (mL/min)	Initial dosage	Maintenance/prevention dosage
≥60	900 mg twice daily	900 mg once daily
40–59	450 mg twice daily	450 mg once daily
25–39	450 mg once daily	450 mg every 2 days
10–24	450 mg every 2 days	450 mg twice weekly
<10 (on hemodialysis)	Not recommended	Not recommended

Alternative adjustment:

GFR >50 mL/min	*900 mg orally twice daily (induction); 900 mg orally once daily (maintenance)*
GFR 10–50 mL/min	*450 mg orally every 24–48 h*
GFR <10 mL/min	*450 mg orally twice weekly*
Hemodialysis	*Minimal data available; preferably avoid (consider IV ganciclovir)*
CAPD	*Minimal data available; preferably avoid*
CVVHF	*450 mg enterally every 48 h (consider IV ganciclovir)*

Note: Following kidney transplantation, preemptive therapy and prophylaxis appear similarly effective for management of cytomegalovirus disease. Preliminary data suggest that prophylactic valganciclovir regimens as low as 450 mg orally once daily may be effective.

Dosage Adjustment of Medications Eliminated by the Kidneys

Vancomycin - Selected References

Barraclough K, Harris M, Montessori V, Levin A. An unusual case of acute kidney injury due to vancomycin—lessons learnt from reliance on eGFR. Nephrol Dial Transplant. 2007;22:2391–4.

Böhler J, Reetze-Bonorden P, Keller E, Kramer A, Schollmeyer PJ. Rebound of plasma vancomycin levels after haemodialysis with highly permeable membranes. Eur J Clin Pharmacol. 1992;42:635–40.

Bunke CM, Aronoff GR, Luft FC. Pharmacokinetics of common antibiotics used in continuous ambulatory peritoneal dialysis. Am J Kidney Dis. 1983;3:114–7.

Cook FV, Farrar WW Jr. Vancomycin revisited. Ann Intern Med. 1978;86:813–8.

Cutler NR, Narang PK, Lesko LJ, Ninos M, Power M. Vancomycin disposition: the importance of age. Clin Pharmacol Ther. 1984;36:803–10.

Farber BF, Moellering RC Jr. Retrospective study of the toxicity of vancomycin preparations of vancomycin from 1974 to 1981. Antimicrob Agents Chemother. 1983;23:138–41.

Freeman CD, Quintilani R, Nightingale CH. Vancomycin therapeutic drug monitoring: is it necessary. Ann Pharmacother. 1993;27:594–8.

Golper TA, Noonan M Elzinga L, et al. Vancomycin pharmacokinetics, renal handling, and nonrenal clearance in normal human subjects. Clin Pharmacol Ther. 1988;43:565–70.

Hazelwood KA, Brouse SD, Pitcher WD, Hall RD. Vancomycin-associated nephrotoxicity: grave concern or death by character assassination? Am J Med. 2010;123:182.e1–182.e7. doi:10.1016/j.amjmed.2009.05.031.

Hidayat LK, Hsu DI, Quist R, Shriner KA, Wong-Beringer A. High-dose vancomycin therapy for methicillin-resistant *Staphylococcus aureus* infections: efficacy and toxicity. Arch Intern Med. 2006;166:2138–44.

Hierholzer WJ Jr, Garner JS, Adams AB, et al. Recommendations for preventing the spread of vancomycin resistance. Infect Control Hosp Epidemiol. 1995;16:105–13.

Jeffres MN, Isakow W, Doherty JA, et al. Predictors of mortality for methicillin-resistant *Staphylococcus aureus* healthcare-associated pneumonia: specific evaluation of vancomycin pharmacokinetic indices. Chest. 2006;130:947–55.

Kullar R, Leonard SN, Davis SL, et al. Validation of the effectiveness of a vancomycin nomogram in achieving target trough concentrations of 15–20 mg/L suggested by the Vancomycin Consensus Guidelines. Pharmacotherapy. 2011;31:441–8.

Liu C, Cosgrove SE, Daum RS, et al. Clinical practice guidelines by the Infectious Diseases Society of America for the treatment of methicillin-resistant *Staphylococcus aureus* infections in adults and children. Clin Infect Dis. 2011;52:e18–55. doi:10.1093/cid/ciq146.

Liu C, Cosgrove SE, Daum RS, et al. Clinical practice guidelines by the Infectious Diseases Society of America for the treatment of methicillin-resistant *Staphylococcus aureus* infections in adults and children: executive summary. Clin Infect Dis. 2011;52:285–92.

Matzke GR, McGory RW, Halstenson CE, Keane WF. Pharmacokinetics of vancomycin in patients with various degrees of renal function. Antimicrob Agents Chemother. 1984;25:433–7.

Matzke GR, Zhanel GG, Guay DRP. Clinical pharmacokinetics of vancomycin. Clin Pharmacokinet. 1986;11:257–82.

McClellan SD, Whitaker CH, Friedberg RC. Removal of vancomycin during plasmapheresis. Ann Pharmacother. 1997;31:1132–6.

Minejima E, Choi J, Beringer P, Lou M, Tse E, Wong-Beringer A. Applying new diagnostic criteria for acute kidney injury (AKI) to facilitate early identification of nephrotoxicity in vancomycin-treated patients. Antimicrob Agents Chemother. 2011. Epub ahead of print. doi:10.1128/AAC.00173-11.

Moellering RC Jr, Krogstad DJ, Greenblatt DJ. Vancomycin therapy in patients with impaired renal function: a nomogram for dosage. Ann Intern Med. 1981;94:343–6.

Moellering RC Jr, Krogstad DJ, Greenblatt DJ. Pharmacokinetics of vancomycin in normal subjects and in patients with reduced renal function. Rev Infect Dis. 1991;3(Suppl):S230–5.

Rybak MJ, Lomaestro BM, Rotschafer JC, et al. Vancomycin therapeutic guidelines: a summary of consensus recommendations from the Infectious Diseases Society of America, the American Society of Health-System Pharmacists, and the Society of Infectious Diseases Pharmacists. Clin Infect Dis. 2009;49:325–7.

UCH Vancomycin Dosing Protocol; Aurora: University of Colorado Hospital; 2011.

Dosage Adjustment of Medications Eliminated by the Kidneys

Vancomycin/Vancocin® (IV)   {Antibacterial, glycopeptide bacterial cell wall biosynthesis inhibitor}

Usual initial dose:	25–30 mg/kg actual body weight IV
Usual maintenance dose:	15–20 mg/kg IV every 8–12 h
Typical maximum dose:	60 mg/kg/day
Proportion eliminated unchanged:	90 %

Adjustment for Kidney Disease

FDA-approved product labeling: *Vancomycin dosage for patients with impaired renal function*

CrCL (mL/min)	Dose
100	1,545 mg per 24 h
90	1,390 mg per 24 h
80	1,235 mg per 24 h
70	1,080 mg per 24 h
60	925 mg per 24 h
50	770 mg per 24 h
40	620 mg per 24 h
30	465 mg per 24 h
20	310 mg per 24 h
10	155 mg per 24 h

Alternative adjustment: *Vancomycin initial dosage regimens for patients with impaired renal function*

eGFR (mL/min/1.73 m2)	Actual body weight (kg) <60	60–80	81–100	>100
>90	750 mg q8h	1,000 mg q8h	1,250 mg q8h	1,500 mg q8h
50–90	750 mg q12h	1,000 mg q12h	1,250 mg q12h	1,000 mg q8h
15–49	750 mg q24h	1,000 mg q24h	1,250 mg q24h	1,500 mg q24h
<15, CRRT, hemodialysis	750 mg	1,000 mg *See below for dosing frequency*	1,250 mg	1,500 mg

Intermittent hemodialysis:

Give one dose at 15 mg/kg actual body weight (rounded to nearest 250 mg).

Check a random vancomycin level 2 h after hemodialysis.

If random level is ≤20 mcg/mL, repeat dose.

If random level is >20 mcg/mL, do not re-dose; repeat level after next dialysis.

Patients with eGFR <15, CRRT, or unstable renal function (e.g., acute renal failure):

Give one dose at 15 mg/kg actual body weight (rounded to nearest 250 mg).

Check a random vancomycin level 24 h after the dose.

If random level is ≤20 mcg/mL, repeat dose.

If random level is >20 mcg/mL, do not re-dose; repeat random level in 12 h.

Therapeutic monitoring:

Goal trough is 10–20 mcg/mL in general inpatient population.

Patients with pulmonary and CSF infections require higher troughs of 15–20 mcg/mL.

For patients dosed every 8–12 h, check trough 30 min prior to fourth dose.

For patients dosed every 24 h, check trough 30 min prior to third dose.

Vandetanib - Selected References

Caprelsa® tablet [package insert]. Wilmington: AstraZeneca Pharmaceuticals LP; 2011.

Drappatz J, Norden AD, Wong ET, et al. Phase I study of vandetanib with radiotherapy and temozolomide for newly diagnosed glioblastoma. Int J Radiat Oncol Biol Phys. 2010;78:85–90.

Gustafson DL, Frederick B, Merz AL, Raben D. Dose scheduling of the dual VEFGR and EGFR tyrosine kinase inhibitor vandetanib (ZD6474, Zactima®) in combination with radiotherapy in EGFR-positive and EGFR-null human head and neck tumor xenografts. Cancer Chemother Pharmacol. 2008;61:179–88.

Lyros O, Mueller A, Heidel F, et al. Analysis of anti-proliferative and chemosensitizing effects of sunitinib on human esophagogastric cancer cells: synergistic interaction with vandetanib via inhibition of multi-receptor tyrosine kinase pathways. Int J Cancer. 2009;127:1197–208.

Martin P, Oliver S, Kennedy S-J, et al. Pharmacokinetics of vandetanib: three phase I studies in healthy subjects. Clin Ther. 2011;Epub ahead of print. doi:10.1016/j.clinthera.2011.11.011.

Robinson BG, Paz-Ares L, Krebs A, Vasselli J, Haddad R. Vandetanib (100 mg) in patients with locally advanced or metastatic hereditary medullary thyroid cancer. J Clin Endocrinol Metab. 2010;95:2664–71.

Weil A, Martin P, Smith R, et al. Pharmacokinetics of vandetanib in subjects with renal or hepatic impairment. Clin Pharmacokinet. 2010;49:607–18.

Wells SA Jr, Gosnell JE, Gagel RF, et al. Vandetanib for the treatment of patients with locally advanced or medullary hereditary medullary thyroid cancer. J Clin Oncol. 2010;28:767–72.

Zhang L, Li S, Zhang Y, et al. Pharmacokinetics and tolerability of vandetanib in Chinese patients with solid, malignant tumors: an open-label, phase I, rising multiple-dose study. Clin Ther. 2011;33:215–27.

Zheng L-S, Wang F, Li Y-H, et al. Vandetanib (Zactima, ZD6474) antagonizes ABCC1- and ABCG2-mediated multidrug resistance by inhibition of their transport function. PLoS One. 2009;4:e5172. doi:10.1371/journal/pone.0005172.

Dosage Adjustment of Medications Eliminated by the Kidneys

<u>Vandetanib</u>/Caprelsa®	**{Antineoplastic, tyrosine kinase [including epidermal growth factor receptor (EGFR), vascular endothelial growth factor (VEGF), and rearranged during transfection (RET)] inhibitor}**

Usual initial dose: 300 mg orally

Usual maintenance dose: 300 mg orally once daily; tablets should be swallowed whole (not crushed) or, if they cannot be taken whole, tablets may be dispersed in a glass containing 60 mL of non-carbonated water and stirred for approximately 10 min (will not completely dissolve, no other liquids should be used, dispersion should be swallowed or instilled through nasogastric or gastrostomy tubes immediately, and any residues in the glass should be mixed again with an additional 120 mL of non-carbonated water and swallowed)

Typical maximum dose: 1,200 mg/day (increases in prevalence of QTc prolongation and other serious adverse effects are observed with doses >300 mg/day with minimal efficacy differences)

Proportion eliminated unchanged: 25 %

Adjustment for Kidney Disease

    FDA-approved product labeling: *CrCL <50 mL/min*   *Starting dose should be reduced to 200 mg orally once daily.*

    Alternative adjustment: *Data not available*

Dosage Adjustment of Medications Eliminated by the Kidneys

Varenicline - Selected References

Aveyard P, Begh R, Parsons A, West R. Brief opportunistic smoking cessation interventions: a systematic review and meta-analysis to compare advice to quit and offer of assistance. Addiction. 2011. Epub ahead of print. doi:10.1111/j.1360-0443.2011.03770.x.

Benowitz NL. Clinical pharmacology of nicotine: implications for understanding, preventing, and treating tobacco addiction. Clin Pharmacol Ther. 2008;83:531–41.

Benowitz NL. Clinical pharmacology of nicotine: addiction, smoking-induced disease, and therapeutics. Annu Rev Pharmacol Toxicol. 2009;49:57–71.

Bird ML, Vesta KS. Varenicline-associated renal failure. Ann Pharmacother. 2008;42:1908–11.

Burstein AH, Fullerton T, Clark DJ, Faessel HM. Pharmacokinetics, safety, and tolerability after single and multiple oral doses of varenicline in elderly smokers. J Clin Pharmacol. 2006;46:1234–40.

Chantix® tablet film coated [package insert]. New York: Pfizer Laboratories Inc; 2011.

Faessel HM, Gibbs MA, Clark DJ, et al. Multiple-dose pharmacokinetics of the selective nicotinic receptor partial agonist, varenicline, in healthy smokers. J Clin Pharmacol. 2006;46:1439–48.

Faessel HM, Obach RS, Rollema H, Ravva P, Williams KE, Burstein AH. A review of the clinical pharmacokinetics and pharmacodynamics of varenicline for smoking cessation. Clin Pharmacokinet. 2011;49:799–816.

Faessel HM, Ravva P, Williams K. Pharmacokinetics, safety, and tolerability of varenicline in healthy adolescent smokers: a multicenter, randomized double-blind, placebo-controlled, parallel-group study. Clin Ther. 2009;31:177–89.

Faessel HM, Smith BJ, Gibbs MA, et al. Single-dose pharmacokinetics of varenicline, a selective nicotinic receptor partial agonist, in healthy smokers and nonsmokers. J Clin Pharmacol. 2006;46:991–8.

Feng B, Obach RS, Burstein AH, Clark DJ, de Morais SM, Faessel HM. Effect of human renal cationic transporter inhibition on the pharmacokinetics of varenicline, a new therapy for smoking cessation: an in vitro-in vivo study. Clin Pharmacol Ther. 2008;83:567–76.

Harrison-Woolrych M, Maggo S, Tan M, Savage R, Ashton J. Cardiovascular events in patients taking varenicline: a case series from intensive postmarketing surveillance in New Zealand. Drug Saf. 2012;35:33–43.

Jiménez-Ruiz C, Berlin I, Hering T. Varenicline: a novel pharmacotherapy for smoking cessation. Drugs. 2009;69:1319–38.

Kikkawa H, Maruyama N, Fujimoto Y, Hasunuma T. Single- and multiple-dose pharmacokinetics of the selective nicotinic receptor partial agonist, varenicline, in healthy Japanese adult smokers. J Clin Pharmacol. 2011;51:527–37.

King DP, Paciga S, Pickering E, et al. Smoking cessation pharmacogenetics: analysis of varenicline and bupropion in placebo-controlled clinical trials. Neuropsychopharmacology. 2011. Epub ahead of print. doi:10.1038/npp.2011.232.

Kortmann GL, Dobler CJ, Bizarro L, Bau CHD. Pharmacogenetics of smoking cessation. Am J Med Genet B Neuropsychiatr Genet. 2010;153B:17–28.

Manley HJ, Stack NM. Smoking cessation therapy considerations for patients with chronic kidney disease. Nephrol Nurs J. 2008;35:357–63, 394.

Moore TJ, Furberg CD, Glenmullern J, Maltsberger JT, Singh S. Suicidal behavior and depression in smoking cessation treatments. PLoS One. 2011;6:e27016. doi:10.1371/journal.pone.0027016.

Ravva P, Gastonguay MR, French JL, Tensfeldt TG, Faessel HM. Quantitative assessment of exposure-response relationships for the efficacy and tolerability of varenicline for smoking cessation. Clin Pharmacol Ther. 2010;87:336–44.

Ravva P, Gastonguay MR, Tensfeldt TG, Faessel HM. Population pharmacokinetic analysis of varenicline in adult smokers. Br J Clin Pharmacol. 2009;68:669–81.

Rennard S, Hughes J, Cinciripini PM, et al. A randomized placebo-controlled trial of varenicline for smoking cessation allowing flexible quit dates. Nicotine Tob Res. 2011. Epub ahead of print. doi:10.1093/ntr/ntr220.

Zhao Q, Schwam E, Fullerton T, O'Gorman M, Burstein AH. Pharmacokinetics, safety, and tolerability following multiple oral doses of varenicline under various titration schedules in elderly nonsmokers. J Clin Pharmacol. 2011;51:492–501.

Dosage Adjustment of Medications Eliminated by the Kidneys

<u>Varenicline</u>/Chantix®   {**Smoking cessation aid, nicotine $\alpha_4\beta_2$-receptor partial agonist**}

Usual initial dose:	0.5 mg orally once daily after meals
Usual maintenance dose:	Following a 1 week titration, 1 mg orally twice daily after meals
Typical maximum dose:	2 mg/day
Proportion eliminated unchanged:	92 %

Adjustment for Kidney Disease

FDA-approved product labeling:	*CrCL <30 mL/min*	*0.5 mg once daily titrated as needed to 0.5 mg twice daily*
	Hemodialysis	*0.5 mg once daily*
Alternative adjustment:	*Data not available*	

Dosage Adjustment of Medications Eliminated by the Kidneys

Venlafaxine - Selected References

Amsterdam JD, Hooper MB, Amchin J. Once- versus twice-daily venlafaxine therapy in major depression: a randomized, double-blind study. J Clin Psychiatry. 1998;59:236–40.

Aronoff GA, Bennett WM, Berns JS, et al. Drug prescribing in renal failure: dosing guidelines for adults and children. 5th ed. Philadelphia: American College of Physicians; 2007.

Crone CC, Gabriel GM. Treatment of anxiety and depression in transplant patients: pharmacokinetic considerations. Clin Pharmacokinet. 2006;43:361–94.

DeVane CL. Pharmacokinetics of the newer antidepressants: clinical relevance. Am J Med. 1994;97(Suppl 6A):13–23S.

Effexor® tablet [package insert]. Philadelphia: Wyeth Pharmaceuticals Subsidiary of Pfizer Inc; 2010.

Effexor® XR capsule extended release [package insert]. Philadelphia: Wyeth Pharmaceuticals Subsidiary of Pfizer Inc; 2011.

Fantaskey A, Burkhart KK. A case report of venlafaxine toxicity. J Toxicol Clin Toxicol. 1985;33:359–61.

Fukuda T, Nishida Y, Zhou Q, Yamamoto I, Kondo S, Azuma J. The impact of the CYP2D6 and CYP2C19 genotypes on venlafaxine pharmacokinetics in a Japanese population. Eur J Clin Pharmacol. 2000;56:175–80.

Fukuda T, Yamamoto I, Nishida Y, et al. Effect of the CYP2D6*10 genotype on venlafaxine pharmacokinetics in healthy adult volunteers. Br J Clin Pharmacol. 1999;47:450–3.

Gex-Fabry M, Balant-Gorgia AE, Balant LP, Rudaz S, Veuthey J-L, Bertschy G. Time course of clinical response to venlafaxine: relevance of plasma level and chirality. Eur J Clin Pharmacol. 2004;59:883–91.

Hawton K, Bergen H, Simkin S, et al. Toxicity of antidepressants: rates of suicide relative to prescribing and non-fatal overdose. Br J Psychiatry. 2010;196:354–8.

Holliday SM, Benfield P. Venlafaxine: a review of its pharmacology and therapeutic potential in depression. Drugs. 1995;49:280–94.

Howell C, Wilson AD, Waring WS. Cardiovascular toxicity due to venlafaxine poisoning n adults: a review of 235 consecutive cases. Br J Clin Pharmacol. 2007;64:192–7.

Klamerus KJ, Maloney K, Rudolph RL, Sisenwine SF, Jusko WJ, Chiang ST. Introduction of a composite parameter to the pharmacokinetics of venlafaxine and its active O-desmethyl metabolite. J Clin Pharmacol. 1992;32:716–24.

Klamerus KJ, Parker VD, Rudolph RL, Derivan AT, Chiang ST. Effects of age and gender on venlafaxine and O-desmethylvenlafaxine pharmacokinetics. Pharmacotherapy. 1996;16:915–23.

Nichols AI, Richards LS, Behrle JA, Posener JA, McGrory SB, Paul J. The pharmacokinetics and safety of desvenlafaxine in subjects with chronic renal impairment. Int J Clin Pharmacol Ther. 2011;49:3–13.

Raymond CB, Wazny LD, Honcharik PL. Pharmacotherapeutic options for the treatment of depression in patients with chronic kidney disease. Nephrol Nurs J. 2008;35:257–63.

Saletu B, Grüneberger J, Anderer P, Linzmayer L, Semlitsch HV, Magne G. Pharmacodynamics of venlafaxine evaluated by EEG brain mapping, psychometry and psychophysiology. Br J Clin Pharmacol. 1992;33:589–601.

Whyte IM, Dawson AH, Buckley NA. Relative toxicity of venlafaxine and selective serotonin reuptake inhibitors in overdose compared to tricyclic antidepressants. Q J Med. 2003;96:369–74.

Dosage Adjustment of Medications Eliminated by the Kidneys

| <u>Venlafaxine</u>/Effexor® | {Antidepressant; serotonin and norepinephrine reuptake inhibitor (SNRI)} |

Usual initial dose: 75 mg/day administered in two or three divided doses or (XR capsules) once daily taken with food

Usual maintenance dose: 150–225 mg/day administered in two or three divided doses or (XR capsules) once daily taken with food

Typical maximum dose: 350 mg/day

Proportion eliminated unchanged: 5 % plus 29 % of each dose as active metabolite

Adjustment for Kidney Disease

FDA-approved product labeling:	*CrCL 10–70 mL/min*	*112.5–150 mg/day in two to three divided doses (25 % decrease)*
	Hemodialysis	*75–112.5 mg/day in two to three divided doses (50 % decrease)*
Alternative adjustment:	*GFR >50 mL/min*	*37.5–225 mg (ER) orally every 24 h (~25 % decrease)*
	GFR 10–50 mL/min	*37.5–187.5 mg (ER) orally every 24 h (50 % decrease)*
	GFR <10 mL/min	*37.5–187.5 mg (ER) orally every 24 h (50 % decrease)*
	Hemodialysis	*37.5–187.5 mg (ER) orally every 24 h (50 % decrease)*
	CAPD	*37.5–187.5 mg (ER) orally every 24 h (50 % decrease)*
	CRRT	*37.5–187.5 mg (ER) orally every 24 h (50 % decrease)*

Dosage Adjustment of Medications Eliminated by the Kidneys

Vigabatrin - Selected References

Aronoff GA, Bennett WM, Berns JS, et al. Drug prescribing in renal failure: dosing guidelines for adults and children. 5th ed. Philadelphia: American College of Physicians; 2007.

Bachman D, Ritz R, Wad N, Haefeli WE. Vigabatrin dosing during haemodialysis. Seizure. 1996;5:239–42.

Browne TR, Mattson RH, Penry JK, et al. A multicenter long-tem study of vigabatrin [abstract]. Neurology. 1990;40(Suppl 1):158.

Dodrill CB, Arnett JL, Sommerville KW, Sussman NM. Evaluation of the effects of vigabatrin on cognitive abilities and quality of life in epilepsy. Neurology. 1993;43:2501–7.

Dodrill CB, Arnett JL, Sommerville KW, Sussman NM. Effects of differing dosages of vigabatrin (Sabril) on cognitive abilities and quality of life in epilepsy. Epilepsia. 1995;36:164–73.

Durham SL, Hoke JF, Chen T-M. Pharmacokinetics and metabolism of vigabatrin following a single oral dose of [^{14}C] vigabatrin in healthy male volunteers. Drug Metab Dispos. 1993;21:480–4.

Elwes RDC, Binne CD. Clinical pharmacokinetics of newer antiepileptic drugs: lamotrigine, vigabatrin, gabapentin and oxcarbazepine. Clin Pharmacokinet. 1996;30:403–15.

French JA, Mosier M, Walker S, Sommerville K, Sussman N. A double-blind, placebo-controlled study of vigabatrin three g/day in patients with uncontrolled complex partial seizures. Neurology. 1996;46:54–61.

Frisk-Holmberg M, Kerth P, Meyer P. Effect of food on the absorption of vigabatrin. Br J Clin Pharmacol. 1989;27(Suppl 1):23–5S.

Gram L, Sabers A, Dulac O. Treatment of pediatric epilepsies with γ-vinyl GABA (vigabatrin). Epilepsia. 1992;33(Suppl 5):S26–9.

Grant SM, Heel RC. Vigabatrin: a review of its pharmacodynamic and pharmacokinetic properties, and therapeutic potential in epilepsy and disorders of motor control. Drugs. 1991;41:889–926.

Grove J, Alken RG, Schecter PJ. Assay of γ-vinyl-γ-aminobutyric acid (4-amino-hex-5-enoic acid) in plasma and urine by automatic amino acid analysis. J Chromatogr. 1984;306:383–7.

Haegele KD, Huebert ND, Ebel M, Tell GP, Schechter PJ. Pharmacokinetics of vigabatrin: implications of creatinine clearance. Clin Pharmacol Ther. 1988;44:558–65.

Haegele KD, Schechter PJ. Kinetics of the enantiomers of vigabatrin after an oral dose of the racemate or the active S-enantiomer. Clin Pharmacol Ther. 1988;40:581–6.

Hoke JF, Yuh L, Antony KK, Okerholm RA, Elberbeld JM, Sussman NM. Pharmacokinetics of vigabatrin following single and multiple oral doses in normal volunteers. J Clin Pharmacol. 1993;33:458–62.

Ifergane G, Masalha R, Ziguinski R, Merkin L, Wirguin I, Herishanu YO. Acute encephalopathy associated with vigabatrin monotherapy in patients with mild renal failure. Neurology. 1998;51:314–5.

Jacqz-Aigrain E, Guillonneau M, Rey E, et al. Pharmacokinetics of the S(+) and R(−) enantiomers of vigabatrin during chronic dosing in a patient with renal failure. Br J Clin Pharmacol. 1997;44:183–8.

Lacerda G, Krumel T, Sabourdy C, Ryvlin Hirsch E. Optimizing therapy of seizures in patients with renal or hepatic dysfunction. Neurology. 2006;67(Suppl 4):S28–33.

Petroff OA, Rothman DL, Behar KL, Mattson RH. Initial observations on effect of vigabatrin on in vivo ^{1}H spectroscopic measurements of γ-aminobutyric acid, glutamate, and glutamine in human brain. Epilepsia. 1995;36:457–64.

Rimmer EM, Richens A. Double-blind study of γ-vinyl GABA in patients with refractory epilepsy. Lancet. 1984;1:189–90.

Sabril® tablet film coated and powder for solution [package insert]. Deerfield: Lundbeck; 2011.

Schecter PJ. Clinical pharmacology of vigabatrin. Br J Clin Pharmacol. 1989;27(Suppl 1):19–22S.

Schecter PJ, Hanke NFJ, Grove J, Huebert N, Sjoerdsma A. Biochemical and clinical effects of γ-vinyl GABA in patients with epilepsy. Neurology. 1984;34:182–6.

Sivenius J, Matilainen R, Riekkinen P, Murros K. Efficacy of gamma-vinyl GABA (vigabatrin) in long-term therapy in patients with partial epilepsy [abstract]. Neurology. 1990;40(Suppl 1):187.

Sivenius J, Ylinen A, Murros K, Mumford JP, Riekkinen PJ. Vigabatrin in drug-resistant partial epilepsy: a 5-year follow-up study. Neurology. 1991;41:562–5.

Tassarini CA, Michelucci R, Ambrosetto G, Salvi F. Double-blind study of vigabatrin in the treatment of drug-resistant epilepsy. Arch Neurol. 1987;44:907–10.

Tolman JA, Faulkner MA. Treatment options for refractory and difficult to treat seizures: focus on vigabatrin. Ther Clin Risk Manag. 2011;7:367–75.

Dosage Adjustment of Medications Eliminated by the Kidneys

Vigabatrin/Sabril®   {Antiepileptic, γ-aminobutyric acid transaminase (GABA-T) inhibitor}

Usual initial dose:	500 mg twice orally daily
Usual maintenance dose:	1,500 mg orally twice daily
Typical maximum dose:	6,000 mg/day
Proportion eliminated unchanged:	65 %

Adjustment for Kidney Disease

FDA-approved product labeling:	*Renal impairment*	*A lower dose is necessary in patients with mild, moderate, and severe renal impairment.*
	CrCL >50 to 80 mL/min	*1,125 mg orally twice daily (25 % decrease)*
	CrCL >30 to 50 mL/min	*750 mg orally twice daily (50 % decrease)*
	CrCL >10 to <30 mL/min	*375 mg orally twice daily (75 % decrease)*
Alternative adjustment:	*GFR >50 mL/min*	*1,000–2,000 mg orally every 24 h*
	GFR 10–50 mL/min	*1,000–2,000 mg orally every 48 h*
	GFR <10 mL/min	*1,000–2,000 mg orally every 48–72 h*
	Hemodialysis	*500 mg orally every 72 h; administer after hemodialysis on dialysis days*
	CAPD	*1,000–2,000 mg orally every 48–72 h*
	CRRT	*1,000–2,000 mg enterally every 48 h*

Dosage Adjustment of Medications Eliminated by the Kidneys

Voriconazole - Selected References

Abel S, Allan R, Gandelman K, Tomaszewski K, Webb DJ, Wood ND. Pharmacokinetics, safety and tolerance of voriconazole in renally impaired subjects: two prospective, multicentre, open-label, parallel-group volunteer studies. Clin Drug Invest. 2008;28:409–20.

Bruggemann RJ, Donnelly JP, Aarnoutse RE, et al. Therapeutic drug monitoring of voriconazole. Ther Drug Monit. 2008;30:403–11.

Burkhardt O, Thon S, Burhenne J, Welte T, Kielstein JT. Sulphobutylether-beta-cyclodextrin accumulation in critically ill patients with acute kidney injury treated with intravenous voriconazole under extended daily dialysis. Int J Antimicrob Agents. 2010;36:93–4.

Eiden C, Cociglio M, Hillaire-Buys D, et al. Pharmacokinetic variability of voriconazole and N-oxide voriconazole measured as therapeutic drug monitoring. Xenobiotica. 2010;40:701–6.

Fuhrmann V, Schenk P, Jaeger W, et al. Pharmacokinetics of voriconazole during continuous venovenous haemodiafiltration. J Antimicrob Chemother. 2007;60:1085–90.

Hafner V, Czock D, Burhenne J, et al. Pharmacokinetics of sulfobutylether-beta-cyclodextrin and voriconazole in patients with end-stage renal failure during treatment with two hemodialysis systems and hemodiafiltration. Antimicrob Agents Chemother. 2010;54:2596–602.

Koch M, Trapp R, Goepel M. Successful maintenance of continuous ambulatory peritoneal dialysis in a patient after fungal peritonitis and dialysate leakage. Clin Nephrol. 2006;65:294–8.

Luke DR, Tomaszewski K, Damle B, Schlamm HT. Review of the basic and clinical pharmacology of sulfobutylether-β-cyclodextrin (SBECD). J Pharm Sci. 2010;99:3291–301.

Lutsar I, Hodges MR, Tomaszewski K, Troke PF, Wood ND. Safety of voriconazole and dose individualization. Clin Infect Dis. 2003;36:1087–8.

Myrianthefs P, Markantonis SL, Evaggelopoulou P, et al. Monitoring plasma voriconazole levels following intravenous administration in critically ill patients: an observational study. Int J Antimicrob Agents. 2010;35:468–72.

Pascual A, Calandra T, Bolay S, Buclin T, Bille J, Marchetti O. Voriconazole therapeutic drug monitoring in patients with invasive mycoses improves efficacy and safety outcomes. Clin Infect Dis. 2008;46:201–11.

Pasqualotto AC, Xavier MO, Andreolla HF, Linden R. Voriconazole therapeutic drug monitoring: focus on safety. Expert Opin Drug Saf. 2010;9:125–37.

Peng LW, Lien Y-HH. Pharmacokinetics of single, oral-dose voriconazole in peritoneal dialysis patients. Am J Kidney Dis. 2005;45:162–6.

Purkins L, Wood N, Ghahramani P, Greenhalgh K, Allen MJ. Kleinermans D. Pharmacokinetics and safety of voriconazole following intravenous to oral-dose escalation regimens. Antimicrob Agents Chemother. 2002;46:2546–53.

Quintard H, Papy E, Massias L, et al. The pharmacokinetic profile of voriconazole during continuous high-volume venovenous hemofiltration in a critically ill patient. Ther Drug Monit. 2008;30:117–9.

Radej J, Krouzecky A, Shehlik P, et al. Pharmacokinetic evaluation of voriconazole treatment in critically ill patients undergoing continuous venovenous hemofiltration. Ther Drug Monit. 2011;33:393–7. doi:10.1097/FTD.0b013e3182205d93.

Robatel C, Rusca M, Padoin C, Marchetti O, Liaudet L, Buclin T. Disposition of voriconazole during continuous venovenous haemodiafiltration (CVVHDF) in a single patient. J Antimicrob Chemother. 2004;54:269–70.

Scott LJ, Simpson D. Voriconazole: a review of its use in the management of invasive fungal infections. Drugs. 2007;67:269–98.

Teranishi J, Nagatoya K, Kakita T, et al. Voriconazole-associated salt-losing nephropathy. Clin Exp Nephrol. 2010;14:377–80.

Theuretzbacher U, Ihle F, Derendorf H. Pharmacokinetic/pharmacodynamic profile of voriconazole. Clin Pharmacokinet. 2006;45:649–63.

VFEND® injection [package insert]. New York: Pfizer Inc; 2011.

von Mach MA, Burhenne J, Weilemann LS. Accumulation of the solvent vehicle sulphobutylether beta cyclodextrin sodium in critically ill patients treated with intravenous voriconazole under renal replacement therapy. BMC Clin Pharmacol. 2006;6:6. doi:10.1186/1472-6904-6-6.

Dosage Adjustment of Medications Eliminated by the Kidneys

Voriconazole/VFEND®   **{Antifungal; triazole ergosterol biosynthesis inhibitor}**

Usual initial dose: 6 mg/kg IV every 12 h for the first 24 h or 200 mg orally

Usual maintenance dose: 4 mg/kg IV or 200 mg orally every 12 h

Typical maximum dose: 12 mg/kg/day

Proportion eliminated unchanged: <2 %

Adjustment for Kidney Disease

FDA-approved product labeling: *CrCL <50 mL/min*   *Accumulation of the IV vehicle, sulfobutylether 7-beta-cyclodextrin (SBECD), occurs. Oral voriconazole should be administered to these patients, unless an assessment of the benefit/risk to the patient justifies the use of IV voriconazole. Serum creatinine levels should be monitored closely in these patients, and, if increases occur, consideration should be given to changing to oral voriconazole therapy.*

Because standard doses result in highly variable voriconazole exposure, monitoring plasma concentrations in seriously ill patients may be recommended to assure attainment of trough levels above inhibitory concentrations for most pathogenic fungi (≥1 mg/L) and avoid toxicity.

Alternative adjustment: *GFR >50 mL/min*   *6 mg/kg IV for the first 24 h followed by 4 mg/kg IV every 12 h or 200 mg enterally every 12 h*

     GFR ≤50 mL/min   *200 mg enterally every 12 h (avoid IV administration)*

     Hemodialysis   *200 mg enterally every 12 h (IV administration not recommended)*

     CAPD   *200 mg enterally every 12 h (avoid IV administration)*

     CVVH   *400 mg enterally every 12 h for the first 24 h, then 4 mg/kg or 200 mg orally every 12 h or 6 mg/kg IV for the first 24 h followed by 4 mg/kg IV every 12 h (limited data suggest IV administration is safe, although possible vehicle accumulation was not studied)*

     CVVHD or CVVHDF   *400 mg enterally every 12 h for the first 24 h, then 4 mg/kg or 200 mg orally every 12 h (IV administration not clinically confirmed as safe)*

Note: Patients weighing <40 kg should receive half the usually recommended dose.

Z

L.K. Golightly et al. (eds.), *Renal Pharmacotherapy*,
DOI 10.1007/978-1-4614-5800-5_21, © Springer Science+Business Media New York 2013

Zalcitabine - Selected References

Adams JM, Shelton MJ, Hewitt RG, et al. Zalcitabine population pharmacokinetics: application of radioimmunoassay. Antimicrob Agents Chemother. 1998;42:409–13.

Adkins JC, Peters DH, Faulds D. Zalcitabine: an update of its pharmacodynamic and pharmacokinetic properties and clinical efficacy in the management of HIV infection. Drugs. 1997;53:1054–80.

Aronoff GA, Bennett WM, Berns JS, et al. Drug prescribing in renal failure: dosing guidelines for adults and children. 5th ed. Philadelphia: American College of Physicians; 2007.

Broder S. Pharmacodynamics of 2′,3′-dideoxycytidine: an inhibitor of human immunodeficiency virus. Am J Med. 1990;88(Suppl 5B):2–7S.

Devineni D, Gallo JM. Zalcitabine: clinical pharmacokinetics and efficacy. Clin Pharmacokinet. 1995;28:351–60.

Gupta SK, Eustace JA, Winston JA, et al. Guidelines for the management of chronic kidney disease in HIV-infected patients: recommendations of the HIV Medicine Section of the Infectious Diseases Society of America. Clin Infect Dis. 2005;40:1559–85.

Gustavson LE, Fukuda EK, Rubio FA, Dunton AW. A pilot study of the bioavailability and pharmacokinetics of 2′,3′-dideoxycytidine in patients with AIDS or AIDS-related complex. J Acquir Immune Defic Syndr. 1990;3:28–31.

Hivid® tablet film coated [package insert]. Nutley: Roche Pharmaceuticals Inc; 2002.

Massarella JW, Nazareno LA, Passe S, Min B. The effect of probenecid on the pharmacokinetics of zalcitabine in HIV-positive patients. Pharm Res. 1996;13:449–52.

Nazareno LA, Holazo AA, Limjuco R, et al. The effect of food on pharmacokinetics of zalcitabine in HIV-positive patients. Pharm Res. 1995;12:1462–5.

Roberts WL, Buckley TJ, Rainey PM, Jatlow PI. Solid-phase extraction combined with radioimmunoassay for measurement of zalcitabine (2′,3′-dideoxycytidine) in plasma and serum. Clin Chem. 1994;40:211–5.

Terasaki T, Pardridge WM. Restricted transport of 3′-azido' 3′deoxythymidine and dideoxynucleosides through the blood–brain barrier. J Infect Dis. 1988;158:630–2.

Vanhove GF, Kastrissios H, Gries J-M, et al. Pharmacokinetics of saquinavir, zidovudine, and zalcitabine in combination therapy. Antimicrob Agents Chemother. 1997;41:2428–32.

Williams PEO, Muirhead GJ, Sereni D, Rousseau FS, Edelman K, Hooker M. Pharmacokinetics of 2-fluorodideoxycytidine (2FddC) in patients infected with human immunodeficiency virus. Br J Clin Pharmacol. 1993;35:255–60.

Dosage Adjustment of Medications Eliminated by the Kidneys

Zalcitabine/Hivid®, ddC   {**Antiretroviral, nucleoside analog reverse transcriptase inhibitor**}

Usual initial dose:	0.75 mg orally
Usual maintenance dose:	0.75 mg orally every 8 h
Typical maximum dose:	2.25 mg/day
Proportion eliminated unchanged:	80 %

Adjustment for Kidney Disease

FDA-approved product labeling:	*CrCL 10–40 mL/min*	*0.75 mg orally every 12 h*
	CrCL <10 mL/min	*0.75 mg orally every 24 h*
Alternative adjustment:	*GFR >50 mL/min*	*0.75 mg orally every 8 h*
	GFR 10–50 mL/min	*0.75 mg orally every 12 h*
	GFR <10 mL/min	*0.75 mg orally every 24 h*
	Hemodialysis	*Data not available*
	CAPD	*Data not available*
	CRRT	*0.75 mg orally every 12 h*

Dosage Adjustment of Medications Eliminated by the Kidneys

<u>Zidovudine</u> - Selected References

Aronoff GA, Bennett WM, Berns JS, et al. Drug prescribing in renal failure: dosing guidelines for adults and children. 5th ed. Philadelphia: American College of Physicians; 2007.

Cooper DA, Gatell JM, Kroon S, et al. Zidovudine in persons with asymptomatic HIV infection and CD4[+] cell counts greater than 400 per cubic millimeter. N Engl J Med. 1993;329:297–303.

Dalakas M, Leon-Monzon ME, Bernardini I, Gahl WA, Jay CA. Zidovudine-induced mitochondrial myopathy is associated with muscle carnitine deficiency and lipid storage. Ann Neurol. 1994;35:482–7.

Fischl MA, Richman DD, Grieco MH, et al. The efficacy of azidothymidine (AZT) in the treatment of patients with AIDS and AIDS-related complex. N Engl J Med. 1987;317:185–91.

Fischl MA, Parker CB, Pettinelli C, et al. A randomized controlled trial of a reduced daily dose of zidovudine in patients with the acquired immunodeficiency syndrome. N Engl J Med. 1990;323:1009–14.

Frem GJ, Rennke HG, Sayegh MH. Late renal allograft failure secondary to thrombotic microangiopathy-human immunodeficiency virus nephropathy. J Am Soc Nephrol. 1994;4:1643–8.

Garraffo R, Cassuto-Viguier E, Barillon J, Chanalet L, Lapalus P, Duplay H. Influence of hemodialysis on zidovudine (AZT) and its glucuronide (GAZT) pharmacokinetics: two case reports. Int J Clin Pharmacol Ther Toxicol. 1989;27:535–9.

Grau JM, Masanés F, Casademont J, Fernández-Solá J, Urbano-Márquez A. Human immunodeficiency virus type 1 infection and myopathy: clinical relevance of zidovudine therapy. Ann Neurol. 1993;34:206–11.

Gupta SK, Eustace JA, Winston JA, et al. Guidelines for the management of chronic kidney disease in HIV-infected patients: recommendations of the HIV Medicine Section of the Infectious Diseases Society of America. Clin Infect Dis. 2005;40:1559–85.

Ifudu O, Rao TK, Tan CC, Fleischman H, Chirgwin K, Friedman EA. Zidovudine is beneficial in human immunodeficiency virus associated nephropathy. Am J Nephrol. 1995;15:217–21.

Klecker RW Jr, Collins JM, Yarchoan R, et al. Plasma and cerebrospinal fluid pharmacokinetics of 3'-azido-3'-deoxythymidine: a novel pyrimidine analog with potential application for the treatment of patients with AIDS and related diseases. Clin Pharmacol Ther. 1987;41:407–12.

Kremer D, Munar MY, Kohihepp SJ, et al. Zidovudine pharmacokinetics in five HIV seronegative patients undergoing continuous ambulatory peritoneal dialysis. Pharmacotherapy. 1992;12:56–60.

Niu MT, Bethel J, Holodniy M, Standiford HC, Schnittman SM. Zidovudine treatment in patients with primary (acute) human immunodeficiency virus type 1 infection: a randomized, double-blind, placebo-controlled trial. J Infect Dis. 1998;178:80–91.

Ostrop NJ, Burgess E, Gill MJ. The use of antiretroviral agents in patients with renal insufficiency. AIDS Patient Care STDS. 1999;13:517–26.

Pachon J, Cisneros JM, Castillo JR, Garcia-Pesquera F, Cañas E, Viciana P. Pharmacokinetics of zidovudine in end-stage renal disease: influence of haemodialysis. AIDS. 1992;6:827–30.

Paoli I, Dave M, Cohen BD. Pharmacodynamics of zidovudine in patients with end-stage renal disease [letter]. N Engl J Med. 1992;326:839–40.

Retrovir® capsule, tablet film coated, syrup [package insert]. Research Triangle Park: GlaxoSmithKline; 2010.

Retrovir® IV infusion [package insert]. Research Triangle Park: GlaxoSmithKline; 2006.

Ruhnke M, Bauer FE, Seiffert M, Trautmann M, Hille H, Koeppe P. Effects of a standard breakfast on pharmacokinetics of oral zidovudine in patients with AIDS. Antimicrob Agents Chemother. 1993;37:2153–8.

Singlas E, Pioger J-C, Taburet A-M, Colin J-N, Fillastre J-P. Zidovudine disposition in patients with severe renal impairment: influence of hemodialysis. Clin Pharmacol Ther. 1989;46:190–7.

Stellbrink H-J, Averdunk R, Stoehr A, Albrecht H. Zidovudine half-life in haemodialysis patients [letter]. AIDS. 1993;7:141–2.

Takeda M, Khamdang S, Narikawa S, et al. Human organic anion transporters and human organic cation transporters mediate renal antiviral transport. J Pharmacol Exp Ther. 2002;300:918–24.

Tourret J, Tostivint I, Tézenas Du Montcel S, et al. Antiretroviral drug dosing errors in HIV-infected patients undergoing hemodialysis. Clin Infect Dis. 2007;45:779–84.

Wilde MI, Langtry HD. Zidovudine: an update of its pharmacodynamic and pharmacokinetic properties, and therapeutic efficacy. Drugs. 1993;46:515–78.

Yarchoan R, Mitsuya H, Myers CE, Broder S. Clinical pharmacology of 3'-azido-2',3'-dideoxythymidine (zidovudine) and related dideoxynucleosides. N Engl J Med. 1989;321:726–38.

Dosage Adjustment of Medications Eliminated by the Kidneys

Zidovudine/Retrovir® {**Antiretroviral, nucleoside analog reverse transcriptase inhibitor**}

Usual initial dose: 300 mg orally or 1 mg/kg IV over 1 h

Usual maintenance dose: 600 mg/day orally in divided doses (preferably fasting) or 1 mg/kg IV over 1 h every 4 h (five to six times daily)

Typical maximum dose: 600 mg/day orally or 6 mg/kg/day IV

Proportion eliminated unchanged: 14–29 % (plus 62 % of 2′, 3′-dideoxy-5′-glucuronylthymidine metabolite [devoid of antiviral activity but perhaps associated with unwanted adverse effects])

Adjustment for Kidney Disease

FDA-approved product labeling:	*CrCL <15 mL/min*	*100 mg orally or 1 mg/kg IV every 6–8 h*
	Hemodialysis	*100 mg orally or 1 mg/kg IV every 6–8 h*
	CAPD	*100 mg orally or 1 mg/kg IV every 6–8 h*
Alternative adjustment:	*GFR >50 mL/min*	*200 mg orally every 8 h*
	GFR 10–50 mL/min	*200 mg orally every 8 h*
	GFR <10 mL/min	*100 mg orally every 8 h*
	Hemodialysis	*100 mg orally every 8 h*
	CAPD	*100 mg orally every 8 h*
	CRRT	*200 mg enterally every 8 h*

Dosage Adjustment of Medications Eliminated by the Kidneys

Zoledronic Acid - Selected References

Balla J. The issue of renal safety of zoledronic acid from a nephrologist's point of view [letter]. Oncologist. 2005;10:306–8.

Black DM, Delmas PD, Eastell R, et al. Once-yearly zoledronic acid for treatment of postmenopausal osteoporosis. N Engl J Med. 2007;356:1809–22.

Brufsky AM, Harker WG, Beck JT, et al. Final 5-year results of Z-FAST trial: adjuvant zoledronic acid maintains bone mass in postmenopausal breast cancer patients receiving letrozole. Cancer. 2011. Epub ahead of print. doi:10.1002/cncr.26313.

Chang JT, Green L, Beitz J. Renal failure with the use of zoledronic acid [letter]. N Engl J Med. 2003;349:1676–8.

Chen T, Berenson J, Vescio R, et al. Pharmacokinetics and pharmacodynamics of zoledronic acid in cancer patients with bone metastases. J Clin Pharmacol. 2002;42:1228–36.

De Cock E, Hutton J, Canney P, et al. Cost-effectiveness of oral ibandronate versus IV zoledronic acid or IV pamidronate for bone metastases in patients receiving oral hormonal therapy for breast cancer in the United Kingdom. Clin Ther. 2005;27:1295–310.

Gnant M, Mlineritsch B, Stoeger H, et al. Adjuvant endocrine therapy and zoledronic acid in premenopausal women with early-stage breast cancer: 62-month follow-up from the ABCSG-12 randomised trial. Lancet. 2011;12:631–41.

Guarneri V, Donati S, Nicolini M, Giovanelli S, D'Amico R, Conte PF. Renal safety and efficacy of i.v. bisphosphonates in patients with skeletal metastases treated for up to 10 years. Oncologist. 10:842–8.

Haas M, Leko-Mohr Z, Roschger P, et al. Zoledronic acid to prevent bone loss in the first 6 months after renal transplantation. Kidney Int. 2003;63:1130–6.

Henley D, Kaye J, Walsh J, Cull G. Symptomatic hypocalcemia and renal impairment associated with bisphosphonate treatment in multiple myeloma. Intern Med J. 2005;35:726–8.

Henry DH, Costa L, Goldwater F, et al. Randomized, double-blind study of denosumab versus zoledronic acid in the treatment of bone metastases in patients with advanced cancer (excluding breast and prostate cancer) or multiple myeloma. J Clin Oncol. 2011;29:1125–32.

Lee Y-K, Nho J-H, Koo K-H. Persistence with intravenous zoledronate in elderly patients with osteoporosis. Osteoporos Int. 2011. Epub ahead of print. doi:10.1007/s00198-011-1881-x.

Markowitz GS, Fine PL, Stack JI, et al. Toxic acute tubular necrosis following treatment with zoledronate (Zometa). Kidney Int. 2003;64:281–9.

MedWatch the FDA Safety Information and Adverse Event Reporting Program. Reclast (zoledronic acid): Drug safety communication – new contraindication and updated warning on kidney impairment. Available at: http://www.fda.gov/Safety/MedWatch/SafetyInformation/ucm239914.htm. Accessed 1 Sept 2011.

Miller PD. The kidney and bisphosphonates. Bone. 2011;49:77–81.

Munier A, Gras V, Andrejak M, et al. Zoledronic acid and renal toxicity: data from French Adverse Effect Reporting database. Ann Pharmacother. 2005;39:1194–7.

Perry CM, Figgitt DP. Zoledronic acid: a review of its use in patients with advanced cancer. Drugs. 2004;64:1197–211.

Räkel A, Boucher A, Ste-Marie L-G. Role of zoledronic acid in the prevention and treatment of osteoporosis. Clin Interv Aging. 2011;6:89–99.

Reclast® injection [package insert]. East Hanover: Novartis Pharmaceuticals Corp; 2011.

Rosen LS, Gordon D, Kaminski M, et al. Zoledronic acid versus pamidronate in the treatment of skeletal metastases in patients with breast cancer or osteolytic lesions of multiple myeloma: a phase III, double-blind, comparative trial. Cancer J. 2001;7:377–87.

Schwarz C, Mitterbauer C, Heinze G, Woloszczuk W, Haas M, Oberbauer R. Nonsustained effect of short-term bisphosphonate therapy on bone turnover three years after renal transplantation. Kidney Int. 2004;65:304–9.

Skerjanec A, Berenson J, Hsu CH, et al. The pharmacokinetics and pharmacodynamics of zoledronic acid in cancer patients with varying degrees of renal function. J Clin Pharmacol. 2003;43:154–62.

Tanvetyanon T, Choudhury AM. Hypocalcemia and azotemia associated with zoledronic acid and interferon alfa. Ann Pharmacother. 2004;38:418–21.

Weide R, Köppler H, Antràs L, et al. Renal toxicity in patients with multiple myeloma receiving zoledronic acid vs ibandronate: a retrospective medical records review. J Cancer Res Ther. 2010.6:31–5.

Zometa® injection [package insert]. East Hanover: Novartis Pharmaceuticals Corp; 2011.

Dosage Adjustment of Medications Eliminated by the Kidneys

Zoledronic Acid/Reclast®, Zometa®   {Anti-osteoporotic, hypocalcemic agent; bisphosphonate}

Usual initial dose:	4–5 mg IV
Usual maintenance dose:	4 mg IV once weekly (hypercalcemia) or 4 mg IV every 3–4 weeks (bone metastases) or 5 mg IV once a year (osteoporosis/Paget's disease of bone)
Typical maximum dose:	5 mg/dose
Proportion eliminated unchanged:	39 %

Adjustment for Kidney Disease

FDA-approved product labeling: *Recommended zoledronic acid dose for patients with multiple myeloma and metastatic bone lesions with mild-to-moderate renal function impairment*

CrCL (mL/min)	Recommended dose
>60	4 mg IV every 3–4 weeks
50–60	3.5 mg IV every 3–4 weeks
40–49	3.3 mg IV every 3–4 weeks
30–39	3 mg IV every 3–4 weeks
<30 and/or acute renal impairment	Not recommended
Osteoporosis/Paget's disease	
CrCL ≥35 mL/min	5 mg IV over 15 min once a year
CrCL <35 mL/min and/or evidence of acute renal impairment	Contraindicated

Alternative adjustment: *Definitive data not available* — *For osteoporosis, anecdotal data suggest that for patients with stage 3–5 chronic kidney disease (GFR <30 mL/min), dosages should be reduced by half (i.e., 2 mg IV once yearly), infusion rates should be slowed (i.e., infuse each dose over 60 min), and duration of treatment should be limited to not more than 3 years.*

Dosage Adjustment of Medications Eliminated by the Kidneys

Zonisamide - Selected References

Aronoff GA, Bennett WM, Berns JS, et al. Drug prescribing in renal failure: dosing guidelines for adults and children. 5th ed. Philadelphia: American College of Physicians; 2007.

Berg MJ, Gross RA, Tomaszewski KJ, Zingaro WM, Haskins LS. Generic substitution in the treatment of epilepsy: case evidence of breakthrough seizures. Neurology. 2008;71:525–30.

Bermejo PE, Anciones B. A review of the use of zonisamide in Parkinson's disease. Ther Adv Neurol Disord. 2009;2:313–7.

Frampton JE, Scott LJ. Zonisamide: a review of its use in the management of partial seizures in epilepsy. CNS Drugs. 2005;19:347–67.

Gadde KM, Franciscy DM, Wagner HR, Krishman KRR. Zonisamide for weight loss in obese adults: a randomized controlled trial. JAMA. 2003;289:1820–5.

Hammond EJ, Perchalski RJ, Wilder BJ, McLean JR. Neuropharmacology of zonisamide, a new antiepileptic drug. Gen Pharmacol. 1987;18:303–7.

Ieiri I, Morioka T, Kim S, Nishio S, Fukui M, Riguchi S. Pharmacokinetic study of zonisamide in patients undergoing brain surgery. J Pharm Pharmacol. 1996;48:1270–5.

Ijiri Y, Inoue T, Fukuda F, et al. Dialyzability of the antiepileptic drug zonisamide in patients undergoing hemodialysis. Epilepsia. 2004;45:924–7.

Inoue T, Kira R, Kaku Y, Ikeda K, Gondo K, Hara T. Renal tubular acidosis associated with zonisamide therapy. Epilepsia. 2000;41:1642–4.

Johannessen SI, Tomson T. Pharmacokinetic variability of newer antiepileptic drugs: when is monitoring needed? Clin Pharmacokinet. 2006;45:1061–75.

Kimura M, Tanaka N, Kimura Y, et al. Factors influencing serum concentration of zonisamide in epileptic patients. Chem Pharm Bull (Tokyo). 1992;40:193–5.

Kochak GM, Page JG, Buchanan RA, Peters R, Padgett CS. Steady-state pharmacokinetics of zonisamide, an antiepileptic agent for treatment of refractory complex partial seizures. J Clin Pharmacol. 1998;38:166–71.

Kossoff EH, Pyik PL, Furth SL, Hladky HD, Freeman JM, Vining EPG. Kidney stones, carbonic anhydrase inhibitors, and the ketogenic diet. Epilepsia. 2002;43:1168–71.

Leppik IE. Zonisamide: chemistry, mechanism of action, and pharmacokinetics. Seizure. 2004;13(Suppl 1):S5–9.

Marson AG, Kadir ZA, Chadwick DW. New antiepileptic drugs: a systematic review of their efficacy and tolerability. BMJ. 1996;313:1169–74.

Mohammadianinejad SE, Abbasi V, Sajedi, et al. Zonisamide versus topiramate in migraine prophylaxis: a double-blind randomized clinical trial. Clin Neuropharmacol. 2011;34:174–7.

Okada Y, Seo T, Ishitsu T, et al. Population estimation regarding the effects of cytochrome P450 2C19 and 3A5 polymorphisms on zonisamide clearance. Ther Drug Monit. 2008;30:540–3.

Oommen KJ, Mathews S. Zonisamide: a new antiepileptic drug. Clin Neuropharmacol. 1999;22:192–200.

Perucca E, Bialer M. The clinical pharmacokinetics of the newer antiepileptic drugs: focus on topiramate, zonisamide and tiagabine. Clin Pharmacokinet. 1996;31:29–46.

Peters DH, Sorkin EM. Zonisamide: a review of its pharmacodynamic and pharmacokinetic properties, and therapeutic potential in epilepsy. Drugs. 1993;45:760–87.

Richards KC, Smith MC, Verma A. Continued use of zonisamide following development of renal calculi. Neurology. 2005;64:763–4.

Sills GJ, Brodie MJ. Pharmacokinetics and drug interactions with zonisamide. Epilepsia. 2007;48:435–41.

Villani V, Ciuffoli A, Prosperini L, Sette G. Zonisamide for migraine prophylaxis in topiramate-intolerant patients: an observational study. Headache. 2011;51:287–91.

Zachry WM III, Doan QD, Clewell JD, Smith BJ. Case–control analysis of ambulance, emergency room, or inpatient hospital events for epilepsy and antiepileptic drug formulation changes. Epilepsia. 2009;50:493–500.

Zonegran® capsule [package insert]. Woodcliff Lake: Esai Inc; 2011.

Dosage Adjustment of Medications Eliminated by the Kidneys

Zonisamide/Zonegran® {Antiepileptic; sodium channel and voltage-dependent T-type Ca²⁺ channel blocker}

Usual initial dose:	100 mg orally once daily
Usual maintenance dose:	200–400 mg/day orally in one or two divided doses
Typical maximum dose:	600 mg/day
Proportion eliminated unchanged:	35 %

Adjustment for Kidney Disease

FDA-approved product labeling:

Marked renal impairment (CrCL <20 mL/min) is associated with an increase in zonisamide exposure (AUC) of 35 %. Zonisamide therapy has been associated with a mean 8 % increase SCr and BUN over from baseline. Zonisamide should be discontinued in patients who develop acute renal failure or a clinically significant sustained increase in the SCr/BUN concentration. Patients with renal disease should be treated with caution and might require slower titration and more frequent monitoring.

Alternative adjustment:

GFR >50 mL/min	*50–300 mg orally twice daily (0–25 % decrease)*
GFR 10–50 mL/min	*50–200 mg orally twice daily (25 % decrease)*
GFR <10 mL/min	*25–150 mg orally twice daily (50 % decrease)*
Hemodialysis	*4–8 mg/kg/day orally once daily in the evening; administer after hemodialysis on dialysis days*
CAPD	*25–150 mg orally twice daily (50 % decrease)*
CRRT	*50–200 mg enterally twice daily (25 % decrease)*

Index

L.K. Golightly et al. (eds.), *Renal Pharmacotherapy*,
DOI 10.1007/978-1-4614-5800-5, © Springer Science+Business Media New York 2013